Pearson's Surgical Technology Exam Review

Emily H. Boegli, RN, BS, MA
Director (retired), Surgical Technology Program
Savannah Technical Institute
Savannah, Georgia

Emily W. Rogers, CST, RN, BS, CNOR
Head, Surgical Technology Department
Spartanburg Technical College
Spartanburg, South Carolina

Kat LaRue, CST
Program Chair, Surgical Technology Program
Brown Mackie College-Greenville
Greenville, South Carolina

PEARSON

Boston   Columbus   Indianapolis   New York   San Francisco   Upper Saddle River
Amsterdam   Cape Town   Dubai   London   Madrid   Milan   Munich   Paris   Montreal   Toronto
Delhi   Mexico City   Sao Paulo   Sydney   Hong Kong   Seoul   Singapore   Taipei   Tokyo

Library of Congress Cataloging-in-Publication Data

Boegli, Emily H.
  Pearson's surgical technology exam review / Emily H. Boegli, Emily
W. Rogers, Kat LaRue. — 3rd ed.
    p. cm.
  Rev. ed. of: Prentice Hall's complete review of surgical technology.
© 2006. 2nd ed.
  Includes bibliographical references and index.
  ISBN-13: 978-0-13-500048-9
  ISBN-10: 0-13-500048-3
  1. Surgical technology—Outlines, syllabi, etc. I. Rogers, Emily W.
II. LaRue, Kat. III. Boegli, Emily H., 1932– Prentice Hall's complete
review of surgical technology. IV. Title.
  RD32.3.B64 2013
  617'.023076—dc23

                                        2011038678

Notice:
The authors and the publisher of this volume have taken care that the information and technical recommendations contained herein are based on research and expert consultation and are accurate and compatible with the standards generally accepted at the time of publication. Nevertheless, as new information becomes available, changes in clinical and technical practices become necessary. The reader is advised to carefully consult manufacturers' instructions and information material for all supplies and equipment before use and to consult with a health care professional as necessary. This advice is especially important when using new supplies or equipment for clinical purposes. The authors and publisher disclaim all responsibility for any liability, loss, injury, or damage incurred as a consequence, directly or indirectly, of the use and application of any of the contents of this volume.

Publisher: Julie Levin Alexander
Assistant to Publisher: Regina Bruno
Editor-in-Chief: Mark Cohen
Executive Editor: John Goucher
Assistant Editor: Nicole Ragonese
Editorial Assistant: Rosalie Hawley
Media Editor: Amy Peltier
Media Project Manager: Lorena Cerisano
Managing Production Editor: Pat Walsh
Production/Manufacturing: Pat Brown

Creative Director: Jayne Conte
Cover Designer: Bruce Kenselaar
Director of Marketing: David Gesell
Executive Marketing Manager: Katrin Beacom
Marketing Specialist: Michael Sirinides
Composition: Munesh Kumar/Aptara®, Inc.
Printer/Binder: LSC Communications
Cover Printer: LSC Communications
Cover Credits: Shutterstock/Tyler Olson

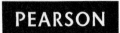

ISBN-10: 0-13-500048-3
ISBN-13: 978-0-13-500048-9

Brief Contents

Contents

Introduction

About the Book

- *Study Questions: Pearson's Surgical Technology Exam Review 3/e*. The book has been designed to help the student prepare for the national certification exam. There are over 700 multiple-choice questions which cover the topics on the exam and follow the exam format, as well as anatomy labeling exercises in several chapters. Working through these questions will help you assess your strengths and weaknesses in each area of study. Correct answers and comprehensive rationales are included.

- *Outline Format:* Unlike some review books that only contain questions and answers, *Pearson's Surgical Technology Exam Review 3/e* contains valuable review information in an easy-to-read outline format.

Certification

The NBSTSA (National Board of Surgical Technology and Surgical Assisting) is responsible for administering the national certification exam for surgical technologists. The NBSTSA will determine a candidate's eligibility to sit and is responsible for granting, denying, renewing and revoking certification of surgical technologists and surgical assistants. The NBSTSA provides a handbook for prospective candidates that outlines the process of scheduling, administering, and renewing certification. To obtain a handbook, you may contact the NBSTSA at

NBSTSA
6 West Dry Creek Circle, ste 100
Littleton, CO 80120-8031
Phone: 800-707-0057
www.nbstsa.org

Phone: 800-707-0057
Fax: 719-328-0801

About the Exam

The national certifying examination for Surgical Technologists is given year round, through independent testing agencies located throughout the United States. Once eligibility has been validated by the NBSTSA, you will be given the information to contact the testing agency to select a test date and time.

The certifying exam is computer-based. The test center manager along with a computerized tutorial will help you become familiar with computerized testing before you begin the actual exam.

The exam consists of 250 multiple-choice questions. Each question has four choices listed, only one of which is correct. You will be allowed 4 hours to take the examination. Once you have completed the exam, scoring will take place within 5 minutes and you will receive your printed pass/fail report before you leave the testing center.

Effective January 1, 2003, the exam is based on the Exam Content Outline developed from the 2002 job analysis. The exam content outline includes the following three broad functional areas:

I. Peri-Operative Patient Care (54%)
   a. Pre-Operative Preparation (18%)
   b. Intra- and Post-Operative Procedures (36%)

II. Ancillary Functions (Materials Management, Sterilization, Other) (13%)

III. Basic Sciences (33%)
   a. Anatomy and Physiology (20%)
   b. Microbiology (7%)
   c. Surgical Pharmacology (6%)

Effective January 1, 2003, certification must be renewed every 4 years. Renewal of the Certified Surgical Technologist certification can be accomplished by taking and passing the national certifying examination prior to your certification expiration date or by providing proof of completing 60 continuing education credits that meet the requirements of the NBSTSA and the AST during the 4-year certification period. There is a formal list of accepted continuing educational courses available through the AST.

Study Tips
Review Materials

Save time by making sure that you are studying the correct material. Refer to the content outline in the candidate handbook and mark those areas in which you are least comfortable. Study those areas first. Before the exam, the best study preparation would be to use this review to identify your strengths and weaknesses. If you need more in-depth study than provided in this text, the bibliography will direct you to additional resources.

Set a Study Schedule

The certification exam is not like other tests you have taken. In addition to reviewing the information and practicing by taking sample exams, preparation for the certification exam requires planning. It is best to begin studying months ahead rather than waiting until the last minute.

Use your time-management skills to create a preparation schedule. Take into consideration the amount of information you know and what you will need to review in-depth. Also, determine the amount of time you can devote to studying on a daily or weekly basis. Once these are identified and a tentative or actual exam date is selected, plan out a schedule of goals and activities, put your plan in writing, and follow it. Remember to give yourself extra time to study information that remains challenging and for unexpected obstacles such as emergencies. Choose and write down two or three dates during your preparation schedule to review your goals to be sure that you are on track with your preparation activities.

It is recommended that you take the certification exam as soon as possible upon graduation. Studies show that the longer you wait the lower your score.

Following a study schedule will allow you to be as ready as possible when the time comes to take the exam, will decrease your general anxiety related to the test-taking process, and will optimize your ability to be successful in passing the exam.

Take Practice Tests

Practice as much as possible, using the questions in this book and the accompanying website at www.myhealthprofessionskit.com. These questions are designed to follow the format used for the questions appearing on the certification exam. The more you practice using this question format, the more comfortable you will be answering these types of questions. Familiarity with the test question format should help to decrease test anxiety during the certification exam.

The practice test on the website will give you an opportunity to simulate the certification exam in a familiar environment. When you take this practice test, try to do it under the same conditions you will encounter when taking the certification exam. Take this practice test in a quiet environment without any disturbances. Do not use any of your textbooks or notes during the test. Allow yourself 4 hours to answer the questions.

When you are done, use the information to identify the areas that need further study and review.

Prepare Physically and Mentally

Being prepared physically and mentally to take the examination is as important as studying the information.

On the day before the examination, do not plan a last-minute studying marathon session. Instead, plan to engage in a pleasurable and relaxing activity to help reduce anxiety and stress. If necessary, plan to spend 30–45 minutes reviewing those points of information that remain a challenge.

Eat a nutritious dinner the evening before the exam to prepare your body for the stressors of exam day. Eat a light, well-balanced meal before you go to the test center,

being sure to include some protein and carbohydrates to give you energy throughout the exam.

Be sure to plan for a full night's sleep the night before the exam, so that you will be rested and alert. Avoid stimulants or using any medications you do not commonly use.

Dress in comfortable, casual clothing for the exam. Wearing something that makes you feel positive and comfortable will boost your self-esteem and confidence. Wear clothing in layers to allow for adjustments to the temperature of the testing center.

Be positive and confident about your knowledge and skills. Use the exam as an opportunity to recognize your abilities and professional behaviors.

The Testing Center

Be sure to obtain specific directions to both the testing center and parking facilities before the day of the test. If you are unfamiliar with the location, you may want to make a trial run before the actual test date. Be sure to bring your admissions information, identification, any other documentation required by the testing center, and money for parking fees, if necessary. Thoroughly review all the information and instructions sent to you regarding the examination to be sure that you have everything you need for taking the exam. Organize these items ahead of time to be sure that they travel with you to the testing center. If required documentation is missing when you arrive at the test center, you may forfeit your examination opportunity and any associated fees.

On the day of the exam, allow yourself ample time for getting to the testing center. Remember to plan for such travel delays as detours, construction, and rush-hour traffic issues.

Taking the Examination

Read the examination directions thoroughly! A tutorial program will help you become familiar with the computer before you actually begin the exam. A test center manager is available to answer any questions you may have. If you are given a test booklet or blank paper, it is acceptable to jot down any facts that you are afraid you might forget once the test starts.

If you feel yourself becoming anxious during the exam, close your eyes, take several deep breaths, and readjusting your sitting position. These activities will help you regain your focus and self-control.

Selecting the Right Answer

Keep in mind that only one answer is correct. First carefully read the stem of the question with *each* possible choice provided and eliminate choices that are obviously incorrect. Be cautious about choosing the first answer that *might* be correct; all possibilities should be considered before the final choice is made; the *best* answer should be selected.

If a question is complicated, try to break it down into small sections that are easy to understand or put it in your own words. Pay special attention to qualifiers such as *only, except,* and so on. For example, negative words in a question can confuse your understanding of what the question asks ("Which of the following is *not . . .*"). When numbers are involved, be very careful, especially with decimals.

Intelligent Guessing

If you don't know the answer, eliminate those answers that you know or suspect are wrong. Your goal is to narrow down your choices. Here are some things to consider:

- Is the choice accurate in its own terms? If there's an error in the choice—for example, a term that is incorrectly defined—the answer is wrong.

- Is the choice relevant? An answer may be accurate, but it may not relate to the essence of the question.

- Are there any distractors, such as *always, never, all, none,* or *every?* Qualifiers make it easy to find an exception that makes a choice incorrect.

- Often, the longest answer is the correct choice.

- Do not spend more than 30 to 60 seconds on any one question.

Mark answers you aren't sure of, and go back to them at the end of the test when you may be more relaxed. Ask yourself whether you would make the same guesses again. Chances are that you will leave your answers alone, but you may notice something that will make you change your mind—a qualifier that affects meaning or a remembered fact that will enable you to answer the question without guessing. You may discover the answer in another question. Answer all questions. An unanswered question will count the same as an incorrect one.

Watch the Clock

Keep track of how much time is left and how you are progressing. With the current computerized format, there is a "time remaining" box at the top of your screen. Wear a watch or bring a small clock with you to the test room in case the time remaining function is not working and there is no clock in the room.

Some students are so concerned about time that they rush through the exam and have time left over. In such situations, it's tempting to leave early. The best approach, however, is to take your time. Stay until the end so that you can check your answers.

Keys to Success Across the Boards

- Study, review, and practice.
- Keep a positive, confident attitude.
- Follow all directions on the examination.
- Do your best.

Good luck!

You are encouraged to visit http://www.internettime.com/Learning for additional tips on studying, test taking, and other keys to success. At this state of your education and career, you will find these tips helpful.

Some of the study and test-taking tips were adapted from *Keys to Effective Learning, second edition,* by Carol Carter, Joyce Bishop, and Sarah Lyman Kravits.

Preface

In the years since Emily Boegli first published *Surgical Technology Review,* the world of the operating room has changed dramatically. Today's OR requires that Surgical Technologists develop the knowledge, skills, and behaviors that permit them to be an active, integral part of the surgical team. The technological advances—including minimally invasive approaches to traditional surgical procedures and the use of robotics—require Surgical Technologists to work with complex equipment and supplies, to think on their feet, and to serve as a resource to the surgeon. The Surgical Technologist is becoming the expert at the sterile field and is expected to manage every facet of this complex and fast-paced role.

The need to educate Surgical Technologists to an appropriate level for functioning, not only in today's surgical arena but also in the operating room of the future, requires that their texts and review books aid them in that preparation. With publication of the Association of Surgical Technologists' 5th edition of the *Core Curriculum for Surgical Technology* in 2002, the need to revise and update this review book became critical—critical in that the availability of materials written for Surgical Technologists by professionals in the field directly involved with surgical technology education is greatly needed.

With a combined 45 years of experience in surgical technology education, we have joined our knowledge, expertise, and skills to provide the surgical technology educational community with a current source of materials to challenge and promote growth within this exciting profession. It is our hope that through our work, the Surgical Technologist—student, novice, and experienced practitioner alike—will gain a more secure knowledge base in the essentials of the profession.

How to Use This Book

Imagine the perfect set of class notes. You've gone to class every day, you've written down all the essential notes on the material that your instructor has taught, and you have even added some illustrations where appropriate. What could be better? *This book is that complete set of notes!*

Despite its streamlined appearance, this is an all-inclusive book. Every attempt has been made to include the important points in the course while eliminating much of the extraneous material that often is included. To make it easy for you to use, the book is presented in outline format.

All the books in this series have been developed by analyzing the existing textbooks in the field and the requirements of the specific accrediting organizations. From this analysis, we have determined the key areas and topics to be included in this book. What this means is that if you are a student in California, Georgia, Maine, or Minnesota—any state in the country—and regardless of what textbook you are using, this book will review the key material. This is important because you will want to use this book to help you review what you have learned as you prepare to enter the profession of Surgical Technology.

There is a step-by-step process involved in using any type of review book. First, you attend classroom lectures. What happens, however, when you have attended class, read your textbook, but still find the information somewhat unclear? It's time to call on this outline book.

With this book's easy-to-use format, you can quickly identify the important ideas, concepts, and facts that are presented. Important terms are defined where necessary, and illustrations are included in the procedures chapters for review. Find the chapter in this book that corresponds to the topic in your textbook or to what you are covering in class. Read through the chapter quickly, skimming the material until you find the section that has given you difficulty. Now read through that part slowly. Underline or highlight words or phrases that you feel are important. It may be helpful to rewrite the information in your own words so that it becomes even clearer to you. You might want to make notes in the margins. Finally, compare this outline with your own class notes.

The concept of any review book is to make it easier to understand information you have learned elsewhere. The purpose of presenting this outline format is to make it even easier! These are your class notes—to read, to memorize, to annotate, and to help you understand everything you will need to be successful in your educational classes.

Emily W. Rogers and Kat LaRue

Acknowledgments

As I begin my 30th year of teaching Surgical Technology at Spartanburg Technical College, I am amazed at all of the changes that have taken place in the operating room. I dedicate this text to my past and future students who I hope I have positively influenced in some way. I would not have been able to complete it without them. I also want to thank my husband, Randy, and two sons, Andy and Mark, for sharing me with my students and my profession.

Emily W. Rogers

I would like to thank Nicole Ragonese, who graciously allowed me to be a part of this review book. She has been an invaluable resource as I undertook a new endeavor. I would like to dedicate my work to my students: past, present, and future, who will use this book as part of their study regime in preparation for the exam. Finally, I would like to thank my son, Jacob LaRue, for his understanding that "Mommy is working on something very important right now," and my parents Walter and Margaret Wren.

Kat LaRue

Reviewers

Dorothy Connolly, BSN, CNOR, CST
Bridgeport Hospital
Bridgeport, CT

Dana E. Earnest, CST
Daytona State College
Daytona Beach, Florida

Linda Harrison, CST, F-AST
Edgecombe Community College
Tarboro, North Carolina

Suzanne A. Jackson, AS, CST
Flowers Hospital
Dothan, AL

Teri Junge, CST, CSFA, FAST, BS
San Joaquin Valley College
Fresno, California

Deborah Smith, RN, CNOR
Southeastern Technical College
Vidalia, Georgia

Sally M. Smith, ST, RN, BSEd, MEd
Okefenokee Technical College
Waycross, Georgia

Sue H. Stallings, RN, CNOR, CST
Sentara College of Health Science
Chesapeake, Virginia

Gretchen Bates, CST
Baptist Health Schools
Little Rock, Arkansas

Bibliography

AORN *Standards and Recommended Practices for Perioperative Nursing.* Denver, CO: Association of peri-Operative Registered Nurses, Inc., 2003.

Association of Surgical Technologists, Inc., *Surgical Technology for the Surgical Technologist,* 2nd ed. Clifton Park, NY: Delmar, 2004.

Core Curriculum for Surgical Technology, Inc., 5th ed. Littleton, CO: Association of Surgical Technologists, Inc., 2002.

Da Vinci surgical systems. Online: http://www.intuitive-surgical.com/products/da_vinci.html (accessed 2/04).

Deitch, E., *Tools of the Trade and Rules of the Road, A Surgical Guide,* Philadelphia, PA; Lippincott-Raven, 1997.

Dorland's Illustrated Medical Dictionary, 27th ed. Philadelphia, PA: W. B. Saunders, 1988.

Ehrlich, A., *Medical Terminology for Health Professions.* Albany, NY: Delmar, 1988.

Five Stages of Group Dynamics. Online: http://www.gmu.edu/student/csl/5stages.html (accessed 4/04)

Fuller, J. R., *Surgical Technology: Principles and Practice,* 3rd ed. Philadelphia, PA: W. B. Saunders, 1994.

Goldman M. A., *Pocket Guide to Operating Room,* 2nd ed. Philadelphia, PA: F. A. Davis, 1996.

Gruendemann, B., and Mangum, S., *Infection Prevention in Surgical Settings,* Philadelphia, PA: W. B. Saunders, 2001.

Heat transfer. Online: http://theory.uwinnipeg.ca/mod_tech/node74.html (accessed 2/04)

Leadership styles. Online: http://www.elixiran.com/English/virtual/management%20courses/leadership/Leadership%20Styles2.htm (accessed 4/04)

Mader S., *Understanding Anatomy and Physiology.* Dubuque, IA: Wm. C. Brown, 1991.

Marieb, E., *Essentials of Human Anatomy and Physiology,* 6th ed. San Francisco, CA: Benjamin/Cummings, 2000.

McGuiness, A. "Technology for the 21st Century." *The Surgical Technologist.* October 2003.

McMurtrie, H., and Rikel, J. K., *The Coloring Review Guide to Human Anatomy.* Dubuque, IA: Wm. C. Brown, 1991.

Miller-Keane, B. *Encyclopedia and Dictionary of Medicine, Nursing, and Allied Health,* 7th ed. Philadelphia, PA: W. B. Saunders, 2003.

Mosby's Medical, Nursing, and Allied Health Dictionary, 4th ed. St. Louis, MO: CV Mosby, 1986.

Newton's law of gravity. Online: http://www.glenbrook.k12.il.us/gbssci/phys/Class/newtlaws/u2l1a.html (accessed 2/04)

Newton's Law of Motion. Online: http://theory.uwinnipeg.ca/mod_tech/node54.html (accessed 2/04)

Nursing Care of the Patient in the O.R., 2nd ed. Somerville, NJ: Ethicon, 1987.

Phillips, N., *Berry & Kohn's Operating Room Technique,* 10th ed. St. Louis, MO: Mosby-Year Book, 2004.

Rothrock, J. C., *Alexander's Care of the Patient in Surgery,* 12th ed. St. Louis, MO: Mosby-Year Book, 2001.

Snyder, K., and Keegan, C., *Pharmacology for the Surgical Technologist,* Philadelphia, PA: W. B. Saunders, 1999.

State of matter. Online: http://www.krysstal.com/states.html (accessed 2/04)

Taber's Cyclopedic Medical Dictionary, 19th ed. Philadelphia, PA: F. A. Davis Co, 2001.

Lecture notes collected over the years from a variety of sources: journal articles, surgeons' lectures, workshops, and national conferences.

Medical Terminology

Medicine has a language all its own. Most of the words used to discuss procedures, diagnosis, and all other medically related topics have their basis in this language. The majority of the words are of Latin or Greek origin, and are built around a "core" word, or root word. Once this language is mastered, you can dissect most surgery schedules. To understand this language, you must know the commonly used root words. Once that is understood, the suffixes and prefixes are added to change the meaning, describe the procedure, or build new terms. For example, if a nephrectomy is scheduled for 7:00 A.M., you must know what this term means before you can plan for the case. Using the root word "nephr" and the suffix "ectomy," you are able to dissect the word to come up with the meaning. Nephr is the root word for kidney, and ectomy is the suffix used for surgical removal. If you add these together, it is understood that the 7:00 A.M. case is the surgical removal of a kidney. This same concept can be used for other words commonly used in medicine.

CHAPTER OUTLINE

TIP   How to Answer Medical Terminology Questions

First, make sure that you understand the question being asked. Some certification questions have multiple parts that can be confusing. Once you have established what the question is, dissect the word that you need to define. You must identify and define the root word in order to come up with the correct meaning. Next, examine the prefix and suffix. Do they change the meaning of the word? If so, how? Once you have identified all the components of the word, you are ready to define what the word means. Remember, some words combine several root words.

Practice Question:
What does a bilateral salpingo-oopherectomy entail?

a. Surgical removal of the uterus
b. Surgical fixation of the ovary and fallopian tube
c. Surgical removal of both fallopian tubes and ovaries
d. Surgical repair of a genetic anomaly of the fallopian tube and ovary

Answer and Rationale:
What is the question asking?

• The question is what is involved in the procedure

What word(s) needs to be defined?

• Bilateral and salpingo-oopherectomy

What is the root word or words?

• For *bilateral*, the word "lateral" or "side" is being used. Adding the prefix *bi-* changes the meaning to both sides. So now, you know that this procedure is involving two sides.
• For *Salpingo-oopherectomy*, you must define both *salping/o* and *oopher/o*. Remembering the root words that were studied, you should be able to define these two words. They are fallopian tube and ovary. You now know that the procedure involves both fallopian tubes and ovaries.

What are the prefix and suffix, and how do they impact the word?

• In this case, you only need to decipher the suffix. The suffix *–ectomy* is used to describe what the procedure is. *–ectomy* means the surgical removal.

When you add all of the elements together, you know that the patient will be having both fallopian tubes and ovaries removed.

Medical Word Parts and Combining Forms*

1. The prefix comes before the main part (root) of the word and alters the meaning.
    Example: Antiemetic: anti- (against) plus emesis (vomit); thus, an antiemetic is an agent used to prevent or stop vomiting.
2. The suffix comes at the end of the root word and alters the meaning.
    Example: Thoracotomy: thorax (chest) plus -otomy (cut into); thus, thoracotomy is cutting (incision) into the chest.
3. The root word is the main part of the word.
    Example: Splenectomy: splen- (spleen) plus -ectomy (surgical removal); thus, splenectomy is the surgical excision of the spleen.

4. Some words are compound words (they have more than one root word).
   Example: Nephrolithotripsy: nephr- (kidney) plus lith- (stone) plus -tripsy (crushing); thus, nephrolithotripsy is the crushing of a kidney stone.

5. To facilitate the connection of word parts, the combining form is used. To add a suffix to myrinx, modification is necessary. The combining form is myring/o. It is now easy to add a suffix.
   Example: Myring/o/centesis: puncturing to aspirate fluid from the eardrum.

6. Once the word parts are known, medical terms may be analyzed and/or built. Practice with the following list of word parts will refresh your memory and prepare you for the chapters that follow.

Frequently Used Prefixes

Prefixes are added to the beginning of a word or words and frequently change the meaning. It is important to remember that some commonly used medical terms contain prefixes that change the root word, and thus the meaning of the term. This is a concern when breaking the word down to the components. An example of this is *atrophy*. The term "atrophy" means wasting away. When broken down into the components, the meaning is opposite. Trophy means nourishment or development. It is only with the addition of the prefix *a-*, meaning without, that we get the full picture: without nourishment or development. Because we are familiar with the term "atrophy," we sometimes forget that this is a root word with an added prefix.

Prefix	Meaning	Example
a-, an-, in	without, negative	a/men/orrhea: without a monthly flow
ab-	from, away from	ab/normal: away from normal
ad-, ac-, as-, at-	to, toward	ad/duct: carry toward
ante-	before, in front	ante/natal: before birth
anti-, ant-	against	anti/bacteri/al: pertaining to against bacteria
bi-	two	bi/lateral: two sides
bio-	life	bio/logy: study of life
brachy-	short	brachy/dactylism: short fingers/toes
brady-	slow	brady/cardia: slow heart rate
cent-	hundred	centi/meter: one one-hundredth of a meter
circum-	around	circum/cis/ion: cutting around
co-, com-, con-	with, together	con/genital: born with
contra-	against	contra/indicated: against indication
de-	down from	de/hydrate: lose water
dextr-	right	dextr/o/gastria: stomach displaced to right
dia-	through	dia/rrhea: flow through
dis-	apart	dis/sect: to cut apart
dys-	bad, difficult	dys/pnea: difficult breathing
e-, ex-	out, out from	ex/cise: to cut out
ecto-, exo-, extra-	outside	extra/corpore/al: pertaining to outside the body
en-	in, on	en/capsulated: in a capsule
end-, endo-	within	endo/scopy: visualization within
epi-	upon	epi/dermis: upon the skin
eu-	good	eu/phonic: good sound
hemi-, semi-,	half	hemi/gastr/ectomy: surgical removal of half the stomach
hyper-	over, above	hyper/kinetic: overactive

hypo-	under, below	hypo/glossal: under the tongue
infra-	beneath	infra/mammary: beneath the breast
inter-	between	inter/cellular: between the cells
intra-	within	intra/crani/al: pertaining to within the cranium (skull)
kil-, kilo-	thousand	kilo/gram: one thousand grams
macr-, macro-	large	macro/cyte: large cell
mal-	bad	mal/nutrition: bad nourishment
mes-	middle	mes/entery: middle of intestine
meta-	after, beyond	meta/carpals: beyond the carpals (wrist)
micr-, micro-	small	micro/cephal/ic: having a small head
milli-	one one-thousandth	milli/liter: one one-thousandth of a liter
multi-	many	multi/para: one who has many children
neo-	new	neo/plasm: new growth
olig-	scanty, few	olig/uria: scanty amount of urine
onc-	tumor	onc/ology: study of tumors
para-	beside	para/median: beside the median
per-	through	per/cutaneous: through the skin
peri-	around	peri/tonsillar: around the tonsil
poly-	much, many	poly/cystic: having many cysts
post-	after	post/mortem: after death
pre-	before	pre/nat/al: pertaining to before birth
presby-	old	presby/opia: old vision
primi-	first	primi/gravida: woman in first pregnancy
pro-	before	pro/gnosis: foreknowledge, prediction of outcome
re-	back, again	re/generate: produce or develop again
retr-, retro-	behind	retro/stern/al: pertaining to behind the sternum
sub-	under, below	sub/lingu/al: pertaining to under the tongue
super-, supra-	above	supra/pelvic: above the pelvis
syn-, sym-	with, together	syn/ergism: working together
tachy-	fast	tachy/phasia: fast speech
trans-	across, beyond	trans/urethr/al: pertaining to across the urethra
uni-	one	uni/lateral: one side

Frequently Used Root Words

The root words are the heart of medical terminology. Many root words are familiar to surgical technology students. For the words that are unfamiliar, try to find a common context to use the word. For example, the root word "arthr/o" means joint. For students who are unfamiliar with this, consider arthritis—inflammation of a joint. Once the word is in a familiar context, it becomes easier to remember.

Note: Words that are the same as anatomical terms used in English have been omitted (i.e., pancreas and tonsil).

Root Word	Meaning	Example
acr-	extremity, peak	acro/megaly: enlarged extremities
		acro/phobia: abnormal fear of heights
aden-	gland	adeno/pathy: disease of a gland

angi-	vessel	angi/oma: tumor of a vessel
anter-	front	anter/ior: toward the front
arthr-	joint	arthr/algia: pain in a joint
blephar-	eyelid	blepharo/plegia: paralysis of an eyelid
brachi-	arm	brachi/al: pertaining to the arm
carcin-	cancer	adeno/carcin/oma: cancerous tumor of a gland
cardi-	heart	myo/cardi/tis: inflammation of the heart muscle
carp-	wrist	carpo/ptosis: wrist drop
caud-	tail	caud/al: pertaining to tail
cephal-	head	hydro/cephalus: head enlarged by water
cerebr-	brain	cerebro/spin/al: pertaining to the brain and spine
cervic-	neck	cervic/al: pertaining to the neck
cheil-	lip	cheilo/plasty: shaping of the lip
cheir, chir-	hand	chiro/megaly: large hands
chol-	bile, gall	chole/cyst/ectomy: surgical removal of the gallbladder
cholecyst-	gallbladder	chole/cyst/itis: inflammation of the gallbladder
chondr-	cartilage	osteo/chondr/itis: inflammation of cartilage and bone
chrom-	color	poly/chrom/atic: having many colors
chron-	time	syn/chron/ous: occurring at the same time
col-	large intestine, colon	mega/colon: enlarged colon
colp-	vagina	colp/orrhaphy: suturing of the vagina
cost-	rib	inter/cost/al: pertaining to between the ribs
crani-	skull	crani/otomy: incision into the skull
cry-	cold	cryo/philic: attracted to cold
crypt-	hidden	crypt/orchid/ism: hidden (undescended) testicle
cutan-, cut-	skin	sub/cutaneous: below the skin
cyan-	blue	acro/cyan/osis: abnormal condition of blueness of the extremities
cyst-	bladder	cysto/cele: bladder hernia
cyt-	cell	thrombo/cyte: clotting cell (platelet)
dacry-	tear	dacryo/cysto/rhin/ostomy: creating an opening between the tear sac and nose
dactyl-	finger, toes	poly/dactyl/ism: too many fingers or toes
dent-, odont-	tooth	peri/odont/al: pertaining to around the teeth
derm-, dermat-	skin	intra/derm/al: pertaining to within the skin
dextr-	right	dextro/cardia: heart displaced to the right
dips-	thirst	poly/dipsia: excessive thirst
dors-	back	dorsi/flex: bend backwards
duct-	carry	ovi/duct: tube to carry ova (egg)
encephal-	brain	encephalo/cele: hernia of the brain
enter-	intestine	gastro/enter/itis: inflammation of the stomach and the intestine
erythr-	red	erythro/cyto/penia: deficiency of red cells
esthe- fasci-	Sensation fascia	an/esthe/tic: agent to eliminate sensation fasci/itis: inflammation of the fascia
febr-	fever	a/febrile: without fever
flex-	bend	latero/flexion: bending to the side

gastr-	stomach	gastro/scopy: visualization of the stomach
gen-	produce	patho/genic: agent which produces disease
gingiv-	gums	gingiv/ectomy: removal of the gums
gloss-	tongue	glosso/dynia: pain in the tongue
gnath-	jaw	micro/gnath/ism: small jaw
gynec-	female	gyneco/logy: study of female conditions
hem-, hemat-	blood	hemat/emesis: vomiting blood
hepat-	liver	hepato/rrhexis: ruptured liver
heter-	different	hetero/genous: of different origins
hidr-	perspiration	hidro/rrhea: flow of perspiration
hist-	tissue	histo/logy: study of tissue
home-, hom-	same	homeo/stasis: stability in equilibrium
hydr-, hydra-	water	de/hydra/tion: process of losing water
hyster-	uterus	hyster/ectomy: removal of the uterus
iatr-	physician	iatro/genic: produced by the physician
irid-	iris	irid/ectomy: surgical removal of the iris
is-	equal	iso/tonic: equal in tone
kerat-	cornea	kerato/plasty: shape the cornea
kin-, kinesi-	move, movement	kinesio/logy: study of movement
lacrim- lamin-	Tear Lamina (part of the vertebral arch)	lacrima/tion: crying lamin/ectomy: excision of the lamina
lact-, galact-	milk	lacto/genic: producing milk
lapar-	abdomen	lapar/oscopy: visualization of the abdomen
laryng-	larynx	laryngo/scope: instrument to visualize the larynx
later-	side	bi/lateral: having two sides
leuk-, leuc-	white	leuko/rrhea: white discharge
lingu-	tongue	sub/lingu/al: pertaining to under the tongue
lip-	fat	lip/oma: tumor of fat
lith-	stone	litho/tripsy: crushing a stone
mamm-, mast-	breast	mammo/gram: x-ray of the breast mast/itis: inflammation of the breast
melan-	black	melan/oma: black tumor
men-	monthly, menses	dys/meno/rrhea: difficult monthly flow
metr-	uterus	endo/metr/ium: inner lining of the uterus
morph-	shape, form	poly/morphic: having many shapes
my-	muscle	myo/metr/itis: inflammation of the muscle of the uterus
myc-	fungus	onycho/myc/osis: fungus condition of the nails
myel-	marrow, spinal cord	myelo/gram: x-ray of the spinal cord
myring-	eardrum	myringo/tomy: opening into the eardrum
nas-	nose	naso/pharyng/eal: pertaining to the nose and the throat
necr-	dead	necr/opsy: examination of dead bodies; autopsy
nephr-, ren-	kidney	hydro/nephr/osis: abnormal condition of water in the kidney
neur-	nerve	neur/orrhaphy: suturing of a nerve
noct-, nyct-	night	noct/uria: voiding at night
null-	none	nulli/gravida: woman who has had no pregnancies
ocul-	eye	mon/ocular: pertaining to one eye

omphal-	umbilicus	omphalo/rrhea: discharge from the navel
onych-	nail	onycho/crypt/osis: condition of hidden (ingrown) nail
oo-	egg, ova	oo/genesis: production of eggs
oophor-	ovary	oophoro/cyst/ectomy: removal of a cyst from the ovary
ophthalm-	eye	ex/ophthalmia: condition of protruding eyes
or-	mouth	oro/pharynge/al: pertaining to the mouth and the throat
orchid-	testes	orchid/ectomy: removal of the testes
orexia-	appetite	an/orexia: absence of appetite
orth-	straight	orth/odont/ist: one who straightens teeth
oste-, oss-	bone	osteo/chondr/oma: tumor of bone and cartilage
ot-, aur- palat-	ear palate	ot/itis: inflammation of the ear palate/plasty: surgical repair of the palate
para-	to bear	primi/para: woman bearing her first child
path-	disease	patho/physio/logy: study of effects of diseases on body functions
pect-	chest	pect/oralis: chest muscle
ped-	child	ped/iatr/ician: physician who specializes in children's care
phag-	swallow, eat	a/phagia: inability to swallow
pharmac-	drug	pharmaco/logy: study of drugs
pharyng-	throat	pharyng/itis: inflammation of the throat
phas-	speak, say	tachy/phasia: fast speech
phleb-	vein	phlebo/thromb/osis: condition of clot in a vein
phon-	voice	a/phonic: absence of voice
phren-	diaphragm	phreno/hepatic: pertaining to the liver and the diaphragm
pneum-	air, breath	pneumo/thorax: air in the chest
pneumon-	lung	pneumon/ectomy: surgical removal of the lung
pod-	foot	pod/iatr/ist: physician specializing in foot problems
proct-	rectum	procto/scopy: visualization of the rectum
pseud-	false	pseudo/cyesis: false pregnancy
psych-	mind	psycho/somatic: pertaining to the mind and the body
pulmo(n)-	lung	cardio/pulmonary: pertaining to the heart and the lungs
py-	pus	py/uria: pus in the urine
pyel-	kidney pelvis	pyelo/nephr/itis: inflammation of the renal pelvis
pyr-	fire, fever	anti/pyretic: agent used against fever
quadri-	four	quadri/plegia: paralysis of all four extremities
rhin-	nose	rhino/plasty: surgical revision of the nose
salping-	fallopian tube	salping/itis: inflammation of the fallopian tube
sanguin-	blood	ex/sanguina/tion: process of bleeding out (bleeding to death)
scler-	hard	arterio/scler/osis: condition of hardening of arteries
sect-	cut	dis/section: cutting apart
sept-	contamination	anti/septic: agent used against contamination
sial-	saliva	sial/ogram: x-ray of salivary gland
sten-	narrow, constricted	pyloric sten/osis: condition of narrowing of the pylorus
stomat-	mouth	stomat/itis: inflammation of the mouth
strict-	draw tight	vaso/con/strict/or: agent that compresses vessels
tax-	order, arrange	a/taxic: uncoordinated
ten-	tendon	teno/rrhaphy: suturing a tendon

therm-	heat	hyper/thermia: high body temperature
thorac-	chest	thoraco/centesis: puncturing to aspirate fluid from the chest
thromb-	clot	phlebo/thromb/osis: condition of clot in a vein
tox-	poison	tox/emia: poison in the blood
trache-	windpipe	trache/ostomy: opening into the trachea
trachel	neck	trachel/ectomy: surgical removal of the cervix (neck of the uterus)
traumat-	wound	traumat/ology: study of wounds or injuries
tri-	three	tri/geminal: having three beginnings or origins
trop-	turn	ec/tropion: turned out
troph-	nurture, nutrition	a/trophy: without growth (wasting away)
ur-	urine	ur/emia: excess of urine constituents in the blood
vas-	vessel	vaso/dilat/ion: dilating of a vessel
vert-	turn	retro/vert/ed: turned backward
vesic-	bladder	vesico/cele: hernia of the bladder
viscer-	internal organs	e/viscera/tion: organs protruding from the abdominal wall
vita-	life	vital: necessary for life

Frequently Used Suffixes

Most suffixes are added to words to add meaning to the word. The most commonly used suffixes in surgery pertain to the action being taken. For example, *-ectomy* which means surgical removal or excision, or *–scopy* which means visualization. Other suffixes are used in diagnosis, such as *–itis* and *–malacia*. Suffixes may also change the meaning of the root word.

Suffix	Meaning	Example
-al	pertaining to	spin/al: pertaining to the spine
-algia	pain	an/algia: without pain
-asthenia	weakness	my/asthenia: muscle weakness
-atresia	without an opening	proct/atresia: rectum without an opening
-cele	hernia	omphalo/cele: umbilical hernia
-centesis	puncturing to aspirate fluid	arthro/centesis: puncturing to aspirate fluid from a joint
-cide, cidal	kill	bacterio/cidal: able to kill bacteria
-cis	cut	ex/cise: cut out
-cyte	cell	erythro/cyte: red cell
-desis	fusion	arthro/desis: fusion of a joint
-dynia	pain	cephalo/dynia: pain in the head
-ectasia	expansion, dilation	cor/ectasia: dilating a pupil
-ectomy	cut out, excise	nephr/ectomy: surgical removal of a kidney
-edema	swelling	lymph/edema: swelling due to stasis of lymph

SURGERY HINT

Many surgeries are referred to by a different name. It is important for the Surgical Technologist to know the alternate names for surgical procedures. For example, gastroduodenostomy may be called a Billroth I, while a gastrojejunostomy may be scheduled as a Billroth II. Two more common alternate names are Miles resection, which is an abdominoperineal resection, and Whipple procedure, which is a pancreaticoduodenectomy.

-emesis	vomiting	hyper/emesis: excessive vomiting
-emia	blood	hyper/glyc/emia: elevated blood sugar
-gnosis	knowledge	dia/gnosis: knowledge through examination (determining the cause of a disease)
-gram	record, x-ray	myelo/gram: x-ray of the spinal cord
-graphy	making a record	angio/graphy: making a record of vessels
-iasis	condition	chole/lith/iasis: the condition of gallstones
-ist	one who	opto/metr/ist: one who measures vision
-itis	inflammation	aden/itis: inflammation of a gland
-lepsy	seizures	narco/lepsy: seizures of numbness (sleep)
-logist	one who specializes	ophthalmo/logist: one specializing in the eyes
-logy	study of	cardio/logy: study of the heart
-lysis, lytic	break down, dissolve	teno/lysis: destruction of tendons
-malacia	abnormal softening	osteo/malacia: abnormal softening of bone
-mania	madness	pyro/mania: madness for setting fires
-megaly	enlargement	spleno/megaly: enlargement of the spleen
-meter	measure	thermo/meter: instrument to measure temperature
-oid	resembling	muc/oid: resembling mucus
-oma	tumor	neur/oma: nerve tumor
-opia	vision	ambly/opia: dim vision
-osis	abnormal condition	nephr/osis: abnormal condition of a kidney
-ostomy	creation of an opening	col/ostomy: creation of an opening in the colon
-otia	ear	macr/otia: large ear
-pathy	disease	encephalo/pathy: disease of the brain
-penia	deficiency, poor	leuko/cyto/penia: deficiency of white cells
-pepsia	digestion	dys/pepsia: bad digestion
-pexy	surgical fixation	nephro/pexy: surgical fixation of the kidney
-phasia	speak, say	a/phasia: without the ability to speak
-philia	love, attraction	thermo/philia: attracted to warmth
-phobia	abnormal fear	agora/phobia: abnormal fear of crowds
-plasia	formation	hyper/plasia: excessive formation
-plasm	substance	proto/plasm: original substance
-plasty	make, shape	rhino/plasty: shaping of the nose
-plegia	paralysis	hemi/plegia: paralysis of one half of the body
-pnea	breathe	tachy/pnea: fast breathing
-ptosis	prolapse, drooping	hystero/ptosis: prolapse of the uterus
-rrhagia	burst forth	metro/rrhagia: hemorrhage from the uterus
-rrhaphy	suture, sew	hernio/rrhaphy: suturing of a hernia
-rrhea	flow, discharge	oto/rrhea: discharge from an ear
-rrhexis	rupture	spleno/rrhexis: rupture of the spleen
-scope	instrument for viewing	oto/scope: instrument to look in the ears
-scopy	visualization	laryngo/scopy: visualization of the larynx
-some, soma	body	lyso/some: body which lyses or dissolves
-spasm	twitching	blepharo/spasm: twitching of an eyelid
-stasis	stop, control	hemo/stasis: control of bleeding
-therapy	treatment	hydro/therapy: treatment with water

-tome	instrument to cut	osteo/tome: instrument to cut bone
-tomy	to cut	laparo/tomy: cutting into the abdomen
-tripsy	crushing	neuro/tripsy: the crushing of a nerve
-trophy	development	hyper/trophy: overdevelopment
-uria	urine	hemat/uria: blood in the urine

Show What You Know

Directions
Each of the numbered items or incomplete statements in this section is followed by answers or by completions of the statement. Select the ONE lettered answer or completion that is BEST in each case.

1. The part of a word that comes after the root word and changes its meaning is the:
   A. prefix
   B. root
   C. suffix
   D. combining form

2. An agent used against fever is:
   A. antiemetic
   B. analgesic
   C. antipyretic
   D. anticholinergic

3. A slow pulse rate is:
   A. bradycardia
   B. tachycardia
   C. myocardium
   D. eucardia

4. An incision made below the breast is:
   A. hypodermic
   B. suprapubic
   C. inframammary
   D. subcutaneous

5. A congenital anomaly is a/an:
   A. normal condition that one has at birth
   B. abnormal condition existing at birth
   C. birthmark
   D. condition acquired after birth

6. An instrument used to view the large intestine is a/an:
   A. gastroscope
   B. endoscopy
   C. colonoscope
   D. bronchoscope

7. Surgical removal of half the stomach is:
   A. hemigastrectomy
   B. hemiglossectomy
   C. gastroscopy
   D. gastropathy

8. You are scheduled to scrub on a cheiloplasty. The anatomical part to be revised is the:
   A. hand
   B. ear
   C. eyelid
   D. lip

9. A record made of a joint is:
   A. arthrodesis
   B. arthrogram
   C. osteopathy
   D. angiography

10. A preoperative diagnosis of cholelithiasis indicates a/an:
    A. infection in the large intestine
    B. abnormal condition of the vagina
    C. abnormal condition of kidney stones
    D. condition of gallstones

11. Hepatomegaly is:
    A. an enlarged liver
    B. a small kidney
    C. cancer of the liver
    D. an abnormal condition of the spleen

12. Inflammation of the brain is:
    A. nephritis
    B. encephalitis
    C. neuroma
    D. hydrocephalus

13. A laparoscope would be used to visualize the:
    A. cranial cavity
    B. abdominal cavity
    C. spinal cavity
    D. joint

14. A patient with chondromalacia would have an abnormal softening of the:
    A. bones
    B. cells

C. ribs

D. cartilage

15. The suffix that means to suture is:

A. -orrhexis

B. -plasty

C. -rrhagia

D. -rrhaphy

16. Intracellular fluid would be found:

A. within the cell

B. between the cells

C. below the cell

D. above the cell

17. A bilateral salpingo-oophorectomy is a surgical procedure to:

A. reconnect a tubal ligation

B. reconnect a vasectomy

C. remove the uterus and ovaries

D. remove both fallopian tubes and ovaries

18. An arthrocentesis is a procedure to:

A. fuse a joint

B. remove plaque from an artery

C. puncture and aspirate fluid from a joint

D. make a recording of an artery

19. A myelogram is:

A. a recording of a muscle

B. an x-ray of the brain

C. an x-ray of the spinal cord

D. a unit of weight in the metric system

20. A cholecystectomy is a procedure to:

A. remove the colon and bladder

B. join the bile duct to the small intestines

C. suture the colon

D. remove the gallbladder

21. A red blood cell is known as a/an:

A. erythrocyte

B. leukocyte

C. thrombocyte

D. cytopenia

22. The term pertaining to a hidden testicle is:

A. omphalocele

B. cryptorchidism

C. orchiopexy

D. onychocryptosis

23. The surgical procedure to crush a stone is a:

A. lithiasis

B. lithectomy

C. lithotripsy

D. lithoptosis

24. A blepharoplasty is a procedure to:

A. remove redundant skin from the face—a facelift

B. repair of the lips

C. separating fused digits

D. repair of the eyelids

25. Hydronephrosis is:

A. a condition of water on the brain

B. a procedure to suture the kidney in place

C. a condition of water in the kidney

D. voiding at night

Answers & Rationales

1. **C. Rationale:** A suffix comes at the end of a word and alters the meaning.

2. **C. Rationale:** Anti- equals against; pyr- equals fever; -ic equals pertaining to.

3. **A. Rationale:** Brady- equals slow; cardia equals heart.

4. **C. Rationale:** Infra- equals below, mammary equals pertaining to the breast.

5. **B. Rationale:** Con- equals with; genital equals birth; a- equals without; nomaly equals normal.

6. **C. Rationale:** Colon equals large intestine; scope equals instrument for visualization.

7. **A. Rationale:** Hemi- equals half; gastr- equals stomach; ectomy -equals surgical removal.

8. **D. Rationale:** Cheil- equals lip; -plasty equals surgical repair or shaping.

9. **B. Rationale:** Arthr- equals joint; -gram equals record.

10. **D. Rationale:** Chole- equals bile; lith- equals stone; -iasis equals condition.

11. **A. Rationale:** Hepat- equals liver; -megaly equals enlarged.

12. **B. Rationale:** Encephal- equals brain (inside head); -it is equals inflammation.

13. **B.** **Rationale:** Lapar- equals abdomen; -scope equals instrument for viewing.

14. **D.** **Rationale:** Chondr- equals cartilage; -malacia equals abnormal softening.

15. **D.** **Rationale:** -rrhaphy equals suture or sew up.

16. **A.** **Rationale:** Intra equals within; inter equals between; supra equals above; sub equals below.

17. **D.** **Rationale:** Bi equals two; lateral equals side; salpingo is the combining form for fallopian tube; oophor equals ovary; ectomy equals removal of.

18. **C.** **Rationale:** Arthro equals joint; centesis equals puncturing to aspirate fluid.

19. **C.** **Rationale:** Myelo equals spinal cord; gram equals record of or x-ray.

20. **D.** **Rationale:** Chole equals bile or gall; cyst equals bladder or fluid-filled sac; ectomy equals removal of.

21. **A.** **Rationale:** Erythro equals red; cyte equals cell.

22. **B.** **Rationale:** Crypt equals hidden; orchid equals testicle.

23. **C.** **Rationale:** Litho is the combining form for stone; tripsy equals crushing.

24. **D.** **Rationale:** Blepharo is the combining form for eyelids; plasty equals repair or shape.

25. **C.** **Rationale:** Hydro equals water; nephr equals kidney; osis equals condition.

Part II: Deciphering a Surgical Schedule

The following mock surgery schedule will be used to answer several questions pertaining to medical terminology. The same schedule, or a similar one, may be used in subsequent chapters to ask questions about the content of the chapter.

Rm. # time	Surgeon	Procedure	Anest.	Rm. # time	Surgeon	Procedure	Anest.
Rm.00				**Rm07**			
OC	Dr. Z	Rt. Knee Arthroscopy	Gen.	7:00	Dr. M	Rhinoplasty	Gen.
OC	Dr. C	Craniotomy	Gen.				
OC	Dr. Z	Angioplasty	Gen.	TF	Dr. M	Lipoma removal	MAC
Rm.01				**Rm08**			
7:00	Dr. X	Lobectomy	Gen.	11:00	Dr. E	Bovine Thrombectomy	MAC
TF	Dr. X	Thoracotomy	Gen.				
TF	Dr. X	Tracheostomy	Gen.				
Rm02				**Rm09**			
7:00	Dr. B	Hemicolectomy	Gen.	8:30	Dr. T	Cholecystectomy	Gen.
TF	Dr. B	Gastrectomy	Gen.	TF	Dr. T	Palatoplasty	Gen.
Rm03				**Rm10**			
7:00	Dr. A	Cystoscopy	MAC	7:00	Dr. K	Nephrectomy	Gen.
TF	Dr. A	Cystoplasty	Gen.	TF	Dr. K	Choledocholithotripsy	MAC
12:30	Dr. F	Pyleogram	MAC				
3:00	Dr. F	Cystocele repair	Gen.	TF	Dr. K	Hepatic resection	Gen.
Rm04				**Rm11**			
7:00	Dr. Y	Valvoplasty	Gen.	7:00	Dr. L	Colposcope	Gen.
TF	Dr. Y	Fasciotomy	Gen.	12:00	Dr. L	Mastectomy	Gen.
Rm05				**Rm12**			
7:00	Dr. G	Trans-sphenoidal Adenectomy	Gen.	7:00	Dr. W	Trans-metatarsal amputation	Gen.
TF	Dr. G	Trans-urethral resection of the prostate	Gen	TF	Dr. W	Osteotomy	Gen.
TF	Dr. G	Bletharoplasty	Gen.	TF	Dr. W	Arthrocentesis	Gen.
Rm06				**Rm13**			
7:00	Dr. R	Lumbar Laminectomy	Gen.	7:00	Dr. O	Hysterectomy	Gen.

The following questions should be answered using the surgery schedule above

1. There is a Lumbar Laminectomy scheduled in Room 6. What will this surgery entail?

   A. Removal of a lobe of the lung
   B. Removal of a tumor on the lower back
   C. Excision of part of the vertebral arch
   D. Creation of a surgical incision for a lumbar puncture

2. What is involved in the surgery scheduled in Room 3 at 7:00?

   A. Visualization of the bladder
   B. Surgical fixation and repair of a herniated bladder
   C. Visualization of the gallbladder
   D. Removal of the cystic duct

3. A Gastrectomy follows a Hemicolectomy in Room 2. What does a Gastrectomy mean?

   A. Creation of an opening in the stomach
   B. Surgical removal of the large intestine
   C. Surgical removal of the stomach
   D. surgical removal of part of the colon

4. A Fasciotomy is scheduled in Room 4. What is a Fasciotomy?

   A. Creation of an opening in the abdominal peritoneum
   B. Excision of the fascia
   C. Creation of an opening in the spinal cord
   D. Creation of an opening in the fascia

5. The surgery scheduled in Room 7 at 7:00 will involve what?

   A. The surgical fixation of the septum
   B. Visualization of the sinus cavities
   C. Fusion of the nasal bones
   D. Reshaping the nose

6. An Arthrocentisis is scheduled to follow the Osteotomy in Room 12. What is an Osteotomy?

   A. Puncture of a joint to remove fluid
   B. A cut into the bone
   C. A cut made in the cartilage
   D. Plating a bone of the leg

7. The Colposcopy scheduled for Room 11 will involve

   A. Reshaping the lips
   B. Visualization of the colon
   C. Visualization of the vaginal vault
   D. Visualization of the middle ear

8. A Hysterectomy, which is scheduled in Room 13, involves

   A. Surgical removal of the fallopian tubes and ovaries
   B. Surgical removal of a breast
   C. Surgical removal of the uterus
   D. Surgical removal of the labia majora

9. There is a Craniotomy on call for Doctor C. What is a Craniotomy?

   A. An incision into the skull
   B. An incision into the ribs
   C. Clipping an aneurysm
   D. Removal of a cranial tumor

10. The palatoplasty in Room 9 is a procedure for
   A. Repair of a cleft lip
   B. Repair of a cleft palate
   C. Repair of a deviated septum
   D. Repair of a defect of the heart muscle

Answers & Rationale

1. **C.** **Rationale:** The medical term *lamin/o* refers to the *lamina*, which is part of the vertebral arch. This surgery is usually done to relieve pain caused by the compression of a spinal nerve. The suffix *–ectomy* refers to excision or removal, so the term *laminectomy* means the removal of part of the vertebral arch. Lumbar is the section of the spine that the surgery will be performed on.

2. **A.** **Rationale:** The term *cyst/o* refers to the urinary bladder. The suffix *–scopy* means to view, or visualization. Therefore, the surgery scheduled for 7:00 would be the direct visualization of the bladder. Be careful not to confuse *cyst/o* with *cholecyst/o*. The term *cholecyst/o* is referring to the gallbladder.

3. **C.** **Rationale:** *Gastr* is the medical term for stomach. Combined with the suffix *–ectomy*, the terms meaning becomes clear. The surgery will involve the surgical removal of part or all of the stomach. This is usually performed due to a malignancy or uncontrollable gastric bleeding.

4. **D.** **Rationale:** *Fasci-* is the root word for fascia, the fibrous membrane that covers and separates muscles. When combined with *–otomy*, the suffix meaning incision or cutting into. This procedure is usually performed due to compartment syndrome, an injury that may result from improper positioning of the patient.

5. **D.** **Rationale:** *Rhin-* is the root word meaning nose, and *–plasty* is the suffix for surgical repair or shaping. The resulting word *rhinoplasty* is the term for reconstruction of the nose for cosmetic or reconstructive purposes.

6. **B.** **Rationale:** Osteotomies are surgical incisions into bone. *Oste-* is the root word for bone, and *–otomy* is the suffix meaning cutting into. An osteotomy may be performed any time a surgical opening into bone is necessary.

7. **C.** **Rationale:** *Colp-* is the root word for vagina. When you add the suffix *–scopy*, meaning to view, the final definition is the visualization of the vaginal vault. This is performed with an instrument called a Colposcope, and is usually done to biopsy or view abnormal tissue.

8. **C.** **Rationale:** Hysterectomy is the combination of *hyster-*, the root word for uterus, and *–ectomy*, the suffix meaning surgical removal. The procedure may be done several different ways. It may be vaginally, abdominally, or with the assistance of a laparoscope.

9. **A.** **Rationale:** A craniotomy is an incision into the skull. It combines *crani-*, the root word for skull, and *–otomy*, meaning incision or cutting into.

10. **B.** **Rationale:** A palatoplasty is the procedure for the repair of a cleft palate. It combines the root word *palat-* and the suffix *–plasty*. This procedure is routinely done to correct congenital deformities.

Anatomy and Physiology

2

From the beginning of time, mankind has been fascinated with how the human body works. Multiple texts and treatises have been published and researched, all dedicated to that one thing all humans have in common. The human body is complex and exciting, and, for anyone in the medical field, a necessary component of study. Surgical Technologists must have an intimate knowledge of human anatomy and physiology. They must know where things are located in the body, what these structures look like, and how they work, both alone and in each system. Without this knowledge, it is impossible to function in the role of Surgical Technologist.

CHAPTER OUTLINE

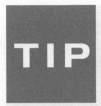

How to Answer Anatomy Questions

First, determine, if possible, the area of the body that the question is targeting. Which system is involved? Once that has been determined, begin the process of elimination. For example, if the question asked is where the gallbladder is located, picture in your mind the relevant anatomy. Once you can visualize the structures involved, you should be able to answer the question.

Example:
Which bone forms the medial Malleolus?

a. The femur
b. The tibia
c. The fibula
d. The radius

To answer this question, first ask yourself what area of the body is being targeted. The bones of the lower leg form the lateral and medial Malleolus, or ankles. Once you have established this, two answers are automatically thrown out. The femur is the long bone of the thigh, and the radius is an arm bone. That leaves you with two possible answers. If you picture the bones of the lower leg, you will see that the tibia, the larger weight bearing bone of the lower leg, makes up the medial Malleolus, while the fibula makes up the lateral Malleolus. Therefore, B would be the correct answer.

How to Answer Physiology Questions:
Again, determine which system the question targets. Once the system has been identified, remember the major organs that comprise the system. Ask yourself several questions pertaining to the system: What does the system do as a whole? What are the components of the system? How do they work together and separately? Chances are, once you have answered these questions, you will be able to identify the correct choice.

Example:
What does the cystic duct do?

a. Allows bile to travel from the liver to the duodenum
b. Allows pancreatic fluids to enter the small intestine
c. Connects the gallbladder to the common bile duct
d. Connects the common bile duct to the pancreas

To answer this question, you must understand the function of the digestive system and know the relevant anatomy. The function of the digestive system is to break down food into particles small enough to be used by the body. Some of the relevant anatomy includes the stomach, liver, gallbladder, small intestine, pancreas and large intestine. This question deals with the movement of digestive fluids into the small intestine. Remembering relevant anatomy, the common bile duct connects to both the cystic and hepatic ducts. Now you can use the process of elimination to answer this question. B can be eliminated, as it does not involve these structures. D can also be eliminated, as can A. This leaves C as the correct answer to this question. The cystic duct allows bile to travel from the liver via the hepatic duct, where it is stored in the gallbladder. The bile then flows down the cystic duct to the common bile duct.

The Body as a Whole

I. In order to direct an individual or team around the body, it is imperative that everyone use the same directional commands. All of these commands must have a starting point, or point of reference. In anatomy, we call this the correct anatomical position. This position is standing erect, with palms facing outward and feet forward. All of the directional terms use this anatomical stance as a starting point. Always remember that when talking about directions, the position is always related to the PATIENT. The following directional terms are commonly used in the medical field.

A. *Superior:* above; *inferior:* below
   Examples: *The femur is superior to the tibia; the pelvis is inferior to the clavicle.*
   - These terms are relative to the structures that are being used as a reference. In this example, the femur is superior. The femur COULD become inferior if it is being compared to the structures located above it.
   - This can also denote two points on the same bone or structure.
   - These terms are most commonly used to denote structures of the trunk.

B. *Cephalic:* toward the head; *caudal:* toward the tail

C. *Anterior (ventral):* front; *posterior (dorsal):* back
   Examples: *The ribs are anterior to the lungs. The pancreas is posterior to the stomach.*

D. *Medial:* nearer the middle; *lateral:* to the side
   Examples: *The ankle is formed by the medial malleolus and the lateral malleolus*

E. *Proximal:* nearest to the point of origin; *distal:* farthest from the point of origin
   Examples: *The phalanges are distal to the carpals. The acetabulum is proximal to the tibia.*
   - These terms tend to confuse. They are simply a means of saying that something is closer to the point of attachment or further away. When used in surgery, it usually refers to points on a structure. For example: the PIP joint. This is the abbreviation for <u>proximal</u> interphalangeal joint, or the joint <u>closest</u> to the point where the finger meets the hand while remaining in the finger (inter-).

F. *Superficial:* near the surface; *deep:* farther from the surface
   Examples: *Superficial fascia is closer to the surface; deep fascia covers muscles.*

G. *Visceral:* organ; *parietal:* wall
   - **These terms are used when describing the double-layered serous membranes of the body.**

II. **Body Planes and Cavities:** Body planes are imaginary divisions of the body, much like the equator divides the earth. Cavities and quadrants are used to narrow points of reference. When dealing with the body, it is easier to narrow the point of reference to the smallest possible area.

A. *Sagittal plane (vertical):* divides the body into right and left; *Midsagittal plane (median):* divides the body into equal halves

B. *Transverse plane (horizontal):* divides the body into superior and inferior

C. *Frontal plane (coronal):* vertical plane that divides the body into anterior and posterior

D. *Dorsal cavities:* cranial and spinal

E. *Ventral cavities:* thoracic and abdomino-pelvic. These cavities are separated by the diaphragm.
   1. *Quadrants of the abdomen:* right upper quadrant (RUQ), left upper quadrant (LUQ), right lower quadrant (RLQ), and left lower quadrant (LLQ)
   2. *Regions of the abdomen:* right and left hypochondriac, right and left iliac, right and left lumbar, umbilical, epigastric, and hypogastric
      - It is important to know where certain organs are located in reference to the quadrants. For example, the gallbladder is located in the upper right quadrant.

III. *Cells* (**cyto-**): Basic unit of structure; a living factory.

   A. *Cell (plasma) membrane:* semipermeable boundary that serves as a doorway to the cell

   B. *Nucleus:* control center that contains chromosomes (23 pairs: 22 body, 1 sex), genes, RNA, and DNA

   C. *Cytoplasm:* cellular material outside the nucleus and inside the cell membrane that contains organelles (little organs)
      1. *Mitochondria:* cell "batteries" that store energy and supply the cell with ATP
      2. *Lysosomes (soma:* **body;** *lyso:* **dissolve**): carry out digestive functions in the cell
      3. *Golgi apparatus:* delivers proteins to the cell
      4. *Endoplasmic reticulum:* transport system and site of protein synthesis
      5. *Ribosomes:* sites of protein synthesis
      6. *Peroxisomes:* disarm free radicals
      7. *Centrioles:* function during cell division
      8. *Cilia:* hairlike extensions responsible for movement of fluid around the cell
      9. *Flagella:* whiplike extension responsible for motility of the cell (sperm)
      10. *Cytoskeleton:* internal framework that determines cell shape

   D. *Transport across the cell membrane:* passive transport occurs without any energy
      1. *Diffusion* (**spreading out**): molecules moving to a less concentrated area, as in oxygen moving from alveoli in the lungs into capillaries
      2. *Osmosis:* diffusion of water molecules across a semipermeable membrane to a concentrated area for the purpose of dilution
      Example: Blood cells placed in a hypertonic solution, such as 5% NaCl, will lose water to the solution and shrink; blood cells placed in a hypotonic solution such as water will gain water from the solution and swell and burst; and blood cells placed in an isotonic solution (0.9% sodium chloride, which is normal saline) will remain unchanged
      3. *Filtration:* movement of molecules through a filter or a semipermeable membrane as a result of pressure
      Example: Because of a higher pressure in blood capillaries than in the nephron (basic unit of structure in the kidney where urine is made), waste products move (are filtered) from the blood capillaries into the nephron
      4. *Active transport:* use of energy to move molecules across a membrane to a higher concentration, such as the sodium-potassium pump between cell membranes
      5. Some cells are also capable of
         a. *Phagocytosis* (cell eating), as in the case of white blood cells engulfing bacteria
         b. *Pinocytosis* (cell drinking), as in the case of proximal kidney tubules reabsorbing filtered proteins

   E. *Cell division (mitosis):* some cells, such as RBC and nerve cells, do not divide or reproduce
      1. Five phases of mitosis
         a. **Interphase:** phase in which the cell grows and carries on its usual metabolic activities
         b. **Prophase**
         c. **Metaphase**
         d. **Anaphase**
         e. **Telophase:** the division of the cytoplasm (cytokinesis) is complete

IV. **Body Tissues:** Collections of specialized cells designed for a special function

   A. *Epithelial tissue*
      1. Lines (cavities, vessels), covers (body and body organs), and secretes (glandular)

2. Named by shapes
    a. *Squamous*
        Simple squamous: covers surface of pleura, peritoneum, and pericardium, and lines blood vessels
        Stratified squamous: skin, lines mouth and esophagus
    b. *Cubodial:* lines surface of kidney tubules and covers ovaries
    c. *Columnar:* lines stomach, intestines, and part of respiratory tract
3. Named by arrangement of cells
    a. *Simple:* one layer of cells
    b. *Stratified:* many layers; named for the shape of the outer layer
    c. *Pseudostratified:* appears to be two layers, but is only one
4. May be ciliated (contain hairlike cilia designed to move fluid) or nonciliated
5. Regenerates readily and heals quickly
6. Innervated (capable of sensations)
7. In surgery, it is generally sutured with absorbable sutures (exception: skin)
8. Cancer of epithelial tissue is carcinoma (basal cell or squamous cell)
9. Makes up membranes
    a. *Mucous:* lines passageways leading to outside, such as the gastrointestinal tract, genitourinary tract, and respiratory tract
    b. *Serous:* lines closed ventral cavities, includes peritoneum (lines abdomen), pericardium (sac that encloses heart), and pleura (lines chest). These membranes are double sided, made up of a visceral layer and a parietal layer.
10. Glandular epithelium; two types of glands
    a. *Exocrine:* secretions that travel through a duct to another area. Example: swat glands
    b. *Endocrine:* ductless glands that secrete hormones into the bloodstream. Example: the thyroid gland

B. *Connective tissue:* most variable and widespread tissue in the body
    1. Binds, protects, supports
    2. Types
        a. *Adipose (fat):* connective tissue that has a poor blood supply and is generally sutured with absorbable materials
            • Adipose tissue has a high possibility for surgical site infections because it is avascular.
        b. *Fibrous (fascia):* dense connective tissue—composes sheaths covering joints, muscles, meninges (coverings of brain and spinal cord), synovium (lining of synovial joints), scar tissue, tendons (connects muscles to bones), and ligaments (connects bone to bone)
        c. *Cartilage (chondro):* elastic tissue (gristle) that has little blood supply
        d. *Bone (osseous tissue)*
            i. *Cortical (compact):* bone cells arranged in concentric circles around central (haversian) canals; make up "shell" of bone to provide strength and support; and covered by periosteum
            ii. *Cancellous (spongy):* bone contains spaces with red marrow for making blood cells
        e. *Reticular (netlike):* blood and lymph tissue
        f. *Areolar:* loose connective tissue that fills spaces and helps to hold organs in place
    3. *Matrix:* intercellular substance in connective tissue

C. *Muscle tissue*
    1. *Skeletal (found attached to bones):* striated, voluntary. Example: biceps
    2. *Smooth:* (found in internal organs such as blood vessels and bladder) visceral, involuntary
    3. *Cardiac (found only in the heart):* striated, involuntary; contains intercalcated disks

    D. *Nerve tissue:* most highly specialized tissue
      1. **Found in nerves, brain, and spinal cord**
      2. *Neurons (nerve cells):* basic unit of structure in the nervous system; made up of dendrites (cell extensions that receive impulses), cell body, and axon (extension of the cell that conducts impulses away from the cell body)
      3. *Neuroglia (Schwann cells):* nonconductive covering of peripheral nerves which provide nutrition and protection; make up the myelin sheath of the neurons and give nerves a white, glistening appearance; supporting cells
      4. **Coordinates and integrates body function**

  V. **Organs:** Composed of different types of tissue and perform specific functions
    Examples: liver, heart

 VI. **System:** Composed of different organs working together to perform specific functions
    Example: circulatory system, which is composed of heart and blood vessels

VII. **Abnormalities**

    A. *Aplasia:* failure of an organ to develop normally
    B. *Hypoplasia:* underdevelopment of an organ
    C. *Atrophy:* without development, a decrease in the size of an organ
    D. *Hypertrophy:* overdevelopment, an increase in the size of an organ
    E. *Hyperplasia:* excessive proliferation of cells; body cells increase in number
    F. *Dysplasia:* abnormal development of tissue or an organ
    G. *Anaplasia:* loss of cell function

Terminology

1. *Anabolism:* production and maintenance of living tissue
2. *Carbohydrates:* organic compounds used by the body to produce heat and energy
3. *Catabolism:* transformation or breaking down of substances for energy production
4. *Element:* one type of atom, such as hydrogen (H), oxygen (O), carbon (C), calcium (Ca), phosphorus (P), sodium (Na), chloride (Cl), potassium (K), magnesium (Mg), or nitrogen (N)
5. *Homeostasis:* the body's system of checks and balances to maintain a constant internal environment
6. *Hydrolysis:* dissolution of substances by water
7. *Hypertonic solution:* one with a greater concentration than found in cells, thereby increasing osmotic pressure
8. *Hypotonic solution:* one less concentrated than body cells, thereby decreasing osmotic pressure
9. *Isotonic solution:* same concentration as body cells (0.9% NaCl) and therefore the same osmotic pressure
10. *Lipids (fats):* organic compounds that are insoluble in water and are used by the body for heat and energy
11. *Metabolism:* sum of all chemical and physical activity of living tissue
12. *Molecule:* two or more elements formed by a reaction, such as water (H_2O), sodium chloride (NaCl), potassium chloride (KCl), or carbon dioxide (CO_2)
13. *pH scale:* a scale of 1 to 14 to measure acidity (below 7.0); and alkalinity (over 7.0); 7.0 = neutral
14. *Proteins:* organic (living) compounds necessary to build and repair tissue

15. *Solution:* homogeneous mixture of a substance(s) (solutes) in a dissolving medium (solvent) such as water

16. *Synthesis:* putting together of molecules

The Body Systems

I. Integumentary System (the body covering, including skin, hair, and nails)

A. Medical prefixes for skin are *derm-, dermat-, cut-, cutan-*

B. Functions of the skin
1. Acts as a mechanical barrier to microorganisms (body's first line of defense)
2. Acts as a sensory organ, to keep us in touch with our environment
3. Regulates body temperature by the process of evaporation (sweating) and radiation (blood close to the body surface to give off heat)
4. Protects against physical trauma and fluid loss
5. Synthesizes vitamin D
6. Absorption of certain drugs

C. Structure of the skin (largest organ of the body)
1. *Epidermis:* outer layer of the skin composed of stratified squamous epithelium
   a. Composed of five strata (layers); regenerates from the bottom strata and forces cells outward, packing them closely together
   b. The outer strata (corneum) is composed of tough (keratinized) dead cells, which are constantly being shed
   c. Contains no nerve endings or blood vessels
   d. Provides a protective, waterproof covering due to a substance in the skin called keratin
   e. Contains fingerprints, ridges unique to each individual
   f. Contains melanocytes (pigment cells) for protection from sunlight
   g. Protected by normal body flora (bacteria), which serve as a natural protection
   h. Regenerates readily
2. *Dermis (true skin):* made up of dense connective tissue
   a. Contains collagen (gluelike fibers that run parallel to the skin and are the source of body lines) *(Note:* When the surgeon makes an incision, he or she attempts to follow body lines that results in a less pronounced scar)
   b. Blood vessels are in excellent supply; they dilate to bring blood near the surface for cooling and constrict to prevent the loss of heat; and they provide for effective healing.
   c. Sudoriferous (sweat) glands lie deep in the dermis and send secretions through ducts to the skin for evaporation and cooling. These glands are classified as exocrine glands.
   d. Sebaceous (oil) glands open into hair follicles and secrete sebum to keep hair and skin lubricated and provide protection against both bacteria and drying. Sebaceous glands are only present at sites where there are follicles.
   e. Sensory receptors for pain, cold, heat, touch, and vibration are located in the dermis.
   f. Arrector pili muscles (attached to hair) contract to make hair stand up and produce "goosebumps".
3. *Subcutaneous tissue (below the skin)*
   a. Made up of adipose tissue (fat)
   b. Provides insulation and gives the body a rounded appearance
   c. Because of good blood supply, it is surgically closed with an absorbable suture; it provides an area for hypodermic injection of medication intended to be absorbed slowly

> **SURGERY HINT**
>
> When entering the abdominal cavity, the tissue layers are as follows:
>
> - Skin
> - Subcuticular
> - Subcutaneous tissue and adipose/superficial fascia
> - Deep fascia
> - Muscle
> - Extraperitoneal fat
> - Peritoneum

    D. **Appendages of the skin (extensions of the epidermis)**
       1. *Hair:* produced by hair follicle; root part of hair enclosed in follicle, shaft part of hair projected from surface of skin; its color is derived from melanocytes, and it is kept pliable by oil from sebaceous glands; excess hair may be removed prior to surgery
       2. *Nails:* provide protection but may harbor microorganisms; the surgical scrub includes special attention to the subungual areas (under the nails), and nails should be short and free of polish

II. **Skeletal System**

    A. **Functions**
       1. Support/framework
       2. Protection of internal structures
       3. Movement (along with muscles)
       4. Storage of minerals (calcium and phosphorus)
       5. Blood cell formation (hematopoiesis)

    B. **Anatomy of a long bone**
       1. *Periosteum:* covering of bone that contains nerves and blood vessels and provides nourishment for growth and regeneration; may be separated from bone during surgery with muscles attached; repositioned and immobilized after surgery for healing; and surgically closed with absorbable sutures
       2. *Epiphyses:* ends of long bone
       3. *Epiphyseal plate located at the metaphysis:* cartilage disk near the end of long bones, which provides for growth in length until ages 15 to 17; may slip out of place and require a fusion (epiphysiodesis). Breaks along the epiphyseal plate may cause the bone to fuse, resulting in stunted growth along that bone.
       4. *Diaphysis:* shaft of a long bone
       5. *Cortical bone (compact bone):* forms the hard shell of bone because of deposits of calcium, phosphorus, and mineral salts
       6. *Cancellous bone (spongy bone):* contains pores and red marrow that makes blood cells
       7. *Articular cartilage:* protective layer covering articulating surfaces of bone
       8. *Medullary canal:* cavity that runs through the center of a long bone and is filled with yellow marrow; lined with endosteum

    C. **Types of bone, according to shape**
       1. *Long bones (longer than they are wide):* found in extremities (arms and legs) and serve as levers for movement
       2. *Short bones (cube shaped):* small bones in the wrists and ankles that provide for a variety of small movement
       3. *Flat bones (two thin layers of compact bone sandwiching a layer of spongy bone):* protective bones such as ribs and cranium
       4. *Irregular bones (those that do not fit into the previous categories):* variable in shape, such as vertebrae

D. Joints
  1. *Synarthroses:* immovable joints that are fused, such as sutures in the cranium
     a. *Fontanel:* "soft spot" at junctions of bones of the fetal skull prior to fusion; evident in children under 2 years of age
  2. *Amphiarthroses:* cartilage joints that are slightly movable: found between vertebrae, costochondral (rib cartilage) junctions, symphysis pubis, and epiphyseal lines
  3. *Diarthroses:* freely movable joints lined with synovium (tough connective tissue), which secretes synovial fluid as a lubricant; held together by ligaments
     a. *Ball and socket:* gives the widest range of motion
        Examples:
        Shoulder: head of the humerus fits into the glenoid cavity formed by the acromion and coracoid processes of the scapula and clavicle
        Hip: head of the femur fits into the acetabulum (deep fossa in the pelvis)
     b. *Hinge joint:* provides for flexion (bending) and extension (straightening), as at the elbow and knee
     c. *Condyloid joint:* oval-shaped rounded surface that fits into an elliptical cavity and provides movement in different planes, as seen between metacarpals and phalanges
     d. *Pivot joint:* projection through a ring that provides for rotation, as the cranium on the atlas and axis
     e. *Gliding joint:* flat surfaces sliding or twisting in various planes, as seen in the wrists and ankles
     f. *Saddle joint:* saddle-shaped bone fitting into another saddle that provides a variety of movements, as found in the thumb

E. Bones in the body (Total: 206)
  1. *Axial skeleton (80 bones):* head, vertebrae, ribs, and sternum
     a. *Skull (cranium) 8 bones:* frontal, temporal (2), parietal (2), occipital, ethmoid, and sphenoid
     b. *Face:* mandible, zygomatic, lacrimal, nasal, palatine, maxilla, vomer, and nasal conchae
     c. *Middle ear (3 auditory ossicles):* malleus, incus, and stapes
     d. *Hyoid bone:* U-shaped free-floating bone in the neck to which the tongue and other muscles are attached (essential during swallowing to bring the larynx forward to be closed off by the epiglottis). It is the only bone of the body that does not articulate directly with any other bone
     e. *Vertebral column:* 7 cervical, 12 thoracic, 5 lumbar, 1 sacrum, and 1 coccyx
     f. *Thorax:* sternum and 12 pairs of ribs (7 true ribs attached directly to sternum, 5 false ribs—last 2 are called floating ribs)
  2. *Appendicular skeleton* (126 bones): limbs and girdles
     a. *Pectoral girdle:* clavicle (collarbone) and scapula (shoulder blade)
     b. *Upper extremity:* humerus, ulna, and radius; wrist (8 carpals): scaphoid, lunate, triquetrum, pisiform, trapezium, trapezoid, capitate, and hamate; metacarpals (5); and phalanges (14)
     c. *Pelvic girdle (os coxa):* ilium, ischiuim, and pubis; attached to symphysis pubis anteriorly and to sacrum and coccyx posteriorly
     d. *Lower extremity:* femur, patella (knee cap), tibia, and fibula; ankle the medial and lateral malleolus of the tibia and fibula make up the ankle. (7 tarsals): navicular, talus, calcaneus (heel), cuneiforms (3), and cuboid; metatarsals (5); and phalanges (14)

F. Bone markings
  1. *Fossa:* depression (acetabulum, glenoid)
  2. *Sinus:* air-filled cavity in a bone lined with mucous membranes (4 paranasal sinuses: maxillary, sphenoid, ethmoid, frontal)

3. *Foramen (window):* opening through a bone, as the foramen magnum in the occipital bone for passage of the spinal cord. The largest foramen is the foramen magnum, located at the base of the skull.
4. *Projections for muscle attachment:* trochanter on the femur, crest of the tibia, and spinous processes on the vertebrae

G. Movement of joints
- It is essential that the Surgical Technologist is familiar with the terms related to movement of joints.
    1. *Abduction:* move away from the midline (to "abduct" someone is to take them away)
    2. *Adduction:* move toward the midline ("add" it back to the body)
    3. *Flexion:* bending; decreases the angle between articulating bones
    4. *Extension:* straightening; increases the angle between articulating bones
    5. *Inversion:* turning in
    6. *Eversion:* turning out
    7. *Supination:* palm up; supine: face up
    8. *Pronation:* palm down; prone: face down
    9. *Circumduction:* moving the distal end of an extremity to make a circle
    10. *Dorsiflexion:* toes pointed upward
    11. *Plantarflexion:* toes pointed downward

H. Terms
    1. *Bursa:* a fluid-filled synovial membrane sac that reduces friction and cushions tendons where they cross bones
    2. *Callus:* a bony collar that forms around a fracture site and is replaced by bone during the healing process
    3. *Haversian system:* a system of canals and matrix rings found in compact bone that allows blood vessels and nerves to be carried to all areas of the bone
    4. *Ligament:* tough connective tissue that secures bone to bone
    5. *Ossification:* bone development, two types
        a. *Intramembraneous ossification:* occurs within a fibrous membrane, in flat bones such as the skull
        b. *Endochondral ossification:* bone development that uses hyaline cartilage as models that are replaced by bone
    6. *Osteoblast:* bone-building cell
    7. *Osteoclast:* bone-destroying cell; helps to shape bone.
    8. *Osteocyte:* mature bone cell
    9. *Tendon:* tough connective tissue that connects muscles to bone

III. Muscular System

A. *Functions:* movement, maintenance of posture, and production of heat
B. Characteristics of muscle tissue
    1. *Irritability:* will respond to a stimulus
    2. *Extensibility and elasticity:* can stretch and resume former length

---

SURGERY HINT

When placing plates during open reduction internal fixations (ORIF), the order for instrumentation is as follows:

- Drill
- Depth gauge
- Tap
- Screw

---

   3. *Contractibility:* can shorten and thicken to exert pull
   4. *Tone:* slight tension
   5. *Fatigue:* loss of ability to respond to a stimulus

C. Muscle contraction
   1. *Steps*
      a. Stimulus from a motor neuron
      b. Release of acetylcholine at the myoneural junction for transmission
      c. Calcium ions released for actin and myosin (protein filaments which slide into place to cause contraction)
      d. **Acetylcholinesterase:** an enzyme to counteract acetylcholine
   2. *Concepts*
      a. Energy for muscle activity may be derived from
         i. *Aerobic respiration:* food source + oxygen equals energy plus water + carbon dioxide (which is expelled by respiration)
         ii. *Anaerobic respiration:* use of stored energy from mitochondria; has a waste product, creatinine, which is excreted in the urine
      b. The presence of waste, such as lactic acid buildup as a result of oxygen debt, causes more irritability of muscles. This results in muscle soreness and fatigue after exercise.
      c. Prolonged contractions can cause muscle cramps and impaired movement
      d. Rest is essential to allow blood to carry off waste and replenish glucose, oxygen, and protein for restoration

D. Naming of muscles
   1. *Shapes:* Examples: deltoid (triangular), serratus (sawtooth), and trapezius (trapezoid)
   2. *Sizes:* Examples: magnus (large, great), minus (small), brevis (short), and maximus (greatest)
   3. *Point of attachment:* Example: sternocleidomastoid
   4. *Location:* Examples: femoral (thigh), brachial (arm), pectoral (chest), gluteal (buttock), external (outermost), and lateral (side)
   5. *Action:* Examples: flexor, extensor, adductor, levator, depressor, and masseter
   6. *Direction of muscle fibers:* Examples: rectus (straight), oblique (slanted), and transverse (across)
   7. *Number of origins:* Examples: biceps (2); triceps (3)

E. Terminology related to muscles
   1. *Origin:* where the muscle is attached to a fixed or more fixed bone; the place the muscle originates or starts
   2. *Insertion:* where the muscle is attached to a movable bone
   3. *Agonist/prime mover:* the main muscle responsible for moving a part
   4. *Antagonist:* a muscle that has the opposite action as the agonist
   5. *Synergist:* a muscle or muscles that assist the agonist with moving the part

F. Skeletal muscles of the head
   1. *Facial expression:* frontalis (raise eyebrows), orbicularis oculi (close eyes), orbicularis oris (pucker mouth), buccinator (whistle, blow), and zygomaticus (smile)
   2. *Chewing (mastication):* masseter and temporalis

G. Muscles that move the head
   1. *Sternocleidomastoid:* flex the head
   2. *Trapezius:* hold up and extend the head
   3. *Platysma:* on anterior portion of neck, must be dissected to perform anterior neck procedures (tracheotomy)

H. Muscles that move the arm
   1. *Deltoid:* abduct the arm; used for intramuscular (IM) injections
   2. *Pectoralis major and minor:* extend and abduct the arm

3. *Serratus anterior:* pulls the scapula down and forward
4. *Latissimus dorsi:* extends and helps adduct the upper arm
5. *Biceps brachii:* flexes the lower arm and supinates the hand
6. *Triceps brachii:* extends the lower arm (forearm)

I. Muscles of respiration
   1. *Diaphram:* major muscle of breathing; separates the abdominal from the thoracic cavity; moves downward during inspiration
   2. *Intercostals:* located between the ribs; raises rib cage during inspiration

J. Muscles of the abdominal wall (used to tense the abdominal wall, expel abdominal contents, and flex the spine)
   1. *Rectus abdominis:* paired, straplike, superficial muscles; they extend from the rib cage to the pubis
   2. *External oblique:* paired, slanted, superficial muscles that make up the lateral wall of the abdomen
   3. *Internal oblique:* paired, slanted muscles located beneath the external obliques; their fibers run at right angles to the external obliques
   4. *Transverse abdominis:* deepest muscle of the abdominal wall; fibers run horizontally across the abdomen

K. Muscles of the lower limbs
   1. *Iliopsoas:* flexes the thigh
   2. *Gluteus maximus:* extends the leg
   3. *Gluteus medius:* abducts the thigh (area for IM injections)
   4. *Adductor longus, gracilis, and adductor magnus:* adduct the thigh
   5. *Quadriceps (rectus femoris, vastus lateralis, vastus intermedias and the vastus medialis):* extend the leg
   6. *Hamstring group (biceps femoris, semitendinosus, and semimembranous):* flex the leg
   7. *Sartorius:* longest muscle in the body; used to cross the legs
   8. *Gastrocnemius:* calf muscle; used for plantar flexion (stand on tiptoe); attached to bone by the Achilles tendon.
   9. *Tibialis anterior:* dorsiflexes the foot
   10. *Peroneus:* used for eversion of the foot

IV. Nervous System

A. Basic unit of structure is the neuron
   1. *Cell body:* main portion of neuron; contains the nucleus
   2. *Dendrites:* extensions that receive impulses and take them to the cell body
   3. *Axon:* extension that carries impulses away from the cell body; protected by
      a. *Myelin sheath:* white, fatty material that provides insulation
      b. *Neurilemma:* (exposed membrane of the Schwann cell; gives nerves a white glistening appearance)
      c. *Nodes of Ranvier:* gaps between Schwann cells; increase speed of transmission of impulse
   4. *Types of neurons*
      a. *Sensory (afferent):* carry messages to the central nervous system (CNS) from sensory receptors
      b. *Motor (efferent):* carry messages away from the CNS to the viscera, muscles, or glands (effectors)
      c. *Interneurons:* carry impulses within the CNS. They connect the sensory and motor neurons
   5. *Nerve impulse:* requires sodium (Na) and potassium (K); a deficiency or excess will affect nervous system function
   6. *Neurotransmitter chemicals (i.e., acetylcholine):* carry impulses across a synapse (gap between the axon of one nerve fiber and the dendrites of another); absence results in neurological disorders

B. Reflex arc (automatic, involuntary response)
   1. *Example:* knee-jerk reflex
   2. *Pathway:* receptor (receives stimuli), to sensory neuron (afferent), to dorsal root of the spinal cord, to interneuron in the gray matter of spinal cord to brain (for information), and to motor neuron (ventral root) to effect an action or reflex
   3. Surgical interruption of the reflex arc may be done to
      a. Stop intractable pain by severing the dorsal root (Rhizotomy)
      b. Improve circulation by the removal of a lumbar sympathetic ganglion from the ventral root (Lumbar Sympathectomy)

C. **Central nervous system (brain and spinal cord)**
   1. Made up of gray matter (does not regenerate) and white matter
      a. Gray matter of the brain is in the cortex (outer portion)
      b. Gray matter of the spinal cord surrounds the canal (inner portion, H-shaped)
   2. *Meninges:* 3-layered membrane covering the brain and spinal cord
      a. *Dura mater:* tough outer covering. Epidural hematomas are bruises to the brain above the dura. Subdural hematomas occur underneath the dura. It is important to differentiate the two during surgeries to evacuate hemotomas.
      b. *Arachnoid:* middle layer
      c. *Pia mater:* inner layer; the subarachnoid space is filled with cerebrospinal fluid (CSF)
   3. *Ventricles:* 4 cavities inside the brain where CSF is made. These are major structures in the brain. There are two lateral ventricles and the third and fourth ventricles. The third ventricle is of particular importance as it separates the right and left thalamus and is above the hypothalamus.
   4. *Cerebrospinal fluid:* a colorless fluid that provides a protective cushion for the brain, is constantly being produced in the choroid plexus of the ventricles, circulates around the brain and spinal cord, and is absorbed from the arachnoid villi into the venous circulation. Obstruction in the flow of CSF results in increased intracranial pressure and severe pain and can be surgically drained via a shunt between the ventricles and the peritoneuin (VP shunt) or the atria of the heart (VA shunt). If this obstruction occurs in a newborn prior to the fusion of the skull bones, the resulting hydrocephalus will cause the head to enlarge.
   5. **Divisions of the brain**
      a. *Cerebrum:* largest part of the brain; occupies the upper part of the cranium, has two hemispheres united by the corpus callosum, and controls body movement, reason, memory, and emotions
         Generally divided into four lobes: frontal (motor and speech), parietal (sensory), temporal (auditory and olfactory), and occipital (visual). Divided into two hemispheres by a deep fissure (longitudinal fissure).
         Cortex: outer surface made up of gray matter
         Corpus callosum: a connecting link between the two hemispheres
      b. *Cerebellum* (little brain): separated from the cerebrum with a deep fissure (tentorium); controls muscle tone, coordination, and equilibrium
      c. *Brain stem:* connects the spinal cord with the cerebrum and cerebellum
         Medulla oblongata: "vital center" that controls respiration, heartbeat, and blood pressure
         Midbrain and Pons: contain reflex centers and connect with other parts of the brain
      d. *Diencephalon:*
         Hypothalamus: control center for homeostasis, hunger, thirst, sleep, body temperature, water balance, and the pituitary gland/hypophysis
         Thalamus: central relay station

6. *Spinal cord:* 16 to 18 inches long and extends from the brain stem to the first lumbar vertebra; protected by the vertebral column
    a. Ends with extension of nerves (cauda equina)
    b. 31 pairs of nerves branch off from the cord, one pair for each intervertebral space
    c. *Plexus:* group of spinal nerves joined together which give off branches—cervical (C1–C4), brachial (C5–T1), and lumbosacral (T12–S5)
    d. *Sciatic nerve:* largest nerve in the body, formed from lumbosacral nerves and extends down the leg
    e. *Function:* carry information to and from the brain and body parts not served by the cranial nerves
7. *Peripheral nervous system (PNS):* made up of spinal nerves (31 pairs), cranial nerves (12 pairs), and ganglia (nerve cell bodies in the PNS)
    Cranial Nerves
    a. CN I: *Olfactory* (smell), sensory
    b. CN II: *Optic* (vision), sensory
    c. CN III: *Oculomotor* (controls movement of the intrinsic muscles of the eye and four pairs of extrinsic eye muscles), motor
    d. CN IV: *Trochlear* (controls the superior oblique muscle to move the eye down and to the side), motor
    e. CN V: *Trigeminal* (three branches): ophthalmic; maxillary; and mandibular, sensory, and motor
    f. CN VI: *Abducens* (controls the lateral rectus muscle to move the eye to the side), motor
    g. CN VII: *Facial* (motor and sensory to the face)
    h. CN VIII: *Vestibulocochlear* (hearing and equilibrium), sensory (old name is acoustic or auditory)
    i. CN IX: *Glossopharyngeal* (taste, swallowing), sensory and motor
    j. CN X: *Vagus* (internal organs; parasympathetic), sensory and motor
    k. CN XI: *Spinal accessory* (neck and back muscles), motor
    l. CN XII: *Hypoglossal* (move tongue), motor
8. *Autonomic nervous system (ANS):* controls automatic functions to keep the body in homeostasis; innervates all smooth muscles, heart muscle, and glands
    a. Sympathetic nerves arise from the thoracolumbar area of the spinal cord and function with epinephrine to prepare for "fight or flight," release of epinephrine increases during stress, danger, emotional crisis, or strenuous exercise
    b. Parasympathetic nerves arise from the cranial nerves and fibers from sacral area and work with the vagus to slow down body functions (except gastrointestinal activity); they take over when we sleep

---

SURGERY HINT

Surgery on the spine may be done by either an orthopedic surgeon or a neurosurgeon. Most surgical interventions on the spine are due to chronic pain from pinched or compressed nerve roots.

*An easy way to remember the number of vertebra in each region is **Breakfast, Lunch, and Dinner:** Eat breakfast at 7 (seven cervical vertebra), Lunch at 12 (twelve thoracic vertebra), and Dinner at 5 (five lumbar vertebra).

V. **Special Senses**
  A. **Sense of vision (eye, Cranial Nerve II, and the occipital lobe of the cerebrum)**
    1. *Eyelids (blephar-):* cover eyes
       a. Controlled by orbicularis oculi and levator palpebra superioris muscles and the ophthalmic branch of the trigeminal nerve
       b. Lined with a mucous membrane (conjunctiva) that reflects back to cover the front of the eye, except cornea. Inflammation of this membrane is conjunctivitis. "Pink eye" is a highly contagious, infectious form of conjunctivitis caused by a bacteria or virus
       c. Blink reflex is designed for protection
       d. Eyelashes serve as protection
       e. Meibomian glands are modified sebaceous glands associated with the eyelid edges and produce an oily secretion that lubricates the eye
    2. *Orbital cavity:* protective bony socket, composed of seven cranial and facial bones, in which most of the globe rests
    3. *Extrinsic eye muscles:* six pairs (medial, lateral, superior, and inferior rectus; superior and inferior oblique) controlled by Cranial Nerves III, IV, and VI; hold the globe in place and provide for movement
    4. *Lacrimal (tear) apparatus:* consists of a lacrimal gland situated on the superior lateral aspect of the eye; the gland secretes tears which flow across the eye to keep the conjunctiva clean and moist; tears are then discharged into the lacrimal sac (dacryocyst) on the medial aspect of the eye and into the nasolacrimal duct in the nose, where they help moisten the air we breathe
    5. *Eye (ocul-, ophthalm-)* is composed of three layers
       a. *Sclera (outer layer):* white, fibrous protective covering; the front portion (cornea) is transparent, bends (refracts) light rays, and serves as the "window of the eye"
       b. *Choroid (middle layer):* thin, pigmented vascular coat of the eye which absorbs stray light; it changes in the anterior section of the eye to make up two smooth intrinsic muscle structures, the ciliary body and the iris
          Ciliary body: ring-shaped structure inside the globe which contains suspensory ligaments attached to the lens; it is innervated by Cranial Nerve III (oculomotor) with control over accommodation for near and distant vision; secretes aqueous humor
          Iris: pigmented membrane between the cornea and lens which controls the amount of light entering the eye by controlling pupil size
          Lens: oval-shaped, solid, but flexible transparent structure, held in place by suspensory ligaments (zonules) attached to the ciliary body; it provides for accommodation for near and distant vision by rounding up or flattening out; and refracts light to focus on the retina; opacity (clouding) of the lens is a cataract
          Anterior cavity: made up of the anterior chamber (space between the iris and the cornea) and posterior chamber (space between the iris and suspensory ligaments and lens)
          Aqueous humor: watery fluid produced by the ciliary body (5 to 6 ml/day) that empties into the posterior chamber, passes through the pupil into the anterior chamber, and then passes into a small venous sinus (canal of Schlemm) into the venous circulation; maintains an intraocular pressure of about 20 mm Hg to push the interior of the globe to its periphery and bring oxygen and nutrients to anterior structures of the eye
          Posterior cavity: contains the vitreous humor, a jellylike substance which keeps the retina in close contact with the choroid, bends light rays, and helps maintain the shape of the globe

  c. *Retina (inner layer):* contains rods (black-and-white vision) and cones (color vision); rods and cones are distributed over the entire retina except where the optic nerve leaves the eye (optic disk or blind spot); lateral to the blind spot is the fovea centralis that contains only cones and is the area of greatest visual acuity; receives visual images and converts them into electrical impulses, which are then transmitted through the optic nerve to the optic chiasm (where nerves cross) and then to the occipital lobe of the cerebrum for interpretation and storage

 B. Sense of hearing (ear, cochlear branch of Cranial Nerve VIII (vestibulocochlear), and temporal lobes of the cerebrum)

  1. *External ear (ot/o-)*

   a. *Pinna (auricle):* expanded portion on the side of the head, composed of cartilage and covered with skin; contains folds for collecting sound waves and directing them inward

   b. *External auditory canal:* lined with a mucous membrane, fine hairs, and ceruminous (wax) glands for protection

   c. *Tympanic membrane (myring, tympan):* the eardrum separates external from the middle ear and vibrates from sound waves

  2. *Middle ear:* air-filled cavity

   a. *Eustachian (auditory) tube:* connects the middle ear with nasopharynx; equalizes air pressure on both sides of the eardrum

   b. *Auditory ossicles:* three small bones (malleus, incus, and stapes) that amplify and conduct sound waves from the eardrum to the oval window

   c. *Mastoid sinus:* connected to the posterior wall

  3. *Inner ear*

   a. *Osseous labyrinth (series of fluid-filled canals):* contains organs for hearing and equilibrium; located in the temporal bone

   b. *Vestibule:* space between the cochlea and semicircular canals

   c. *Semicircular canals (three at right angles to each other):* contain receptors for equilibrium; filled with perilymph

   d. *Cochlea:* snail-shaped bony structure containing receptor cells for hearing (organ of Corti); filled with perilymph

   e. *Vestibulocochlear nerve (Cranial Nerve VIII):* has two branches; carries impulses from the cochlea to the temporal lobe of the cerebrum for hearing, and from the vestibule to the cerebellum for equilibrium

 C. Other senses

  1. *Olfactory (smell):* receptor cells located in the superior part of the nasal cavity, respond to chemical stimuli and transmit sensory messages through the olfactory (Cranial Nerve I) to the temporal lobe of the cerebrum

  2. *Gustatory (taste):* receptor cells (responding to chemical stimuli) located in the taste buds of the tongue (sweet, sour, salty, bitter) transmit sensory impulses through the glossopharyngeal (Cranial Nerve IX) and facial (Cranial Nerve VII) nerves and through the medulla and thalamus to the parietal lobe of the cerebrum

  3. *Somatic (body):* receptors located in the skin for pain, touch (tactile), vibration, pressure, heat, and cold; carried through peripheral nerves to the parietal lobe of the cerebrum

  4. *Proprioceptors:* sensory nerve endings that respond to changes in the tension of joints, tendons, and muscles; sometimes referred to as the kinesthetic sense

VI. **Endocrine System**

 A. Group of ductless glands scattered throughout the body that secrete hormones (chemicals) directly into the blood; each gland has specific functions and works with the nervous system to integrate and coordinate body functions

B. **Endocrine glands**
   1. *Pituitary gland (hypophysis):* located in a depression of the sphenoid bone (sella turcica); called the master gland
      a. *Anterior pituitary (adenohypophysis):* stimulated by releasing hormones from the hypothalamus; secretes tropic hormones that stimulate other glands to produce hormones, controlled by a negative feedback mechanism
         Thyroid stimulating hormone (TSH): stimulates the thyroid gland
         Adrenocorticotropic hormone (ACTH): stimulates the cortex of the adrenal gland
         Growth hormone (GH): stimulates growth, especially of bones and muscles
         Gonadotropic hormones (follicle stimulating [FSH] and luteinizing [LH] hormones): stimulate the sex glands to produce sperm or eggs and other sex hormones
         Prolactin (PRL): stimulates the production of milk
      b. *Posterior pituitary (neurohypophysis)*
         Antidiuretic hormone (ADH): promotes retention of water by kidneys
         Oxytocin (OXT): causes uterine contractions
   2. *Pineal gland:* located in the brain; secretes melatonin, which is involved in establishing the day/night cycle
   3. *Thymus gland:* located in the mediastinum, largest during childhood; secretes thymosin, which regulates the development and function of the immune system
   4. *Thyroid gland:* located in the neck in front of the trachea and below the larynx; composed of a right and a left lobe connected by a bridge of tissue (isthmus); has an excellent blood supply; and secretes
      a. *Thyroxine:* hormone that controls cellular metabolism; requires iodine for synthesis
      b. *Calcitonin:* a hormone needed to store calcium in bones and teeth
   5. *Parathyroid glands:* four very small glands embedded on the posterior surface of the thyroid gland; they produce parathormone or parathyroid hormone, a hormone that maintains proper calcium and phosphorus levels in the blood by "pulling it" from bones and teeth
   6. *Adrenal glands (suprarenal):* pair of glands located retroperitoneally over the kidneys; these glands have two divisions
      a. *Adrenal medulla (inner portion):* secretes epinephrine and norepinephrine, which work with the sympathetic nervous system to prepare for "fight or flight"
      b. *Adrenal cortex (outer portion):* secretes sex hormones and steroid (corticoids) hormones (cortisol, cortisone, and aldosterone) that protect during stress by regulating fluid and electrolyte balance and by converting stored energy to a usable form; influences sexual development
   7. *Pancreas (gland lying in the arms of the duodenum):* both an exocrine (produces pancreatic juices and enzymes to digest all types of food and sends them by ducts to the duodenum) and an endocrine gland; the two hormones secreted by islet of Langerhans cells in the pancreas and which empty directly into the blood are
      a. *Insulin:* secreted by beta cells; needed to metabolize and carry sugar into cells, thereby decreasing blood sugar levels; lack of this hormone results in the disease diabetes mellitus
      b. *Glucagon:* secreted by alpha cells; increases blood sugar levels
   8. *Testes (orchi-):* two male sex glands located in the scrotum; responsible for spermatogenesis and the production of *testosterone* by interstitial cells; a hormone influencing male characteristics

9. *Ovaries (oophor-):* two female sex glands located in the pelvis that produce eggs and two hormones
   a. *Estrogens:* influence female characteristics
   b. *Progesterone:* maintains pregnancy

VII. **Digestive System**

   A. **Made up of the alimentary canal or gastrointestinal (GI) tract (food tube from mouth to anus) and accessory organs (teeth, salivary glands, tongue, liver, gallbladder, and pancreas)**

   B. *Functions:* **breakdown and absorption of food; elimination of solid waste**

   C. **Alimentary canal (gastrointestinal tract)**
      1. *Mouth (oral cavity):* lined with a vascular mucous membrane; begins the process of digestion and includes cheeks, lips, roof (palate), uvula (tissue suspended from soft palate which keeps food out of the nasopharynx), and lingual tonsils (mounds on the back of the tongue)
         a. *Tongue (gloss-, lingua):* skeletal muscle attached anteriorly to the floor of the mouth by a frenulum and posteriorly to the hyoid bone; covered by mucous membrane; innervated by the hypoglossal (Cranial Nerve XII) and glossopharyngeal (Cranial Nerve IX) nerves; it is the organ for speech, taste, and swallowing
         b. *Salivary glands:* three pairs of exocrine glands which produce and carry saliva through ducts into the mouth to soften foods; saliva contains an enzyme (amylase) that begins the digestion of starches
            i. *Parotid glands:* below and in front of the ear; inflammation of these glands is the "mumps." The parotid gland is the largest of the salivary glands
            ii. *Submaxillary glands:* below the jaw
            iii. *Sublingual glands:* beneath the tongue
         c. *Teeth:* needed to break up and grind food in preparation for digestion
            i. *Two sets:* 20 deciduous (baby teeth) and 32 permanent
            ii. *Incisors (four upper and four lower):* sharp and designed for cutting and biting
            iii. *Canine (two upper and two lower):* for tearing
            iv. *Premolars (four upper and four lower):* for grinding
            v. *Molars (six upper and six lower):* for grinding
            vi. *Structure:* root(s) in a socket (alveolar); dental pulp; cementum (covers dentin of root); crown, neck, dentin, and enamel (hardest substance in the body); gingiva (gums); periodontal membrane (around teeth)
      2. *Pharynx (throat):* passageway for food and air. Three divisions
         a. *Nasopharynx:* above the soft palate; connects with the nares and contains adenoids (pharyngeal tonsils) and the opening of the eustachian tubes
         b. *Oropharynx:* from soft palate to hyoid bone; contains palatine tonsils
         c. *Laryngopharynx:* from hyoid bone to larynx
      3. *Walls* of GI tract; from esophagus to colon is made up of four layers
         a. *Mucosa:* inner layer; secretes mucus
         b. *Submucosa:* contains blood vessels, nerve endings, and lymph vessels
         c. *Muscularis externa:* contains smooth muscles that contract to propel food (peristalsis)
         d. *Serosa:* outer layer; secretes serous fluid
      4. *Esophagus:* muscular tube extending from pharynx to stomach; has alkaline pH; passes through the mediastinum directly behind the trachea and heart; and penetrates the diaphragm at the hiatus. A hernia occurring at the hiatus is a hiatal hernia
      5. *Stomach (gastr-):* muscular elastic pouch located in the epigastrium
         a. *Divisions:* fundus (top), body, and pylorus (lower portion)

b. *Sphincters:* circular muscles at the top (cardiac) and lower end (pyloric) to control the entry and exit of contents (chyme)

c. Lined with a mucous membrane containing gastric glands that secrete mucin (protects lining), hydrochloric acid (stimulates pepsin, breaks down connective tissue in meats, and kills bacteria), and enzymes (pepsin, which breaks down protein, and lipase, which works on fat)

d. Contains rugae: folds that allow for expansion

6. *Small intestines (enter-):* about 1 inch in diameter, in excess of 20 feet long, and divided into three sections: duodenum, jejunum, and ileum

   a. *Duodenum:* major organ of digestion; receives bile from the gallbladder at Ampulla of Vater for emulsification of fats; and digestive juice with enzymes from the pancreas—lipase (fat), amylase (carbohydrates), and trypsin (protein)

   b. *Jejunum:* begins at ligament of Treitz

   c. *Ileum:* both jejunum and ileum are designed for absorption of food; the end products of carbohydrates, proteins, and fats are glucose, amino acids, and fatty acids and glycerol, respectively

   d. *Villi:* fingerlike structures projecting from the mucosa of the intestinal tract through which food products are absorbed

   e. Amino acids and glucose are absorbed into the portal circulation and taken to the liver

   f. Fats are absorbed through the lacteals in the villi into the lymphatic circulation

   g. Lymph with fats is known as chyle

7. *Large intestines (col-):* 5 to 6 feet long and about 2½ inches in diameter; designed for absorption of water, electrolytes, and some vitamins; and elimination of waste; the walls of the colon contain strips of muscle (teniae coli) and outpouches (haustras)

   a. **Divisions**

      Cecum: first portion (to which the appendix is attached)
      Ascending colon: on the right, attached at hepatic flexure
      Transverse colon: crosses the abdomen just below the stomach
      Descending colon: on the left, attached at splenic flexure
      Sigmoid colon: S-shaped portion in the pelvis
      Rectum: straight portion at the end
      Anal canal and sphincter: opening at the end
      Colon is populated with coliform bacteria (fermentative gram-negative rods, such as *Escherichia, Citobacter, Enterobacter, Klebsiella,* and *Serratia*).

      (*Note:* During surgery on the colon, extreme care must be taken to avoid the transfer of these opportunistic pathogens to other areas of the body.)

D. **Accessory organs**

1. *Pancreas:* fish-shaped organ lying in the "arms" of the duodenum and divided into a head, body, and tail

   a. *Function:* manufacture pancreatic juice for digestion, insulin for carbohydrate metabolism, and glucagon as an antagonist for insulin

   b. Pancreatic juices are carried through the pancreatic duct of Wirsung, which joins with the bile duct to enter the duodenum at the ampulla of Vater which is controlled by the sphincter of Oddi

2. *Liver (hepat-):* largest gland in the body; located in the right hypochondriac region; divided into two lobes; connected to the diaphragm and abdomen by falciform and four other ligaments; and has two major blood supplies entering (portal vein and hepatic artery) and one exiting (hepatic vein, which empties into the inferior vena cava)

   a. *Bile channel:* right and left hepatic ducts from each lobe join to form the common hepatic duct, which joins with the cystic duct (from the

SURGERY HINT

Surgical entry into the gastrointestinal tract is considered a "dirty" part of the procedure. All instrumentation and equipment that come into contact with the GI tract should be considered contaminated and thus should be isolated from the other instruments. Gloves and sometimes gowns will be changed once this portion of the surgery has been completed.

If the surgeon will need specific instruments after this portion, the tech should ensure that they are not used during the entry into the bowel or that replacements are available.

Many surgeons will want to irrigate with antibiotic irrigation after this part of the procedure.

Irrigation should be warm to prevent lowering core body temperature.

gallbladder) to form the common bile duct, which in turn joins with the pancreatic duct to enter the duodenum

  b. *Functions of the liver include*

Destruction of worn-out red blood cells (RBCs) (iron kept for storage or sent back to bone marrow to make more RBCs)

Production of bile (from hemoglobin): used for fat emulsification (works like a dish detergent when emulsifying grease)

Storage of glucose in the form of glycogen for quick conversion in a stress situation; storage of iron and fat-soluble vitamins (A, D, E, and K)

Production of urea from the breakdown of proteins

Manufacture of blood-clotting proteins (fibrinogen and pro-thrombin) *(Note:* Vitamin K, a fat-soluble vitamin, is necessary for the production of prothrombin)

Regulation of blood volume and the production of body heat

Detoxification of harmful substances (anesthesia, drugs, and poisons)

  3. *Gallbladder (cholecyst-):* a pear-shaped sac that lies in a shallow fossa on the inferior surface of the liver; stores bile until needed for fat digestion

E. **Terms related to the digestive system**

  1. *Anabolism:* the constructive phase of metabolism; larger molecules are built from smaller ones

  2. *Catabolism:* the destructive phase of metabolism; complex substances are broken down to simpler ones

  3. *Constipation:* a decrease in the frequency of defecation resulting in the stool becoming hard and difficult to pass

  4. *Defecation:* the passing of stool from the bowel

  5. *Diarrhea:* the passing of a liquid stool due to the quick passage through the colon and therefore insufficient time to absorb water

  6. *Flatus:* gas in the digestive tract

  7. *Jaundice:* a yellow discoloration of the skin due to a buildup of bile

  8. *Mesentery:* a **fan-shaped** fold of peritoneum that anchors the intestines to the posterior abdominal wall

  9. *Metabolism:* a broad term that refers to all physical and chemical changes that take place within an organism

  10. *Omentum:* an **apron-shaped** fold of peritoneum that attaches to the transverse colon and stomach and hangs loosely anteriorly over the abdominal organs; the "watchdog of the abdomen"

  11. *Reflux:* backward flow; gastroesophageal reflux disease (GERD) is the regurgitation of stomach acid into the esophagus causing heartburn and esophagitis

12. *Regurgitation:* a backward flow, the passing of stomach contents back into the mouth through the esophagus
13. *Ulcer:* a craterlike erosion in the mucosa of the gastrointestinal tract caused by hydrochloric acid and pepsin

VIII. Blood

A. *Medical terms: hem-, hemat-, emia, sangui-*

B. *Amount:* average adult, approximately 5 L (approximately 70 ml/kg of body weight)

C. *Composition*
   1. *Plasma (55% of blood):* liquid part of blood (about 92% water)
      a. *Plasma proteins:* albumin (for osmotic pressure), globulin (antibodies for infection control), and fibrinogen and prothrombin (clotting factors)
      b. Plasma also contains waste (urea and ammonia), electrolytes, nutrients, and hormones
   2. Formed elements are erythrocytes, leukocytes, and thrombocytes
      a. *Erythrocytes (red blood cells):* made in red bone marrow with iron; contain hemoglobin (essential as a transport medium for oxygen and other gases, normal: hemoglobin is 13–18 grams per 100 ml of blood for males, 12–16 grams per 100 ml of blood for females); average life of 120 days, after which they are filtered out by the spleen and sent to the liver for breakdown; give blood the red color; normal range is 4.5 to 5.5 million/cubic ml of blood; hematocrit is the percentage of red blood cells in a given volume of blood: normal is 45%.
      b. *Leukocytes (white blood cells):* normal range 5000 to 10,000/cubic ml of blood; needed to fight infection; differential white count as follows:
         Neutrophils: 40% to 70%; made in bone marrow and are phagocytic (engulf microbes)
         Eosinophils: 1% to 4%; help detoxify foreign substances and secrete enzymes that break down clots
         Basophils: less than 1%; release histamine (increases capillary permeability)
         Lymphocytes: 20% to 45%; made in lymphatics; and make antibodies to provide immune response
         Monocytes: 4% to 8%; develop into macrophages and serve as scavenger cells that engulf microbes
      c. *Thrombocytes (platelets):* clotting cells; normal count is about 300,000 per cubic ml of blood

D. **Function of blood**
   1. Transportation of nutrients and oxygen to cells and wastes away from cells
   2. Combat infection
   3. Control body temperature

E. *Blood clotting:* injured thrombocytes release serotonin, which causes blood vessels to spasm and narrow; injured tissues release thromboplastin, which combines with prothrombin in the presence of calcium to form thrombin; thrombin combines with fibrinogen to form fibrin (basis of a clot)

F. *Blood types (determined by certain antigens attached to RBCs)*
   1. *Type A:* A antigen and anti-B antibody
   2. *Type B:* B antigen and anti-A antibody
   3. *Type AB:* both A and B antigens, and no antibodies (universal recipient)
   4. *Type 0:* absence of antigens, and both anti-A and anti-B antibodies (universal donor)

G. *Rh factor:* antigen found in about 85% to 90% of the population; problem may be created in an Rh-negative mother with an Rh-positive fetus (erythroblastosis fetalis), which can be corrected by the administration of RhoGam around the 28th week of pregnancy

H. **Blood typing and crossmatching are essential to prevent reactions (hemolysis of RBC and allergic) from the administration of whole blood or red blood cells**

IX. **Circulatory System:** The circulatory system is a complex, yet fascinating, method of pickup, transportation, and delivery of numerous items over miles of tiny "roadways" operating under one major force, the heart

A. *Heart:* four-chambered hollow muscle located in the mediastinum near the center of the chest; protected anteriorly by the sternum and posterior by the thoracic spine; apex rests on the diaphragm, with the base (area where great vessels emerge) just below the second rib

1. Layers of the heart wall
   a. *Endocardium:* endothelial lining
   b. *Myocardium:* thick muscular layer composed of cardiac muscle
   c. *Epicardium:* visceral layer of pericardium (a double sac of serous membrane, which secretes a fluid to provide for lubrication); parietal pericardium is the fibrous layer that anchors the heart to surrounding structures

2. Chambers of the heart
   a. *Right atrium:* upper chamber that receives deoxygenated venous blood from the superior and inferior vena cava
   b. *Right ventricle:* lower chamber that pumps deoxygenated blood to the lungs through the pulmonary artery
   c. *Left atrium:* upper chamber that receives oxygenated blood from the lungs via the pulmonary veins
   d. *Left ventricle:* lower chamber that pumps oxygenated blood into systemic circulation (all parts of the body via the aorta); does the most work and has the thickest wall

3. Valves direct the flow of blood in the heart
   a. Two atrioventricular valves are secured by tendinous cords (chordae tendineae) attached to papillary muscles
      Tricuspid: between the right atrium and the right ventricle
      Bicuspid (mitral): between the left atrium and the left ventricle
   b. Two semilunar valves
      Pulmonary: at the opening to pulmonary artery
      Aortic: at the opening to aorta

4. *Blood supply:* coronary arteries that arise from the ascending aorta
   a. Right coronary and its branches (posterior descending and marginal arteries) supply the right atrium, right ventricle, and left ventricle
   b. Left coronary and its branches (anterior descending and circumflex arteries) supply the left atrium, left ventricle, and right ventricle
   c. Venous blood, drained by cardiac veins, returns through the coronary sinus to the right atrium

5. *Nerve supply (autonomic nervous system):* both sympathetic and parasympathetic

6. Electrical conduction pathway
   a. *Pacemaker:* sinoatrial (SA) node initiates each heartbeat, located in the right atrium
   b. Atrioventricular (AV) node: at the junction of atria and ventricles
   c. Bundle of His
   d. Right and left bundle branches
   e. *Purkinje fibers:* found in the ventricles of the myocardium; stimulate contraction of the heart
      (Note: Potassium, calcium, and sodium are essential electrolytes in regulating muscular activity)

7. *Function of the heart:* a double pump separated by a muscle wall (interatrial and interventricular septum)
    a. *Double pump:* right heart receives and sends blood out for oxygen; left heart receives and sends oxygenated blood out to all parts of the body
    b. Blood fills both atria simultaneously and passes through the atrioventricular valves into ventricles while the heart is in diastole (semilunar valves are closed); when the ventricles contract to force blood out of the heart (systole), the semilunar valves are open and AV valves are closed
    c. *Stroke volume:* amount of blood ejected from the heart with each contraction (beat) is approximately 60 to 70 ml; the average number of beats is 70 to 80 per minute, with a regular rhythm
    d. *Pulmonary circulation:* the route of blood from the heart to lungs and back
    e. *Systemic circulation:* the route of blood from the heart to all parts of the body and back
8. Circulation of blood through the heart
    a. Enters the right atrium from superior and inferior vena cava and coronary sinus
    b. Tricuspid valve to the right ventricle
    c. Pulmonary valve to pulmonary artery to lungs for oxygenation and elimination of carbon dioxide
    d. Pulmonary veins to the left atrium
    e. Bicuspid valve to the left ventricle
    f. Aortic valve to aorta into systemic circulation
9. *Blood pressure:* pressure exerted against the walls of arteries when the heart contracts
    a. *Systolic:* pressure when blood is being forced out; normal is 90 to 130 mm Hg
    b. *Diastolic:* pressure when heart is filling; normal is 60 to 80 mm Hg
    c. *Heart rate and blood pressure are affected by:*
       Blood volume
       Blood viscosity (thickness)
       Diameter of the vessels and peripheral resistance
       Pressure receptors in the aortic arch and carotid sinus
       Chemoreceptors that are sensitive to the lack of oxygen, increase in carbon dioxide, and increase in hydrogen ion concentration in the blood
       External stimuli: pain (slows), cold (slows), and heat (accelerates)

B. **Blood vessels**
    1. *Arteries:* carry blood away from the heart; carry oxygenated blood (except pulmonary and umbilical); have thicker walls for higher pressure from the force of the pump; and layers are endothelium (tunica intima) (lining), muscle layer (tunica media) (smooth), and outer layer (tunica externa) (connective tissue); smallest arteries are arterioles
    2. *Veins (phleb-, ven-):* carry blood toward the heart, carry deoxygenated blood (except umbilical and pulmonary); have thinner, less elastic walls because of less pressure and one-way valves; dependent upon contraction of skeletal muscles to force blood back to the heart; smallest veins are venules
    3. *Capillaries:* smallest vessels; connect arterioles to venules; carry blood to cells; have one-cell-thick membranes to allow for movement of nutrients and oxygen into the cells and waste products and carbon dioxide out of the cells

C. **Major arteries and their branches, carry blood away from the heart**
    1. *Aorta*
       a. *Ascending aorta:* coronary arteries; to heart muscle

      b. *Aortic arch:* brachiocephalic (innominate) which divides into the right common carotid and right subclavian; left common carotid, and left subclavian

          Common carotid: head and neck divides into

            i. *Internal carotid:* brain, eye, and orbit

           ii. *External carotid:* face, scalp, muscles of head and neck

          Subclavian branches into

            i. *Vertebral:* brain

           ii. *Axillary:* at the armpit, in the arm becomes the brachial, at bend of elbow becomes the radial, ulnar, volar arches, and digital arteries in hand

          iii. *Circle of Willis:* at base of brain, common place for cerebral aneurysms

      c. *Descending aorta*

          Thoracic aorta: until it passes through the diaphragm

            i. *Intercostals:* muscles, breasts, pleura, vertebral column, and spinal cord

           ii. *Superior phrenic:* diaphragm

          iii. *Esophageal:* esophagus

          iv. *Bronchial: lungs*

          Abdominal aorta: once it passes through the diaphragm

            i. *Inferior phrenic:* diaphragm

           ii. *Lumbar:* muscles of abdomen and trunk

          iii. *Celiac:* branches into: hepatic (liver), gastric (stomach), and splenic (spleen)

          iv. *Superior and inferior mesenteric:* to intestines

           v. *Renal: kidneys*

          vi. *Testicular or ovarian:* to gonads

          Branches into the common iliacs that divide into the internal iliac, which supplies the pelvic organs, and external iliac, which passes through the femoral rings and extends down the leg

    2. *Leg:* external iliac, femoral, popliteal, anterior and posterior tibial, peroneal, dorsalis pedis, and plantar arch

D. *Main veins:* carrying deoxygenated blood toward heart

    1. *Leg:* plantar venous arch, anterior and posterior tibial, great saphenous (superficial), femoral, external iliac, common iliac, inferior vena cava

    2. *Arm:* radial, ulnar, cephalic, basilic, median cubital, brachial, axillary, subclavian, brachiocephalic, superior vena cava

    3. *Head:* external and internal jugular, subclavian, and superior vena cava

    4. Veins generally run alongside arteries and carry the same name

---

SURGERY HINT

During peripheral vascular procedures, the Surgical Technologist may have multiple medications on the back table. Careful labeling and handling of these medications are of the utmost importance during these procedures. These medications may include:

- Heparin
- Thrombin (with gel-foam cut in strips as directed)
- Papaverine
- Lidocaine
- Contrast media
- Antibiotic irrigation

E. Fetal circulation
   1. *Placenta:* filtering device between mother's and fetus' blood stream
   2. *Umbilical vein:* located within umbilical cord and carries oxygen and nutrients from mother to fetus
   3. *Umbilical arteries:* two arteries located within umbilical cord and carry waste products and carbon dioxide from the fetus to the mother
   4. *Ductus venosus:* vein connecting the umbilical vein to the inferior vena cava bypassing the fetus' immature liver
   5. *Foramen ovale:* a flaplike opening in the interatrial septum that allows fetal blood to travel from the right atrium directly into the left atrium bypassing the fetal lungs
   6. *Ductus arteriosus:* artery that connects the pulmonary artery to the aorta bypassing the fetal lungs

X. **Lymphatic System:** The lymphatic system is considered to be a part of the circulatory system as it picks up plasma which has seeped through capillaries to bathe the cells, cleans it up, and gets it back into circulation; it holds the key to our immunity; the lymphatic system is made up of lymph, lymphatic vessels, nodes, and glands

   A. *Lymph vessels:* a network of vessels that covers the body; it begins with lymphatic capillaries lying alongside blood capillaries and merges with other capillaries to form larger vessels
      1. Drains toward the heart
      2. Similar in makeup to veins; thin walls
      3. Contain one-way valves
      4. Depend a great deal upon skeletal muscle action or gravity to force lymph toward the heart
      5. Thoracic duct: largest lymph channel; drains the lower right half of the body and the entire left side and empties into the left subclavian vein
      6. Right lymphatic duct is a short channel that collects lymph from the right upper half of the body and empties it into the right subclavian vein
      7. *Edema:* collection of lymph fluid in the tissues (swelling)

   B. *Lymph nodes:* bean-shaped enlargements along the course of lymph vessels
      1. Functions
         a. Filter out bacteria, and cancer cells and destroy some foreign particles
         b. Make lymphocytes and macrophages (large monocytes) that destroy foreign substances
         c. Produce antibodies
      2. Located in groups or clusters; some examples are
         a. *Floor of the mouth:* drain face
         b. *Neck (cervical):* drain head
         c. *Bend of the elbow (cubital):* drain forearm
         d. *Axilla:* drain arm, chest, and breast
         e. *Subclavian:* drain lungs
         f. *Groin:* drain legs and genitals
         g. *Mesenteric:* drain intestines and contain fat (chyle) absorbed from lacteals in intestinal villi
         h. *Lumbar:* drain pelvic organs
      3. May become enlarged with cancer and certain infections

   C. *Lymph glands*
      1. *Spleen:* a brownish organ located in the left hypochondriac region, behind the stomach and below the diaphragm; functions much like a lymph node
         a. Makes lymphocytes and monocytes
         b. Purifies blood by removing worn-out cells and foreign debris
         c. Stores blood (about 350 ml)
         d. Produces antibodies

2. *Thymus gland:* located in the superior anterior mediastinum; larger in children but decreases in size after puberty; and secretes thymosin (a hormone essential in immunity) and contributes to maturing T cells (special types of lymphocyte)

3. *Tonsils:* two palatine tonsils located in the oropharynx; two pharyngeal tonsils (adenoids) located in the nasopharynx; two lingual tonsils at base of the tongue; larger in children

XI. **Respiratory System:** The respiratory system permits an exchange of essential life gases between the environment and the blood and consists of the nasal cavity, pharynx, larynx, trachea, and the bronchi, bronchioles, and alveoli within the lungs

A. **Functions**
1. Provide oxygen and remove carbon dioxide
2. Produce sound
3. Muscles of respiration assist with abdominal compression for micturition (urination), defecation (bowel elimination), and parturition (childbirth)
4. Coughing and sneezing (protective reflexes)

B. **Air passage**
1. *Nose (rhin-, nas-):* made up of soft tissue, cartilage, and bone; contains two nares (nostrils) separated by a septum; lined with ciliated mucous membrane; communicates with the middle ear through the eustachian tube; contains three conchae (turbinates) which provide more surface to accommodate warming, moisturizing, and filtering the air we breathe; receives its blood supply from branches of the internal and external carotid arteries; innervated by the trigeminal nerve (CN V) and provides for the sense of smell (olfactory nerve, CN I)
   a. Purposes for breathing through the nose are to warm, moisten, and filter air
      Warmed by blood, which is well supplied in the nose
      Moistened by fluid from tears through the nasolacrimal duct, mucous membranes lining the nose and sinuses which drain into the nose
      Filtered by hairs and cilia
   b. Separated: from the oral cavity by the soft and hard palate
2. *Paranasal sinuses:* four-paired cavities in bone; lined with a mucous membrane; contribute to resonance of sound and make bone lighter; drain into the nose
   i. Maxillary—the largest
   ii. Frontal
   iii. Ethmoid
   iv. Sphenoid
3. *Pharynx (throat):* Three parts of the pharynx
   a. *Nasopharynx:* area between the nose and throat
      i. Houses the adenoids (pharyngeal tonsils)
      ii. Eustachian tube connects to middle ear
   b. *Oropharynx:* at mouth
      i. passageway for food and air
      ii. houses palatine tonsils at the end of soft palate and lingual tonsils at the base of tongue
   c. *Laryngopharynx:* at opening to voice box
4. *Larynx (voice box):* made up of cartilages; contains cough reflex
   a. *Epiglottis:* cartilage "lid" that covers the glottis (opening between the vocal cords) during swallowing
   b. *Thyroid cartilage (Adam's apple):* largest cartilage; shaped like a signet ring; and lies superior and posterior to the thyroid gland
   c. *Cricoid cartilage:* first ring of the trachea, which encircles it completely; pressure on the cricoid cartilage can close off the esophagus,

which is just behind it; and cricoid pressure may be used to prevent regurgitation of contents from the stomach into the lungs of an unconscious patient (Sellick's maneuver)

      d. Larynx is innervated by a branch of the vagus nerve (CN X recurrent laryngeal); if this nerve is damaged during a tracheotomy, speech will be affected

  5. *Trachea (windpipe)*

      a. Air passage from the larynx to the carina, where it branches (bifurcates) into the right and left bronchi

      b. Kept open by C-shaped cartilage rings

      c. Lined with a ciliated mucous membrane that traps particles and sweeps them up to larynx to be coughed up

  6. *Bronchi:* two air passages between the trachea and bronchioles (smaller branches) kept patent (open) by cartilage rings; right primary bronchus is wider, shorter, and straighter than the left and is the more common location for an aspirated foreign object to become lodged

  7. *Bronchioles:* smaller air tubes encircled by smooth muscle, capable of constricting and dilating

C. *Lungs (pneumon-, pulmon-):* paired respiratory organs within the thoracic cavity, separated by the mediastinum

  1. Three lobes in the right lung and two in the left

  2. Base rests on the diaphragm and apex under the clavicle

  3. *Alveoli (air sacs):* functional units in the lungs where exchange of gases occurs (external respiration); contain surfactant (chemical film that lowers surface tension to enhance diffusion of gases)

  4. *Pleura:* serous membrane covering of the lungs; double layered

      a. *Visceral pleura:* close contact with the lungs

      b. *Parietal pleura:* continuous with visceral pleura; lines the walls of the thoracic cavity

      c. *Pleural space:* potential space between the two serous membranes (visceral and parietal pleura) which contains a lubricating fluid and less pressure than in the lungs

  5. *Functions:* exchange of gases

      a. *Pulmonary circulation:* deoxygenated blood from the heart comes to the lungs, gives up the waste gas (carbon dioxide) and picks up oxygen, and carries it back to the heart to be circulated throughout the body

  6. *Blood supply:* bronchial artery

  7. *Innervation:* both sympathetic and parasympathetic (intercostals and phrenic nerves)

D. Physiology of respiration

  1. *Inspiration (breathing in):* intercostal muscles contract to raise the chest; the diaphragm (major muscle of respiration) is pulled downward, increasing the space and decreasing pressure; and therefore the air flows in. This process is dependent upon a negative intrapleural pressure.

  2. *Expiration (breathing out):* muscles relax, space is decreased, pressure is increased, and air is forced out

  3. *External respiration:* exchange of gases between the alveoli (air sacs) and blood capillaries (by diffusion)

  4. *Internal respiration:* exchange of gases between blood capillaries and body cells

  5. Controlled by the respiratory center in the medulla oblongata, on the basis of blood levels of oxygen and carbon dioxide and other factors

  6. Terms related to the respiratory system

      a. *Tidal volume:* amount of air we take in with a normal breath (approximately 500 cc)

b. *Vital capacity:* maximum amount of air that can be moved with effort (approximately 4500 cc)

c. *Total lung volume:* total amount the lung will hold (approximately 6000 cc)

d. *Residual capacity:* amount that remains in lungs after expiration

e. *Normal respiration (eupnea):* 14 to 20 per minute; a 1:5 ratio of breaths to heartbeats

f. *Normal values for arterial blood gases:* PO_2 (partial pressure of oxygen) 95 to 100%; PCO_2 (partial pressure of carbon dioxide) 35% to 40%, pH 7.35 to 7.45

g. *Apnea:* without breathing

h. *Bradypnea:* slow breathing

i. *Cheyne-Stokes respirations:* a breathing pattern of periods of apnea followed by gradual increasing depth and frequency, often indicative of a patient near death

j. *Cyanosis:* a bluish discoloration of the skin due to lack of oxygen

k. *Dyspnea:* painful or difficult breathing

l. *Hypercapnia:* an increased amount of carbon dioxide in the blood

m. *Hyperventilation:* excessive number of breaths

n. *Hypoxia:* low oxygen

o. *Tachypnea:* rapid breathing

XII. **Urinary System:** The function of the urinary system is to extract waste products from the blood and excrete them through the kidneys

A. *Urinary system:* consists of two kidneys, two ureters, one bladder, and one urethra

1. *Kidneys:* paired, bean-shaped organs, about the size of a fist, which lie on either side of the vertebral column next to the posterior abdominal wall retroperitoneal and near the level of the 12th thoracic vertebra (left kidney is several centimeters higher)

a. *Blood supply:* renal arteries arise from the abdominal aorta; renal veins empty into the inferior vena cava; these blood vessels connect with the kidney at the hilum (central notch)

b. *Capsule (Gerota's fascia):* tough membrane protecting the kidney

c. *Cortex:* outer portion of the kidney, which houses the nephrons (functional units within the kidney)

d. *Medulla (just beneath the cortex):* contains the loops of Henle, renal pyramids (triangular-shaped masses), and calyces (tubes that empty urine into the kidney pelvis)

e. *Renal pelvis (kidney basin; pyel-):* funnel-shaped area in the kidney which receives urine, through branches called calyces, before it passes into the ureter

f. *Hilum (kidney pedicle):* notch through which vessels, nerves, and ureters enter or leave

g. *Nephrons:* numerous functional units of the kidney (over 1 million in each kidney); responsible for the production of urine, regulating blood volume, adjusting pH, and maintaining fluid and electrolyte balance
Parts of Nephron:

i. *Glomerulus:* networks of blood capillaries bringing blood to nephrons, nestled in Bowman's capsule

ii. *Bowman's capsule:* cup-shaped depression with semipermeable membrane, receiving water and waste products from the blood by processes of filtration, osmosis, and diffusion

iii. *Proximal convoluted (twisted) tubules:* designed for selective reabsorption of nutrients and some electrolytes

iv. *Loop of Henle:* sodium extruded and water reabsorbed

v. *Distal convoluted tubule:* tubular excretion

vi. *Collecting duct:* reabsorption of water, empties into calyces

2. *Urine:* excretion from the kidney
   a. *Normal composition:* 95% water, 5% organic wastes (urea, creatinine, ammonia, and uric acid), and ions (sodium, potassium, magnesium, calcium, chlorides, sulfates, and phosphates)
   b. *Amount:* approximately 1 ml/min or 1500 ml/day
   c. *Regulated by hormones:* aldosterone and antidiuretic
   d. *Color:* straw, yellow
   e. *pH:* 6.0
   f. *Specific gravity:* 1.001–1.035. A high specific gravity indicates concentrated urine and dehydration.
3. *Ureters:* fibromuscular tubes which propel urine by peristaltic waves from the kidney pelvis to the urinary bladder
   a. Long tubes (about 27 cm long and 4 to 5 mm in diameter) running retroperitoneally to the posterior floor of the bladder
   b. Narrow areas where obstructions are more likely to occur are the ureteropelvic junction, crossing over iliac vessels, and the ureterovesicle junction
4. *Urinary bladder:* collapsible muscular pouch that serves as a reservoir for urine
   a. Situated extraperitoneally in front of the sigmoid colon and protected by the symphysis pubis; innervated by the autonomic nervous system; and receives blood from branches of the internal iliac arteries
   b. Size varies; contains rugae, which provide for expansion; capacity for 750 to 800 cc, with urge to void at 250 to 300 cc
   c. Empties by voluntary contraction of muscle wall
   d. *Trigone area:* triangular area of the bladder floor formed by three openings—right ureter, left ureter, and urethra
   e. Sterile area (catheters must always be sterile)
5. *Urethra:* membranous tube that conveys urine from the bladder to the outside
   a. *Female urethra:* 4 cm (1 ½ inches in length and 6 mm in diameter), embedded in the anterior vaginal wall protected by the pubic bone; meatus located between the clitoris and vagina—exits just anterior to the vagina
   b. *Male urethra:* 20 to 25 cm (8 inches) long and divided into three portions (prostatic, membranous, and cavernous) with lining continuous with that of the bladder
      i. *Prostatic:* passes through the prostate gland (widest portion) and contains openings of ejaculatory ducts
      ii. *Membranous:* passes through the pelvic wall
      iii. *Cavernous:* extends through the penis and lies within the corpus spongiosum
      Serves as passageway for semen and urine.

XIII. **Male Reproductive System:** The function of the male reproductive system is to manufacture the male gametes (sperm) and deliver them into the female reproductive tract

   A. *Testes (orchid-):* two oval-shaped gonads
      1. Begin development in the pelvis; descend about 2 months before birth into the scrotum; cryptorchidism: hidden (undescended) testicle

---

SURGERY HINT

Many urology cases are done with the use of fluoroscopy. The Surgical Technologist should protect himself or herself with a lead apron and thyroid shield which should be donned before the case begins. He or she should be ready to accept contrast media to the table.

Always test the balloon for indwelling catheters before placement.

---

2. Located in the scrotum: a muscular sac suspended between the thighs and separated by a septum; lined with glistening tissue (tunica vaginalis) that contracts when cold to bring testes to the warmth of the body and becomes flaccid and pendulous when warm to provide for cooling
3. *Functions:* spermatogenesis and the production of testosterone

B. *Epididymis:* tightly coiled tube on the superior aspect of the testes which holds sperm for maturation

C. *Vas deferens:* long tubes (34 cm) that convey semen (sperm-containing fluid) from the epididymis to the ejaculatory ducts
1. *Pathway of vas deferens:* begins at the epididymis, progresses upward over the pubic bone, through the abdominal wall (inguinal rings), behind the bladder, and joins with seminal vesicles to form ejaculatory duct, which penetrates the prostate gland to empty into the prostatic urethra
2. *Spermatic cord:* vas deferens, spermatic artery, vein, nerve, and lymphatics encased in the cremaster muscle
   (Note: The spermatic cord is carefully retracted during an inguinal herniorrhaphy, often with a penrose drain)

D. *Seminal vesicles:* two accessory reproductive glands lying behind the lower part of the bladder; unite with vas deferens on each side to form ejaculatory duct, which enters the urethra; and provide nutrition (protein and fructose) for sperm

E. *Prostate gland:* walnut-sized gland which completely encircles the male urethra just below the bladder; consists of six lobes (posterior lobe palpable during rectal examination); is covered by a capsule (fibrous sheath) which separates it from the seminal vesicles and forms the internal sphincter and secretes an alkaline fluid to protect the sperm from acid environment of the vagina

F. *Penis:* pendulous organ suspended by ligaments from the pubic symphysis; contains three vascular spongelike bodies (right and left corpus cavernosum and corpus spongiosum surrounding the urethra) which fill with blood during erection; and serves as organ of copulation (sexual intercourse)
1. *Glans:* tip, which contains sensory nerve endings
2. *Prepuce:* foreskin that covers the glans
3. *Urethra:* traverses full length of the penis
4. Rich blood supply accommodates enlargement and rigidity for erection

G. *Cowper's glands (bulbourethral):* two pea-sized glands below the prostate on either side of the membranous urethra which produces mucus that empties through ducts into the urethra; this secretion is the first to pass down the urethra during sexual excitement and cleanses the urethra of any acid **urine and serves** as a lubricant

H. *Hormonal regulation*
1. Gonadotropic hormones (produced by anterior pituitary gland)
   FSH: follicle stimulating hormone for spermatogenesis
   LH: luteinizing hormone for production of testosterone
2. *Testosterone (produced by testes):* promotes the development and maintenance of male sexual characteristics

XIV. **Female Reproductive System:** The function of the female reproductive system is to produce female gametes (ova), to prepare the body for pregnancy, contain and support the fetus, and return the organs to normal following delivery of an infant

A. *Ovaries (oophor):* two oval-shaped glands lying near the pelvic brim connected to uterus by ovarian ligament, secured to lateral walls of the pelvis by suspensory ligaments, produce sex hormones and eggs (oogenesis)
1. Active from puberty (menarche) until menopause
2. Extrude one egg per month during active years
3. *Follicles:* sacs in the ovary with varying stages of developing eggs (oocyte)

4. *Graafian follicle:* mature follicle
5. *Corpus luteum:* the ruptured follicle becomes this gland-like structure after the egg is released (ovulation)

B. *Female hormones*
1. *Estrogen:* responsible for female sex characteristics; produced by follicles
2. *Progesterone:* prepares the uterine lining for pregnancy and maintains pregnancy; produced by the corpus luteum
3. *Human chorionic gonadotropin (HCG):* produced by the placenta to maintain the corpus luteum (*Note:* Present in the urine during pregnancy [common pregnancy test])
4. *Oxytocin:* from posterior pituitary; contracts the uterus
5. *Prolactin:* from anterior pituitary; simulates the production of milk (after childbirth)

C. *Fallopian tubes (salpingo-):* two oviducts that extend from uterus to ovaries
1. *Muscular wall with peristaltic waves:* move ova through the tubes
2. *Infundibulum:* funnel-shaped distal opening
3. *Fimbriae:* fingerlike projections that sweep over the ovary to catch the egg and direct it into the tube
4. *Area of fertilization:* sperm meet the egg usually at distal third of tube
5. *Function:* to transport eggs and/or fertilized egg (zygote) to the uterus

D. *Uterus (hyster-, metr-)*
1. Thick-walled pear-shaped organ capable of tremendous expansion
2. Made up of three layers (endometrium, myometrium, and epimetrium)
   a. *Endometrium:* inner layer of mucous membrane which builds up every month and is discharged with menstruation
   b. *Myometrium:* thick, smooth, middle layer of involuntary muscle under the control of the hormone oxytocin
   c. *Epimetrium:* outer layer of serous membrane (also called visceral peritoneum)
   d. *Portions of the uterus*
      i. *Fundus:* upper, rounded portion
      ii. *Body:* main part of the uterus
      iii. *Cervix:* neck of the uterus
   e. *Uterine ligaments*
      i. *Broad:* transverse folds of the peritoneum extending from the uterus to the lateral pelvic wall
      ii. *Uterosacral:* connects to the sacrum
      iii. *Round:* anchors the uterus to tissues beneath the labia majora; keeps the uterus tilted forward
      iv. *Cardinal:* attach to lateral vaginal fornices
      v. *Lateral cervical:* connects the cervix to the pelvic diaphragm
      vi. *Ovarian:* connects the ovaries to the uterus

E. *Vagina (colp-):* birth canal and organ of copulation
1. Muscular, expandable tube, which extends from the cervix to the vaginal meatus and opens anteriorly between the urethra and the rectum
2. Three layers: mucous membrane lining, muscular middle layer, and outermost layer of thick connective tissue
3. Well supplied with blood
4. *Rugae:* folds in lower two-thirds that allow for expansion
5. *Fornix:* enlarged proximal portion surrounding the cervix
6. *Cul-de-sac of Douglas:* retro uterine pouch (extension of the peritoneal cavity) which lies between the rectum and posterior wall of the uterus; may be approached surgically through the vagina; culdocentesis may be performed to determine blood in the pelvic cavity

F. *External genitalia:* vulva (pudendum)
1. *Hymen:* highly vascular membranous ring of tissue surrounding vaginal opening; may be absent or completely occlude the orifice
2. *Mons pubis:* fatty tissue overlying the symphysis pubis
3. *Labia majora:* hair-covered folds of skin surrounding other genitalia
4. *Labia minora:* hair-free folds of tissue surrounding the vestibule
5. *Vestibule:* area within the labia minora that contains the urethral meatus, orifices of the Bartholin's glands, and vaginal introitus
6. *Bartholin's glands:* two glands that provide lubrication for coitus (sexual intercourse); open into the vaginal orifice
7. *Clitoris:* erectile structure anterior to the urethral meatus
8. *Paraurethral (Skene's) glands:* open into urethra; and secrete fluid to moisten and lubricate the vestibule

G. *Mammary glands (mast-, mamm-):* milk-producing glands
1. *Areola:* pigmented ring around the nipple
2. *Nipple:* rounded protuberance on breast
3. *Lobes:* subdivisions in the breast
4. *Alveoli:* milk-producing units
5. *Lactiferous ducts:* carry milk from alveoli to nipple
6. *Milk:* rich in immunoglobulins and nutrients
7. *Colostrum:* watery, nutritious secretion preceding milk

H. *Menstrual cycle:* alternating periods of building up and tearing down of uterine lining in preparation for pregnancy
1. *Proliferative phase:* the ovarian follicles are growing and cause estrogen levels to rise; the endometrium is repaired with an increased blood supply
2. *Ovulation:* the mature egg is released from the ovary (day 14 of the cycle)
3. *Progestational phase:* the ruptured follicle (corpus luteum) produces progesterone and further increases the blood supply of the endometrium. If fertilization does not occur, the corpus luteum degenerates which causes the endometrial cells to die due to the lack of blood supply
4. *Menstrual phase:* the endometrial lining is sloughed off and the blood and tissue pass through the vagina in the menstrual flow

I. *Terms related to pregnancy*
1. *Fertilization:* the joining of the ovum and sperm
2. *Implantation:* when the fertilized egg (zygote) attaches to the endometrial lining of the uterus
3. *Placenta:* the organ that serves as a filter between the mother's and fetus' blood; also acts as a temporary endocrine gland by secreting progesterone
4. *Amnion:* the thin transparent sac that houses the fetus and protects it with amniotic fluid, the "bag of waters"
5. *Chorion:* an extraembryonic membrane that gives rise to the chorionic villi which connect to the endometrium and form the placenta
6. *Embryo:* the stage of prenatal development between day 15 and the 8th week
7. *Fetus:* the stage of prenatal development between the 9th week and delivery
8. *Gestation:* the length of time a woman is pregnant, normal is 40 weeks, 280 days, 10 lunar months
9. *Gravidity:* the total number of times a woman has been pregnant
10. *Parity:* having carried a pregnancy to a point of infant viability regardless of whether the infant was alive at birth
11. *Abortion:* the loss of the fetus, either spontaneous (miscarriage) or induce

Show What You Know

Directions
Each of the numbered items or incomplete statements in this section is followed by answers or by completions of the statement. Select the ONE lettered answer or completion that is BEST in each case.

1. The part or organelle of the cell considered to be the powerhouse is the:
   A. nucleus
   B. chromosomes
   C. mitochondria
   D. ribosomes

2. The building blocks of all living matter are called:
   A. tissues
   B. cells
   C. organs
   D. systems

3. The thymus gland is located in the _____ cavity.
   A. cranial
   B. dorsal
   C. abdominal
   D. thoracic

4. The umbilicus is located on the _____ surface of the body.
   A. ventral
   B. dorsal
   C. distal
   D. proximal

5. The hormones produced by the adrenal cortex to protect one during a stressful situation are:
   A. corticoids
   B. adrenalin
   C. adrenocorticotropic
   D. insulin

6. The medial malleolus is a projection at the ankle of the:
   A. radius
   B. fibula
   C. femur
   D. tibia

7. The outermost layer of the eye that is commonly called the white of the eye is the:
   A. retina
   B. cornea
   C. choroid
   D. sclera

8. The parotid gland secretes:
   A. cerumen
   B. hormones
   C. saliva
   D. bile

9. Muscles are attached to bones by:
   A. ligaments
   B. tendons
   C. bursae
   D. aponeurosis

10. The large opening located in the occipital bone is called the:
    A. maxillary sinus
    B. foramen magnum
    C. foramen mentalis
    D. sella turcica

11. The liquid part of the blood is:
    A. lipids
    B. plasma
    C. hemoglobin
    D. platelets

12. The mineral essential for the formation of red blood cells is:
    A. sodium
    B. iodine
    C. iron
    D. calcium

13. The myocardium is the:
    A. sac surrounding the heart
    B. lining of the heart
    C. thick muscular wall of the heart
    D. major blood vessel supplying the heart

14. The name of the artery that arises from the ascending aorta and carries blood to the heart muscle is the:
    A. jugular
    B. carotid
    C. cardiac
    D. coronary

15. The largest artery in the body is the:
    A. saphenous
    B. carotid
    C. aorta
    D. renal

16. The membrane that lines the chest cavity and reflects back to cover the lungs is the:
    A. peritoneum
    B. conjunctiva
    C. pericardium
    D. pleura

17. The amount of air taken in with a normal breath is about 500 cc and is referred to as:

    A. tidal volume
    B. vital capacity
    C. ventilatory rate
    D. sigh reflex

18. The auditory nerve receives sound waves from a shell-like structure called the:

    A. semicircular canal
    B. cornea
    C. stapes
    D. cochlea

19. An inflammation of the conjunctiva involves the:

    A. glands that produce tears
    B. delicate membrane lining the eyelids and covering the front of the eyeball
    C. portion of the eye that contains the optic nerve
    D. opaque lens

20. One of the most important glands in the body, often referred to as the "master gland," is the:

    A. thyroid
    B. pituitary
    C. pineal
    D. adrenal

21. Within the kidneys, there are millions of microscopic units that carry out the functions of producing urine. These functional units are called:

    A. alveoli
    B. nephrons
    C. neurons
    D. renal pyramids

22. The long narrow tubes that drain urine from the kidneys to the bladder are called:

    A. renal tubules
    B. ureters
    C. urethras
    D. fallopian tubes

23. Water is absorbed mostly in the:

    A. colon
    B. mouth
    C. stomach
    D. small intestines

24. The pancreas is both an endocrine and an exocrine gland. The hormone secreted by the pancreas directly into the blood is:

    A. trypsin
    B. lipase
    C. amylase
    D. insulin

25. The male reproductive organ(s) that manufactures the male sex cells is (are) called the:

    A. prostate gland
    B. testes
    C. epididymis
    D. Cowper's gland

26. The nerves that control the release of epinephrine during "fight or flight" are the:

    A. sympathetic nerves
    B. parasympathetic nerves
    C. cranial nerves
    D. lumbar nerves

27. An example of reticular tissue is:

    A. bone
    B. fascia
    C. blood
    D. muscle

28. The muscle that flexes the head is the:

    A. masseter
    B. temporalis
    C. trapezius
    D. sternocleidomastoid

29. The middle layer of the meninges is the:

    A. pia
    B. arachnoid
    C. dura
    D. subdural

30. The section of the brain that controls temperature and thirst is the:

    A. thalamus
    B. pons
    C. medulla oblongata
    D. hypothalamus

31. How many pairs of extrinsic eye muscles are there:

    A. 6
    B. 10
    C. 8
    D. 5

32. The jelly-like substance that maintains the shape of the globe is:

    A. aqueous humor
    B. vitreous humor
    C. perilymph
    D. endolymph

33. The descending colon is attached at this anatomical feature:

    A. hepatic flexure
    B. anterior diaphragm
    C. splenic flexure
    D. cecum

34. The function of the liver include all of the following *except:*
    A. storage of glucose
    B. storage of bile
    C. destruction of RBCs
    D. production of urea

35. The normal range for lymphocytes is between:
    A. 10,000 and 13,000
    B. 5000 and 10,000
    C. 7000 and 14,000
    D. 2000 and 5000

36. The valve to the right ventricle is the:
    A. tricuspid
    B. bicuspid
    C. semilunar
    D. pulmonary

37. A superficial vein of the leg is the:
    A. femoral
    B. posterior tibial
    C. saphenous
    D. popliteal

38. The first ring of tracheal cartilage, utilized during Sellick's maneuver is the:
    A. thyroid cartilage
    B. cricoid cartilage
    C. laryngeal cartilage
    D. hyoid cartilage

39. The most likely tough capsule that protects the kidney is:
    A. Gerota's fascia
    B. Renal Cortex
    C. Henle fascia
    D. Galea

40. Fertilization occurs in the:
    A. fimbriae
    B. oviduct
    C. ovary
    D. uterus

Answers & Rationales

1. **C.** **Rationale:** The mitochondria store energy in the form of ATP and are considered to be the powerhouses of the cell.

2. **B.** **Rationale:** Cells are the building blocks of all living tissue. A group of similar cells makes up tissue and a group of specialized tissues makes up organs.

3. **D.** **Rationale:** The thymus gland is a part of both the endocrine and lymphatic systems and is located in the upper mediastinum in the thoracic cavity.

4. **A.** **Rationale:** The umbilicus is on the ventral (anterior) surface of the body.

5. **A.** **Rationale:** Corticoids are produced by the adrenal cortex and protect us in stress by conserving what we need and transforming stored energy to a ready source.

6. **D.** **Rationale:** The large bone in the lower medial aspect of the leg is the tibia, which has a projection at the ankle called the medial malleolus. The lateral malleolus is part of the smaller bone, the fibula.

7. **D.** **Rationale:** The hard white covering of the eye is the sclera. The cornea, although a part of the sclera that covers the front of the eye, is clear.

8. **C.** **Rationale:** The parotid gland is a salivary gland located near the ear and secretes saliva.

9. **B.** **Rationale:** Tendons are tough connective tissues that connect muscles to bones.

10. **B.** **Rationale:** The foramen magnum is the large opening in the occipital bone through which the spinal cord passes.

11. **B.** **Rationale:** Plasma is the liquid part of the blood and makes up about 55% of the blood volume.

12. **C.** **Rationale:** Iron is essential in the formation of hemoglobin, found in RBCs. When the erythrocytes are worn out and broken down, the iron is removed by the liver and either stored or returned to the bone marrow to make more RBCs.

13. **C.** **Rationale:** *Myo-* equals muscle and *cardi-* equals heart.

14. **D.** **Rationale:** The coronary arteries arise from the ascending aorta and supply blood to the heart muscles.

15. **C.** **Rationale:** The aorta is the chief systemic artery and the largest in the body.

16. **D.** **Rationale:** The pleura is a serous membrane that lines the chest (parietal) and covers the lung (visceral).

17. **A.** **Rationale:** Tidal volume is the amount of air we take in with a normal breath and is usually about 500 cc.

18. **D.** **Rationale:** The cochlea is a shell-shaped organ in the inner ear that contains the organ of Corti (receptor cells for hearing).

19. **B.** **Rationale:** The conjunctiva is a mucous membrane that lines the lids and reflects back to cover the front of the eye.

20. **B.** **Rationale:** The pituitary gland (hypophysis) is located at the base of the brain, is divided into two sections, and secretes hormones that control other glands.

21. **B.** **Rationale:** Nephrons are the functional units of the kidneys.

22. **B.** **Rationale:** Urine is carried from the kidneys to the bladder by ureters and from the bladder to the outside by the urethra, a process we refer to as voiding, micturition, or urination.

23. **A.** **Rationale:** One of the chief functions of the large intestine (colon) is absorption of water and electrolytes.

24. **D.** **Rationale:** Insulin is a hormone secreted by the islet cells in the pancreas for the metabolism of sugar. Trypsin, lipase, and amylase are enzymes secreted by the pancreas and carried through ducts to the duodenum.

25. **B.** **Rationale:** The testes produce sperm and testosterone.

26. **A.** **Rationale:** The sympathetic and parasympathetic nerves are part of the autonomic nervous system. The sympathetic nerves control the release of epinephrine (adrenalin) during highly stressful situations, while the sympathetic nerves work to slow down responses.

27. **C.** **Rationale:** Blood and lymph both fall into the category of reticular tissue category. Bone is classified as osseous tissue; fascia and muscle are considered fibrous.

28. **D.** **Rationale:** The sternocleidomastoid muscle runs through the neck and allows for flexing the head. The masseter and temporalis muscles function in chewing, and the trapezius muscle allows for extension.

29. **B.** **Rationale:** The meninges are composed of three layers. The outermost layer is the dura, the middle layer is the arachnoid, and the last is the pia mater. The space between the dura mater and the arachnoid is the subdural space.

30. **D.** **Rationale:** The portion of the brain that controls temperature, thirst, and hunger is the hypothalamus. The medulla oblongata controls basic functions such as heartbeat and respiration. The thalamus is a "relay center" for directing impulses, and the pons is a reflex center.

31. **A.** **Rationale:** There are six pairs of extrinsic eye muscles. They are controlled by several cranial nerves and provide movement to the eye.

32. **B.** **Rationale:** The eye is composed of several chambers and layers. The aqueous humor is located in the anterior cavity and is produce by the ciliary body. The posterior chamber contains vitreous humor, which helps maintain the shape of the globe. Endolymph and perilymph are contained in the ear.

33. **C.** **Rationale:** The splenic flexure is where the colon begins its downward path to the sigmoid colon. The cecum is the first part of the large intestine, and the hepatic flexure is where the ascending colon becomes the transverse colon.

34. **B.** **Rationale:** The liver does not store bile. It produces bile, which is then stored in the gallbladder.

35. **B.** **Rationale:** Normal ranges for white blood cells are between 5000 and 10,000. A higher count would likely indicate an infectious process, which may delay surgery.

36. **A.** **Rationale:** The valve separating the right atrium from the right ventricle is the tricuspid. The aortic semilunar or aortic valve separates the left ventricle and the aorta. The pulmonary valve is located at the pulmonary artery, and the mitral, or bicuspid valve separated the left atrium and ventricle.

37. **C.** **Rationale:** The great Saphenous vein is a superficial vein of the leg. It is commonly used as a grafting vein when needed.

38. **B.** **Rationale:** The cricoid cartilage is the first ring of the larynx. This cartilage is manually depressed during intubation to facilitate the endotracheal tube insertion and to depress the gag reflex. This is referred to as Sellick's maneuver. The thyroid cartilage is often referred to as the Adam's apple.

39. **A.** **Rationale:** The kidney is protected by a fibrous capsule called Gerota's fascia. The cortex and medulla are the outer and inner layers of the kidney, and the galea is located in the scalp.

40. **B.** **Rationale:** Fertilization commonly occurs in the fallopian tube or oviduct. Once the egg has been fertilized, it implants in the endometrial lining of the uterus.

Part II: Deciphering a Surgical Schedule

The following mock surgery schedule will be used to answer several questions pertaining to anatomy. The same schedule, or a similar one, may be used in subsequent chapters to ask questions about the content of the chapter.

Rm. # time	Surgeon	Procedure	Anest.	Rm. # time	Surgeon	Procedure	Anest.
Rm.00				**Rm07**			
OC	Dr. Z	Rt. Knee Arthroscopy	Gen.	7:00	Dr. M	Rhinoplasty	Gen.
OC	Dr. C	Craniotomy	Gen.				
OC	Dr. Z	Angioplasty	Gen.	TF	Dr. M	Lipoma removal	MAC
Rm.01				**Rm08**			
7:00	Dr. X	Lobectomy	Gen.	11:00	Dr. E	Bovine Thrombectomy	MAC
TF	Dr. X	Thoracotomy	Gen.				
TF	Dr. X	Tracheostomy	Gen.				
Rm02				**Rm09**			
7:00	Dr. B	Splenectomy	Gen.	8:30	Dr. T	Cholecystectomy	Gen.
TF	Dr. B	Gastrectomy	Gen.	TF	Dr. T	Palatoplasty	Gen.
Rm03				**Rm10**			
7:00	Dr. A	Cystoscopy	MAC	7:00	Dr. K	Nephrectomy	Gen.
TF	Dr. A	Cystoplasty	Gen.	TF	Dr. K	Choledocholithotripsy	MAC
12:30	Dr. F	Pyleogram	MAC				
3:00	Dr. F	Cystocele repair	Gen.	TF	Dr. K	Hepatic resection	Gen.
Rm04				**Rm11**			
7:00	Dr. Y	Carpal tunnel release	Gen.	7:00	Dr. L	Colposcope	Gen.
TF	Dr. Y	Fasciotomy	Gen.	12:00	Dr. L	Mastectomy	Gen.
Rm05				**Rm12**			
7:00	Dr. G	Trans-sphenoidal Adenectomy	Gen.	7:00	Dr. W	Trans-metatarsal amputation	Gen.
TF	Dr. G	Trans-urethral resection of the prostate	Gen	TF	Dr. W	Osteotomy	Gen.
TF	Dr. G	Bletharoplasty	Gen.	TF	Dr. W	Arthrocentesis	Gen.
Rm06				**Rm13**			
7:00	Dr. R	Lumbar Laminectomy	Gen.	7:00	Dr. O	Hysterectomy	Gen.

The following questions should be answered using the surgery schedule above

1. The right knee arthroscopy that is on call will involve which anatomical structures?

   A. The femur and the fibula
   B. The tibia and the fibula
   C. The femur and the tibia
   D. The femur and the acetabulum

2. Which procedure is done on the foot?

   A. Lumbar laminectomy
   B. Palatoplasty
   C. Trans metatarsal amputation
   D. Carpal tunnel

3. Which procedure will involve entering a cavity?

   A. Osteotomy
   B. Nephrectomy
   C. Tracheostomy
   D. Lobectomy

4. Applying what you know from the chapter, which procedure will involve the right upper quadrant?

    A. Hepatic resection
    B. Nephrectomy
    C. Hysterectomy
    D. Mastectomy

5. Which procedure is likely to be done by a vascular surgeon?

    A. Cystoscopy
    B. Cholecystectomy
    C. Bovine thrombectomy
    D. Fasciotomy

6. Which procedure will NOT involve entering a cavity?

    A. Hemicolectomy
    B. Mastectomy
    C. Cholecystectomy
    D. Lobectomy

7. Which surgery involves repair of facial bone deformities?

    A. Fasciotomy
    B. Palatoplasty
    C. Angioplasty
    D. Craniotomy

8. When performing the splenectomy in Room 2, which quadrant will be entered?

    A. Right lower
    B. Right upper
    C. Left lower
    D. Left upper

9. Room 5 has a transurethral resection of the prostate (TURP) scheduled. Which two body systems are involved?

    A. Urinary and digestive
    B. Digestive and male reproductive
    C. Urinary and male reproductive
    D. Only the reproductive system is involved

10. The Trans-Sphenoidal Adenectomy involves which systems?

    A. Skeletal, nervous, and endocrine
    B. Skeletal, urinary, and endocrine
    C. Endocrine and urinary
    D. Skeletal and endocrine

Answers & Rationales

1. **C. Rationale:** A knee arthroscopy will involve the femur and the tibia. This surgery involves an arthroscope, or an instrument to view a joint, and is most commonly performed for diagnostic purposes or to repair tears in the meniscus.

2. **C. Rationale:** The trans-metatarsal amputation will be done on the foot. In this surgery, the distal portion of the foot is removed by amputating at the metatarsals.

3. **D. Rationale:** The only surgical procedure listed that actually enters a cavity is a lobectomy. The nephrectomy will not enter the peritoneal cavity, as the kidney is located in the retroperitoneal space, or behind the peritoneum. The kidney is usually removed via a transcostal incision in the flank. The osteotomy, while not specified as to which location, is unlikely to involve entering a cavity, and a tracheostomy is also outside a cavity. This leaves the

lobectomy as the only surgery to be performed by entering a cavity, in this case the thoracic cavity.

4. **A.** **Rationale:** The liver is located in the right upper quadrant. Therefore, the hepatic resection is the only surgery that will be performed in this quadrant.

5. **C.** **Rationale:** This question can be answered by the process of elimination. The cystoscopy would be performed by either a general surgeon or a urologist, not by a vascular surgeon. The cholecystectomy would also be performed by a general surgeon, not a vascular. A fasciotomy may be performed by several different specialists, but a bovine thrombectomy will most likely be done by a vascular surgeon. This procedure is done to remove a clot that has formed in a bovine graft, and is routinely done by vascular surgeons.

6. **B.** **Rationale:** A hemicolectomy and cholecystectomy will both involve the peritoneal cavity, and a lobectomy will enter the thoracic cavity. That leaves the mastectomy as the only surgery that will not enter a cavity.

7. **B.** **Rationale:** A palatoplasty involves the repair of a cleft palate. While a craniotomy is performed on the bones of the skull, it is not done on a facial bone.

8. **D.** **Rationale:** The spleen is located in the upper left quadrant, posterior to the stomach. Because of its location, the spleen may be damaged during motor vehicle accidents. The spleen is not a vital organ, and can be removed. However, a person without a spleen may be more susceptible to infections.

9. **C.** **Rationale:** This procedure includes the urinary system, as the procedure is being performed through the urethra, as well as the male reproductive system, of which the prostate is a part. This procedure is usually done to remove the prostate due to abnormalities.

10. **A.** **Rationale:** A trans-sphenoidal adenectomy involves the skeletal, nervous, and endocrine systems. The surgery will be done to remove a diseased portion of the pituitary gland, which will be reached by going through the sphenoid sinus. As the pituitary gland rests on the groove of the sella turcica, the bone that makes up part of the cranial floor, and is connected to the hypothalamus by a narrow stalk called the infundidulum, this will involve both the skeletal and nervous systems.

3 Microbiology and Infection Control

M icrobes have been in existence since long before the beginning of humankind. They are ubiquitous—in the soil, in the air, in the water, and harbored on everything both living and dead. Most microbes serve a useful purpose. Only a small percentage of microorganisms are pathogenic and even those, in order to cause disease in humans, must be able to gain entrance, overcome human barriers, adapt, and multiply. Yet these microbes have claimed more lives than have legions of armies. Understanding how pathogenic microbes work and how they affect the human body is vital in understanding the reasoning behind sterile principles. It is only through knowing how microbes live that we are able to protect our patients from them.

 **How to Answer Microbiology Questions**

Answering microbiology questions can be difficult for some students. The easiest way to overcome difficulties in microbiology is to first classify the microbe in question. Is it bacteria, virus, rickettsiae, or another microbe? Once you have established which microbe that is the subject of the question, you should be able to remember certain characteristics of that group. Remember that there are four classifications of viruses, bacteria are identified by morphology, rickettsiae are commonly transmitted by tick, and antibiotics are not effective in treating viruses. At this point, you should be able to determine the correct answer to the question.

Example:
Staphylococcal bacteria are recognized by

a. Spherical bacteria arranged in chains
b. Spherical bacteria arranged in clusters
c. Rod-shaped bacteria arranged in chains
d. Rod-shaped bacteria arranged in clusters

To answer this question, first remember that bacteria are classified by morphology, or shape. There are several different common shapes that bacteria take, among them are robs, spheres, and spirals. Rod-shaped bacteria are called bacilli. This will immediately remove answers C and D. Coccid bacteria are spherical shaped, meaning that the answer must be A or B. Breaking the answers down further, you should be able to eliminate A, as the arrangement in chains is a characteristic of streptococci. Therefore, the correct answer must be B.

Terminology

1. *Microbiology:* study of microscopic life forms
2. *Microorganisms (microbes):* life forms too small to be seen with the naked eye
   a. Can be found in and on body areas that lead to the outside (normal flora)
   b. Contain intracellular DNA (except viruses and prions); are eukaryotic (DNA is enclosed in a nuclear membrane, i.e., protozoa, fungi, algae) or prokaryotic (DNA is loose in the cytoplasm, i.e., bacteria)
   c. Most serve useful purposes, such as in the nitrogen fixation in soil, the making of certain foods, decomposition, and in medicine (nonpathogenic: do not cause disease)
   d. Some are pathogenic (disease producing)
3. *Microscope:* instrument developed by Anton van Leeuwenhoek in the seventeenth century, used to demonstrate the existence of life forms not visible to the naked eye
4. *Parts of a compound light microscope*
   a. *eyepiece*—magnifies 10x (times)
   b. *low-power objective*—magnifies 10x; combined with the eyepiece, the total magnification is 100x (10 × 10)
   c. *high-power objective*—magnifies 40x; combined with the eyepiece, the total magnification is 400x (10 × 40)
   d. *oil immersion objective*—magnifies 100x; combined with the eyepiece, the total magnification is 1000x (10 × 100); this objective is used for viewing bacteria and requires that a drop of oil be placed on the cover slip to reduce the scattering of light

Microbiology

I. Types of Microorganisms

   A. *Parasitic worms (helminths)*
1. Usually macroscopic, but eggs and larvae are microscopic
2. Often acquired through fecal-oral ingestion, soil contaminated with feces such as in rural farmlands
3. Preventable through cleanliness
4. Treated with antihelmintic drugs
5. Examples: roundworms *(Ascaris),* tapeworms, pinworms, and hookworms

   B. *Protozoa:* one-celled motile animals, the largest microbe
1. Prefer to live in a water environment; transmission is through ingestion, the fecal-oral route, insect bite, or direct contact with the genitourinary tract
2. Cause such diseases as amebic dysentery, trichomoniasis vaginalis, and malaria

   C. *Fungi:* large group of simple plants that lack chlorophyll
1. Some cause diseases (mycotic infections) in the absence of normal body flora (microscopic organisms residing in a given area of the body during health)
2. *Yeast:* single celled; reproduces by budding; used commercially for making beer, wine, and bread; capable of causing infections in mucous membranes such as thrush (caused by *Candida albicans*) vaginitis, and respiratory fungal diseases such as histoplasmosis
3. *Molds:* multicellular plants which may be seen on breads, cheese, etc.; capable of causing ringworm and athlete's foot (*Tinea pedis*); a species of mold *penicillin* was discovered as an antibiotic by Alexander Fleming in the early twentieth century

   D. *Rickettsiae:* true parasites which grow only in living tissue (obligate intracellular parasite); transmitted by vectors (insects which transmit disease) and produce diseases such as Rocky Mountain spotted fever and typhus fever. Most of the rickettsial diseases are contracted through tick bites.

   E. *Viruses:* submicroscopic, can be seen only with an electron microscope; are obligate intracellular parasites that use the host cell for replication; are capable of mutations (alteration in genetic structure of a cell); and are extremely resistant to treatment. There are four broad classifications of viruses. All viruses may be categorized into one of the four categories: pneumotropic viruses that affect the respiratory system, Neurotropic viruses that affect the nervous system, Dermatropic viruses that affect the integumentary system, and Viscerotropic viruses that affect multiple or all body systems. There are few, if any, treatments for viral infections. Most are treated with palliative care. Antibiotics are not a viable treatment for viruses.
1. *Bacteriophages:* viruses that attach to and invade a bacterium
2. During viral infection, host cells produce the inflammatory response, antibodies, and interferon to prevent the replication of the virus in other cells
3. Transmitted by contact, blood or body secretions and excretions, droplets or aerosol spray, animal bites, or arthropod vectors
4. Produces such diseases as
   a. *Hepatitis A to G:* Hepatitis A is the most common type of viral hepatitis and is spread by ingestion of contaminated food and water and by fecal contamination; Hepatitis B is transmitted by blood, saliva, semen, and other body fluids that may contain microscopic traces of blood; health care workers who are exposed to these body fluids, especially blood, are at high risk as the HBV surface antigen can be transmitted through needle sticks, an opening in the skin, or a splash to the

eyes, nose, and mouth; Hepatitis C is a blood-borne pathogen and a concern for health care workers and patients who receive numerous blood transfusions

b. *Human immunodeficiency virus (HIV) infection and acquired immunodeficiency syndrome (AIDS):* The HIV attacks the body's white blood cells (macrophages) and T cells which compromise the immune system

c. *Herpes infection:* Carried by the herpes simplex virus and causes cold sores on the lips or mouth and genital herpes in the perianal region; Herpes zoster virus causes shingles

d. *Human papillomavirus infection:* HPV causes venereal warts (condylomas)

e. *Cytomegalovirus infection:* Causes enlargement of affected organs and can be spread by direct contact with body fluids and transmitted from an infected mother to the fetus

f. *Other viral diseases:* Poliomyelitis, influenza, measles, mumps, rubella, and chickenpox

g. *Prion diseases:* While actually small bits of protein and not technically classified as viral, prions act like a virus. Prions contain no detectable DNA or RNA but have abnormal forms of neurologic cellular protein; prions are resistant to routine methods of sterilization (heat, chemicals, radiation, etc.), and special protocols for the care of instruments should be followed; they cause a group of diseases known as transmissible spongiform encephalopathies (TSEs), including Creutzfeldt-Jakob disease; approximately 90% of these cases have no known source of transmission, but 1% have been traced to a medically related exposure (i.e., use of contaminated surgical instruments, transplantation of neurological tissue such as dura, corneal transplants, and injections of human growth hormone)

F. *Bacteria:* unicellular; distributed throughout nature; reproduce asexually by binary fission (split into half); Gram stain is used to identify bacteria; are classified by shapes (taxonomy by morphology)

1. *Cocci:* round (spherical) nonmotile

a. *Streptococci:* appear in chains, most are gram positive, non-spore forming, and can live with or without free oxygen (facultative); commonly found in the upper respiratory, gastrointestinal (GI), and genitourinary (GU) tracts; some are capable of hemolyzing blood (*Hemolytic streptococcus*); Group A streptococci: cause most streptococcal infections (e.g., *Streptococcus pyogenes*) and cause such diseases as scarlet fever, septicemia (infection in the blood), puerperal (after childbirth) sepsis, septic sore throat, sinusitis, wound infection, pneumonia (*Streptococcus pneumoniae*), gonorrhea (*Neisseria gonorrhoeae*), and rheumatic fever: generally sensitive to penicillin, vancomycin is the drug of choice

b. *Staphylococci:* appear in clusters; are gram negative and may be saprophytic (living on dead or decaying matter) or parasitic (living at the expense of the host); may grow under aerobic (with oxygen) or anaerobic (without oxygen) conditions; and are part of normal body flora (*Staphylococcus epidermis,* on the skin); *Staphylococcus aureus* is the most virulent (powerful) of all species; it gains access to the body through the respiratory tract, breaks in skin, and mucous membranes; it is the most common cause of surgical site infections (SSI) and is found in the nasal passages of about half the population

2. *Spirochetes:* spiral shaped, motile, and cause syphilis *(Treponema pallidum)*

3. *Bacilli:* rod shaped, may be aerobic or anaerobic; may be a spore former such as *Clostridium tetani,* which causes tetanus, or *Clostridium perfringens,* which causes gas gangrene; may be classified as gram positive (diphtheria), gram negative, like *Escherichia coli* (enterococci, normal intestinal flora), or acid fast, as *Mycobacterium tuberculosis* (causes tuberculosis); includes the proteus and pseudomonas species

II. **The Bacterial Cell**

A. *Basic parts and functions*
1. *Cell wall:* confines and protects
2. *Cytoplasmic membrane:* serves as the doorway to the cell and a site of enzyme production; semipermeable, nutrients enter by osmosis
3. *Cytoplasm:* jellylike substance inside the cell, where proteins are made
4. *Nuclear material:* responsible for cell division and hereditary characteristics

B. *Specialized structures of bacteria that enhance their virulence (power to cause disease)*
1. *Flagella:* projecting strands of protein, which enhance motility (movement)
2. *Capsule:* thick layer around the cell that is a defense mechanism against white blood cells (WBCs)
3. *Endospore:* tough, resistant "shell" found in about 150 types of gram-positive bacilli; extremely resistant to destruction; nonpathogenic forms are used to test sterilizer efficiently; when conditions are right for growth, the endospore returns to its vegetative, active growth state

C. *Virulent factors of bacteria*
1. *Endotoxins:* poisons secreted by gram-negative rods *(Salmonella typhosa* and *Shigella dysenteriae)* which are contained within the bacterial cell wall and are liberated at the death of the organism and enter the bloodstream of the host, producing septicemia
2. *Exotoxins:* potent poisons secreted by gram positive spore-forming rods; diseases include clostridia, diphtheria, and tuberculosis
3. *Hyaluronidase:* proteolytic (breaks down protein) enzyme, secreted by such organisms as streptococci and *Clostridium perfringens,* which hydrolyzes (breaks down) the body's hyaluronic acid (intercellular adhesive), allowing the organism to spread
4. *Fibrinolysin:* enzyme produced by some virulent organisms (i.e., hemolytic streptococci) that breaks down fibrin (basis for blood clot) and is a major factor in wound infection
5. *Coagulase:* enzyme produced by some bacteria that speeds up the blood clotting mechanism and induce thrombus formation
6. *Leukocidin:* enzyme produced by some bacteria that destroys WBCs, the second line of defense against bacterial invasion

D. *Drug-resistant bacteria:* These bacteria represent one of the greatest threats in health care today. As a society, we have grown confident that antibiotics can cure any infections. The bacterial world, through adaptation, has proven us wrong. The overuse of antibiotics, patient non-compliance in prescription dosage, and other factors have led to an increase in resistant strains of bacteria.
1. *Methicillin-resistant* **staphylococcus aureus** *(MRSA):* transmitted by contact; strict perioperative protocols must be followed
2. *Vancomycin-resistant enterococci* *(VRE):* transmitted by contact; strict contact precautions should be followed
3. *Vancomycin-intermediate resistant* **staphylococcus aureus** *(VISA):* first seen in the United States in 1997
4. *Multi-drug-resistant mycobacterium tuberculosis (MDR-TB):* the Centers for Disease Control and Prevention (CDC) has published guidelines for preventing the transmission of this bacterium

E. *Environmental requirements*
1. Most pathogens thrive best in a neutral pH range (7.0) or similar to that of the body (slightly alkaline 7.35–7.45); hence, chemicals that are extremely acid (<7) or alkaline (>7) may be used to inhibit the growth of bacteria
2. *Temperature:* most pathogens are mesothermophilic (thrive best in a temperature similar to that of the body (37°C or 98.6°F); hence, extremes in

---

SURGERY HINT

Many surgeons will take cultures during a procedure. These may be anaerobic, aerobic, or both. It is important to ask if the surgeon will require both as there are different tubes for each culture. These cultures are generally passed off the back table to the circulator who will document the cultures and send them to the laboratory. Cultures may be taken in addition to specimens or washings.

---

temperature are often used to inhibit or stop the growth of pathogenic organisms

3. Moisture is necessary for the growth of microbes as they are 75% to 80% water; hence, desiccation (drying) is frequently used as a means of inhibiting the growth of microbes

4. Oxygen is essential for the existence of some microbes (obligate aerobes) and will kill others (obligate anaerobes); some microbes may thrive either in the presence or in the absence of oxygen (facultative); some (microaerophilic) require an oxygen level lower than that in air

5. Most pathogenic bacteria thrive best in darkness, and most are killed by ultraviolet light

6. *Energy source:* autotrophic (self-feeding) bacteria obtain energy from atoms of carbon dioxide in inorganic matter and are nonpathogenic; some heterotrophic bacteria (i.e., clostridia) require dead organic matter (saprophytes), and some require living matter (parasites) to survive

7. Microbial relationships: symbiosis is the living together of two unrelated organisms and can be of three types:
   a. *Mutualism:* beneficial to both organisms, as seen in the relationship of *E. coli* in the intestinal tract to human health
   b. *Commensalism:* one organism benefits but the other organism is neither benefited or harmed
   c. *Parasitism:* one organism lives completely at the expense of the host; understanding the enemy (pathogens) is the first step toward control

F. *Cultures and sensitivity*
   1. *Cultures:* sample of fluid or tissue collected under aseptic conditions: used to identify the microorganism causing a disease
   2. Different collecting and transport mediums may be used for aerobic and anaerobic cultures
   3. Bacteria are grown in a culture medium (i.e., broth, agar, blood) under ideal conditions (proper temperature, darkness, etc.)
   4. A pure culture, taken from an isolated colony, is used to grow out only one type of bacteria in a single dish
   5. *Sensitivity:* antibiotic impregnated disks are placed in the pure culture to determine which antibiotic is most effective in the destruction of the specific organism; if the culture is sensitive to the antibiotic disk, then an area of no growth will appear around it

Infection Control

The human body maintains a system of internal and external security in a manner comparable to the efforts of nations to defend against foreign invasion. Surgery is an invasion of body defenses, thereby necessitating meticulous aseptic technique.

I. Human Defenses

   A. *First line of defense against bacterial invasion*
      1. *Skin:* the largest organ, covered with a resistant layer of epithelium and secretes oils and perspiration, which have antiseptic properties

   2. *Mucous membranes:* line all body cavities leading to the outside (natural portals of entry from outside); thick mucus film traps bacteria
   3. *Body fluid:* tears and mucus secretions provide liquids for "washing out"; fluids (i.e., perspiration, oil, tears) have antiseptic properties and are pH specific for certain areas (i.e., alkaline for the mouth, acid for the vagina)
   4. *Cilia:* hairlike structures which line the respiratory tract and constantly sweep up dust, bacteria, etc., to be "coughed up"
   5. *Normal flora:* generally harmless organisms which under certain conditions may gain access to deeper tissue and cause infection (opportunistic pathogen); transient flora that are easily removed with cleansing; and resident flora that are more fixed and may be altered temporarily through surgical scrubs or the use of broad spectrum antibiotics

B. *Second line of defense:* inflammatory response and phagocytosis
   1. WBCs are mobilized at the site of injury, causing an elevation in the leukocyte count (leukocytosis) and increased production of defense material
   2. WBCs are called phagocytes (*phag-:* to eat; *cyte-:* cell)
   3. Blood supply to the injured area is increased, and capillary walls become dilated and more permeable to WBCs and fluid
   4. Used-up phagocytes may be carried through lymphatics to lymph nodes for filtration or collected with dead tissue cells and fluid as pus (suppuration); pathogens getting past the second line of defense may enter the bloodstream to produce septicemia (contamination in the blood)
   5. Five signs of inflammation (a local tissue reaction to injury)
      a. *Redness:* vessels dilate to bring more blood to the area
      b. *Heat:* due to increased blood supply in area
      c. *Swelling:* due to fluid seeping from dilated capillary walls
      d. *Pain:* swelling puts pressure on nerve endings
      e. *Disturbance of function:* pain causes decreased movement of area

C. *Third line of defense:* antigen–antibody reaction
   1. *Antigen:* foreign substance or microbe entering the body
   2. *Antibody:* protein substance, produced by the body in response to a specific antigen, which serves to provide immunity (protection)
   3. *Immunoglobulins:* family of plasma proteins that contain antibodies; tested to determine immunity
   4. *Classes of antibodies based on action*
      a. *Antitoxins:* neutralize toxins
      b. *Agglutinins:* cause clumping of bacteria
      c. *Lysins:* cause bacteria to dissolve
      d. *Opsonins:* increase vulnerability of pathogens to phagocytosis
      e. *Precipitens:* cause bacteria to settle out of blood for filtration by lymph nodes
   5. *Interferon:* chemical produced by a cell that has been attacked by a virus to prevent replication in similar cells
   6. *Vaccines:* contain antigens; given to produce immunity by stimulating production of antibodies
      a. *Sources:* nonpathogenic strains, closely related microbes, weakened (attenuated) living organisms, killed pathogens, extracts of pathogens, toxoids (inactivated bacterial toxins), and recombinant DNA
      b. *Most common vaccines:* diphtheria, pertussis, tetanus (DPT); measles, mumps, rubella (MMR); poliomyelitis (TOPV); hepatitis B; and varicella (chickenpox)

D. *Types of immunity (the ability to resist disease)*
   1. *Acquired immunity:* that which is obtained during a lifetime
      a. *Active immunity:* antibodies are formed (actively) following exposure to antigens, long lasting; there are two types:
         i. *Naturally acquired active immunity:* results from having had a disease and recovering

ii. *Artificially acquired active immunity:* produced by receiving a vaccine (which contains antigens)
b. *Passive immunity:* antibodies from an outside source are supplied, the immunity is borrowed (your body is passive), short lived; there are two types:
   i. *Naturally acquired passive immunity:* antibodies are passed from the mother to fetus through the placenta or to the infant through the mother's milk
   ii. *Artificially acquired passive immunity:* antibodies from another source (immune serum) are injected, usually after exposure to a disease (antigen)

E. *Overactive immune systems*
   1. *Allergy:* unusual susceptibility to an antigen (examples of allergens are pollen, dust, or eggs) that is ordinarily harmless to others (hypersensitivity)
   2. *Anaphylaxis (without protection):* severe and sometimes fatal reaction to a foreign substance (antigen) such as penicillin
      a. *Symptoms of anaphylaxis:* irritability, dyspnea (difficult breathing), swelling (edema), urticaria (rash, itching, redness), hypotension (low blood pressure), and headache
      b. *Treatment for anaphylaxis:* vasopressor drugs (i.e., epinephrine), antihistamines, oxygen, and corticosteroids
   3. *Autoimmunity:* a system that forms antibodies against its own tissues, destroying those tissues; examples are rheumatoid arthritis, rheumatic fever, and lupus erythematosus
   4. *Rejection syndrome:* results from a transplanted organ
      a. Patient is first crossmatched for transplant tissue
      b. Anti-inflammatory agents are administered to prevent rejection

II. **Process of Infection:** Members of the medical profession are dedicated to the prevention of illness, maintenance of health, and treatment of disease. We must remember: First, do no harm.

A. *Disease is any deviation from a normal, healthy state*
   1. *Endemic:* diseases that are present continually in the community
   2. *Epidemic:* the appearance of an infectious disease that attacks many people at one time in the same geographical area
   3. *Pandemic:* an infectious disease that affects many people in multiple regions around the globe. Most pandemics are respiratory in nature. Example: Influenza

B. *Disease may result from*
   1. *Malnutrition* (i.e., iron-deficiency anemia)
   2. *Congenital anomalies* (i.e., clubfeet or hydrocephalus)
   3. *Degenerative processes* (i.e., arthritis or arteriosclerosis)
   4. *Neoplasms (new growth)* (i.e., benign or malignant tumors)
   5. *Metabolic disorders* (i.e., diabetes or hyperthyroidism)
   6. *Physical or chemical agents* (i.e., burns, trauma, or accidents)
   7. *Infectious organisms (pathogens)* (i.e., wound infection or pneumonia)

C. *Pathology:* study of the cause of disease

D. *Community-acquired infection:* natural disease process that was present or incubating before the patient was admitted to the hospital or health care facility

E. *Nosocomial infection:* infection acquired in a hospital or health care facility with serious implications for all hospital personnel because of patient suffering, rising health care costs, and malpractice liability. Most common sites for nosocomial infections: genitourinary system (due to urinary catheterization), surgical wounds, respiratory tract, and venous access points

F. *Superinfection:* secondary infection that develops during or following antibiotic therapy and is caused by a different microorganism

G. *Sources of infection*
  1. *Exogenous:* acquired from sources outside the body, particles in the air, soil, water, fomites (contaminated objects), carriers (humans harboring organisms without symptoms of disease), human sources (visitors and staff), and vectors (living organisms that carry disease)
  2. *Endogenous:* develops from sources within the body (patient's own flora, exudates, and excretions); control by practices such as
    a. Patient's skin is cleansed prior to injection or incision
    b. Scalpel used to dissect the colon is not used on "cleaner" tissue
    c. Skin knife should likewise not be used on other tissue because of endogenous flora

H. *Transmission of pathogens:* their only way of travel is to be carried
  1. *Direct contact:* hands, aerosol droplets, blood, body fluids; control by
    a. Proper hand washing is the most common and most important practice of asepsis
    b. Appropriate use of surgical attire, personal protective equipment (PPE), and aseptic barriers such as sterile gowns and gloves
    c. Strict implementation of aseptic technique and Standard Precautions
  2. *Indirect contact:* airborne; may be contracted by touching contaminated objects (fomites) and then touching mouth or nose; control by
    a. Air-conditioning systems that allow a minimum of 15–20 air exchange per hour, with air inlet vents high (ceiling) and outlets low (floor), maintaining positive pressure
    b. Damp dusting and wet mopping to remove particles
    c. Filtering out particles with a proper use of high-efficiency particulate air (HEPA) filters
    d. Decreasing air currents (avoiding swinging doors, throwing linen, etc.); keeping doors closed
    e. Decreasing traffic in and out of sterile environments
  3. *Cross-infection:* from patient to patient
  4. People are the major source of microorganisms in the environment (especially the skin, hair, and nasopharynx)

I. *Portals of entry:* microbes enter the body through breaks in the skin (cuts, abrasions, bites, needle sticks) and mucous membranes (alimentary canal, respiratory tract, or genitourinary system)

J. *Portals of exit:* body secretions and excretions, and openings in the skin

K. *Factors that determine whether one exposed to a disease will contract it*
  1. Resistance of the host
  2. Virulence of the microorganism
  3. Number of organisms present (dose)
  4. Duration of exposure

L. *Factors lowering host resistance*
  1. Presence of another disease process
  2. Hormone imbalance
  3. Destruction of lymphatics by antineoplastic (cancer) drugs or radiation therapy
  4. Poor circulation (ischemia)
  5. Poor nutritional state
  6. Use of anti-inflammatory drugs (steroids)
  7. Extremes of age (very young and very old)
  8. Destruction of normal flora
  9. Emotional depression

M. *Body's response to generalized (systemic) infection*
  1. Leukocytosis (elevated WBCs)
  2. Elevated body temperature

3. Elevated metabolic rate (metabolism increases approximately 7% for every degree Fahrenheit rise in temperature) leads to increased pulse, respiration, and oxygen/water/nutrition requirements
4. Malaise (unfit feeling) and fatigue
5. Anorexia (loss of appetite), headache, backache, vomiting, diarrhea, diaphoresis (sweating), chills, fever, delirium, highly colored scanty urine, flushed face, and thick-coated tongue

N. *Terminology related to infection*
   1. *Primary infection:* original infection
   2. *Secondary infection:* follows another infection and is generally caused by opportunistic pathogens
   3. *Latent infection:* inactive or hidden stage in disease, as in the case of tuberculosis, syphilis, or malaria
   4. *Acute infection:* rapid in the onset and serious in nature
   5. *Chronic infection:* slow in the onset and less severe
   6. *Pus (suppuration):* collection of used-up phagocytes, dead tissue, and fluid; fibrinogen from exudate forms network of fibers to "wall off" and form an abscess

O. *Stages of an acute infection*
   1. *Incubation:* from exposure to first symptom
   2. *Prodromal:* vague symptoms
   3. *Acute:* actual illness
   4. *Convalescence:* recovery period

P. *Treatment for localized infection*
   1. Incise and drain abscess (I&D)
   2. Local application of heat (hot, wet compress)
   3. Topical antibiotic
   4. Immobilization of injured part (rest favors healing)
   5. Elevation of injured part facilitates drainage

III. **Isolation Precautions:** Patients may be isolated by diagnosis or by the mode of transmission of pathogenic microorganisms. Protective isolation may be used for the immunocompromised, burned, or organ transplant patient. The CDC Guidelines for Isolation Precautions in Hospitals should be used to determine the appropriate isolation technique.

IV. **Standard Precautions:** Standard Precautions were implemented to protect health care workers from the risk of blood and body fluids of all patients. This single set of precautions combine both Universal Precautions (UP) and Body Substance Isolation (BSI) that had previously been developed by the CDC.
   1. Implemented when blood or body fluids (except sweat) are encountered (tears, urine, feces, vomit, and semen)
   2. Used when working with mucous membrane and/or nonintact skin
   3. Established by the CDC
   4. Enforced by the Occupational Safety and Health Administration (OSHA)
   5. Protective barriers and personal protective equipment (PPE) to prevent skin and mucous membrane contact with blood and body fluid
      a. Gloves appropriate to the task; double gloving reduces the risk of exposure; wash hands immediately upon removing gloves
      b. Eyewear with side shields, goggles, or face shields when splash is possible
      c. Masks are worn for all invasive procedures
      d. Impervious gowns or aprons
   6. Precautions to prevent puncture injuries
      a. "No touch" technique for scalpels and other sharps
      b. No bending, breaking, resheathing, or recapping used needles by hand (*Note:* When recapping is essential, a recapping safety device or one-hand scoop technique should be used.)

    c. Blades, needles, and other disposable sharp instruments are placed in a puncture-resistant container

    d. Reusable sharp instruments are placed in puncture-resistant containers immediately after use

    e. Scalpel blades are applied and removed with an instrument (needle holder)

    f. Used needles should not be removed from disposable syringes

7. If a glove is torn or punctured, remove needle, blade, or instrument from sterile field, and change glove promptly using open gloving technique; if skin is punctured, remove both gloves immediately, squeeze to release blood, wash under running water with an antiseptic, and report incident immediately; baseline testing may be necessary for the patient and health care provider; follow up with physician or infection control officer; and ensure that appropriate vaccines are current

8. Protection should be available for mouth-to-mouth resuscitation (ambu bags, masks with one-way valves)

9. Specimens are handled as potentially infectious material, placed in leak-proof containers, and sealed in biohazard bag

10. Spills are cleaned up and disinfected promptly and effectively (concurrent disinfection)

11. Laundry is placed in leak-proof bag

12. Contaminated fluids may be poured into a sanitary sewer drain or a solidifying agent can be added to disposable suction containers; infectious waste is placed in color-coded impervious bags and incinerated (local and state regulations must be followed)

13. Hand washing follows every contact with patient, blood, or body fluids

14. Avoid eating, drinking, smoking, handling contact lenses, or applying cosmetics while in the perioperative environment

15. Know HIV/HBV antibody status and report seroconversion to the appropriate authority

Show What You Know

Directions Each of the numbered items or incomplete statements in this section is followed by answers or by completions of the statement. Select the ONE lettered answer or completion that is BEST in each case.

1. Microorganisms that cause disease are known as:
   A. carriers
   B. pathogens
   C. vectors
   D. saprophytes

2. Microorganisms that can be macroscopic and treated with antihelmintic drugs are:
   A. bacteria
   B. rickettsiae
   C. protozoa
   D. parasitic worms

3. Mycotic infections (athlete's foot and ringworm) are caused by:
   A. fungi
   B. viruses
   C. staphylococci
   D. rickettsiae

4. Organisms that cause hepatitis are:
   A. bacteria
   B. streptococci
   C. protozoa
   D. viruses

5. The bacteria that are spherical in shape, appear in clusters, and are the most common cause of postoperative wound infections are:
   A. *Treponema pallidum*
   B. *Clostridium perfringens*
   C. *Escherichia coli*
   D. *Staphylococcus aureus*

6. Bacteria that live only in the presence of oxygen are called:

   A. parasites
   B. anaerobes
   C. pathogens
   D. aerobes

7. Which of the following bacilli are spore-forming anaerobes, found in soil, and capable of causing gas gangrene?

   A. *Clostridium perfringens*
   B. mycobacteria
   C. *Pseudomonas aeruginosa*
   D. *Bacillus subtilis*

8. Which of the following infectious organisms is most likely to be transmitted through a contaminated needle stick?

   A. *Clostridium perfringens*
   B. Hepatitis B (HBV)
   C. *Mycobacterium tuberculosis*
   D. *Streptococcus pneumoniae*

9. A tough, resistant "shell form" of some gram-positive bacilli which is extremely resistant to destruction and toward which all sterilization methods are aimed is a/an:

   A. capsule
   B. endotoxin
   C. endospore
   D. flagellum

10. An enzyme produced by some virulent microorganisms, such as the *hemolytic streptococcus,* that breaks down fibrin and leads to wound infection is:

    A. fibrinolysin
    B. coagulase
    C. leukocidin
    D. exotoxin

11. A microbial relationship in which one organism lives completely at the expense of the host is:

    A. parasitism
    B. commensalism
    C. symbiosis
    D. antibiosis

12. The most widely used method for identifying bacteria by dividing them into two groups is:

    A. Gram stain
    B. acid-fast stain
    C. simple stain
    D. sensitivity study

13. Normal flora of the intestinal tract includes:

    A. *Lactobacillus acidophilus*
    B. *Staphylococcus albus*
    C. *Streptococcus pyogenes*
    D. *Escherichia coli*

14. The most likely portal of entry for the *Treponema pallidum* organism is:

    A. the respiratory tract
    B. a break in the skin
    C. the genitourinary tract
    D. the alimentary canal

15. Which of the following factors would have the *least* effect in determining whether or not one exposed to a disease would contract it?

    A. weight of host
    B. resistance of the host
    C. dose and virulence of the organism
    D. duration of exposure

16. Host resistance to infection may be lowered by all of the following *except:*

    A. poor circulation
    B. presence of another disease process
    C. emotional depression
    D. proper nutritional state

17. When a patient has a generalized (systemic) infection, the white blood cell (WBC) count would:

    A. increase
    B. decrease
    C. stay the same
    D. not be a factor

18. The type of isolation recommended for the immunocompromised, burn, or organ transplant patient is:

    A. protective
    B. strict
    C. enteric
    D. drainage and secretions

19. Pathogens that get past the first line of defense are engulfed by white blood cells, a process known as:

    A. filtration
    B. phagocytosis
    C. antigen—antibody reaction
    D. immunization

20. The immunity received by having had a disease (i.e., measles) is known as:

    A. naturally acquired active immunity
    B. artificially acquired active immunity
    C. naturally acquired passive immunity
    D. artificially acquired passive immunity

21. When a person forms antibodies against his or her own tissues, it is known as:

    A. autoimmunity
    B. rejection syndrome
    C. anaphylaxis
    D. passive immunity

22. An infection acquired while one is being treated in a health care facility is known as:

    A. primary infection
    B. acute infection
    C. community-acquired infection
    D. nosocomial infection

23. When an infection is caused by a patient's own normal flora, the source would be referred to as:

    A. endogenous
    B. exogenous
    C. transient
    D. airborne

24. Airborne contamination in the operating room can be reduced by:

    A. negative air pressure
    B. filtering out particles with high-efficiency particulate air (HEPA) filters
    C. increasing traffic in and out of rooms
    D. sterilization

25. Standard Precautions are to be implemented:

    A. when the patient is immunocompromised
    B. for patients with hepatitis B
    C. when the health care provider has open lesions on the hands
    D. when blood or body fluids may be encountered

Answers & Rationales

1. **B.** **Rationale:** Pathogens are disease-causing microorganisms.

2. **D.** **Rationale:** Parasitic worms (helminths), such as pinworms, round worms, or tapeworms, reproduce in the intestinal tract and may be seen in feces.

3. **A.** **Rationale:** Tinea is a ring-shaped lesion caused by a fungus. *Tinea pedis* is a fungus infection of the foot, known as athlete's foot.

4. **D.** **Rationale:** Hepatitis is caused by a virus.

5. **D.** **Rationale:** *Staphylococcus aureus* is a spherical-shaped *(coccus)* bacterium which appears in clusters *(staphyl-)* and produces coagulase (the enzyme which coagulates plasma), resulting in the formation of pus or abscesses.

6. **D.** **Rationale:** Aerobes are life forms which require air or oxygen for survival.

7. **A.** **Rationale:** *Clostridium perfringens* are anaerobic, found in soil, and cause gas gangrene as the result of a "dirty" or puncture wound.

8. **B.** **Rationale:** Hepatitis B (HBV) is a virus which can be transmitted through contaminated blood. It is because of this fact that health care personnel subjected to blood contamination should be vaccinated against this virus.

9. **C.** **Rationale:** Like seeds, an endospore can survive extreme environmental conditions such as drying, freezing, or boiling and is the most resistant to destruction of any life form.

10. **A.** **Rationale:** Fibrinolysin is an enzyme produced by some virulent microorganisms that break down (lyse) fibrin (the basis of a blood clot), leading to a wound infection.

11. **A.** **Rationale:** Parasitism is a microbial relationship in which one organism lives completely at the expense of the host.

12. **A.** **Rationale:** Dr. Gram discovered that certain bacteria would retain a crystal violet stain (gram positive) after treatment with a fixative (Lugol's iodine) and decolorization with ethanol acetone. Organisms which lose the crystal violet stain by decolorization but stain with a counterstain (usually safranin) are gram negative. This method of differentiating bacteria into two groups can be done in a matter of minutes and is useful in the selection of antibiotics, as most antibiotics are described as being effective against gram-positive and/or gram-negative organisms.

13. **D.** **Rationale:** *Escherichia coli* (a member of the coliform group of bacteria) are gram-negative facultative anaerobic, rod-shaped bacteria found in the large intestines of warm-blooded animals. They are nonpathogenic saprophytes in the colon, but opportunistic pathogens in the bladder or in a wound. Meticulous asepsis is required to contain *E. coli* during surgery of the colon.

14. **C.** **Rationale:** *Treponema pallidum* is the causative agent of syphilis, a sexually transmitted disease.

15. **A.** **Rationale:** The critical factors in determining whether or not one exposed to a disease will contract it are resistance of the host, dose of the organism, virulence of the organism, and duration of exposure.

16. **D.** **Rationale:** Proper nutrition *increases* resistance to disease.

17. **A.** **Rationale:** The white blood cells are phagocytes, which serve as the body's second line of

defense against infectious disease and would increase in number during an infection, when the body is "mobilizing the troops."

18. **A.** **Rationale:** Protective isolation (sometimes referred to as reverse isolation) protects a compromised host (i.e., burn or transplant patient) from being overcome with infection and mimics surgical asepsis, as the goal is to keep infectious organisms away from the patient.

19. **B.** **Rationale:** Phagocytosis is the process of phagocytes (WBCs) engulfing and destroying bacteria.

20. **A.** **Rationale:** Naturally acquired active immunity is protection provided by the body actively producing antibodies in response to specific antigens. This type of immunity is naturally acquired as a result of having the disease and is long lasting.

21. **A.** **Rationale:** Autoimmunity is a condition characterized by a specific humoral or cell-mediated immune response against constituents of the body's own tissues.

22. **D.** **Rationale:** A nosocomial infection is one that originates while a patient is in the hospital (health care institution) and may be referred to as iatrogenic.

23. **A.** **Rationale:** The source of an infection caused by the patient's own normal flora would come from within (endogenous).

24. **B.** **Rationale:** Airborne contamination can be reduced by using positive air pressure, and high-efficiency filters to clean the air and decreasing air currents and traffic in and out of rooms (air currents spread dust and lint, which may be laden with microbes).

25. **D.** **Rationale:** Standard Precautions are to be implemented anytime blood or body fluids may be encountered.

Part II: Deciphering a Surgical Schedule

The following mock surgery schedule will be used to answer several questions pertaining to microbiology. The same schedule, or a similar one, may be used in subsequent chapters to ask questions about the content of the chapter.

Rm. # time	Surgeon	Procedure	Anest.	Rm. # time	Surgeon	Procedure	Anest.
Rm.00				**Rm07**			
OC	Dr. Z	Rt. Knee Arthroscopy	Gen.	7:00	Dr. M	Rhinoplasty	Gen.
OC	Dr. C	Craniotomy	Gen.				
OC	Dr. Z	BKA	Gen.	TF	Dr. M	Lipoma removal	MAC
Rm.01				**Rm08**			
7:00	Dr. X	Lobectomy	Gen.	11:00	Dr. E	Bovine	MAC
TF	Dr. X	Thoracotomy	Gen.			Thrombectomy	
TF	Dr. X	Tracheostomy	Gen.				
Rm02				**Rm09**			
7:00	Dr. B	Splenectomy	Gen.	8:30	Dr. T	Cholecystectomy	Gen.
TF	Dr. B	Gastrectomy	Gen.	TF	Dr. T	I&D	Gen.
				TF	Dr. T	Debridement	Gen.
Rm03				**Rm10**			
7:00	Dr. A	Cystoscopy	MAC	7:00	Dr. K	Nephrectomy	Gen.
TF	Dr. A	Cystoplasty	Gen.	TF	Dr. K	Choledocholithotripsy	MAC
12:30	Dr. F	Pyleogram	MAC				
3:00	Dr. F	Cystocele repair	Gen.	TF	Dr. K	Colectomy	Gen.
Rm04				**Rm11**			
7:00	Dr. Y	Carpal tunnel release	MAC	7:00	Dr. L	Cervical Cone Biopsy	Gen.
TF	Dr. Y	Fasciotomy	Gen.	12:00	Dr. L	Sentinel Node Biopsy	Gen.
Rm05				**Rm12**			
7:00	Dr. G	Trans-sphenoidal Adenectomy	Gen.	7:00	Dr. W	Trans-metatarsal amputation	Gen.
TF	Dr. G	Trans-urethral resection of the prostate	Gen	TF	Dr. W	Osteotomy Right Knee	Gen.
TF	Dr. G	Bletharoplasty	Gen.	TF	Dr. W	Arthroplasty	Gen.
Rm06				**Rm13**			
7:00	Dr. R	Lumbar Laminectomy	Gen.	7:00	Dr. O	Hysterectomy	Gen.

The following questions should be answered using the surgery schedule above

1. Room 9 has a debridement scheduled to follow an I&D. Why is this procedure being performed?

    A. To remove necrotic or infected tissue
    B. To remove scarred tissue
    C. To culture the wound
    D. To prevent infection

2. The patient undergoing the Colectomy in Room 10 will be at an increased risk of infection from what?

    A. Endogenous bacteria
    B. Nosocomial infection
    C. Viral infection
    D. Exogenous Bacteria

3. The patient in Room 5 was given penicillin and suffered anaphylactic shock. What is the treatment that needs to be followed?

    A. Levophed should be administered
    B. Dantrolene should be given
    C. Epinephrine should be given
    D. Protamine sulfate should be given

4. The patient in Room 12 is having a trans-metatarsal amputation due to clostridium perfringens. What does this patient have?

    A. Tetanus
    B. Gas gangrene
    C. Viral streptococcus
    D. Necrotizing fasciitis

5. The I&D was originally scheduled before the knee replacement in Room 12. Why was it moved?

    A. The surgeon was already scheduled in Room 9
    B. The patient requested an earlier surgery
    C. An infected case should never be performed before a clean orthopedic case
    D. The equipment that has already been placed in Room 9 is more conducive to the procedure

6. There is an on call below knee amputation that needs to be placed in a Room. Where should this surgery be performed?

    A. Room 12
    B. Room 9
    C. Room 6
    D. It should not be performed

7. One room has a possible issue with cases being performed. Which room should be changed?

    A. Room 12
    B. Room 8
    C. Room 11
    D. Room 13

8. Dr. X in Room 1 wants to know if there is an infectious process going on with his patient. What lab test will he want?

    A. C&S
    B. I&D
    C. Frozen section
    D. CBC

9. Sharon, the Surgical Technologist assigned to Room 3 has learned that the patient is HIV positive. What precautions should she take?

    A. Isolation
    B. Standard
    C. Universal
    D. She should refuse to scrub the case

10. The patient undergoing the lumbar laminectomy has severe rheumatoid arthritis. This is an example of what disease process?

    A. Autoimmune
    B. Acquired immunity
    C. Metabolic disorder
    D. Immunosuppression

Answers & Rationales

1. **A. Rationale:** Debridement is commonly done to remove infected or necrotic tissue. There are specific types of bacteria that grow well in necrotic tissue, including Clostridium Perfringens and other anaerobic bacteria. Generally, the surgeon will remove all of the necrosed an infected tissue along with a margin of healthy tissue to ensure that the infection does not spread. The surgeon may also culture the wound to determine the type of infection present, but, while the goal of the surgery may be to prevent the further spread of and determine the type of infection, it is primarily done to remove tissue already damaged.

2. **A. Rationale:** The patient undergoing a surgical procedure involving entry into the digestive tract is at an increased risk of endogenous infections. The bowel contains many types of bacteria that aid in the digestive process. These bacteria are harmless in their natural location, but become extremely pathogenic and aggressive when they are allowed into other areas of the body. The surgeon in this case may request antibiotics in the irrigation to reduce the risk of an infection.

3. **C. Rationale:** Epinephrine is routinely given to patients in anaphylactic shock.

4. **B. Rationale:** Clostridium perfringens is an anaerobic bacterial infection that requires aggressive treatment, including amputation. This bacterium can be found in the soil, and can enter the body through a break in the skin, usually the foot.

5. **C. Rationale:** It is good practice to try to keep infected cases out of rooms that have a sterile case following. In the case of orthopedics, this is an extremely important practice. Orthopedic procedures are easily contaminated, and represent a distinct threat of infection for the patient who may require more surgery, longer hospital stays, and possible amputation. For these reasons, most ORs will not schedule an infected case before a sterile procedure.

6. **B. Rationale:** Most amputations are performed due to infection that has not been contained. Therefore, every effort should be made to place this procedure in a room that is already dealing with contaminated cases.

7. **A. Rationale:** For the reasons stated in questions 5 and 6, the trans-metatarsal surgery should be rescheduled for another room.

8. **A. Rationale:** A culture and sensitivity test will identify the bacteria that cause the infection.

9. **B. Rationale:** Surgical Technologists should treat all patients with Standard Precautions. The CDC adopted these precautions that combine body substance isolation and Universal Precautions after the AIDS epidemic spread. STs may not always know if a person is infected, so they should treat each patient as a possible source of infection and always follow the standard precaution protocol.

10. **A. Rationale:** Rheumatoid arthritis is an autoimmune disease that targets the joints.

PEARSON
myhealthprofessionskit™

Use this address to access the interactive Companion Website created for this book. Simply select "Surgical Technology" from the choice of disciplines. Find this book and click to enter.

4 Pharmacology and Anesthesia

Surgical patients are exposed to a wide variety of drugs with which they are unfamiliar, increasing the responsibility of the entire surgical team. A system of checks and balances ensures that the correct drug in the correct amount and strength is given by the correct route, for the correct purpose, to the correct patient. The patient is then closely monitored for actions and reactions, and appropriate intervention methods are implemented. Surgical Technologists routinely handle medications on the back table, and must be familiar with the uses and contraindications of these medications, as well as the common doses and contraindications.

CHAPTER OUTLINE

How to Answer Pharmacology Questions

Pharmacology can be daunting for students and Surgical Technologists alike. The calculations and medication names can be confusing, but are of the utmost importance for patient safety. Medication errors can harm or even kill a patient, so this subject must be mastered by everyone involved in patient care. Although safeguards are in place to reduce and prevent errors, they sometimes still occur. The Surgical Technologist must remember that he or she is an important link in the communication of medication administration. Answering questions regarding pharmacology can be difficult and confusing as there are generic names, brand names, and different drug actions that must be considered.

Example:
Anectine is considered a/an

a. Neuromuscular blocker
b. Inhalation agent
c. Antianxiety drug
d. Local anesthetic

To answer this question, first you must identify the drug, then the drug action. Anectine is the trade name for succinylcholine hydrochloride. The drug is an injectable agent which rules inhalation agents B. It is not a local agent, so D would also be considered incorrect. Antianxiety medications are commonly given pre-operatively which would rule out C, leaving A as the correct answer to this question. It should also be noted that Anectine is a possible trigger agent for Malignant Hyperthermia, meaning the ST should be prepared to deal with an emergency situation if this medication is given to the patient. Knowing the treatment for this reaction could be lifesaving to a patient.

Systems of Measurement

I. **Metric System**

  A. **There are three basic units in the metric system**
    1. The basic unit of length is the meter (m)
    2. The basic unit of volume is the liter (L)
    3. The basic unit of weight is the gram (gm or g)

  B. **Certain basic prefixes designate either multiples or divisions of the three basic units**
    1. *kilo:* 1000 times the basic unit
    2. *centi:* one-hundredth (0.01) of the basic unit
    3. *milli:* one-thousandth (0.001) of the basic unit
    4. *micro:* one-millionth (0.000001) of the basic unit

  C. **Those units of the metric system most frequently encountered in medicine are as follows**
    1. **Length:**
      a. meter (m)
      b. centimeter (cm) = 0.01 m (100 cm equals 1 m)
      c. millimeter (mm) = 0.001 m (1000 mm equals 1 m)
    2. **Volume:**
      a. liter (L)
      b. milliliter (ml) = 0.001 L (1000 ml = 1 L)
         (*Note:* A milliliter is equivalent to a cubic centimeter [cc])
    3. **Weight:**
      a. gram (gm)
      b. kilogram (kg) = 1000 gm
      c. milligram (mg) = 0.001 gm (1000 mg = 1 gm)
      d. microgram (mcg) = 0.000001 gm or 0.001 mg
         (1,000,000 mcg = 1 gm and 1000 mcg = 1 mg)

II.   Household System

    A.   teaspoon (tsp) = 5 ml

    B.   tablespoon (tbsp) = 15 ml (or 3 tsp)

    C.   cup = 240 ml (or 8 fl oz)

III.   Apothecary System

    A.   Volume

        1.   minim (m) = 1 drop (gtt)
        2.   dram (dr) = 5 ml (1 tsp)
        3.   ounce (oz) = 30 ml (2 tbsp)
        4.   pint (pt) = 500 ml
        5.   quart (qt) = 32 ounces (2 pints)

    B.   Weight
        1.   grain (gr) = 60 mg

IV.   Miscellaneous Equivalents (Approximate)

    A.   Length
        1.   1 meter = 39 inches
        2.   1 inch = 2.54 cm

    B.   Weight
        1.   l gram = 15gr
        2.   1 pound (lb) = 454 gm
        3.   1 kg = 2.2 lb

    C.   Volume
        A. 1 ml = 15 minims

    D.   *Unit (U):* an amount of a drug possessing a defined amount of pharmacological activity (useful for drugs which are not 100% pure)

    E.   *Milliequivalent (mEq):* a way of expressing the dose of electrolytes based on the number of atoms of an element desired

    F.   *Units of temperature:* Celsius and Fahrenheit

	FREEZING	BODY TEMPERATURE	BOILING	THERMAL DEATH (SPORES)
Celsius	0°	37°	100°	121°
Fahrenheit	32°	98.6°	212°	250°

To convert Celsius to Fahrenheit, multiply Celsius by 9/5 and add 32. Formula: $(C \times 9/5) + 32 = F$

To convert Fahrenheit to Celsius, subtract 32 from Fahrenheit and multiply by 5/9. Formula: $(F - 32) \times 5/9 = C$

Terminology

1. *Acupuncture:* intense stimulation to one part of the body to release endorphins and relieve pain

2. *Adverse effect:* an undesired, potentially harmful side effect of a drug

3. *Agonist:* a drug that binds to a receptor and stimulates the receptor's function

4. *Amnesia:* loss of memory

5. *Anesthesia:* without sensation

6. *Antagonist:* a drug that counteracts the action of another drug

7. *Analgesia:* absence of pain

8. *Antiarrhythmic:* drug given to correct cardiac dysrhythmia

9. *Anticonvulsant:* drug that prevents convulsions

10. *Antidote:* drug that neutralizes a poison, prevents its action, or reverses its toxic effects in the body

11. *Antifungal:* drug used to control fungus infections

12. *Antihypertensive:* drug that lowers blood pressure

13. *Antipruritic:* drug that relieves itching

14. *Antispasmodic:* drug that reduces or prevents spasms

15. *Balanced anesthesia:* technique that uses a variety of drugs to achieve homeostasis, analgesia, amnesia, and muscle relaxation

16. *Cathartic:* drug used to produce evacuation of the bowels; a potent laxative

17. *Contraindication:* the reason a specific drug is not used

18. *Controlled substance:* drug with potential for addiction and abuse

19. *Cryoanesthesia:* using marked cooling to block pain sensation

20. *Decongestant:* drug used to open the air passages of the nose, bronchi, and/or sinuses

21. *Emetic:* drug that induces emesis or vomiting

22. *Expectorant:* drug that promotes expulsion of mucus from the lungs or trachea

23. *Fasciculation:* muscular twitching or contraction following the administration of succinylcholine chloride, a depolarizing neuromuscular blocker used in conjunction with general anesthesia

24. *Hypnoanesthesia:* absence of pain sensation due to a trancelike state

25. *Hypnotic:* drug used to induce sleep

26. *Indication:* the reason for giving a specific drug

27. *Intubation:* insertion of an endotracheal tube for the purpose of controlled respiration

28. *Laxative:* drug that stimulates bowel activity and movements

29. *Malignant Hyperthermia:* hypermetabolic crisis triggered by some anesthetic agents and drugs in susceptible persons

30. *Parenteral:* given by injection or a route other than the gastrointestinal tract

31. *Pharmacodynamics:* the interaction of drug molecules with target cells

32. *Pharmacokinetics:* the entire process of the drug within the body (absorption, distribution, metabolism, and excretion)

33. *Placebo:* inactive substance administered purely for its psychological effect

34. *Sedative:* drug used to allay anxiety or excitement, may be used to induce unconscious state

35. *Side effect:* an expected but unintended effect of a drug

36. *Toxicology:* study of poisons and the adverse effects of chemicals or drugs on the body

37. *Tranquilizer:* drug used to allay anxiety without depressing the patient

Pharmacology is the study of drugs and their actions. Drugs may be sold over the counter (OTC) or may require a prescription. Certain prescription drugs with a high potential to cause psychological and/or physical dependence and abuse are controlled substances and are regulated federally. State practice acts further govern the ordering, dispensing, and administration of medications. Hospital policies and procedures regarding drug use and distribution must also be followed. In surgery, medication orders may be a **standing order** or a **verbal order**. Standing orders are listed on the surgeon's preference card. Verbal orders are common in the operating room and are given by the surgeon to either the anesthesia provider or to another member of the surgical team to be administered from the sterile field.

Uses of Drugs

1. Diagnose or investigate (contrast media and dyes)
2. Treat symptoms without curing disease (aspirin)
3. Cure disease (antibiotics)
4. Prevent illness (vaccines)

Drug Nomenclature

1. *Chemical name:* gives chemical formula (used infrequently)
2. *Generic name:* nonproprietary name that is often given by the original developer; (common name)
3. *Trade name or brand name:* drug name chosen by the manufacturer for proprietary purposes; (registered and capitalized)

Sources of Accurate Drug Information

1. *United States Pharmacopedia (USP):* drugs are admitted to this listing on the basis of therapeutic merit or necessity
2. *National Formulary (NF):* (*Note:* USP and NF are the two official reference books under the auspices of the Food and Drug Administration [FDA]; published every 5 years with annual additions; list generic names only; contain limited clinical information; and set standards for manufacture and testing.)
3. *Physician's Desk Reference (PDR):* most popular and most commonly used reference, listed by manufacturers, and includes the same information as package inserts.

Sources of Drugs

1. Plant products (e.g., digitalis)
2. Animal products (e.g., hormones)
3. Minerals (e.g., iron)
4. Laboratory synthesis (e.g., Demerol)
5. Biotechnology (e.g., Heptovax-Hepatitis B vaccine)

Routes of Administration

1. **Oral (PO):** by mouth. This is also known as *enteral*
2. **Parenteral:** IV (intravenous), IM (intramuscular), SC (subcutaneous), ID (intradermal), and Intrathecial
3. **Topical, rectal, vaginal, sublingual** (beneath the tongue), and **buccal** (in the cheek). Administered to mucous membranes
4. **Inhalation**

Drug Forms

1. *Solids:* powder, tablets, capsules, lozenges
2. *Semisolids:* suppositories, ointments, creams, gels, foams
3. *Liquids:* Most drugs administered during surgical procedures are liquid or gas
   a. *Solutions:* drug dissolved in a liquid, i.e., aqueous (in water), tincture (with water and alcohol), syrup (with water and sugar), and elixir (with sugar and alcohol)

    b. *Suspension:* solid particles float in a liquid and must be shaken prior to use

    c. *Emulsion:* combination of two liquids that do not mix

4. **Gases:** may come in a tank, i.e., oxygen and inhalation anesthetic agents (nitrous oxide)

Factors Influencing the Action and Use of Drugs

1. *Individual variation:* all persons show some differences in their reaction to drugs
2. *Idiosyncrasy:* (i.e., allergy)
3. *Tolerance:* the progressive decrease in the effectiveness of a drug
4. *Cumulation:* buildup effect due to poor metabolism, decreased excretion, or the drug being stored in excess adipose tissue
5. *Pregnancy:* many drugs are harmful to the fetus
6. *Age:* smaller doses for children
7. *Dose:* doubling the dose does not necessarily double effectiveness and can even be harmful
8. *Disease:* disease of liver or kidneys may alter effect of drugs
9. *Psychological factors:* may play a role. Anxiety and other factors can affect the amount of medication needed.
10. *Body weight:* dosage may be calculated on the basis of body weight
11. *Time of administration* is related to activities such as meals or sleep; timing is important to keep the blood level of the drug at an appropriate therapeutic level
12. *Route of administration*
    a. Onset of action depends on the time the drug reaches the circulation
    b. Duration of action depends on the length of time the drug is in the circulation before it is excreted
    c. Oral administration provides slow onset with longer duration
    d. IM or SC administration provides generally rapid onset
    e. Some drugs may be destroyed by digestive juices
    f. Some drugs may not be absorbed from gastrointestinal (GI) tract
    g. Some drugs may be painful when given IM or SC
    h. Some drugs are not effective when given IM
    i. Some drugs may be given through multiple routes
    j. Some drugs are incompatible with other drugs, due to precipitation, inactivation, potentiation, or antagonism

Common Abbreviations Used in Medication Orders

Abbreviation	Meaning
aa	of each
ac	before meals
AD	right ear
ad lib	as desired
AM	morning
AS	left ear
AU	both ears
bid	twice a day
c̄	with

Abbreviation	Meaning
caps	capsules
cc	cubic centimeter (ml)
DC	discontinue
gm, g	gram
gr	grain
gtt	drop
h	hour
hs	at bedtime (hours sleep)
IM	intramuscularly
IV	intravenously
L	liter
NPO	nothing by mouth
OD	right eye
OS	left eye
OU	both eyes
pc	after meals
PO or po	by mouth
PRN or prn	as needed
q	every
qAM	every morning
qd	every day
qh	every hour
qid	four times a day
Rx	take, prescription, therapy
$\bar{s}$	without
SC or SQ	subcutaneous
sig	mark on label
stat	immediately
$\overline{\overline{ss}}$	half
tab	tablet
tid	three times a day
tr, tinct	tincture
ung	ointment

Common Symbols

m	minim or drop
ℨ	teaspoon or dram
℥	1 fluid ounce, 2 tablespoons
Ⓛ	left
®	right
ө	none
△	change
>	greater than
<	less than
↓	increase
↑	decrease

Syringes and Needles for Giving Injections

1. Components of a syringe are the plunger and barrel with calibrations in ml (cc) and/or ounces, or units

2. **Types of syringes**

   a. *Standard:* with a plain tip or Luer-loc tip (screw-type locking mechanism for addition of hypodermic needles)

   b. *Turberculin:* 1 cc for doses of less than 1 ml

   c. *Insulin:* calibrated in units up to 100 units (u)

   d. *Tubex:* a metal or plastic device that holds a carpule of medication

   e. *Irrigating:* asepto, ear, or toomey syringe

3. **Hypodermic needles**

   a. *Size (gauge):* ranges from 14 g to 30 g (30 g has smallest lumen and 14 g the largest); larger needles (18 g to 21 g) are used to draw up medicine; smaller needles (22 g to 30 g) for injection, depending on viscosity (thickness) of the drug; 25 g would be appropriate for local infiltration of a drug

   b. *Length:* 5/8 to 3 1/2 inches, short lengths for hypodermic needles and long for spinal injections

   c. *Considerations when selecting a needle for injection:* safety, depth, comfort of patient, rate of flow, and thickness of solution

Methods of Calculating Dosage

I. **Metric Conversions:** The most frequent calculation involves changing from one unit to another within the metric system; since the system was developed in multiples of 10, the quick and easy method to convert is simply a matter of moving the decimal point to the left to divide and to the right to multiply

   A. When changing from a larger unit to a smaller unit, there will be more units, so multiply by moving the decimal to the right.

   B. When changing from a smaller unit to a larger unit, there will be fewer units, so divide by moving the decimal to the left.
   Example 1: If the doctor asks for 500 mg of a drug and the medication label reads "1 gm/cc," the ST is going to a larger unit and will divide by moving the decimal point three places to the left (remember that there are 1000 mg in 1 gm); thus: 500 mg equals 0.5 gm.
   Example 2: The surgeon's preference card calls for Ancef 2 gm in 500 cc of normal saline for irrigation. The label on the vial reads 1000 mg/cc. The ST is going to multiply by moving the decimal three places to the right (remember that there are 1000 mg in 1 gm); thus 2 gm = 2000 mg.

II. **Ratio and Proportion**

   A. *Ratio:* an expression of the relationship that one quantity has to another
   Example: The ratio for ventilations to compressions when performing one-person CPR is 2:15 (2 breaths to 15 compressions).

   B. *Proportion:* an expression of two equal ratios
   Example: Three staff members can run one operating room (ratio of 1:3). How many staff members would be required to run five rooms? The problem would be written

Known		Unknown
1 room: 3 staff members	=	5 rooms: X staff members

   Multiply means and extremes

   1 room: 3 staff members   =   5 rooms: X staff members

   $(1)X = 15$

III.   Dosage Calculation

    A. Calculating medication dosages is necessary when the amount ordered differs from what the label indicates and may be done by ratio and proportion
Example: The preference card calls for papaverine 30 mg. The label on the vial reads "60 mg/2 cc." How many **cubic centimeters** would be prepared?

Known	**Unknown**
available dose: volume =	desired dose: X volume
60 mg: 2 cc =	30 mg: X cc

$$60X = 2 \times 30$$

$$60X = 60$$

$$\frac{60X}{60} = \frac{60}{60}$$

$$X = \frac{60}{60}$$

$$X = 1 \text{ cc}$$

Check your calculation by substituting the answer for X.

$$60{:}2 = 30{:}1$$

$$60 = 60$$

    B. Calculating dosage for injection when reconstituting a powder
       1. Read the label carefully
       2. Add the specified amount of diluent
       3. Dissolve the drug completely
       4. Note concentration (mg/ml) of the solution produced
       5. Calculate the volume to administer
Example: The physician orders 600,000 units of penicillin. The ST has a vial containing 1,000,000 units of penicillin. Directions on the label read "after addition of 4.6 cc of diluent, each cc contains 200,000 units." The ST would measure 4.6 cc of sterile water, add it to the vial, and dissolve completely before withdrawing the desired dose.

Known	**Unknown**
available dose:volume =	*desired dose:X* volume
200,000 U: 1 cc	= 600,000 U: X cc

$$200{,}000X = 600{,}000$$

$$\frac{200{,}000X}{200{,}000} = \frac{600{,}000}{200{,}000}$$

$$X = 3 \text{ cc}$$

    C. *Percentage preparation:* parts per hundred (1 g:100 g; 1 ml to 100 ml; 1 g: 100 ml)
Example: The physician orders 25 g of dextrose. A 50% solution of dextrose comes to you in a 50-cc syringe. How many cc would be needed?

$$50 \text{ g}{:}100 \text{ cc} = 25 \text{ g}{:}X \text{ cc}$$

$$50X = 2500$$

$$\frac{50X}{50} = \frac{2500}{50}$$

$$X = 50 \text{ cc}$$

You would need all of the dextrose.

    D. *Calculating for ratio strength:* Ratio is often used to express the concentration of liquid, the number of grams of a drug in a specified number of milliliters of solution; prostigmine 1:2000 contains 1 g of neostigmine in 2000 ml of solution

Example: The doctor requests 0.5 mg of adrenalin. The label on the vial reads 1:1000 solution. How much would the ST give?

1 g:1000 ml = 0.5 mg:X ml

Convert "1 g" to "1000 mg" before the problem can be worked

1000 mg:1000 ml = 0.5 mg:X ml

1000X = 500

$$\frac{1000X}{1000} = \frac{500}{1000}$$

$$X = \frac{500}{1000}$$

X = 0.5 ml

Care and Handling of Drugs

1. Drugs are frequently given during surgery.

2. Drugs anticipated for a procedure will be listed on the surgeon's preference card.

3. To help prevent medication errors, the "Six Rights" of medication handling must be followed. Team members work together to make sure of the following:

   a. right patient

   b. right drug

   c. right dose

   d. right route

   e. right time

   f. right label and documentation

4. The circulator secures anticipated drugs before an operation begins, checking the label carefully for name, amount, strength, expiration date, color, and integrity of the container. Some states require a registered nurse to dispense medication to the sterile field. Follow the state practice act.

5. The circulator holds the vial of medication for the scrub to observe appearance and verify name, amount, strength and expiration date, and then makes the medication available to the scrub. The circulator pours the medication into a sterile container using a transfer device, or holds the container, after proper cleaning with an alcohol wipe, for the scrub to withdraw the medication with sterile needle and syringe.

6. The circulator holds the vial for the scrub to verify the name, strength, amount, and expiration date.

7. The circulator keeps the vial in the room until the procedure is over.

8. The scrub labels each medication and/or solution immediately. Labels should be placed on all containers, including the medicine cup and the syringe.

9. When presenting medication to the surgeon, the scrub recites the name, strength, and amount of the drug. The scrub should make a note of the amount used.

10. No drug or solution is used when anyone is uncertain of what it is, if its color has changed, or when there is a question of container integrity.

11. Surgical Technologists should be familiar with all drugs handled as to their use, major action, and major adverse effects.

Drugs Commonly Used in Surgery

1. *Adrenergic drugs:* used to work with the sympathetic nervous system to increase blood pressure and dilate bronchioles; useful in shock and anaphylactic reactions; may be used in combination with local anesthetics

(*Note:* Brand names of drugs appear in parentheses)

Examples:

epinephrine (adrenalin)

phenylephrine hydrochloride (Neo-Synephrine), which is also an adrenergic drug and used more commonly in nasal surgery to decrease bleeding and in eye surgery to dilate the pupil

2. *Antiarrhythmic drugs:* given by anesthesiologist to correct a cardiac dysrhythmia
Examples:

lidocaine (Xylocaine)

procainamide hydrochloride (Pronestyl)

3. *Antibiotics/antibacterial drugs:* used to treat or prevent an infection (antibiotic prophylaxis)

   a. *Aminoglycosides:* broad-spectrum antibiotics that may be given IV or used to irrigate wounds when mixed with saline; the most commonly given category of antibiotics in surgery

   Examples:

   kanamycin (Kantrex)

   gentamicin (Garamycin)

   b. *Cephalosporins:* broad-spectrum antibiotics, may be given IV or mixed with saline or lactated Ringer's solution for irrigation of wounds

   Examples:

   cefazolin (Ancef)

   cefotetan (Cefotan)

   c. *Penicillins:* antibiotic available in many natural and semisynthetic forms

   Example:

   ampicillin (Omnipen)

   d. *Tetracyclines:* broad spectrum antibiotic

   Example:

   doxycycline (Vibramycin)

4. *Anticoagulants:* used to prevent or delay the clotting of blood

   a. *heparin sodium:* interferes with clotting, given IV during vascular surgery, and effects may be reversed prior to wound closure; may be given in smaller doses preoperatively or postoperatively to prevent the formation of blood clots; **protamine sulfate** is the reversal agent.

   b. *warfarin (Coumadin):* oral anticoagulant that interferes with synthesis of prothrombin in the liver, used to prevent the formation of clots, has a latent period of 24 hours, and is residual for several days. Generally discontinued prior to surgery or treated with its antidote, vitamin K (Mephyton, Aqua Mephyton)

5. *Antihistamines:* used to prevent or counteract an allergic reaction
Example:

   diphenhydramine (Benadryl)

6. *Antihypertensive drugs:* used for rapid reduction of blood pressure
Example:

   nitroprusside sodium (Nipride, Nitropress)

7. *Antineoplastic chemotherapy agents:* used to inhibit malignant cells. Since these agents are not commonly given in the operating room, examples are not provided

8. *Bronchodilators:* used in the treatment of both asthma and Cheyne-Stokes respiration to dilate bronchioles and enhance respiration

Examples:

aminophylline

ephedrine sulfate

9. *Cardiac glycosides:* used to increase cardiac output and give a stronger, fuller beat; may result in a slowing of the pulse; also used to treat congestive heart failure and certain arrhythmias
   Example:

   digitoxin (Purodigin)

10. *Cholinergic drugs:* used to work with the parasympathetic nervous system and vagus nerve to speed up smooth muscle activity (promote intestinal motility and bladder motility) and to counteract nondepolarizing neuromuscular blockers
    Example:

    prostigmine (Neostigmine)

11. *Contrast media:* outlines walls of hollow tubes or cavities; allows internal structures to be viewed on x-ray; are radiopaque; most contrast media contain iodine, so the patient's history must be checked for allergies to iodine or shellfish
    Example:

    diatrizoate sodium (Hypaque)

12. *Coronary artery dilators:* used to dilate the coronary arteries to increase blood flow to the heart
    Example: nitroglycerine (may be administered sublingually or by a dermal patch)

13. *Cycloplegic:* used to dilate the pupil by paralyzing the ciliary muscle
    Examples:

    Cyclogyl

    Mydriacyl

14. *Diuretics:* used to increase urinary output and control edema and hypertension; used frequently during neurosurgery or ophthalmic surgery
    Examples:

    furosemide (Lasix): referred to as a loop diuretic because it acts at Henle's loop in the kidney tubule to increase renal excretion of fluid and electrolytes; both urinary output and potassium level should be monitored during use

    mannitol (Osmitrol): referred to as an osmotic diuretic because it raises osmotic pressure at the glomeruli level to increase urinary output; given during certain neurosurgical procedures to reduce intracranial pressure

15. *Dyes:* used to enhance visualization of a structure or for marking skin incisions
    Examples:

    Methylene blue

    Indigo carmine

    Brilliant green

    Gentian violet

16. *Hemostatic agents (coagulants):* used to control bleeding in surgery
    Examples:

    Thrombin: a topical powder that may be mixed with a solution but *never* injected; may be used with Gelfoam

    Bone wax: topical hemostatic agent made from beeswax used on bone surfaces

    Absorbable gelatin sponge (Gelfoam): may be moistened with a saline or thrombin solution and placed on bleeders

    Oxidized cellulose (Oxcel, Surgicel): applied dry and is absorbable; the gauze form may be cut into desired shape and size

> ### SURGERY HINT
>
> Many surgeries require the use of multiple medications. Generally, the Surgical Technologist will have localized medications on the field to pass to the surgeon as required. It is extremely important for the ST to keep track of the amounts of medications that are administered during the procedure, as they have important ramifications to patient care. If the ST will be tracking medications, keep a running total on the back table with a sterile marking pen. Generally, a 10 cc syringe will be utilized. It will be easier to track if the ST pulls up a full 10 cc each time he or she fills a syringe.
>
> Make sure to check the preference card for hypo selection.

Microfibrillar collagen (Avitene): absorbable and must be applied dry

Absorbable collagen sponge: cut into desired shape and applied with pressure to the bleeding site. Should not be used with Methyl Methacrylate

Protamine sulfate: given IV to counteract the effects of heparin

17. *Hormones:* used to replace loss or deficiencies
    Examples:

    Insulin: used to promote utilization of glucose to treat diabetes

    Glucagon: used to antagonize insulin or treat hypoglycemia

18. *Miotics:* used to constrict the pupil
    Example:

    acetylcholine chloride (Miochol)

19. *Mydriatics:* used to dilate the pupil
    Examples:

    Atropine

    Cyclogyl

    Mydriacyl

    Neo-Synephrine

    Tropicamide (cycloplegic and mydriatic)

20. *Oxytocic drugs:* used to contract the uterus to induce or facilitate labor or given in larger doses following delivery to contract the uterus and control bleeding
    Examples:

    oxytocin (Pitocin)

    methylergonovine (Methergine); *never* used with labor as it causes tetanic contractions and would cut off oxygen to the fetus

21. *Stains:* used to identify abnormal tissue—usually iodine based
    Examples:

    Schiller's test uses Lugols solution

    Lugol's solution for identifying abnormal cervical cells prior to biopsy

22. *Steroidal anti-inflammatory drugs:* used to decrease cerebral or ocular edema, prevent swelling; useful in arthroscopy, eye, head, and neck surgery; large doses of steroids preoperatively can interrupt the healing process
    Examples:

    dexamethasone (Decadron)

    hydrocortisone (Solu-Cortef)

    methylprednisolone (Solu-Medrol)

23. *Vasodilator:* used to dilate peripheral blood vessels
    Example:

    papaverine hydrochloride: also prevents vascular spasms

24. *Vasopressor:* used to constrict blood vessels to raise blood pressure

    Examples:

    vasopressin (Pitressin)

    norephinephrine (Levophed)

25. *Viscoelastic agents:* thick, jelly-like substances injected into the eye to keep it expanded

    Examples:

    Viscoat/Amvisc

    Healon

26. *Miscellaneous drugs*

    a. *alpha-chymotripsin (Chymar or Zolase):* an enzyme sometimes used during cataract extraction to dissolve zonules that hold the lens in place when performing intra-capsular lens extraction (ICCE)

    b. *dantrolene sodium (Dantrium):* a skeletal muscle relaxant used in the treatment of Malignant Hyperthermia

    c. *hyaluronidase (Wydase):* an enzyme added to a local anesthetic to enhance infiltration/spread

    d. *Rho GAM—Rh(D) immune globulin:* used to prevent isoimmunization in Rh-negative women exposed to Rh-positive blood; given after abortions, miscarriages, amniocentesis, or delivery

27. *Electrolyte replacement*

    a. *Calcium chloride or calcium gluconate:* given as a myocardial stimulant or to enhance blood clotting in the patient with multiple blood transfusions. Calcium ions are essential in transmission of nerve impulses, muscle contractions, blood coagulation, and cardiac function.

       (*Note:* The preservative in stored blood destroys ionizable calcium, a necessary factor in blood clotting.)

    b. *Magnesium sulfate:* used to prevent seizures in patients with eclampsia (toxemia of pregnancy); also quiets a contracting uterus

    c. *Potassium chloride:* added to the intravenous fluids in hypokalemic patients to correct cardiac dysrhythmias; also used as a cardioplegic in open heart surgery

       (*Note:* Potassium is an essential intracellular electrolyte for regulating neuromuscular excitability and muscle contractions.)

    d. *Sodium bicarbonate:* given to combat metabolic acidosis in a cardiac arrest patient

       (*Note:* Sodium is the chief interstitial [between cells] electrolyte and is essential in maintaining osmotic pressure.)

28. *Intravenous solutions and blood products*

    a. *Water solutions:* used to provide hydration and enhance renal function

       Examples:

       Dextrose 5% in water (D5W)

       Dextrose in normal saline (D5NS)

       0.9 NaCl

       0.45 NS

    b. *Balanced solutions:* used to treat and correct electrolyte imbalances; similar to plasma

       Examples:

       Ringer's solution

       Lactated Ringer's solution

c. *Hyperalimentation solutions:* given through subclavian cannula to patients who cannot eat or drink for long periods of time; includes amino acids, glucose, and water

d. *Whole blood:* given following the loss of blood; sodium citrate and CPDA-1 are anticoagulants used to prolong the storage life of blood

e. *Packed red blood cells:* given for patients with red blood cell deficiency

f. *Plasma:* used for patients in shock, for burn patients or for patients who have had multiple blood transfusions

g. *Plasma expanders:* given when plasma is not available

Example:

Dextran (artificial plasma)

h. *Albumin:* may be used for patients in shock to pull water into the intravascular space

i. *Irrigation solutions:* used in surgical wounds; medications may be added

Examples:

Sterile normal saline; most common

Lactated Ringer's solution

Sterile distilled water; special cases

Anesthesia

Anesthesia means "without sensation," and the anesthetized patient may be conscious or unconscious. The major types of anesthesia are general and regional nerve conduction block (spinal/intrathecal, caudal, epidural, nerve block, bier block, local injection, and topical). The selection of the type of anesthesia is made based on the following factors:

1. American Society of Anesthesiologists (ASA) patient risk classification

2. Patient factors such as age, size, general health, comorbid conditions, current medications, allergies, substance abuse, emergency conditions, and psychological and emotional state

3. Type of procedure, duration, and position

4. Surgeon, anesthesia provider, and patient preference

The intraoperative phases of general anesthesia are

1. *Induction*—Induction agents are administered usually followed by a muscle relaxant. The patient's respirations are controlled with ventilation by inserting an endotracheal tube (ET) (intubation) or a laryngeal mask airway (LMA). A rigid or flexible fiberoptic laryngoscope is used to expose the glottis for intubation, and a stylet may be used to stiffen the endotracheal tube; McGill forceps may also be needed.

2. *Maintenance*—Begins after the insertion of an airway and continues until the operation is completed.

3. *Emergence*—At the end of the surgical procedure, the anesthetic agents are discontinued and allowed to wear off. When the patient is breathing on his or her own, the endotracheal tube is removed (extubation).

4. *Recovery*—When vital signs are stable, the patient is taken to the post-anesthesia care unit (PACU) for the recovery phase.

There are four stages to describe the depth of general anesthesia:

1. *Stage I (amnesia stage)/induction*—Begins with the initial administration of the anesthetic agent and ends with the loss of consciousness.

2. *Stage II (excitement stage)*—Begins with the loss of consciousness and ends with the return of regular breathing and the loss of eyelid reflex. This stage can be very short with the administration of an IV induction agent.

3. *Stage III (surgical anesthesia stage)/maintenance*—The patient is unresponsive to painful stimuli and sensations.

4. *Stage IV (overdose stage)*—If uncorrected, this stage will lead to patient death. It is characterized by dilated or nonreactive pupils and a major drop in blood pressure.

Anesthetic Agents

(*Note:* Brand names of drugs appear in parentheses.)

1. *Preoperative drugs*
   a. *Anticholinergics:* used to block secretions, prevent laryngospasms, and prevent reflex bradycardia; they cause excessive dry mouth and are not recommended for glaucoma patients

      Examples:

      atropine sulfate

      glycopyrrolate (Robinul)

   b. *Antianxiety drugs:* reduce anxiety, are antiemetic and antihistamine, and potentiate anesthesia, thereby lessening anesthesia requirements

      Examples:

      hydroxyzine hydrochloride (Vistaril)

      promethazine hydrochloride (Phenergan)

      diazepam (Valium); also has amnesic qualities lorazepam (Ativan)

      midazolam (Versed)

   c. *Antiemetics:* reduce nausea and prevent vomiting

      Examples:

      metoclopramide (Reglan)

      droperidol (Inapsine)

      ondansetron (Zofran)

   d. *Histamine 2/Antacid:* receptor antigen that decreases gastric acidity and volume

      Examples:

      cimetidine (Tagamet)

      ranitidine (Zantac)

      sodium citrate (Bicitra) given orally

   e. *Narcotic analgesics:* controlled substances given to minimize perception of pain and to potentiate anesthesia; given 1 hour before surgery in order that its action may peak before anesthesia is begun

      Examples:

      meperidine hydrochloride (Demerol)

      morphine sulfate

   f. *Sedative/hypnotics:* promote sleep and reduce anxiety

      Example:

      phenobarbital sodium

2. *Common inhalation anesthetic agents:* produce general (systemic) anesthesia
   a. *nitrous oxide:* a gas used as adjunct to intravenous anesthesia and volatile liquid agents; occasional induction; has analgesic properties; included in balanced anesthesia for most patients; and comes in a blue tank or may be piped in

　　　b. *halothane (Fluothane):* a volatile liquid used for rapid, smooth induction; used for maintenance anesthesia; causes bronchodilation, and may cause shivering or liver toxicity; contraindicated for cesarean section because it relaxes smooth muscle

　　　c. *enflurane (Ethrane):* rapid induction and recovery; used for maintenance anesthesia; and acts similarly to halothane

　　　d. *isoflurane (Forane):* similar to halothane and enflurane

　　　e. *desflurane (Suprane):* has a pungent aroma; has a more rapid onset and recovery; safe to use with liver disease

　　　f. *sevoflurane (Ultane):* used for pediatric anesthesia because it has a rapid induction and recovering

　3. *Common intravenous anesthetic agents:* produce general anesthesia

　　　a. *thiopental sodium (Pentothal):* older agent and is rarely used; rapid, smooth, and pleasant anesthesia induction; quick recovery, and causes respiratory depression

　　　b. *propofol (Diprivan):* sedative/hypnotic used for quick induction and/or short procedures

　　　c. *midazolam (Versed):* may be used for induction during balanced anesthesia

　　　d. *ketamine hydrochloride (Ketalar):* a dissociative anesthesia, used for induction and for superficial procedures of short duration; care must be taken to avoid stimulating the patient (such as loud noises), which could result in hallucinations

　　　e. *droperidol (Inapsine):* an IV tranquilizer and antiemetic used for rapid, smooth induction and quick recovery; may cause increase in pulse rate and drop in blood pressure (BP)

　　　f. *fentanyl citrate (Sublimaze):* potent IV narcotic used for rapid, smooth induction; metabolizes slowly and may cause respiratory depression

　　　g. *etomidate (Amidate):* used for induction for trauma patients or patients with compromised heart function who cannot tolerate a drop in blood pressure

　　　h. *Innovar:* a neuroleptanalgesic combination of droperidol (tranquilizer) and fentanyl (narcotic); given IV for short procedures while the patient is awake

　4. *Common neuromuscular blockers:* used to produce total muscle relaxation by paralyzing every muscle in the body except the heart; require controlled respiration. There are two basic types of muscle relaxants: depolarizing and nondepolarizing.

　　　a. *succinylcholine hydrochloride (Anectine):* may cause fasciculation or trigger malignant hyperthermia; is given to facilitate endotracheal intubation or control laryngospasm; has a duration of 4 to 6 minutes, has no known antagonist or reversal agent, and is the only depolarizing (stimulates autonomic receptors) muscle relaxant commonly used

　　　b. A group of nondepolarizing neuromuscular blockers, which take longer to act, have a longer duration, and are reversible with prostigmine (Neostigmine) and endrophonium (Tensilon); include atracurium besylate (Tracrium), pancuronium bromide (Pavulon), vecuronium bromide (Norcuron), rocuronium bromide (Zemuron), and mivacurium chloride (Mivacron)

　5. *Narcotic reversal/antagonist agents:* used to reverse the sedative effects

　　　a. *naloxone (Narcan)* a narcotic antagonist

　　　b. *flumazenil (Mazicon)* reversal agent for Versed

　6. *Common local and regional anesthetics* (effects are limited)

　　　a. *cocaine hydrochloride:* a vasoconstrictor for topical use only; shrinks congested mucous membrane, used in ear, nose, and throat (ENT) procedures but *not* used with epinephrine, as both are powerful vasoconstrictors

SURGERY HINT

Local anesthetics come in many strengths and may include epinephrine (denoted in RED). It is important for the ST to know the trade names and generic names for each of these medications to reduce errors. Make sure that the name and strength are voiced aloud to the surgeon before handing over the syringe each and every time. The anesthesia care provider will need an exact amount of medication used intraoperatively.

b. *lidocaine hydrochloride (Xylocaine):* an amide, popular, short-acting; may be used for local infiltration or given IV for ventricular arrhythmias; comes in a container with a red label if mixed with epinephrine or with a blue label if plain; and is available in 0.5% to 4% strengths.

(*Note:* Epinephrine is to be avoided in local infiltrations of fingers, toes, penis, or nose, as the blood supply to terminal organs would be severely inhibited.)

c. *bupivicaine hydrochloride (Marcaine, Sensorcaine):* long-acting, four times more potent than lidocaine, available in 0.25%, 0.5%, and 0.75% strengths with or without epinephrine; used for local infiltration, spinal, and/or epidural anesthesia; allergic reactions are rare

d. *mepivacaine (Carbocaine, Polocaine):* two times as potent as lidocaine with slightly longer duration, comes in 1% to 3% strengths.

Show What You Know

Directions   Each of the numbered items or incomplete statements in this section is followed by answers or by completions of the statement. Select the ONE lettered answer or completion that is BEST in each case.

1. The prefix that designates 1000 times the basic unit in the metric system is:
   A. milli-
   B. centi-
   C. kilo-
   D. micro-

2. The basic unit of measurement for weight in the metric system is the:
   A. gram
   B. liter
   C. grain
   D. ounce

3. The number of milliliters in an ounce is:
   A. 100
   B. 30
   C. 240
   D. 16

4. The number of milliliters in a cup is:
   A. 500
   B. 30
   C. 1000
   D. 240

5. Medication used to relieve pain is a/an:
   A. diuratic
   B. analgesic
   C. amnesic
   D. hypnotic

6. A drug with a high potential for addiction and abuse is a/an:
   A. agonist
   B. antagonist
   C. controlled substance
   D. antidote

7. Anesthesia produced by marked cooling is:
   A. cryoanesthesia
   B. hypnoanesthesia
   C. acupuncture
   D. balanced anesthesia

8. An example of a type of drug used to prevent disease is a/an:
   A. sedative
   B. vaccine
   C. anesthetic
   D. contrast medium

9. The route of administration which produces the most immediate action is:

   A. PO
   B. IV
   C. IM
   D. sublingual

10. Saying that a drug is to be given hs means that:

    A. it can be taken as the patient desires
    B. it should be taken at bedtime
    C. it should be placed in both ears
    D. it is to be taken before meals

11. The needle gauge most appropriate for local infiltration is:

    A. 16 g
    B. 18 g
    C. 20 g
    D. 25 g

12. The surgeon's preference card calls for 250 mg of Ancef. The vial you have is labeled "1 g/2 cc." You would draw up:

    A. 0.5 cc
    B. 1 cc
    C. 1.5 cc
    D. 2 cc

13. For a vein graft procedure, you are instructed to draw up 0.3 ml of a drug. The syringe you will use is:

    A. standard
    B. local
    C. 5 cc
    D. tuberculin

14. The physician asks for 30 mg of papaverine and the label on the bottle reads "60 mg/2 ml." How much would you draw up?

    A. 1.5 ml
    B. 1 ml
    C. 0.5 ml
    D. 2 ml

15. After following instructions on the penicillin label for reconstitution, you note that the concentration is "250,000 U/ml." The preference card calls for 500,000 U of penicillin to be added to 500 ml of NS. How many milliliters of penicillin would you draw up?

    A. 2 ml
    B. 1.5 ml
    C. 1 ml
    D. 0.5 ml

16. A 50% solution of dextrose in water means that:

    A. the solution is one-half dextrose
    B. there are 50 g of dextrose in 100 ml of water
    C. there are 50 g of dextrose in 1000 ml of water
    D. there are 50 g of dextrose in 50 ml of water

17. When receiving drugs from the circulator, the scrub should:

    A. clean the top of the vial before inserting the needle
    B. ask the circulator to read the label before withdrawing the solution
    C. keep the medication vial on the back table until the procedure is over
    D. read aloud the name of the drug, strength and/or amount of the drug, and the expiration date

18. When passing a prepared drug to the surgeon, the scrub would:

    A. ask the physician to repeat the request
    B. recite the name, amount, and/or strength of the drug
    C. ask the circulator to read the label from the medication vial
    D. ask the anesthesia provider to recite the name of the drug

19. Anticholinergic medications such as atropine or glycopyrrolate (Robinul) are given preoperatively to:

    A. reduce anxiety and stress
    B. reduce pain and nausea
    C. reduce the output of bile
    D. block secretions and prevent reflex bradycardia

20. Which of the following drugs is a narcotic analgesic?

    A. nitroprusside sodium (Nipride)
    B. meperidine hydrochloride (Demerol)
    C. cimetidine (Tagamet)
    D. propofol (Diprivan)

21. A drug commonly used to reduce vascular spasms during vascular surgery is:

    A. papaverine
    B. prostigmine (Neostigmine)
    C. gentamicin (Garamycin)
    D. heparin sodium

22. A local anesthetic that is *only* used topically is:

    A. lidocaine hydrochloride (Xylocaine)
    B. cocaine hydrochloride
    C. bupivicaine hydrochloride (Marcaine)
    D. procaine hydrochloride (Novocaine)

23. A local anesthetic drug that may also be used to treat ventricular arrhythmias is:

    A. nitroprusside sodium (Nipride)
    B. nitroglycerine
    C. lidocaine hydrochloride (Xylocaine)
    D. cocaine hydrochloride

24. An adrenergic drug that increases blood pressure, dilates bronchioles, constricts blood vessels, and may be added to local anesthetics is:

    A. epinephrine (adrenalin)
    B. phenylephrine hydrochloride (Neo-Synephrine)
    C. atropine
    D. prostigmine (Neostigmine)

25. An absorbable hemostatic agent that *must* be handled dry is:

    A. microfibrillar collagen (Avitene)
    B. absorbable gelatin sponge (Gelfoam)
    C. thrombin
    D. protamine sulfate

26. An anticoagulant used during vascular surgery that can be reversed with protamine sulfate is:

    A. warfarin (coumadin)
    B. heparin sodium

    C. epinephrine (adrenalin)
    D. aminophylline

27. An enzyme sometimes added to a local anesthetic to enhance infiltration/spread is:

    A. acetylcholine chloride (Miochol)
    B. alpha-chymotripsin (Zolase)
    C. dantrolene sodium (Dantrium)
    D. hyaluronidase (Wydase)

28. A contrast medium used when performing a cholangiogram is:

    A. methylene blue
    B. Schiller's solution
    C. diatrizoate sodium (Hypaque)
    D. gentian violet

Answers & Rationales

1. **C.** **Rationale:** *Kilo-* is the prefix that means 1000 times the basic unit.

2. **A.** **Rationale:** The gram is the basic unit of weight in the metric system.

3. **B.** **Rationale:** There are 30 ml in an ounce.

4. **D.** **Rationale:** The average cup is 8 ounces; 8 ounces × 30 ml/ounce = 240 ml.

5. **B.** **Rationale:** A medication to relieve pain is called an analgesic (*an:* without; *algia:* pain).

6. **C.** **Rationale:** Drugs with addictive properties are controlled substances. They are closely controlled by the FDA and are categorized on basis of addictive properties.

7. **A.** **Rationale:** Cryoanesthesia is the absence of sensation produced by extreme cooling.

8. **B.** **Rationale:** Vaccines are killed or attenuated pathogens (antigens), which when injected into the body stimulate the formation of antibodies specific to the antigen (pathogen) and protect against future invasion of that particular antigen.

9. **B.** **Rationale:** The intravenous route (IV) provides the quickest action of any type of drug administration, as the drug is placed into the circulation and can reach its target immediately.

10. **B.** **Rationale:** hs is the abbreviation for at bedtime.

11. **D.** **rationale:** A small needle, such as a 25 g, is more appropriate for local infiltration of drugs since it would cause less pain, less damage to tissue, and less bleeding.

12. **A.** **Rationale:** Formula:

Known	Unknown
Available dose: volume	= desired dose: X volume
1 g: 2 cc	= 250 mg: X cc
1000 mg: 2 cc	= 250 mg: X cc
$1000X$	= 500
$\dfrac{1000X}{1000}$	$= \dfrac{500}{1000}$
X	$= 500/1000 = 1/2$ or 0.5 cc

You would draw up 0.5 cc or 0.5 ml.

13. **D.** **Rationale:** The tuberculin syringe holds 1 cc and is designed for measuring in increments of less than 1 cc.

14. **B.** **Rationale:** Formula:

Known	Unknown
Available dose: volume	= desired dose: X volume
60 mg: 2 mc	= 30 mg: X ml
$60X$	= 60
$\dfrac{60X}{60}$	$= \dfrac{60}{60}$
X	= 1 ml

You would draw up 1 ml.

15.   A.   Rationale: Formula:

Known	Unknown
Available dose: volume	= desired dose: X volume
250,000 U: 1 ml	= 500,000 U: X ml
250,000X	= 500,000

$$\frac{250,000X}{250,000} = \frac{500,000}{250,000}$$

X = 2 ml (500,000/250,000)

You would add 2 ml of penicillin to the 500 ml of NS.

16.   B.   Rationale: A percent solution is g/100 ml or ml/100 ml. A 50% solution of dextrose would be one made by adding 50 g of dextrose (solute) to every 100 ml of solution (solvent).

17.   D.   Rationale: When receiving drugs from the circulator, it is important for the scrub to read aloud the name, amount, and/or strength of a drug as well as the expiration date. The circulator is responsible for cleaning the top of the vial and keeping the container in the room until the procedure is complete.

18.   B.   Rationale: When passing drugs to the surgeon, it is essential that the scrub recite the name, amount, and/or strength of the drugs.

19.   D.   Rationale: Anticholingergic drugs block the parasympathetic/vagal response, which results in blocking secretions and preventing reflex bradycardia and laryngospasms.

20.   B.   Rationale: Meperidine hydrochloride (Demerol) is a narcotic analgesic frequently given to the surgical patient to reduce pain.

21.   A.   Rationale: Papaverine is the drug used during vascular surgery, such as vein grafts, to control vascular spasms. Prostigmine is used as an antagonist for a nondepolarizing muscle blocker. Gentamicin is an antibiotic. Heparin is an anticoagulant.

22.   B.   Rationale: Cocaine hydrochloride is a local anesthetic which is always administered topically. Cocaine is used mostly for ENT surgery because of its anesthetizing and vasoconstricting effect.

23.   C.   Rationale: Lidocaine hydrochloride (Xylocaine) is the most widely used local anesthetic and is frequently used as a bolus or as an IV drip to control ventricular arrhythmias.

24.   A.   Rationale: Epinephrine (adrenalin) works with the sympathetic nervous system to prepare us for "fight or flight" by vasoconstriction, increasing cardiac output, and dilating bronchioles.

25.   A.   Rationale: Microfibrillar collagen (Avitene) is a hemostatic agent that is handled in the dry state with forceps and placed directly on capillary bleeding points. Gelfoam may be moistened with normal saline or thrombin solution and placed directly on bleeders. Protamine sulfate is an anticoagulant that neutralizes heparin when given IV.

26.   B.   Rationale: Heparin sodium can be injected directly into a vessel to prevent clotting during surgery or given SC after surgery to avoid the formation of clots. The effects of heparin sodium can be reversed with protamine sulfate which is generally administered by the anesthesiologist. Warfarin (Coumadin) is a slow-acting anticoagulant that can be reversed with vitamin K.

27.   D.   Rationale: Hyaluronidase (Wydase) may be added to a local anesthetic to enhance spread by breaking down the hyaluronic acid between cells.

28.   C.   Rationale: Diatrizoate sodium (Hypaque) is a contrast medium used for x-ray procedures, as it is opaque to x-rays. Schiller's solution is an iodine preparation used to stain the cervix to differentiate abnormal from normal tissue. Methylene blue and gentian violet are dyes.

Part II: Deciphering a Surgical Schedule

The following mock surgery schedule will be used to answer several questions pertaining to pharmacology. The same schedule, or a similar one, may be used in subsequent chapters to ask questions about the content of the chapter.

Rm. # time	Surgeon	Procedure	Anest.	Rm. # time	Surgeon	Procedure	Anest.
Rm.00				**Rm07**			
OC	Dr. Z	Rt. Knee Arthroscopy	Gen.	7:00	Dr. M	Rhinoplasty	Gen.
OC	Dr. C	Craniotomy	Gen.				
OC	Dr. Z	Angioplasty	Gen.	TF	Dr. M	Lipoma removal	MAC
Rm.01				**Rm08**			
7:00	Dr. X	Lobectomy	Gen.	11:00	Dr. E	Bovine Thrombectomy	MAC
TF	Dr. X	Thoracotomy	Gen.				
TF	Dr. X	Tracheostomy	Gen.				
Rm02				**Rm09**			
7:00	Dr. B	Splenectomy	Gen.	8:30	Dr. T	Cholecystectomy	Gen.
TF	Dr. B	Gastrectomy	Gen.	TF	Dr. T	Palatoplasty	Gen.
Rm03				**Rm10**			
7:00	Dr. A	Cystoscopy	MAC	7:00	Dr. K	Nephrectomy	Gen.
TF	Dr. A	Cystoplasty	Gen.	TF	Dr. K	Choledocholithotripsy	MAC
12:30	Dr. F	Pyleogram	MAC				
3:00	Dr. F	Cystocele repair	Gen.	TF	Dr. K	Colectomy	Gen.
Rm04				**Rm11**			
7:00	Dr. Y	Carpal tunnel release	MAC	7:00	Dr. L	Cervical Cone Biopsy	Gen.
TF	Dr. Y	Fasciotomy	Gen.	12:00	Dr. L	Sentinel Node Biopsy	Gen.
Rm05				**Rm12**			
7:00	Dr. G	Trans-sphenoidal Adenectomy	Gen.	7:00	Dr. W	Trans-metatarsal amputation	Gen.
TF	Dr. G	Trans-urethral resection of the prostate	Gen.	TF	Dr. W	Osteotomy	Gen.
TF	Dr. G	Bletharoplasty	Gen.	TF	Dr. W	Right Knee Arthroplasty	Gen.
Rm06				**Rm13**			
7:00	Dr. R	Lumbar Laminectomy	Gen.	7:00	Dr. O	Hysterectomy	Gen.

The following questions should be answered using the surgery schedule above

1. Dr. R, who is performing a lumbar laminectomy in Room 6, has asked for an absorbable gelatin sponge hemostatic for this procedure. What should the Surgical Technologist expect on the back table?

   A. Monsel's solution
   B. Surgicel
   C. Gelfoam
   D. Avitene

2. Which medication will likely be found on the back table in Room 8?

   A. Gentamicin
   B. Heparin
   C. Propofol
   D. Isosulfan blue

3. Which surgery would most likely utilize radiopaque dye?

   A. Lumbar laminectomy
   B. Hysterectomy
   C. Cystoscopy
   D. Tracheotomy

4. Dr. M, who is performing a rhinoplasty, has requested a topical anesthetic to shrink the mucous membranes. What is the most likely medication to be given?

   A. Cocaine
   B. Polocaine
   C. Marcaine
   D. Xylocaine

5. The patient in Room 5 is experiencing malignant hyperthermia. What drug will be used to control this anesthetic emergency?

   A. Sulfonamide
   B. Plasmalyte
   C. Dantrolene
   D. Anectine

6. Dr. K in Room 10 will require antibiotic irrigation for the colectomy he will be performing. What type of antibiotic should the ST expect?

   A. Penicillin
   B. Aminoglycoside
   C. Cephalosporin
   D. Tetracycline

7. Dr. W is doing a knee replacement in Room 12 and is using methyl methacrylate. Which hemostatic agent should NOT be used in this surgery?

   A. Absorbable Collagen Sponge
   B. Oxidized Cellulose
   C. Bone Wax
   D. Absorbable Gelatin

8. Which diagnostic agent will likely be used in Room 11 during the sentinel node biopsy?

   A. Methylene Blue
   B. Gentian Violet
   C. Isosulfan Blue
   D. Isovue

9. The surgeon in Room 5 needs solution for the TURP. What type of solution should the ST retrieve?

   A. NaCl
   B. Glycine
   C. Sorbitol
   D. Sterile Water

10. Dr. E in Room 8 is concerned that the patient may have been given too much Heparin. What medication will he use to reverse the effects?

    A. Dantrolene
    B. Protamine Sulfate
    C. Lidocaine
    D. Diazepam

Answers & Rationales

1. **C.** **Rationale:** Gelfoam is an absorbable gelatin sponge that is routinely used in orthopedic and neurosurgeries. Monsel's solution is used primarily to stop bleeding during cervical cone biopsies. Surgicel and Avitene are not absorbable gelatin sponges. Avitene is a microfibrillar collagen hemostatic, and Surgicel is oxidized cellulose.

2. **B.** **Rationale:** Heparin is used during bovine thrombectomies to prevent clotting. Propofol is an anesthetic agent, Isosulfan Blue is a diagnostic agent that is used to locate the sentinel nodes during biopsies, and Gentamicin is an antibiotic.

3. **C.** **Rationale:** Cystoscopies are generally performed with the addition of a radiopaque dye that allows visualization of the ureters. Lumbar laminectomies, hysterectomies, and tracheotomies would not require the use of this diagnostic agent.

4. **A.** **Rationale:** Cocaine is a vasoconstrictor and anesthetic agent that may be applied topically

to reduce the swelling of mucous membranes during nasal surgeries. Polocaine, Marcaine, and Xylocaine are commonly injected local anesthetics.

5. **C.** **Rationale:** Dantrolene is the agent used to treat malignant hyperthermia (MH). While MH is rare, it must be recognized and treated as quickly as possible to avoid fatal consequences. Sulfonamide is an antibiotic, Plasmalyte is an electrolyte solution, and Anectine is a paralytic agent.

6. **B.** **Rationale:** Aminoglycosides may be added to irrigation fluids for colorectal cases to prevent postoperative infections. While cephalosporins are also occasionally added to irrigation fluids, they are not used as often as aminoglycosides for abdominal procedures.

7. **A.** **Rationale:** Absorbable collagen sponges are contradicted when using bone cement. It may reduce the bonding strength of bone cement and should be avoided when using cemented implants.

8. **C.** **Rationale:** Sentinel node biopsies will routinely require the use of Isosulfan blue. This agent is absorbed into lymphatic pathways, making the nodes more visible. Methylene blue is commonly used to view the patency of anatomical structures such as fallopian tubes or ureters. Gentian violet is generally used in skin marking and Isovue is a radiopaque agent.

9. **C.** **Rationale:** In TURPs, irrigation is commonly used to visualize structures and bleeders. Because many solutions are conductive, the irrigation used in these procedures must be carefully chosen. Sterile water and saline are not routinely used in TURPs because of the complications that can occur. Glycine is used for TURPs, but may result in several serious conditions if overabsorbed by the patient. Therefore, Sorbitol is the best choice for the procedure.

10. **B.** **Rationale:** Protamine Sulfate is used to counteract the effects of heparin. Dantrolene is used in the treatment of MH, Lidocaine is a local anesthetic agent, and Diazepam is a sedative.

PEARSON
myhealthprofessionskit™

Use this address to access the interactive Companion Website created for this book. Simply select "Surgical Technology" from the choice of disciplines. Find this book and click to enter.

chapter

5 Biomedical Sciences and Technology

As operating room practice continues to incorporate an increased number of technology-based supplies, instrumentation, and equipment, Surgical Technologists need to have a foundation in the biomedical sciences that support that technology. Without this foundation, the Surgical Technologist will be unable to adapt to the increasing demands for newer technology.

CHAPTER OUTLINE

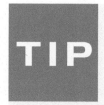

TIP

Most students are comfortable with the basic technology that is used in everyday life. Computers, printers, scanners, and faxes are used by most Americans on a daily basis. It is only when faced with newer technologies and their applications that we get intimidated. This chapter will explain the principles behind biomedical science, lasers, and robotics. Remember that this is a quickly growing field that Surgical Technologists must master in order to stay on the cutting edge of surgery.

When faced with a question regarding biomedical sciences, remember the basic concepts that you know, and then apply these components to the question. While the use of these newer technologies is limited, the growing trend seems to be pointing to the increased utilization of robotics and other cutting-edge technology in the operating room. That means that Surgical Technologists must learn these newer sciences to keep up with the continuing changes that occur in how surgeries are performed.

I. Energy

   A. Electrical energy
      1. *Atom*
        a. **Definition:** smallest piece of an element that keeps its chemical properties
        b. Composition
          i. *Nucleus:* center of an atom
            • *Protons:* carry a positive electrical charge
            • *Neutrons:* carry a neutral charge
          ii. *Valence shell:* pathways around the nucleus where electrons flow
            • *Electrons:* carry a negative charge
      2. *Electrical energy:* the movement of electrons from one atomic valence shell to the valence shell of an adjacent atom
        a. *Free electrons:* "moving" electrons
        b. When electrons leave their base atoms and move to adjacent atoms, the charges of the atoms are changed
          i. Those having fewer electrons than protons become positively charged
          ii. Those with more electrons than protons become negatively charged
      3. *Electricity:* like charges repel each other and unlike charges attract each other during electron movement
        a. *Conductivity:* the ability of materials to carry an electrical charge
          i. The greater the number of free electrons involved in electron movement, the greater the conductivity of the substance or material
          ii. **Conductors:** materials that allow the flow of free electrons
            • *Metal conductors:* copper, silver, aluminum, and brass
            • *Non-metal conductors:* water, salt water, and carbon
          iii. **Insulators:** materials that inhibit the flow of free electrons; include rubber and plastic casing material
        b. *Current:* measurement of the rate of flow of the electrons
          i. Definitions
            • *Amperes (amps):* measurement of the amount of current flowing past a given point in a circuit in one second
            • *Voltage (V):* the force or push that moves free electrons from one atom to another; indicates the strength or energy of electricity; the force that will cause one amp to flow through one ohm of impedance or resistance

- *Frequency:* the number of energy waves that pass through a specific point over a specific amount of time; measured in hertz (Hz) or cycles per second
    1. Radiofrequency cycles approximately 100,000 times per second
    2. Household current cycles at 60 cycles per second
- *Power:* the rate at which the electrical movement is accomplished; measured in watts

    ii. Types of current
- AC or alternating current
    1. The electrons flow back and forth along a single pathway due to changes in polarity (negative and positive charges)
    2. Household alternating current changes directions approximately 60 times per seconds
    3. AC current is the most common type of current used in powering operating room (OR) equipment
- DC or direct current
    1. Flows in one direction but loses voltage when it travels through conductors over long distances
    2. Examples of DC current include batteries

  c. *Circuit:* pathway of electron flow; created when the electrical energy flows from and returns to its point of origin

    i. Electricity flows along the path of least resistance and will find the easiest route to return to ground or its electron reservoir

    ii. *Impedance:* materials that either facilitate or obstruct the flow of electricity

    iii. *Resistance:* a property of substances that obstructs the flow of free electrons
- Measured in ohms; indicates the ease or difficulty in which a current can flow through that substance
- As electron flow encounters impedance, heat builds

4. *Technology applications*

  a. *Electrosurgery*

    i. Involves the use of electric current to seal blood vessels, achieve hemostasis, and cut or dissect tissue

    ii. Types of current
- Dampened interrupted current resulting in tissue desiccation and coagulation
- Undampened or continuous current resulting in tissue cutting
- Blend mode combines the two currents in quick alteration, providing both effects simultaneously

    iii. Pathway of current flow
- Electrosurgical unit (ESU) generator
- Active or positive electrode: contacts the patient tissues at the point of desired effect
- Tissue
- Patient inactive or return electrode: returns energy to the generator
    1. "Grounding pad"
    2. Capacitance pad

    iv. Types of flow
- *Monopolar:* the flow of electricity occurs in one direction; the active and inactive electrodes are separated by a significant distance; results in the need for the electrical energy to pass through adjacent body tissues before contacting the return electrode; may inadvertently damage unintended tissues causing an alternate site burn

- • *Bipolar:* the active and return electrodes are contained within the same delivery device; the current flows from one jaw of the instrument to the opposite jaw of the instrument
  - v. *Monitoring systems:* assist in the prevention of alternate pathway burns
    - • *Remote electrode monitoring (REM) return patient electrode:* utilizes a divided, disposable return electrode pad that can sense the amount of electrical impedance/resistance at the contact point between the pad and the patient's body; the sensor will interrupt power delivery if the quality of the contact is compromised
    - • *Active electrode monitoring system:* permits measurement of the amount of current delivered to the active electrode in comparison to the amount of current returned to the generator; if the difference between the two amounts exceeds pre-set parameters, the generator will shut down and alarm
  - b. *LigaSure™:* bipolar forcep device that uses force and energy to cause the collagen matrix in vessel walls and connective tissue to reform into a permanently fused tissue matrix
  - c. *Argon-enhanced coagulation:* a stream of argon gas is used to deliver the electrical current to the target tissues using a "no-touch" technique; used to cauterize, cut, or seal large areas of non-specific, oozing, friable tissue, such as liver or kidney parenchyma; it is not a LASER
- B. *Mechanical energy:*
  1. The energy found in moving objects
  2. Definitions
     - a. *Force:* any agent that causes a change in movement; the energy that causes acceleration
     - b. *Speed:* a measurement of how fast an object is moving regardless of the direction of that movement
     - c. *Velocity:* the direction and speed of an object when moving in a straight line
     - d. *Acceleration:* a change in velocity, including a change in direction, in speeding up, or in slowing down
     - e. *Friction:* the resistance of the movement of one surface as it passes another
  3. Types of mechanical energy
     - a. *Kinetic energy:* the energy an object has while in motion or during activity; overcomes friction and resistance to produce movement
     - b. *Potential energy:* the energy an object has at rest or stores for use when resistance is lowered or removed
  4. Mechanical laws
     - a. *Newton's Laws of Motion*
       - i. *Law of inertia:* an object at rest tends to stay at rest and an object in motion tends to stay in motion with the same speed and in the same direction unless acted upon by an unbalanced force
       - ii. The acceleration of an object is dependent upon two variables: the net force acting upon the object and the mass of the object
       - iii. For every action, there is an equal and opposite reaction
     - b. *Newton's Law of Gravity:* every particle attracts another particle with a force that is proportional to the product of their masses and inversely proportional to the distance between them
  5. Technology applications
     - a. *Cavitational Ultrasonic Suction Aspirator (CUSA):* an ultrasonic vibrating tip used to "break up" and vacuum away tissue
     - b. *Harmonic Scalpel®:* delivers ultrasonic sound waves to target tissues that simultaneously cut tissue and seal blood vessels; a piezoelectric transducer creates mechanical friction energy at up to 55,500 times a minute

  c. *Morcellator:* a mechanical device that fragments tissue into long strips that can be extracted through the barrel of the instrument

C. **Light energy**

 1. A series of photons given off by an object in the forms of both waves and particles

  a. *Photons:* light particles given off by an electron; created when an electron is moved to a higher orbit or valence shell and permitted to return to its preferred lower orbit or valence shell; the photons generated have the same wavelength and waveform as the original electron

 2. Characteristics of light energy

  a. *Reflection:* the ability to bounce light rays off a particular object

  b. *Refraction:* the ability to bend or redirect light rays as the light passes through an object

  c. *Color:*

   i. Determined by the height and distance of a light waveform

   ii. Light waves:

    • Invisible to the human eye

     1. Infrared waves

     2. Ultraviolet waves

    • Waves of the human visual spectrum: include red, orange, yellow, green, blue, indigo, and violet

 3. Technology applications

  a. *LASER*

   i. Definition

    • Light amplification by the stimulated emission of radiation

    • Creation of an intense light capable of tissue dissection and vaporization

   ii. Characteristics

    • *Coherence:* light waves are in phase; peak and trough together

    • *Collimation:* light waves travel parallel to one another

    • *Monochromatic:* light is composed of only one pure light wavelength

   iii. **Radiant exposure:** the effect on the tissue

    • *Thermal dissolution:* light energy causes intracellular water to heat, creating steam causing cell wall lysis

    • *Photodynamic destruction:* light energy interacts with chemically sensitized cells that lead to a disruption of the cell's basic metabolic processes, resulting in cell destruction

   iv. Common OR LASER mediums

    • **Solid**

     1. *Yttrium-aluminum-garnet (YAG)*

      a. *Neodymium (Nd:YAG):* No visible beam is emitted, so it is used in conjunction with a helium neon beam. Often used in the removal of bladder tumors and in cystoscopies and hysteroscopies

      b. *Holmium (Holmium:YAG):* May be used in orthopedic/arthroscopic, ENT, urologic, GYN, and general surgery

      c. *Erbium (erbium:YAG)*

     2. *KTP:* Nd:YAG light that is then passed through a potassium titanyl phosphate crystal

    • **Gas**

     1. *Carbon dioxide (CO_2):* Invisible beam, used in conjunction with a red helium laser beam to produce a visible red light. Used for plastic surgery, cervical ablations, neurosurgery, and other surgical procedures. The most commonly used laser.

        2. *Argon:* Blue-green beam, used in ophthalmic and dermatologic procedures
        3. *Krypton:* Used in retinal surgeries
        4. *Excimer:* Extremely precise beam, extremely toxic gas
- **Liquid**
        1. Tunable dye
        Vascular lesions and PDT

II. Introduction to Physics

A. Matter

1. States/properties
   a. Solid
      i. Have a fixed volume
      ii. Have a fixed shape
      iii. Arrangements
         - Crystals: organized
         - Amorphous: random
   b. Liquid
      i. Fixed volume
      ii. Take the shape of the container
      iii. Solution
         - *Solvent:* medium used to dissolve other substances
         - *Solute:* substance dissolved by the liquid solvent
   c. Gas
      i. No fixed volume
      ii. No fixed shape: expand to fill all available space
   d. Plasma
      i. A gas that is so hot that it has ionized; the gas is electrically charged and is affected by magnetic and electric fields

B. Heat transfer

1. *Conduction:* loss of heat due to collision of molecules at different temperatures; examples include the body's heat loss due to contact with a cool solution during irrigation
2. *Convection:* loss of heat due to heat rising into a cooler gas; examples include heat loss due to air currents moving over exposed body surfaces
3. *Radiation:* energy carried by waves; examples include radiant warmers used for neonates during surgery or immediately after delivery

III. Robotics

A. Terminology

   a. *Articulated:* sectioned with joints. These allow the robotic components to move in certain planes. Like the human body, there are degrees of articulation depending on the type of joint.
   b. *Binaural hearing:* this robotic component functions like the human ears, allowing it to locate the direction that a sound is coming from.
   c. *Degrees of freedom:* this term is used to describe the number of ways that a manipulator can move
   d. *Degrees of rotation:* defines the degree that a component can rotate
   e. *Manipulators:* term generally applied to robotic arms
   f. *Pitch:* up and down movement
   g. *Roll:* rotating movement
   h. *Telechir:* remotely controlled robot
   i. *Yaw:* right and left movement

B. Technologies

1. **Single robotic arm**
   a. Device attached to the bed rail of the operating table that manipulates surgical instrumentation under the surgeon's direct guidance

            b. Functions
               i. Manipulate endoscopic telescopes
              ii. Perform dissection, suturing, and manipulation of internal tissues and structures

    2. **Voice-activated control system**
        a. Directs the robotic arm
        b. Controls room functions in an integrated OR suite
            i. Lights
           ii. Insufflator
         iii. Pumps
         iv. Recording technologies

    3. **Remote surgical manipulator**
        a. Multiple-armed robotic device
        b. Guided by surgeon seated at a remote manipulator console
        c. Translates actions of surgeon's hand movements to robotic arms

    4. **DaVinci Surgical System by Innovative Surgical**
        a. Robotic system in 3DHD
        b. allows surgeon to experience feedback from the field to adjust the surgery from the consol
        c. Surgeon sits at a consol during procedure
        d. minimally invasive
        e. multiple surgical procedures, including prostate, cardiovascular, and general procedures
        f. multiple arms

IV. Information Management

  A. Computers

    1. **Components**
        a. Drives
            i. Hard drive
           ii. Floppy drive
         iii. CD-ROM drive
         iv. Other
        b. Monitor
        c. Input devices
            i. Keyboard
           ii. Mouse
         iii. Scanner
        d. Output devices
            i. Printer
           ii. Burners
         iii. Modem

    2. **Applications**
        a. Word processing
        b. Documentation
            i. Charting
           ii. Procedural documentation
         c. Research

Show What You Know

Directions
Each of the numbered items or incomplete statements in this section is followed by answers or by completions of the statement. Select the ONE lettered answer or completion that is BEST in each case.

1. In an atom, the negatively charged particles are called:

    A. electrons
    B. neutrons
    C. photons
    D. protons

2. Which particles are found in the nucleus of an atom?

    A. electrons and photons
    B. neutrons and photons
    C. protons and electrons
    D. protons and neutrons

3. Which particles are found in the valence shell of an atom?

    A. electrons
    B. neutrons
    C. photons
    D. protons

4. Which of the following materials is NOT a conductor of electrical energy?

    A. carbon
    B. rubber
    C. copper
    D. water

5. The force or push that moves free electrons from one atom to another is referred to as:

    A. amperes
    B. frequency
    C. power
    D. voltage

6. Which of the following electrical energy concepts is measured in Hertz?

    A. amperes
    B. frequency
    C. power
    D. voltage

7. Which of the following electrical energy concepts is measured in Watts?

    A. amperes
    B. frequency
    C. power
    D. voltage

8. Which of the following electrical energy concepts is measured in Ohms?

    A. frequency
    B. impedance

    C. power
    D. resistance

9. Which of the following concepts of electrical energy is true?

    A. radiofrequency cycles at approximately 60 cycles per second
    B. radiofrequency cycles at approximately 100,000 cycles per second
    C. household current cycles at approximately 100,000 cycles per minute
    D. household current cycles at approximately 60 cycles per minute

10. Which of the following statements concerning current is true?

    A. Direct current flows in one direction and gains voltage when it travels through conductors over long distances.
    B. AC current is used in batteries.
    C. Alternating current flows back and forth along a single pathway due to changes in polarity.
    D. Household direct current changes directions approximately 60 times per seconds

11. Which of the concepts of electrosurgical unit (ESU) electrical energy flow is correct?

    A. Use of monopolar energy flow may result in alternate site burns.
    B. During the use of monopolar electrical energy, the energy passes through the tissue and returns through the same instrument used to deliver the energy.
    C. Use of bipolar energy flow may result in alternate site burns.
    D. Use of bipolar energy flow requires the use of a return electrode pad.

12. The electrical energy device that causes the collagen matrix in vessel walls and connective tissue to reform into a permanently fused tissue matrix is the:

    A. argon-enhanced coagulator
    B. electrosurgical unit (ESU)
    C. Harmonic Scalpel®
    D. LigaSure™

13. The mechanical energy device that uses a piezo-electric transducer to create mechanical friction energy is called the:

    A. argon-enhanced coagulator
    B. Harmonic Scalpel®

C. LigaSure™
D. morcellator

14. Which aspect of Newton's Law of Inertia is *incorrect*?

A. An object at rest tends to stay at rest unless acted upon by an unbalanced force.
B. An object in motion tends to stay in motion unless acted upon by an unbalanced force.
C. For every action, there is an equal and opposite reaction.
D. The acceleration of an object is dependent upon two variables: speed and velocity.

15. The characteristics of light energy include all of the following *except*:

A. color
B. radiation
C. reflection
D. refraction

16. The characteristics of LASER light include all of the following *except*:

A. coherence
B. collimation
C. divergence
D. monochromatic

17. Solid medium LASERs include which of the following?

A. argon and carbon dioxide
B. carbon dioxide and KTP
C. KTP and Nd:YAG
D. tunable dye and Nd:YAG

18. Which of the following is not a property of solids?

A. have a fixed volume
B. take the shape of the container
C. are found in crystal arrangements
D. are found in amorphous arrangements

19. The state of matter that has no fixed volume or shape and is affected by magnetic and electrical fields is:

A. gas
B. liquid

C. plasma
D. solid

20. The method of heat transfer used in a neonatal warmer is:

A. conduction
B. convection
C. radiation
D. refraction

21. The heat transference that results from contact of internal organs with a cool irrigation solution is:

A. conduction
B. collimation
C. radiation
D. reflection

22. Computer input devices include a:

A. modem
B. monitor
C. printer
D. scanner

23. The single robotic arm:

A. attaches to the bedrail of the OR table
B. is guided by the surgeon seated at a remote console
C. controls the room functions in an integrated suite
D. translates actions of the surgeon's hand movements

24. The mechanical energy device that uses an ultrasonic vibrating tip to "break up" and vacuum away tissue is the:

A. Cavitational Ultrasonic Suction Aspirator
B. Harmonic Scalpel®
C. LigaSure™
D. Morcellator

25. A particle of LASER light energy is called a/an:

A. electron
B. neutron
C. photon
D. proton

Answers & Rationales

1. **A.** **Rationale:** In an atom, the negatively charged particles are called electrons. Protons have a positive charge, neutrons have no charge, and photons are light energy given off to create LASER light.

2. **D.** **Rationale:** Protons and neutrons are found in the nucleus of an atom. Electrons are found in the valence shell.

3. **A.** **Rationale:** Electrons are found in the valence shell. Protons and neutrons are found in the nucleus of an atom.

4. **B.** **Rationale:** Rubber is not a conductor of electricity. Copper is a metal conductor of electricity, and water and carbon are non-metal conductors of electricity.

5. **D.** **Rationale:** Voltage is the force or push that moves free electrons from one atom to another. Amperes is the measurement of the amount of current flowing past a given point in a circuit in one second, frequency is the number of energy waves that pass through a specific point over a specific amount of time, and power is the rate at which the electrical movement is accomplished.

6. **B.** **Rationale:** Frequency is measured in hertz. Amperes is a measurement of the amount of current flowing past a given point in a circuit in one second, power is measured in watts, and voltage is measured in volts.

7. **C.** **Rationale:** Power is measured in watts. Frequency is measured in Hertz, voltage is measured in volts, and amperes is a measurement of the amount of current flowing past a given point in a circuit in one second.

8. **D.** **Rationale:** Resistance is measured in ohms. Frequency is measured in Hertz, power is measured in watts, and impedance is a material that either facilitates or obstructs the flow of electricity.

9. **B.** **Rationale:** Radiofrequency cycles at approximately 100,000 cycles per second. Household current alternates at 60 cycles per second.

10. **C.** **Rationale:** Alternating current flows back and forth along a single pathway due to changes in polarity. Direct current flows in one direction and loses voltage when it travels through conductors over long distances, DC current is used in batteries, and household current is alternating current that changes directions approximately 60 times per second.

11. **A.** **Rationale:** The use of monopolar energy flow may result in alternate site burns. Bipolar energy does not require the use of a return electrode pad, does not result in alternate site burns, and the electrical energy passes through the tissue and returns through the same instrument used to deliver the energy.

12. **D.** **Rationale:** The LigaSure™ is the electrical energy device that causes the collagen matrix in vessel walls and connective tissue to reform into a permanently fused tissue matrix. The argon-enhanced coagulator and electrosurgery unit (ESU) both use electricity to desiccate and coagulate tissue, and the Harmonic Scalpel® uses mechanical energy.

13. **B.** **Rationale:** The Harmonic Scalpel® is the mechanical energy device that uses a piezoelectric transducer to create mechanical friction

energy. The Argon-enhanced coagulator and LigaSure™ use electrical energy and the morcellator fragments tissue into long strips that can be extracted through the barrel of the instrument.

14. **D.** **Rationale:** Aspects of Newton's Law of Inertia include that an object at rest tends to stay at rest unless acted upon by an unbalanced force; that an object in motion tends to stay in motion unless acted upon by an unbalanced force; and that for every action, there is an equal and opposite reaction. The acceleration of an object is dependent upon two variables: the net force acting upon the object and the mass of the object.

15. **B.** **Rationale:** The characteristics of light energy include color, reflection, and refraction.

16. **C.** **Rationale:** The characteristics of LASER light include coherence, collimation, and being monochromatic.

17. **C.** **Rationale:** Solid medium LASERs include KTP and the Nd:YAG LASERs. Carbon dioxide and argon LASERs use a gas medium to create the LASER light, and a tunable dye laser has a liquid medium.

18. **B.** **Rationale:** Solids have a fixed volume and shape and are found in both crystal and amorphous arrangements.

19. **C.** **Rationale:** Plasma is a state of matter that has no fixed volume or shape and is affected by magnetic and electrical fields.

20. **C.** **Rationale:** Radiation is the method of heat transfer used in a neonatal warmer.

21. **A.** **Rationale:** Conduction is the method of heat transference that results from contact of internal organs with a cool irrigation solution.

22. **D.** **Rationale:** A scanner is a computer input device. A modem, monitor, and printer are all output devices.

23. **A.** **Rationale:** The single robotic arm attaches to the bedrail of the OR table. The remote surgical manipulator is guided by the surgeon seated at a remote console and translates actions of the surgeon's hand movements. The voice-activated control system controls the room functions in an integrated OR suite.

24. **A.** **Rationale:** The Cavitational Ultrasonic Suction Aspirator (CUSA) is a mechanical energy device that uses an ultrasonic vibrating tip to "break up" and vacuum away tissue. The Harmonic Scalpel® is the mechanical energy device that uses a piezoelectric transducer to create

mechanical friction energy, the LigaSure™ is the **electrical energy** device that causes the collagen matrix in vessel walls and connective tissue to reform into a permanently fused tissue matrix, and the morcellator fragments tissue into long strips that can be extracted through the barrel of the instrument.

25. **C.   Rationale:** A particle of LASER light energy is called a photon.

Part II: Deciphering a Surgical Schedule

The following mock surgery schedule will be used to answer several questions pertaining to biomedical sciences. The same schedule, or a similar one, may be used in subsequent chapters to ask questions about the content of the chapter.

Rm.# time	Surgeon	Procedure	Anest.	Rm. # time	Surgeon	Procedure	Anest.
Rm.00				**Rm07**			
OC	Dr. Z	Rt. Knee Arthroscopy	Gen.	7:00	Dr. M	Rhinoplasty	Gen.
OC	Dr. C	Craniotomy	Gen.				
OC	Dr. Z	Angioplasty	Gen.	TF	Dr. M	Lipoma removal	MAC
Rm.01				**Rm08**			
7:00	Dr. X	Lobectomy	Gen.	11:00	Dr. E	Bovine Thrombectomy	MAC
TF	Dr. X	Thoracotomy	Gen.				
TF	Dr. X	Tracheostomy	Gen.				
Rm02				**Rm09**			
7:00	Dr. B	Splenectomy	Gen.	8:30	Dr. T	Cholecystectomy	Gen.
TF	Dr. B	Gastrectomy	Gen.	TF	Dr. T	Palatoplasty	Gen.
Rm03				**Rm10**			
7:00	Dr. A	Cystoscopy	MAC	7:00	Dr. K	Nephrectomy	Gen.
TF	Dr. A	Cystoplasty	Gen.	TF	Dr. K	Choledocholithotripsy	MAC
12:30	Dr. F	Pyleogram	MAC				
3:00	Dr. F	Cystocele repair	Gen.	TF	Dr. K	Colectomy	Gen.
Rm04				**Rm11**			
7:00	Dr. Y	Carpal tunnel release	MAC	7:00	Dr. L	Cervical Ablation	Gen.
TF	Dr. Y	Fasciotomy	Gen.	12:00	Dr. L	Sentinel Node Biopsy	Gen.
Rm05				**Rm12**			
7:00	Dr. G	Trans-sphenoidal Adenectomy	Gen.	7:00	Dr. W	Trans-metatarsal amputation	Gen.
TF	Dr. G	Trans-urethral resection of the prostate	Gen.	TF	Dr. W	Osteotomy Right Knee	Gen.
TF	Dr. G	Bletharoplasty	Gen.	TF	Dr. W	Arthroplasty	Gen.
Rm06				**Rm13**			
7:00	Dr. R	Lumbar Laminectomy	Gen.	7:00	Dr. O	Hysterectomy	Gen.

The following questions should be answered using the surgery schedule above

1. The surgeon in Room 11 has requested a LASER for the cervical ablation that is scheduled for 7:00. What type of LASER is the most likely one to be used?

    A. Nd:YAG
    B. Carbon Dioxide
    C. Holmium: YAG
    D. Krypton

2. The surgeon that has an arthroscopy on call will also need to use a LASER. Which one?

   A. Nd:YAG
   B. Holmium: YAG
   C. Krypton
   D. Carbon Dioxide

3. They will also require a LASER in Room 3 for a cystoscopy. Which one will be used?

   A. Nd:YAG
   B. Holminum:Yag
   C. Carbon Dioxide
   D. Krypton

4. Dr. R, who is performing a Lumbar Laminectomy in Room 6, will need an electrosurgical device that allows him to focus current in a small area between the tips. What type of electrocautery will he need?

   A. Monopolar
   B. Footswitch
   C. Bipolar
   D. Morcellator

5. Dr. X wants an instrument that will use ultrasonic sound waves to cut and cauterize tissue. What should the Surgical Technologist request?

   A. Morcellator
   B. Harmonic scalpel
   C. Ligasure
   D. Bipolar

6. The surgeon in Room 2 is using a robotic device for his surgery. Unfortunately, he is encountering some difficulty. The right and left movement of the arm is off. What does the ST need to check?

   A. Yaw
   B. Roll
   C. Telechir
   D. Articulation point

7. The surgeon is now encountering difficulties with the rotation. What should be checked?

   A. Yaw
   B. Roll
   C. Telechir
   D. Articulation point

8. Dr. B has an ophthalmic case that will be on the schedule tomorrow. Which LASER will he need?

   A. Krypton
   B. Nd:YAG
   C. Holmium
   D. Carbon Dioxide

9. Dr. P has a great opportunity to perform a surgery via remote control. What type of robot will he be using to do this?

   A. Binaural
   B. Robotic articulator
   C. Telechir
   D. Yaw and roll

10. Dr. T needs a robotic device that will attach to the table rail to hold an endoscope. What would he require?
    A. Single Robotic Arm
    B. CUSA
    C. FRED
    D. Remote surgical manipulator

Answers & Rationales

1. **B.** **Rationale:** The carbon dioxide LASER is commonly used for cervical ablations.

2. **B.** **Rationale:** Holmium: YAG is commonly used in arthroscopic procedures.

3. **A.** **Rationale:** Cystoscopies will occasionally utilize the Nd:YAG LASER.

4. **C.** **Rationale:** When a surgeon requires an electrocautery device that is able to focus the current in a very small area, the ST should have a bipolar on hand. Many surgeries that are performed on delicate areas, or near nerves, will use this instead of the monopolar.

5. **B.** **Rationale:** The device the surgeon will expect is the Harmonic scalpel.

6. **A.** **Rationale:** Yaw is the term used to describe right and left movement.

7. **B.** **Rationale:** The rotation of the robotic arm is called roll.

8. **A.** **Rationale:** Krypton is the most likely LASER to be used in this case.

9. **C.** **Rationale:** Telechir is the term used for a robot that is controlled via remote control.

10. **A.** **Rationale:** The single robotic arm is used in surgeries that need a "hand" to hold an endoscope.

PEARSON
myhealthprofessionskit™

Use this address to access the interactive Companion Website created for this book. Simply select "Surgical Technology" from the choice of disciplines. Find this book and click to enter.

The Surgical Environment

6 chapter

Patients being rolled through those mysterious double doors into the operating room have given permission for invasion of their most prized possession, their body. Surgery breaks the patient's defenses against disease, interrupts vascular pathways, initiates a stress response, and subjects the patient to numerous potential hazards. The surgical team's awareness of the risks involved for both the patient and the staff is a prerequisite for a safe operating room environment with reduced litigation and a more productive staff.

CHAPTER OUTLINE

TIP How to answer OR environment questions

Questions concerning the operating environment have one thing in common: How will it affect patient care? The patient's safety must always come first. While there are variations in protocol from hospital to hospital, most of these concepts are universal. When dealing with these questions, fall back on the fundamental knowledge that has been gained from both classrooms and practice.

There are several aspects to the questions that come under general OR environment: ethical concepts, the physical layout and setup of the suite, equipment, and safety. First, target which one of these concepts the question is targeting.

Example:
When using LASERs, what is a safety requirement that must be followed?

a. Use dry towels around the operative area to protect patients skin
b. Use scratch-free clear safety goggles
c. Use non-reflective instruments
d. The LASER must remain in the "on" position to prevent loss of energy

To answer this question, first remember what LASERs are and some of the safety precautions that must be taken when using LASERs, both for patient and staff safety. LASERs can ignite fires on drapes and towels and may also damage exposed tissues. Therefore, you would use moist towels around the surgical site to reduce the risk of fire and tissue damage. While safety glasses are required for use in LASER surgery, they must be equipped with specialized lenses to protect the eyes from damage. LASERs should also be kept "off" when not in use like most hazardous equipment. This is to prevent accidents and accidental activation of the machine. When you take these precautions and compare them to the possible answers, the only answer that is correct is C. The use of non-reflective instruments in LASER surgery is to reduce the possibility of unintentional reflection of the beams.

Operating Room Team

I. *Goal of the Team:* The OR team is a group of medical and allied health professionals coordinating efforts to achieve a common goal: efficient and effective delivery of care for patients requiring surgical intervention.

II. *Qualifications for Team Members*

A. *Technical standards:* demonstrate physical stamina; bend, stoop, stand, or sit for long periods of time in one location; lift a minimum of 20 pounds; refrain from nourishment or restroom breaks for up to 6 hours; demonstrate visual acuity to work with fine (10-0) suture and peripheral vision; hear equipment, alarms, and communications from behind masks; detect odors; demonstrate manual dexterity; communicate effectively; be free of communicable disease and chemical abuse; possess immunity to certain diseases; and ambulate without assistive devices

B. *Other:* knowledge of the roles and functions of team members, skilled in own role, conscientious, caring, organized, flexible, perceptive, honest, dependable, motivated, team mentality, possess critical thinking skills, have a strong work ethic, professional, objective, ethical, work quickly and accurately, attention to detail, integrate a number of activities according to priority, work under pressure in stressful situations, consistent attendance, and be a lifelong learner

III. *Sterile Team Members*

   A. *Operating surgeon:* performs the surgical procedure

   B. *Assistant to surgeon:* maintains visibility of the operative site and assists with the procedure as needed; can be a physician or non-physician

   C. *Scrub:* anticipates and responds to the needs of the surgeon. (*Note:* This term has been used throughout this text to denote the person in the scrub role regardless of his or her credentials.)

IV. *Unsterile Team Members*

   A. *Circulator:* liaison for the team and patient advocate, anticipates the needs of sterile team members. (*Note:* This term has been used throughout this text to denote the person in the circulating role regardless of his or her credentials.)

   B. *Anesthesia provider:* administers drugs to alleviate pain and maintains patient homeostasis during surgery; can be an anesthesiologist (MD), nurse anesthetist (CRNA), or anesthesia assistant (AA).

V. *Other Team Members*

   A. *Pathologist* for tissue examination

   B. *Radiologic technologist* to operate x-ray equipment

   C. *Perfusionist* to operate heart–lung machine

   D. *Administrative staff:* supervisor, manager, and clinical coordinator

   E. *Support personnel:* patient care technicians, anesthesia technicians, equipment technicians, secretaries, aides/orderlies, and housekeepers

Operating Room Suite

I. *Physical Layout:* designed on an individual facility basis

II. *Location:* an area accessible to critical care areas and supporting departments; where traffic is limited

III. *Design:* environmentally controlled traffic patterns to prevent infection

   A. **Two common designs are the race track plan and central core design**

   B. **Separate clean from contaminated**

   C. **Traffic patterns for the movement of personnel and patients are established**
      1. *Unrestricted area:* street clothes may be worn; includes offices, front desk, and dressing rooms
      2. *Semirestricted area:* scrub suit, cap, and shoe covers or designated shoes are worn
      3. *Restricted area:* scrub suit, cap, mask, and shoe covers or designated shoes are required; eye protection is required during the surgical procedure

IV. *Exchange Areas:* areas for the entry of patients and personnel from nonrestricted to restricted areas

   A. *Preoperative check-in unit:* same-day surgery admission

   B. *Preoperative holding area:* designated area for patients to wait in the operating room suite and receive final preparation for surgery

   C. *Postanesthesia Care Unit (PACU):* area where patients recover from the anesthesia and surgery

   D. *Dressing rooms and lounges:* area for operating room team to change into surgical attire

V. *Peripheral Support Areas:* unrestricted to semirestricted areas

   A. *Central administrative control:* checkpoint with security system, computers, and centralized communication

   B. *Offices:* areas for operating room management and anesthesia personnel

   C. *Conference room:* semirestricted zone for team conferences, in-service education, and staff meetings

   D. *Laboratory:* for immediate access to pathologist

   E. *Radiology service:* readily accessible for x-ray and imaging

   F. *Pharmacy:* for ready access of medications

   G. *Work and storage areas:* storage areas for equipment

   H. *Utility and decontamination room:* contains sink or ultrasonic cleaner for cleaning of instruments prior to sending them to the central processing area

   I. *Sterile supply rooms:* contains supplies used daily in the OR. Sometimes called materials management

   J. *Instrument room:* for storage of surgical instruments. May be called sterile processing

VI. *Scrub Area:* adjacent to operating room where the surgical hand scrub is performed

VII. *Substerile Room:* immediately adjacent to the OR, contains a sink, steam and/or peracetic acid sterilizers, blanket and solution warmer, and storage cabinets

VIII. *Operating Room*

   A. *Size:* 20 feet by 20 feet by 10 feet, or 400–600 square feet (multipurpose)

   B. *Doors:* sliding (preferred) or swinging (remain closed during surgery)

   C. *Ventilation*
      1. At least 20 air changes per hour; at least 20% of the air change per hour should be fresh outside air.
      2. Laminar unidirectional airflow that provides up to 600 air exchange per hour is installed in some rooms.
      3. Positive air pressure in the operating room
      4. High-efficiency particulate air (HEPA) filters that are cleaned frequently and are separate from the general hospital ventilating system
      5. Relative humidity maintained at 50% to 55%
      6. Room temperature maintained at 68°F to 75°F (20°C to 24.4°C); higher for pediatric, geriatric, and burn patients (up to 80°F)

   D. *Floors:* nonporous for cleaning by flooding and wetvacuuming technique; conductivity is not a prime concern because explosive anesthetic gases are no longer used

   E. *Walls and ceiling:* finishes that are hard, nonporous, fire resistant, waterproof, stainproof, seamless, nonreflective, easy to clean, and soundproof; ceilings are used to mount such equipment as lights, microscopes, monitoring equipment, and x-ray equipment

   F. *Built-in systems*
      1. Vacuum for suction, compressed air, nitrogen, oxygen (green hose), and/or nitrous oxide (blue hose) with outlets on the wall or suspended from the ceiling
      2. X-ray viewing boxes recessed in the walls
      3. Grounded wall outlets installed above the 5-foot level (unless explosion-proof plugs are used); connected to emergency power backup
      4. Code button for emergency response

   G. *Lighting*
      1. General illumination recessed in the ceiling
      2. Overhead operating light must be intense, up to shadowless blue-white color of daylight, be freely adjustable, produce minimal heat, be easily cleaned, and be connected to the emergency backup generator system

H. *Clock with a second hand and a time-elapsed clock:* essential during operations where accurate timing of operative sequences is required

I. *Cabinets or carts for storage of readily accessible sterile items; must be easy to clean*

J. *Furniture and other equipment*
  1. Operating bed with attachments for positioning
  2. Instrument table or back table
  3. Mayo stands
  4. Ring stand(s) for basins
  5. Anesthesia machine
  6. Standing and sitting stools
  7. Suction containers and tubing
  8. Linen hamper frame
  9. IV poles
  10. Kick buckets on wheeled bases
  11. Wastebaskets (hampers)
  12. Writing surface

K. *Communication systems* (vary with different facilities)
  1. Voice intercommunication system/phones
  2. Call light system
  3. Closed-circuit television for surveillance
  4. Two-way audio-video system to provide for immediate consultation with the pathologist or to classroom
  5. Computer terminals in each operating room for ready access to information or data input

L. *Monitoring equipment*

Environmental Hazards and Safety

It is the responsibility of every member of the surgical team to ensure a safe environment for both patients and personnel.

I. *Physical*

  A. *Injury:* sprains and strains from lifting and moving patients and equipment can be minimized by
    1. Using good body mechanics
    2. Keeping objects being moved close to the body
    3. Keeping the back straight, knees slightly flexed, feet apart, and pivoting in direction you are moving; avoid twisting at the waist
    4. Lifting with a slow, even motion using the large muscle groups of the legs and abdomen, not the back
    5. Using a patient lifting frame, Davis roller slide board, or air-transfer device
    6. Using appropriate number of personnel in relation to patient condition
    7. Pushing, rather than pulling, stretchers and tables
    8. Using a wide stance with heels apart and weight evenly distributed on both feet when standing for long periods
    9. Sitting with the back straight from hips to neck and bending forward from the hips
    10. Aligning head and neck with the body when standing or sitting
    11. Changing position, stretching, or walking around occasionally (except for sterile team members)

II. *Ionizing Radiation:* positively and negatively charged particles that can alter enzymes, proteins, cell membranes, and genetic material and cause cancer, cataracts, injury to bone marrow, burns, tissue necrosis, congenital anomalies, and spontaneous abortions.

  A. *Sources:* radioactive elements, x-rays, and fluoroscopy

B. *Patient safety precautions*
1. Turn off the fluoroscope when not in use
2. Reconcile incorrect counts to avoid x-rays
3. Shield body areas from scatter radiation with a thyroid/sternal collar, gonadal shield, or, in the case of pregnancy, a lead shield for the abdominopelvic area
4. Document the location of any beam or type of radioactive implant and the protective measures provided during the operation

C. *Personnel safety precautions*
1. *Time:* decrease time in any beam; rotate assignments; if pregnant, request relief from exposure; turn off machines when not in use; keep radioactive elements in the lead-lined container until ready for use; and quickly contain body fluids from patients with radioactive emissions
2. *Distance:* stay as far from the source of radiation as possible; unsterile team members should leave the room during the single x-ray exposure; sterile team members should stand 6 feet from the patient and out of the direct beam; radiation is reduced by the square of the distance from the source
3. *Shielding:* provided by lead-lined walls, lead aprons, thyroid/sternal collars, gonadal shields, portable lead screens, lead-impregnated surgical gloves, or leaded glasses; lead aprons should be donned before performing the surgical scrub when fluoroscopy is used. (*Note:* Lead aprons should be hung up or laid flat to avoid cracking, which leads to ineffectiveness. Lead shields should be tested routinely for defects.)

D. *Radiation monitors:* should be worn by all personnel with extensive exposure to radiation on prolonged procedures. Film badges are most commonly used.

E. *Nonionizing radiation:* radiant energy from radios, microwave transmitters, television sets, computers, radiant warmers, and light sources such as fiber optics and LASER is not cumulative and does not require monitoring.

III. **LASER (light amplification by stimulated emission of radiation)**

A. **LASERs are used to cut, vaporize, or coagulate tissue, but they present potential hazards for patients and personnel.**

B. **Patient safety precautions**
1. Protect eyes with LASER-specific glasses/goggles, or moistened pads (no ointments)
2. Administer anesthesia and oxygen in a closed system
3. Use nonflammable antiseptics for skin prep. (*Note:* Alcohol and tinctures can produce vapors which can ignite)
4. Use fire-retardant drapes
5. Moisten drapes around target tissue
6. Use special endotracheal tubes when oral/laryngeal LASER procedures are done. (Cuffs should be filled with methylene-blue tinted sterile normal saline and protected with wet compressed cotton; the tubes should be made of red rubber wrapped with metal tape, or flexible ceramic tubes should be used.)
7. For LASER procedures of the perineum or anus, insert a moist sponge in the rectum to prevent escape of flammable methane gas from the intestinal tract

C. **Personnel safety precautions**
1. Wear LASER-specific safety glasses/goggles that include side protection
2. Use lens covers with LASER filters fitted over the optics of endoscopes or microscopes
3. Post warning signs on windows and doors
4. Wear a fire-resistant gown for skin protection
5. Use nonreflective, ebonized, or anodized instruments to avoid burns and fires

6. Turn off the LASER generator when not in use, or keep on "standby" or "shutter-closed"
7. Avoid inhaling LASER plume by using a smoke evacuator and wearing masks that filter 0.1-micron particles
8. Use caution when using certain dyes with some lasers because of possible toxicity
9. Have Halon fire extinguishers available
10. Avoid liquid spills on the LASER generator, which could act as conductors to short circuit the mechanism

IV. *Electricity:* Inadequately trained personnel and improper functioning of equipment can result in fatalities or severe injury to both patients and personnel.

A. **Grounding of all electrical equipment in the operating room is essential. The third prong of an electrical plug provides a return for leakage current through the ground wire to earth.**

B. **Isolation power system**
1. Used in hazardous locations such as the operating room
2. Isolates operating room electrical circuits from grounded circuits in the power main
3. Prevents the flow of current through a person in contact with a hot wire
4. Line isolation monitors; check the hazard current from an isolated circuit to ground
   a. Wall-mounted meter in each operating room
   b. Warning system (alarm and light) alerts personnel to danger
   c. If activated, unplug the last piece of electrical equipment plugged into the power system and continue to unplug equipment to identify faulty equipment; if necessary, close the operating room until biomedical engineers can check for current leakage

C. **Precautions to be taken with electronic devices**
1. Check frequently for frayed or broken power cords and malfunctioning power switches
2. Avoid excess pull on cords or rolling heavy equipment over them
3. Keep liquids away from electrical units
4. Place electrosurgical units on operator's side of the table and away from patient monitoring equipment
5. Ensure proper grounding
6. Turn the machine off before plugging and unplugging
7. Grasp plugs, not cords, when unplugging
8. Have routine preventative maintenance checks made by biomedical engineering department
9. Do not use extension cords with the electrosurgical unit or LASER unit
10. Do *not* use equipment if there is evidence of smoke, smell, or spark
11. When in doubt about the safety of equipment, do not use, take out of circulation, tag for inspection, and notify the appropriate authority
12. In the event of electrical shock, clear the person from the equipment with a nonconductive object, unplug the equipment or turn circuit breakers off, and initiate CPR as appropriate

D. **Static electricity**
1. Develops from friction and accumulates on objects
2. Can ignite flammable material or gases
3. Decreases with a higher humidity (maintained at 50% to 55%)

V. **Fire and Explosions**

A. **The fire triangle consists of fuel (a flammable agent), oxygen, and an ignition source**

B. **To avoid explosion or fire, one part of the triangle must be eliminated**

C. Keep flammable agents (ethylene oxide, oil or grease, alcohol, collodion, ether, and methane gas from the colon) at safe distance from possible ignition sources

D. Ignition sources: electrosurgical units, LASERs, fiber-optic light cables, and static electricity

E. Do not use flammable antiseptics and fat solvents (i.e., alcohol, tinctures) as skin prep before LASER or electrosurgery

F. Use explosion-proof electrical receptacles or locking plugs

G. Oil or grease is not used on oxygen valves or parts of anesthesia machines

H. Requirements are much more stringent around anesthesia equipment and the patient's head; friction against the reservoir bag should be avoided; cover the patient's hair to avoid static electricity

I. *Fire safety*
   1. Prevention is always the first consideration
   2. Fire drills and practice with fire extinguishers are a part of in-service education for all personnel
   3. Priorities should a fire occur: RACE (Rescue, Alarm, Confine, Extinguish)
   4. In the operating room, move burning articles away from anesthesia machine and gases, turn off piped-in gases under the direction of the anesthesia provider, unplug electrical cords, pull fire alarm, extinguish fire in room if possible, move patient from immediate danger, and act quickly and calmly.

J. Classes of fire and extinguishers
   1. *Class A:* wood, paper, cloth—extinguished with pressurized water or water-mist
   2. *Class B:* flammable liquids—extinguished with carbon dioxide or dry chemicals
   3. *Class C:* electrical or laser—extinguished with Halon

K. *Use of the fire extinguisher:* PASS (Pull the pin, Aim the nozzle at the base of the fire, Squeeze the handle, Sweep from side to side)

VI. *Chemicals*

A. *Hazards:* irritation to tissue, toxicity, and presence of carcinogens

B. Use proper labeling

C. Read the label and understand the chemical before using

D. Refer to MSDS (material safety data sheet) on each chemical which lists
   1. Name, composition, properties
   2. Known health effects
   3. Exposure limits and protective measures
   4. Antidote or first-aid measures

E. Anesthetic gases
   1. Use scavenging equipment properly
   2. Use proper anesthesia techniques
   3. Provide proper maintenance of equipment
   4. Provide minimum complete air changes of 20 per hour

F. Sterilizing disinfecting agents
   1. *Ethylene oxide:* can cause dizziness, nausea, and vomiting; is a known mutagen and carcinogen
   2. *Glutaraldehyde:* irritating to eyes, nose, and throat
   3. *Peracetic acid:* can burn skin and mucous membranes on contact
   4. *Disinfectants:* phenol and sodium hypochlorite

G. *Polymethylmethacrylate (bone cement):* vapors are irritating to eyes and respiratory tract, may cause drowsiness, can damage the cornea if splashed in eye, can diffuse through latex gloves to cause allergic dermatitis, and can cause spontaneous abortion; soft contact lenses should not be worn by personnel in the room when mixing; an exhaust system is used during mixing to collect vapors; and vapors are flammable

     H. *Cytotoxic agents:* avoid contact or inhalation; wear gloves, masks, gowns, and eye protection; wash hands after handling; and place all cytotoxic waste in an approved, sealed, leakproof container and incinerate

VII. *Biologic*

     A. *Infectious waste:* segregate from general waste before disposal in marked leakproof container to be incinerated

     B. *Biohazards:* contact with blood, body fluids, and tissues requires careful handling, adequate protection, and handwashing

     C. *Bloodborne diseases:* Standard Precautions
        1. Prevent needle sticks, cuts, and splashes in the eye or mucous membranes
        2. Be immunized against Hepatitis B
        3. If needle stick exposure occurs, immediately express blood, clean the site, report the incident, and follow established protocol

     D. **Surgical plume from LASERs or electrosurgical units: requires use of high filtration masks, face shields or goggles, and a smoke evacuator**

VIII. *Latex Sensitivity/Allergy:* This is a concern for both the patient and health care worker; local and systemic reactions are possible, including skin rash, itching, burning, and anaphylactic shock; sensitization to latex can result from cutaneous absorption, direct mucosal contact, and inhaling airborne allergens; testing procedures are available; health care facilities have policies and procedures for caring for latex-sensitive patients which include the use of alternate synthetic materials and products; a latex allergy cart can be used, and the surgery should be scheduled for the first case of the day to minimize the amount of airborne allergens

Risk Management

  I. *Purpose:* The operating room is a high-risk area for patients and staff; the goal is to prevent harm and minimize financial loss

  II. Preventive Measures

     A. Establish safety practices and provide in-service programs

     B. Require immunizations

     C. Use protective attire and safety equipment

     D. Provide training programs on new equipment

     E. Perform routine preventive maintenance on equipment

     F. Remove malfunctioning equipment from service

     G. Report and follow up on injuries or unsafe conditions

Ethical, Moral, and Legal Issues

  I. Ethical Practices

     A. Honor the American Hospital Association's Patient Bill of Rights

     B. Respect a patient's confidence and comply with HIPAA regulations

     C. Discuss surgical procedures only as required in professional practice

     D. Respect the confidence of co-workers

  II. Ethical Concerns in Clinical Practice

     A. Right to die
        1. Euthanasia
        2. End-of-life decisions

B. Organ donation and transplantation

C. HIV and other infections

D. Genetic engineering

E. Human experimentation

F. Abortion and reproductive technology

G. Gender reassignment

H. Refusal of treatment

III. Moral Issues

A. Honor the trust your patient has placed in you

B. Respect the patient's rights, beliefs, values, and wishes

C. Respect your own religious convictions

IV. Principles Governing Legal Responsibilities

A. Perform only those functions for which you are prepared by experience and training

B. Perform those duties competently

C. You are responsible for being able to do what others in your profession, at your level, can do regardless of geographic location

D. Follow instructions quickly, accurately, and completely

E. Be familiar with the policies and procedures of the institution in which you function and state practice acts and practice within those policies

F. Remember that certain professional responsibilities cannot be delegated

G. Take measures based on observation and follow standing orders, regulations, rules, policies, and procedures. You may be liable for both inaction and inappropriate action.

H. Remember that legally, "if it wasn't documented, it wasn't done"

V. Legal Terms and Doctrines

A. *Res ipsa loquitur:* the thing speaks for itself; the patient's injury obviously came from the incident over which the defendant had control (e.g., a sponge found in a patient's abdomen).

B. *Respondent superior:* master–servant employment relationship; an employer may be held responsible for an employee's negligent acts (i.e., you were assigned to a case for which you were not prepared and the supervisor knew it)

C. *Corporate negligence:* an institution is liable for failure to ensure an acceptable level of care

D. *Informed consent:* the physician and the patient have discussed, and the patient understands the nature of the procedure as well as risks and alternative treatment options

E. *Assault and battery:* unlawful threat to harm and carrying out that threat (i.e., the doctor goes beyond the limits to which the patient consented)

F. *Invasion of privacy:* patient records are confidential and must be held in confidence

G. *Accountability:* every person is accountable to the patient, employer, profession, and self

H. *Doctrine of reasonable man:* everyone is expected to do his or her job as would any reasonable prudent person in similar circumstances
   1. *Negligence:* lack of reasonable care by omission to fulfill a duty
   2. *Malpractice:* professional misconduct, unreasonable lack of skill or judgment, or illegal or immoral conduct

     I. *Borrowed servant rule:* the captain or master is liable for servant's behavior; the surgeon is liable for actions of team members only when he or she has a right to control and supervise the way team members perform

    J. *Iatrogenic medical injury:* injury sustained by the patient from activity of health care professionals

    K. *Primum non nocere:* first, do no harm

    L. *Aeger primo:* the patient first (motto of the Association of Surgical Technologists [AST])

    M. *Liability:* to be legally bound and responsible for personal actions

    N. *Extension doctrine:* the surgeon may extend the surgical procedure to correct or remove any abnormal pathology during the course of the procedure as deemed necessary

    O. *Abandonment:* leaving the patient when the patient's condition warrants the presence of the health care professional

    P. *Defamation:* injury to an individual's character orally (slander) or in writing (libel)

    Q. *Tort:* a civil wrong (intentional or unintentional)

VI. **Operating Room Incidents/Sentinel Events**

    A. Patient misidentification

    B. Use of defective equipment/instruments

    C. Falls resulting in patient injury

    D. Abandonment of patient

    E. Performing an incorrect procedure

    F. Incorrect positioning

    G. Patient burns

    H. Drug errors

    I. Loss of or damage to patient property

    J. Retained items left in a wound due to incorrect counting procedures

    K. Infection due to a break in aseptic technique

    L. Errors in documentation

    M. Improper handling of a specimen

    N. Exceeding authority or violation of a policy

VII. **Surgical Conscience:** The operating room professional's personal moral integrity when it comes to patient care; includes

    A. Professional honesty

    B. Avoiding discriminatory treatment of patients

    C. Patient confidentiality

    D. Accepting responsibility for actions

    E. Commitment to cost containment

    F. Commitment to the application of principles of aseptic technique

Show What You Know

Directions: Each of the numbered items or incomplete statements in this section is followed by answers or by completions of the statement. Select the ONE lettered answer or completion that is BEST in each case.

1. The proper attire for the semirestricted area in the operating room suite, such as a conference room, is:

   A. street clothes
   B. scrub suit, cap, shoe covers
   C. scrub suit, cap, shoe covers, mask
   D. scrub suit, cap, shoe covers, mask, eye protection

2. To decrease airborne contamination and static electricity, the relative humidity of the operating room is maintained at:

   A. 30% to 35%
   B. 40% to 45%
   C. 50% to 55%
   D. 70% to 75%

3. The operating room temperature should be raised from the normal 68°F to 75°F for which of the following patient populations?

   A. the diabetic patient
   B. the female patient
   C. the infant
   D. the adolescent

4. Patient safety in the operating room is the responsibility of the:

   A. surgeon
   B. anesthesiologist
   C. nurse
   D. entire surgical team

5. When lifting heavy objects, you should:

   A. lift with a slow, even motion
   B. keep knees straight
   C. stand as far from the object being moved as possible
   D. keep feet close together

6. Which of the following is not a source of ionizing radiation?

   A. radioactive elements
   B. x-rays
   C. fluoroscopy
   D. LASERs

7. All of the following actions will decrease exposure to ionizing radiation *except*:

   A. decreasing the time in the beam
   B. increasing the distance between you and the source of radiation

   C. using a smoke evacuator and high filtration mask
   D. wearing a lead apron, collar, or gonadal shield

8. A moist sponge is placed in the rectum during a LASER procedure of the perineum or anus to:

   A. prevent seepage of fecal material
   B. prevent the escape of methane gas
   C. keep bacteria out of the field
   D. decrease bad odors

9. If the red light comes on or the alarm from the line isolation monitor sounds, you would *first*:

   A. pull the fire alarm
   B. notify the supervisor
   C. ignore it
   D. unplug the last piece of equipment plugged into the power system

10. All of the following are safeguards to be followed when using electronic devices *except*:

    A. avoid excess pull on cords
    B. disconnect equipment to turn it off
    C. do not place electrosurgical units next to patient monitors
    D. keep liquids off electrical equipment

11. Which of the following is not a part of the fire triangle?

    A. fuel
    B. carbon dioxide
    C. an ignition source
    D. oxygen

12. Which of the following antiseptics is not used as a skin prep when using electrosurgery or LASER?

    A. povidone iodine
    B. hexachlorophene
    C. chlorhexidine gluconate
    D. isopropyl alcohol

13. Pressurized water is most effective in containing:

    A. class A fires
    B. class B fires
    C. class C fires
    D. all of the above

14. Which of the following agents gives off toxic vapors when being mixed?

    A. alcohol
    B. chlorhexidine gluconate

C. polymethylmethacrylate
D. nitrous oxide

15. The legal doctrine which holds the institution liable for failure to ensure an acceptable level of care is:

A. respondent superior
B. doctrine of reasonable man
C. borrowed servant rule
D. corporate negligence

16. The legal term that means "first, do no harm" is:

A. *primum non nocere*
B. *res ipsa loquitur*
C. iatrogenic medical injury
D. respondent superior

17. The legal rule broken when a surgical team member discloses information about a patient which he or she learned in the operating room is:

A. invasion of privacy
B. doctrine of reasonable man
C. iatrogenic injury
D. *primum non nocere*

18. Defamation or injury to an individual's character carried out in writing is called:

A. slander
B. liable
C. libel
D. abandonment

19. The motto of the Association of Surgical Technologists is *Aeger Primo,* which means:

A. first do no harm
B. the thing speaks for itself
C. the patient first
D. do your best

20. If a surgical sponge was left in a patient, this would be an example of which legal doctrine?

A. *res ipsa loquitur*
B. respondent superior

C. extension doctrine
D. assault and battery

21. If a premedicated patient were left unattended and fell from the stretcher and received an injury, this would be a direct example of:

A. abandonment
B. corporate negligence
C. accountability
D. doctrine of the reasonable man

22. Which of the following is a recommended ventilation practice in an individual operating room?

A. at least 20 air exchanges per minute
B. laminar air flow at a rate of 25 air exchanges per hour
C. negative air pressure
D. use of in-line HEPA filters

23. All of the following are safety precautions when using a LASER *except:*

A. use of special endotracheal tubes when performing oral LASER procedures
B. use of moistened drapes around target tissue
C. use of reflective metal instruments
D. wearing of special LASER eyewear by the surgical team

24. Which of the following is not a requirement for an individual operating room?

A. grounded wall outlets 2 feet above the floor
B. x-ray view boxes
C. nonporous floors, walls, and ceilings
D. outlets for vacuum, oxygen, and nitrous oxide

25. Which of the following is not recommended furniture or equipment in an individual operating room?

A. standing and sitting stools
B. computer terminals
C. waste and linen hampers
D. fax machines

Answers & Rationales

1. **B.** **Rationale:** The scrub suit, cap, and shoe covers are donned upon entering the OR suite and would be required in the semirestricted area such as the OR conference room.

2. **C.** **Rationale:** A relative humidity of 50% to 55% serves both to decrease airborne contamination by causing dust and lint to settle and to decrease static electricity by enhancing conductivity.

3. **C.** **Rationale:** The temperature in the OR is raised for infants, geriatric patients, or burn patients because of their ineffective temperature control mechanism. Body heat is lost primarily through the skin. The ratio of body surface to volume is critical when factoring the potential for heat loss in the OR environment.

4. D. **Rationale:** The entire surgical team is responsible for assuring that the OR is safe both for patients and staff.

5. A. **Rationale:** When lifting heavy objects, you should keep the knees flexed and the back straight, bend at the hips, pivot feet in the direction you are moving, keep feet apart, stand near the object being moved, and lift with a slow, even motion.

6. D. **Rationale:** Radiant energy from LASERs, fiber optics, microwaves, computers, television sets, and radiant warmers is nonionizing and does not require the use of radiation precautions taken with x-rays, fluoroscopy, or radioactive elements.

7. C. **Rationale:** Principles of radiation protection are:

    Time (decrease time in beam)

    Distance (radiation received is decreased by the square of the distance from source)

    Shielding (lead blocks radiation)

8. B. **Rationale:** Methane gas, produced by the action of bacteria in the colon, is flammable and must not be permitted near a heat source such as an electrosurgical unit or LASER.

9. D. **Rationale:** A light or alarm from the line isolation monitor in the OR indicates a problem with the grounding system and would alert personnel to unplug the last piece of equipment plugged in.

10. B. **Rationale:** Electrical equipment should be turned off before unplugging and plugged in before activating to prevent a sudden surge of electricity.

11. B. **Rationale:** The fire triangle consists of fuel, oxygen, and an ignition source. Carbon dioxide can be used as an extinguisher, whereas oxygen supports combustion.

12. D. **Rationale:** Alcohol is not recommended as a skin prep for procedures where the LASER or electro surgery unit will be used because of its flammable nature.

13. A. **Rationale:** Class A fires consist of paper, wood, and cloth and are best extinguished with pressurized water or water mist.

14. C. **Rationale:** Polymethylmethacrylate is a type of bone cement that gives off toxic fumes when being mixed and necessitates the use of an exhaust system.

15. D. **Rationale:** The legal doctrine which holds an institution liable for failure to ensure an acceptable level of care is corporate negligence.

16. A. **Rationale:** The legal term *primum non nocere* means "first do no harm".

17. A. **Rationale:** Invasion of privacy is disclosing information about a patient. The patient's record contains confidential information.

18. C. **Rationale:** Libel is written defamation; slander is oral defamation; liable is to be legally bound; abandonment is leaving the patient when the patient's condition warrants the presence of the health care professional.

19. C. **Rationale:** *Aeger primo* means "the patient first".

20. A. **Rationale:** The legal term *res ipsa loqitor* means "the thing speaks for itself".

21. A. **Rationale:** Leaving a premedicated patient unattended would be an example of abandonment. The patient's condition warranted the presence of the health care professional.

22. D. **Rationale:** In-line high-efficiency particulate air (HEPA) filters are used in the operating room ventilation system along with at least 20 air exchanges per hour and positive air pressure; laminar air flow systems provide up to 600 air exchanges per hour.

23. C. **Rationale:** Instruments should be nonreflective, ebonized, or anodized to provide reflection of the LASER beam.

24. A. **Rationale:** Grounded wall outlets should be located above the 5-foot level or should be explosion proof to avoid explosions from anesthetic gases.

25. D. **Rationale:** Fax machines contain too many hard-to-clean surfaces and would not be used in an individual operating room.

Part II: Deciphering a Surgical Schedule

The following mock surgery schedule will be used to answer several questions pertaining to the operating room environment. The same schedule, or a similar one, will be used in subsequent chapters to ask questions about the content of the chapter.

Rm# time	Surgeon	Procedure	Anest.	Rm# time	Surgeon	Procedure	Anest.
Rm00				**Rm07**			
OC	Dr. Z	Rt. Knee Arthroscopy	Gen.	7:00	Dr. M	Rhinoplasty	Gen.
OC	Dr. C	Craniotomy	Gen.	TF	Dr. M	Lipoma removal	
OC	Dr. Z	Angioplasty	Gen.				MAC
Rm01				**Rm08**			
7:00	Dr. X	Lobectomy	Gen.	11:00	Dr. E	Bovine Thrombectomy	MAC
TF	Dr. X	Thoracotomy	Gen.				
TF	Dr. X	Tracheostomy	Gen.				
Rm02				**Rm09**			
7:00	Dr. B	Splenectomy	Gen.	8:30	Dr. T	Cholecystectomy	Gen.
TF	Dr. B	Gastrectomy	Gen.	TF	Dr. T	Palatoplasty	Gen.
Rm03				**Rm10**			
7:00	Dr. A	Cystoscopy	MAC	7:00	Dr. K	Nephrectomy	Gen.
TF	Dr. A	Cystoplasty	Gen.	TF	Dr. K	Choledocholithotripsy	MAC
12:30	Dr. F	Pyleogram	MAC	TF	Dr. K	Hepatic resection	
3:00	Dr. F	Cystocele repair	Gen.				Gen.
Rm04				**Rm11**			Gen.
7:00	Dr. Y	Carpal tunnel release	Gen.	7:00	Dr. L	Colposcope	Gen.
TF	Dr. Y	Fasciotomy	Gen.	12:00	Dr. L	Mastectomy	
Rm05				**Rm12**			
7:00	Dr. G	Trans-sphenoidal Adenectomy	Gen.	7:00	Dr. W	Trans-metatarsal amputation	Gen.
TF	Dr. G	Trans-urethral resection of the prostate	Gen.	TF TF	Dr. W	Osteotomy Arthrocentesis	Gen.
TF	Dr. G	Bletharoplasty	Gen.		Dr. W		Gen.
Rm06				**Rm13**			
7:00	Dr. R	Lumbar Laminectomy	Gen.	7:00	Dr. O	Hysterectomy	Gen.

The following questions should be answered using the surgery schedule above

1. The Surgical Technologist in Room 10 received an emergency phone call from home. If this ST leaves the room before a replacement is found, what could this action be considered?
   A. Breach of Trust
   B. Abandonment
   C. Res Ipsa Loquitor
   D. Malpractice

2. Dr. X will need a specialty instrument for his second case. Where will the Surgical Technologist go to find this item?
   A. Materials management
   B. Sub sterile room
   C. Instrument room
   D. Decontamination

3. A small LASER fire has ignited in Room 3. What class of extinguisher will be used to douse the fire?
   A. Class A
   B. Class B
   C. Class C
   D. Water

4. The Surgical Technologist in Room 13 knows the patient. She decides to send flowers to the woman at her office. What tort would this be a breach of?
   A. Privacy
   B. Defamation
   C. Professionalism
   D. Breach of Trust

5. The ESU cord in Room 4 is frayed. What should the ST do?
   A. Use the machine until a replacement has been brought in
   B. Cancel the surgery
   C. Wrap the cord securely with electrical tape
   D. Do not use the ESU

6. The specimen in Dr. Ks Nephrectomy was accidentally discarded. This would be considered a(n)
   A. Sentinel event
   B. Misconduct
   C. Patient safety issue
   D. Ethical breach

7. The last three patients in Room 5 have suffered complications due to surgical site infections. Which department will investigate the reasons?
   A. Pathology
   B. Risk management
   C. OR supervisor
   D. Hospital board

8. Halfway through the Mastectomy in Room 11, the circulating nurse realizes that a wrapper that contained an instrument set has a small tear in it. What protocol should be followed?
   A. All members of the team should immediately be informed and proper precautions should be implemented
   B. The patients family should be informed post-operatively
   C. Nothing should done, as the surgery is already in progress
   D. The surgeon should be told after surgery is finished so that he can order prophylactic antibiotics

9. The patient scheduled for the Arthrocentisis in Room 12 is latex allergic. What should be done?
   A. Surgery must be cancelled
   B. The surgery should be rescheduled to be the first case of the day
   C. The surgery should be moved to Room 8 following the bovine Thrombectomy
   D. There is no need to alter the schedule as long as precautions are taken

10. The ST in Room 3 has accidentally spilled peracetic acid while processing. What does the ST need to make sure that this spill is handled correctly?
    A. MSDS sheet
    B. Copious amounts of water
    C. The OR manager
    D. The housekeeping department as it is their job to clean areas

Answers & Rationales

1. **B.** **Rationale:** This would fall under abandonment. The patient is in a vulnerable state that is dependent on the presence of health care professionals. The Surgical Technologist must remain with the patient until a suitable replacement is found.

2. **C.** **Rationale:** The ST should find the surgeons instrument in the instrument room. This may be a part of the sterile processing department. Materials management usually has the disposables used in procedures, and the sub sterile room should not be used to house instruments.

3. **C.** **Rationale:** LASER fires are extinguished with Halon, found in class C extinguishers. Class A uses pressurized water or mist, and is used primarily for paper or wood fires, while Class B extinguishers contain Carbon Dioxide or dry chemicals to extinguish flammable liquids.

4. **A.** **Rationale:** This would be a breach of confidentiality. All privileged information should remain confidential, even if the patient is known to a member of the team.

5. **D.** **Rationale:** This is a dangerous situation that should be handled immediately. The ESU cannot be used in this condition, and another one must be located before the surgery can begin.

6. **A.** **Rationale:** Sentinel events include improper handling of a specimen, including loss of a specimen. The incident needs to be reported and documented correctly. The impacts of a lost or mishandled specimen are great and may require the patient to undergo another invasive surgery to retrieve another specimen. It is imperative that the ST handle specimens correctly.

7. **B.** **Rationale:** Risk management may be called into assess this situation and investigate the circumstances. Although the OR supervisor will be informed, the risk management team will undertake the job of finding the source of the infections and take measures to correct any issues.

8. **A.** **Rationale:** In cases where there is a question about sterility if instrumentation or supplies, all of the team members need to be aware so that precautions can be undertaken to protect the patient from infection. The ST should always check the integrity of packages and wrappers before they are opened, but occasionally there is a missed perforation. This is a situation that requires the ST to take responsibility and admit to the mistake. This is one of the cornerstones of surgical conscience.

9. **B.** **Rationale:** Patients with Latex sensitivity and allergies should always be scheduled to be the first case of the day. This is done to ensure that no airborne particles containing latex from a previous case come into contact with the sensitive patient.

10. **A.** **Rationale:** The materials safety data sheets should always be consulted when dealing with a chemical spill. This is especially important when unsure of the proper protocol for containment. Some chemicals are extremely volatile and chemical reactions can occur if they come into contact with other substances, so the ST must always consult these sheets.

PEARSON myhealthprofessionskit

Use this address to access the interactive Companion Website created for this book. Simply select "Surgical Technology" from the choice of disciplines. Find this book and click to enter.

7 Surgical Asepsis

The most critical yet challenging concepts and techniques to be learned and implemented by the surgical team are those related to surgical asepsis. Failure to utilize sterile practices during invasive procedures predisposes the patient to great harm; yet the culprits are invisible and require continuous vigilance and a persistent surgical conscience. The concepts involved in surgical asepsis have evolved over time, and are at a pinnacle for patient safety. Less than one hundred years ago, survival rates in surgery were grim. Through medical breakthroughs, including surgical asepsis, these survival rates have strengthened to the point where routine surgeries are considered as safe as they can possibly become. However, much of this safety depends upon a Surgical Technologists adherence to the principles and applications of sterile techniques. With the increase in antibiotic resistant strains of bacteria, it is becoming even more important that the entire health care team is involved in reducing infections through surgical asepsis.

CHAPTER OUTLINE

 **How to Answer Surgical Asepsis Questions**

Most of the questions regarding surgical asepsis rely on the fundamental knowledge of microbiology and disease transmission. Students and practitioners should have this information in mind in order to answer many of the questions covered in this section. The goal of surgical asepsis is to reduce the possibility of infections to the patient. Most of that relies on the sterilization and disinfection processes used in preparing instruments and materials for use. Another variable is the actual instrument set or supplies that need to be sterilized or processed. Not all instruments can be steam sterilized, and each type of instrument has a preferred manufacturer's specific method for sterilization. Surgical equipment, instruments, and supplies are extremely costly, so these guidelines must be maintained to protect the investment that the hospital has made. Knowing these guidelines is an important part of the Surgical Technologists job.

A large portion of these questions rely on critical thinking skills as well as the understanding of the differences in the types of sterilization methods.

Example:
When sterilizing a Cystoscope, which method would the Surgical Technologist use?

a. Gravity displacement
b. Prevacuum
c. Cobalt 60
d. Glutaraldehyde

To answer this question, you must first take into consideration the object to be sterilized, in this case, a Cystoscope. Can the item be exposed to heat? In this case, the answer is no. Heat will damage the lens of a scope, so it cannot be placed in a sterilizer that relies on heat. This will automatically rule out the two steam sterilizers. That will leave cobalt 60 or Glutaraldehyde. Cobalt 60, or ionizing radiation, is expensive, and is usually restricted to commercial use for sterilization of disposable items. The elimination of these sources of sterilization has left one option. Therefore, the correct answer will be D. Glutaraldehyde is routinely used for objects that will be damaged by heat or pressure. There are other options for sterilization of these items, but they were not given as possible answers.

Terminology

1. *Aerosol:* particulate matter or droplets in the air
2. *Antiseptic:* chemical that inhibits the growth of endogenous microorganisms (resident flora) on skin and mucous membranes
3. *Aseptic:* without infection
4. *Bacteriocidal:* agent that kills bacteria
5. *Bacteriostasis:* inhibition of bacterial growth
6. *Bioburden:* degree of microbial contamination
7. *Contaminated:* soiled; presence of microorganisms
8. *Decontamination:* cleaning and disinfecting or sterilizing to render contaminated items safe
9. *Disinfectant:* agent that kills microorganisms on inanimate objects
10. *Disinfection:* process of destroying pathogenic microorganisms, except spores
11. *Sanitary:* clean
12. *Shelf life:* length of time a package in storage remains sterile
13. *Sporicidal:* agent capable of killing spores
14. *Sterile:* completely free from all microorganisms and spores

15. *Sterilization:* process by which all microorganisms and spores are destroyed
16. *Strike-through contamination:* transmission of microbes through a moisture-permeated sterile barrier
17. *Surgical asepsis:* procedure for creating and maintaining a sterile field
18. *Surgical conscience:* professional commitment to honesty, use of strict aseptic technique, conscientiousness, and respect for others
19. *Surgically clean:* mechanically cleaned, but unsterile
20. *Terminal sterilization and disinfection:* procedure for destroying pathogens at the end of a surgical case. This is performed to protect the health care worker who will be handling the surgical instruments in the sterile processing department.

Decontamination and Sterilization

All items that come in contact with the patient and/or the sterile field are systematically decontaminated.

I. Mechanical Cleansing of Instruments
   A. During a surgical procedure, excess blood or proteins are removed with a wet sponge
   B. Following use of instruments, they are opened and cleaned of any gross debris (bioburden) to prevent blood or protein from hardening and are covered for safe transport to the decontamination area
   C. In the decontamination room, contaminated instruments are run through a washer–sterilizer cycle for cleaning and terminal sterilization
   D. Instruments may be placed in an ultrasonic cleaner: special equipment that uses high-frequency sound waves to dislodge dried proteins from instruments by the process of cavitation (formation of tiny bubbles that expand and implode to create a vacuum which dislodges minute particles of soil from the instrument)
   E. When necessary, soiled instruments may be cleaned manually, giving special attention to box locks and serrated edges while wearing personal protective equipment (PPE) (gown/apron, gloves, and mask with eye shield)
   F. Thorough rinsing and drying should precede storage
   G. Following decontamination and disinfection, the instruments are sent to the clean processing area to be inspected, reassembled in sets, and packaged for sterilization

II. Methods and Principles of Sterilization
   A. Saturated steam under pressure
      1. Recognized as safest, most common thermal means of sterilizing supplies and most instruments (heat- and moisture-stable items)
      2. Destructive to heat-sensitive items
      3. Kills microbes by coagulating the protein
      4. Temperature is raised by increasing pressure (*Note:* The temperature of boiling water at sea level is 100°C/212°F, and the thermal death point for spores is 121°C/250°F, thereby requiring the addition of pressure to raise the temperature high enough to kill spores)
      5. The addition of 15 to 17 psi (pounds per square inch) of pressure can raise the temperature to 250°F/121°C; the addition of 27 psi of pressure will raise the temperature to 270°F/132°C
      6. Exposure time depends on the size and contents of the load and the temperature in the autoclave
      7. Moisture decreases sterilizing time. Moisture is left in lumens to enhance steam sterilization
      8. Air and steam cannot occupy the same space at the same time; therefore, air must be removed either by gravity displacement or vacuum before

steam sterilization can be accomplished; steam enters the top rear of the chamber and air exits the bottom front (*Note:* When packaging items for steam sterilization or loading the sterilizer, it is essential to avoid trapping air [i.e., "nested" basins are separated by a towel and loaded on their sides, tubes are coiled, and plungers are removed from syringes])

9. Tests are done daily to ensure the complete removal of air from the pre-vacuum sterilizer. The Bowie-Dick test and the DART (daily air removal test) are commonly used
10. Critical factors for steam sterilization: Every surface in the package must be reached by the steam at the proper temperature for the proper length of time

B. **Dry heat sterilization**
   1. Air must circulate freely
   2. Longer time and higher temperature required than with steam
   3. Used to sterilize anhydrous oils, petroleum products, and talc, which steam cannot penetrate; this method is not used frequently as most of these items are now commercially sterilized by the manufacturer using ionizing radiation

C. **Ionizing radiation**
   1. Cobalt 60, a radioactive isotope, is the most common
   2. Limited primarily to commercial use

D. **Ethylene oxide (EO) gas sterilization**
   1. Flammable gas, but may be mixed with other agents to decrease flammability
   2. Regarded by OSHA (Occupational Safety and Health Administration) as a potential carcinogen with a potential for causing reproductive defects and chromosomal alteration; irritating to the skin and mucous membranes
   3. Used to sterilize heat- and moisture-sensitive items (plastics, rubber)
   4. Items must be clean, dry (to prevent the formation of ethylene glycol) and free of all lubricants before packaging
   5. Free circulation and penetration of the EO gas must be considered when loading the sterilizer
   6. Careful monitoring, adequate ventilation, and safe work habits are necessary
   7. Sterilization is dependent upon concentration of sterilant, relative humidity, temperature, and exposure time (the time required for sterilization may be 2 to 3 hours, but the entire process can take up to 16 hours because of aeration)
   8. Items sterilized with EO must be properly aerated:
      a. When a combination sterilizer/aerator unit is used, both cycles should be completed before the items are removed
      b. If a separate aerator is used, items should be transported quickly from the EO sterilizer to the aerator, be pulled rather than pushed, remain on the sterilizer cart or in a basket during transportation, and be handled as little as possible and with gloves
      c. Aeration time depends on the type of EO system, type of aeration system, use of the item, composition of the item, and the temperature of the aerator chamber

E. **Activated glutaraldehyde (Cidex)**
   1. The solution is activated by adding a powdered buffer to a liquid
   2. Once mixed, the expiration date is marked on the container and the solution is reusable until this date
   3. Activated glutaraldehyde must be stored in a covered container in a well-ventilated room. Gloves and goggles should be worn when working with the chemical

4. Monitoring is necessary to ensure proper concentration
5. Items must be cleaned and dried before placing in the solution
6. Used for endoscopes and for plastic and rubber items
7. Time required to sterilize (sporicidal) is 10 hours, and, for high-level disinfection, 20–30 minutes
8. Rinsing in sterile distilled water and flushing of lumens is necessary following exposure to glutaraldehyde, which is toxic to tissue

F. Hydrogen peroxide plasma sterilization (Sterrad®)
1. Uses radio frequency waves at a low temperature (104°F), and the process is dry
2. Sterilizes in approximately 1 hour
3. No cellulose-based products can be used with this method
4. Forms radicals that interact with the cell membrane killing the microorganism; the radicals then recombine to form oxygen and water

G. Peracetic acid sterilization (STERIS®)
1. Used to sterilize endoscopes
2. 131°F for 20–25 minutes: cycle takes 30–35 minutes
3. Sterilized items are for immediate use only and cannot be stored
4. Sterilant can be used only for a single sterilization cycle
5. Kills microbes by oxidation to denature proteins

III. Types of Steam Sterilizers

A. Gravity air displacement sterilizer
1. Pressure is preset at 15 to 17 psi
2. Temperature is 250°F (121°C)
3. Used for wrapped items
4. Exposure (sterilizing) time is 15 to 30 minutes
5. Steam enters the top rear; since air is heavier than steam, it is displaced downward and out at the bottom front; a filter and thermometer are located at this outlet
6. Drying time required is dependent upon the size of the package

B. High vacuum (prevacuum)
1. Pressure is preset at 27 psi
2. Temperature is 270°F to 276°F (132°C –135°C)
3. Minimum exposure time is 4 minutes for wrapped items
4. Widely used sterilizer in the central processing area for wrapped instruments, basins, linens, and as a flash autoclave in the OR suite for unwrapped instruments
5. Tested for air removal daily with the Bowie-Dick test
6. Complete cycle takes 15–30 minutes

C. Flash sterilizer
1. Pressure is preset at 27 psi
2. Temperature 270°F (132°C)
3. Used for unwrapped items in emergency situations (i.e., dropped instruments needed to continue a surgical procedure or a few instruments needed for a special procedure)
4. Should not be used for routine sterilization of instrument sets or sterilization of implants
5. Can have a gravity displacement or prevacuum cycle
6. Minimum exposure time is 3 minutes, for unwrapped, nonporous, stainless steel items without a lumen
7. For porous items or instruments with a lumen or instrument marking tape, the exposure time will be increased to 4 minutes in the prevacuum cycle and 10 minutes in the gravity displacement cycle.
8. Sterilized items will be wet with steam and must be carried to a sterile field by the scrub if the sterilizer is located adjacent to the OR in a

substerile room; the circulator may use a special open flash sterilization tray with detachable handle or closed flash sterilization tray

  D. **Care of the sterilizer:** wash the inside of the chamber daily according to the manufacturer's recommendations; clean the filter screen daily; flush the discharge line weekly with an approved solution

IV. **Monitoring Methods**

  A. *Chemical indicators:* method-sensitive tape on outside of package, and strips inside package that change color when the package has been exposed to a specific temperature, humidity, or sterilant; they do not prove sterility of the package, they only indicate exposure to the sterilizing parameters

  B. *Mechanical monitoring:* thermometers, pressure gauges, and charts/print-outs with a record of sterilizing cycles (length and temperature)

  C. *Biological monitoring (spore tests):* ensures sterilization of items
   1. *Bacillus stearothermophilus* is used for steam sterilizers; run at least weekly (preferably daily)
   2. *Bacillus subtilis* is used for EO gas sterilizers and dry heat; run with every load
   3. A commercially prepared spore strip containing either microbe is used to test the peracetic acid sterilizer (STERIS®) and hydrogen peroxide sterilizer (Sterrad®) daily
   4. Loads that contain implantables must always be monitored, and the results of the test known before the implant is used

V. **Preparation of Items for Sterilization**

  A. **Items are cleaned to reduce the bioburden and freed of oil (steam will not penetrate oil)**

  B. **Packaging and wrapping material should**
   1. Be compatible with the sterilizing process
   2. Allow the sterilizing agent to penetrate and reach all surfaces to be sterilized
   3. Provide a barrier to microorganisms
   4. Be durable, cost-effective, flexible, memory free, and allow for easy aseptic presentation
   5. Have seal integrity

  C. **Packaging for sterilization**
   1. *Rigid container system:* filters should remain intact and gaskets remain sealed following sterilization
   2. *Peel packages:* a combination of paper and plastic is used most frequently; can be heat sealed or sealed with adhesive tape; staples should not be used to seal the package and rubber bands, tape, or paper clips should not be used to hold several packages together as the sterilant may not penetrate them
   3. *Woven textiles:* muslin must be at least 140 threads per square inch, must be freshly laundered for rehydration to prevent superheating of fabric, must be allowed to dry before removal from the autoclave, and must be of double thickness and double wrapped sequentially by a square fold or envelope fold
   4. *Single-use disposable nonwoven materials:* double wrapped sequentially and used according to manufacturer's recommendations; paper has "memory" and has a tendency to return to its original position

  D. **All articles in a package are arranged to provide direct exposure of the sterilizing agent to all surfaces for the prescribed time and temperature**
   1. Jointed instruments are opened and/or unlocked, then placed on a rack in a mesh-bottom tray with a towel beneath the instruments and heavy instruments at the bottom

2. Tubing with a lumen is loosely coiled to allow the steam to reach inside; if using a gravity displacement sterilizer, a residual of distilled water should be left in the lumen
3. A rubber sheet must be covered with a piece of fabric and loosely rolled and wrapped; this allows steam to penetrate the package
4. Woven textile drape packs should not exceed 12 by 12 by 20 inches, weigh no more than 12 pounds, be fan folded, and be packaged loosely
5. Weight for package of surgical instruments should not exceed 16 pounds
6. Rubber bands should not be used around solid items because steam cannot penetrate the rubber
7. Wooden items such as tongue blades must be individually wrapped
8. Basins that will be nested should be separated with an absorbent towel; sponges and additional woven fabrics should not be placed in a basin set
9. Each package is labeled to identify content, sterilization date and shelf-life indication, the sterilizer used, the cycle or load number to allow for retrieval in the event of sterilization failure, and the initials of the person who prepared the package

E. **Loading the steam sterilizer**
1. Packs or articles are arranged to allow a full flow of steam and removal of air
2. Mixed loads are not recommended; if basin sets are run with linen packs, they should be placed on a lower shelf to prevent condensation from dripping on the linen
3. Textile packs are loaded on edge (vertical); large packs are separated 2–4 inches. Small packs may be crisscrossed on top of each other; closed containers and instrument trays with mesh bottoms are loaded flat; basins and solid containers are loaded on their side so that if they contained water it would flow out; solutions are sterilized alone and on slow exhaust; packages must not touch the inside walls of the chamber

F. **Unloading the autoclave**
1. Ensure that chamber pressure is at zero before opening the door
2. A load of wrapped packages is left untouched to dry for 15–60 minutes depending on the load and the sterilizer
3. Warm packs are left on racks to cool before moving to storage; warm packs laid on a solid cold surface cause steam condensation and become damp and contaminated
4. Sterilized items are handled carefully and minimally

G. **Storage of sterile supplies**
1. Store in a well-ventilated, limited-access area with controlled temperature and humidity; closed cupboards are preferred
2. Ensure stock rotation (first in/first out)
3. Shelf-life of packaged sterile items is dependent on the handling of the package and the type of packaging and environment, such as cleanliness, temperature, humidity, dust covers, and closed cabinets (event-related/not time-related)

VI. **Chemical Disinfection: The use of a chemical germicide is based on the risk of infection involved in the use of the disinfected item**

A. **Classification of patient care items**
1. *Critical items:* must be sterilized because they contact sterile tissue (e.g., surgical instruments, cardiac catheters, and needles)
2. *Semicritical items:* come in contact with nonintact skin or mucous membranes and require high-level disinfection (e.g., respiratory therapy and anesthesia equipment and gastrointestinal endoscopes)
3. *Noncritical items:* come in contact with intact skin; intermediate or low-level disinfection is adequate (e.g., blood pressure cuffs and furniture)

B. Levels of disinfection
   1. *High-level disinfection:* all bacteria, viruses, and fungi are killed.
   2. *Intermediate-level disinfection:* most bacteria, viruses, and fungi are killed.
   3. *Low-level disinfection:* kills most vegetative bacteria, fungi, and the least resistant viruses (including HIV)

C. Germicides are used according to manufacturers' written guidelines and are registered with the EPA (Environmental Protection Agency) (*Note:* Material Safety Data Sheets [MSDSs] are required for each chemical used in the operating room)

D. Factors influencing chemical disinfection are
   1. Thorough cleaning before disinfection to reduce bioburden
   2. Concentration: instruments must be dry to avoid diluting the solution
   3. Exposure time
   4. Temperature and pH
   5. Active ingredient
   6. Complete immersion is essential, with all surfaces exposed to the germicide
   7. Thorough rinsing with sterile distilled water is necessary following contact with the germicide
   8. Closely monitored expiration date

E. Physical disinfection
   1. **Boiling water:** not a sterilizing process; kills some microorganisms
   2. **Ultraviolet irradiation:** can kill vegetative bacteria, fungi, and some viruses. UV lights have been used in some ORs

F. Safe environments are necessary for personnel using germicides
   1. Keep germicides covered
   2. Store in closed containers in well-ventilated room
   3. Protective attire (eyewear, gloves, and masks) is necessary for skin protection

G. Commonly used disinfectants
   1. *Glutaraldehyde 2%:* a high-level disinfectant useful for endoscopes; requires 10 hours of exposure time for sterilization and 10 minutes of direct contact for high-level disinfection (a 20-minute soak is recommended)
   2. *Isopropyl alcohol:* a housekeeping disinfectant; cannot be used on lensed instruments because it dissolves the cement that holds the lens in place
   3. *Chlorine compounds:* housekeeping disinfectants, used for spot cleaning of blood and body spills
   4. *Iodophor (iodine with detergent):* germicidal in 20 minutes
   5. *Phenolic compounds:* housekeeping disinfectants germicidal in 20 minutes
   6. *Quaternary ammonium compounds (Quats):* Used to sanitize noncritical surfaces, but their use is declining because their effectiveness is easily reversed with contact with soaps, water, or organic debris

VII. **Environmental Sanitation/Terminal Disinfection of the Operating Room**

A. *Purpose:* confine and contain cross-contamination

B. *Procedure*
   1. Handle contaminated material as little as possible
   2. Impervious biohazardous waste receptacles are used for bloody waste
   3. Other trash and linen are put in fluid-impervious bags
   4. Sharps are placed in a rigid, puncture-proof container
   5. Gown and gloves are removed and discarded before leaving the OR after clean-up of all contaminated instruments and supplies
   6. Any spills of blood or body fluid are cleaned immediately (concurrent disinfection)
   7. Fluids are treated and discarded according to hospital policy
   8. Surgical lights and horizontal surfaces of furniture and equipment within and around the perimeter of the sterile field are cleaned with a high-level disinfectant (terminal disinfection)

9. A perimeter of several feet around the surgical field of the floor is mopped with clean mop head and high-level disinfectant or wet vacuum

10. Wheels and casters on mobile furniture are pushed through a disinfectant solution

11. Walls are not considered contaminated and are washed only if splashed with blood or organic debris

12. At the end of the day, every OR, including the furniture, scrub room, and service area, is cleaned using mechanical friction and chemical disinfection

13. A weekly and monthly schedule of cleaning should be established which includes walls, ceiling, air conditioning grills, storage shelves, and peripheral support areas

Principles and Application of Aseptic Technique

I. Surgical Attire

A. Worn by all personnel entering the semirestricted and restricted areas of the OR to protect both the patient and staff

B. Scrub suits must be nonstatic, freshly laundered, and with maximum skin coverage; they should be close fitting to avoid contaminating sterile fields; the scrub suit should be changed whenever it becomes wet or visibly soiled; caps should cover all hair (including long facial hair) and be clean, nonstatic, and free of lint; caps should be donned prior to donning the scrub suit

C. High-filtration masks are worn in restricted areas; masks are either on or off and should not hang around the neck; strings should not be crisscrossed over the head; masks should be handled by the strings, and changed between cases

D. Protective eyewear is worn any time a risk exists of exposure to blood or body fluids

E. Shoe covers are worn unless shoes are dedicated for use in the OR

II. Traffic Pattern in the Surgical Suite

A. Personnel entering the surgical suite follow a special traffic pattern
1. Unrestricted areas: Street clothes are permitted
2. Semirestricted areas (storage areas for clean and sterile supplies): scrub attire is worn
3. Restricted area (areas where sterile procedures are being carried out): scrub attire plus masks and protective eye wear are worn

B. Doors to the OR are kept closed to maintain positive air pressure in the room

C. Traffic is monitored and restricted

D. Movement of the patient to, through, and from surgical suites is by the most direct route to prevent cross-contamination
1. Clean bed/stretcher is used to transport the patient to surgery
2. The patient is freshly bathed, has on clean gown, and is covered with clean bed linen

E. Traffic patterns are designed to separate clean or sterile supplies and equipment from soiled equipment or waste

F. Outside equipment is cleaned prior to being brought into the OR suite

Aseptic Barrier Materials for Gowns and Drapes

1. Surgical gowns and drapes are made of materials that provide an effective barrier to microorganisms

2. Material is resistant to penetration of blood and other fluids

3. Material is resistant to tears and punctures
4. Reusable fabric should maintain barrier quality through multiple laundering, be receptive to sterilization, and be repaired with heat-sealed patches
5. Monitoring the number of times a woven textile gown is laundered is necessary in order to remove the gown from use when it is no longer an effective barrier

The Surgical Scrub

I. Requirements Prior to Beginning a Scrub

   A. Remove jewelry from hands and forearms; jewelry around the neck and ears, if permitted, must be contained within the scrub top and cap

   B. Put on proper attire: scrub suit, cap, high-filtration masks, eye protection, and, if required, shoe covers

   C. Check that hands and forearms are free of lesions or breaks in the skin

   D. Fingernails should be short and free of any artificial devices

II. Scrub Procedure: the surgical scrub renders the hands and arms surgically clean

   A. Standardized for all personnel, with subsequent scrubs following the same procedure as the first scrub of the day

   B. Hands and arms are washed with warm water and antiseptic soap to remove gross soil and transient microbes

   C. Nails and subungual areas (beneath nails) are cleaned with disposable nail cleaner under running water

   D. Sterile brush with antimicrobial soap and water is used to scrub; a vigorous circular motion is used, beginning with the fingertips and progressing to 2 inches above the elbow, not retracing; hands are held higher than elbows to allow water to run from hands (cleanest area) off the elbows; hands and arms are not allowed to touch anything that is not sterile once the scrub begins; avoid getting scrub attire wet; hands and arms are rinsed thoroughly under running water from fingertips to elbows

   E. Friction (mechanical), coupled with the germicidal (chemical) action of the soap and water, renders the hands and forearms surgically clean, removing skin oils and some resident flora

III. Types of Scrubs

   A. Anatomical timed scrub (5 minutes) allots a prescribed amount of time for each anatomical area

   B. The counted brush stroke allots a set of brush strokes to each designated surface of the hands and forearms

   C. A "waterless scrub" is available which consists of rubbing a chemical solution on clean hands and arms and allowing it to dry; follow manufacturer's guidelines for the use of this product

Basic Aseptic Technique

1. Scrubbed persons wear sterile gowns and gloves

   a. Following the surgical scrub, the hands are dried with a sterile towel, bending at the waist to make sure that the towel does not come in contact with scrub suit

   b. The gown is considered sterile in front from the chest to waist level or the level of sterile field

   c. The sleeves are considered sterile from 2 inches above the elbow to the proximal edge of stockinette cuff; gloves should completely cover the nonimpervious cuff

SURGERY HINT

Many people who enter the operating room do not have the same training as Surgical Technologists. It is the duty of STs to watch each of these individuals for possible contaminations.

When draping large equipment, such as microscopes and C-arms for use at the sterile field, the ST may be required to step away from the back able to accomplish this task. Once draped, the item should be viewed as part of the sterile field and should be monitored carefully when not in use.

   d. The neckline, shoulders, areas under the arms, and the back of the gown are considered unsterile

   e. Self-gowning and gloving is performed from a separate sterile surface using the closed gloving technique. The closed gloving technique cannot be used to change a glove once donned. Once the hands have passed through the cuff, the cuffs are considered contaminated

2. **Sterile drapes are used to establish a sterile field**

   a. Placed on the patient and all furniture and equipment to be included in the sterile field

   b. Drapes are not passed over nonsterile areas; it may be necessary to carry the folded drape to the opposite side of the operating bed

   c. Handled as little as possible

   d. Held above waist level in a compact position and draped from the operative site to the periphery

   e. Gloved hands are always protected by creating a cuff of the drape edge

   f. Once placed in position, sterile drapes are not to be moved or shifted; a contaminated drape is removed by the circulator

3. **All items used within a sterile field are sterile**

   a. They are properly packaged

   b. They are properly sterilized, stored, and handled to maintain sterility

   c. Before sterile items are dispensed to a sterile field, the non-sterile person checks the package integrity, the chemical process indicator, and, if present, the expiration date

4. **All items introduced into a sterile field are dispensed by methods that maintain the sterility of the item and the integrity of the sterile field**

   a. A sterile package is opened from the far side first to avoid reaching over the sterile field

   b. All wrapper tails should be secured when supplies are presented to the sterile field to avoid contamination (wrapper edges are considered contaminated)

   c. The inside of envelope and square fold wrapped packages is considered sterile except for a 1-inch margin around the edge

   d. Peel packs are considered sterile to the inside of the heat seal only; the flaps should be peeled back to avoid tearing, and the contents must not be allowed to slide over the edge of the package

   e. Sterile items are presented to the scrubbed person or dispensed on the sterile field; sharp and/or heavy objects are presented to the scrubbed person or dispensed on a separate surface

   f. When dispensing solutions to the sterile field

   The entire content of the bottle is poured, or the remainder is discarded.

   The solution receptacle is placed near the edge of the table or held by the scrubbed person to avoid the unsterile person reaching over the sterile field

   Splashing is avoided to prevent strike-through contamination

5. **A sterile field should be constantly monitored and maintained**

   a. The sterile field should be prepared as close as possible to the scheduled time of use and not covered

   b. Unguarded sterile fields are considered contaminated

   c. Every team member watches for events which may compromise the sterile field and initiates corrective action if needed

   d. Tables are considered sterile only at the table level. Anything falling over the table edge is unsterile; gloved fingers/hands should not go over the edge of a draped table to move it

   e. Whenever a sterile barrier is permeated, contamination has occurred; the item should be removed from the sterile field, and the barrier must be removed or covered

   f. Conversation is kept to a minimum in the OR

   g. Tubing and cables for equipment are secured on the sterile field with a non-perforating device

   h. Items of doubtful sterility are considered unsterile and discarded. "When in doubt, throw it out"

6. **All personnel moving around or within a sterile field do so in a manner to maintain the integrity of the sterile field**

   a. Scrubbed persons keep arms and hands within the parameters of the sterile field

   b. Scrubbed team members move from sterile areas to sterile areas; if they must change positions, they turn back to back or face to face while maintaining a safe distance

   c. Scrubbed team members stay close to the sterile field and do not leave the room

   d. Scrubbed persons avoid changing levels and are seated only when the entire surgical procedure will be performed at this level

   e. Unscrubbed team members move from unsterile areas to unsterile areas, maintaining an awareness of the need for distance from the sterile field. Unsterile members should maintain a distance of at least 12–18 inches

   f. Scrubbed and unscrubbed persons approach sterile areas facing them and do not walk between two sterile areas

   g. Sterile dressing materials are applied prior to the removal of surgical drapes to avoid contaminating the wound

Show What You Know

Directions
Each of the numbered items or incomplete statements in this section is followed by answers or by completions of the statement. Select the ONE lettered answer or completion that is BEST in each case.

1. A chemical agent used to inhibit the growth of microorganisms on skin and mucous membranes is a/an:

    A. sporicide
    B. disinfectant
    C. antihistamine
    D. antiseptic

2. The process of destroying microorganisms on inanimate (nonliving) objects is:

    A. sanitation
    B. sterilization
    C. disinfection
    D. decontamination

3. The procedure for destroying pathogens at the end of the procedure is:

    A. surgical asepsis
    B. surgical conscience
    C. terminal sterilization
    D. sterilization

4. The safest, most practical means for sterilizing heat- and moisture-stable items is:

    A. saturated steam under pressure
    B. ethylene oxide gas
    C. activated glutaraldehyde
    D. boiling water

5. The minimal temperature required to kill bacterial spores is:

    A. 212°F (100°C)
    B. 250°F (121°C)
    C. 270°F (132°C)
    D. 32°F (0°C)

6. The Bowie-Dick test must be run daily in which of the following types of sterilizers?

    A. ethylene oxide gas
    B. hydrogen peroxide plasma
    C. peracetic acid
    D. Prevacuum

7. Which of the following types of sterilizers would require a drying cycle?

    A. peracetic acid
    B. gravity displacement
    C. ethylene oxide gas
    D. ionizing radiation

8. Aeration is essential following sterilization by:

    A. ionizing radiation
    B. hydrogen peroxide plasma
    C. activated glutaraldehyde
    D. ethylene oxide gas

9. In the middle of the surgical procedure, a critical stainless steel instrument is contaminated and there is no sterile replacement. Which time setting would be selected for the flash autoclave?

    A. 3 minutes
    B. 10 minutes
    C. 15 minutes
    D. 30 minutes

10. The most reliable means of monitoring the effectiveness of the sterilizer that ensures sterilization parameters have been met is:

    A. biological
    B. mechanical
    C. chemical
    D. none, monitoring is not required

11. When packaging instruments for sterilization, instruments should be:

    A. fully assembled
    B. lubricated
    C. placed in closely nested section
    D. left open and placed on a rack

12. When storing sterile packs, you should place them:

    A. in open cabinets near a vent
    B. behind packs with older dates
    C. on their sides
    D. in areas of high humidity

13. Items that contact sterile tissue and must be sterilized are considered:

    A. critical
    B. semicritical
    C. noncritical
    D. restricted

14. When disinfecting instruments for use, you would do all of the following except:

    A. rinse immediately before putting in the germicide
    B. clean to reduce the bioburden
    C. ensure that all surfaces are exposed to the germicidal agent
    D. rinse thoroughly with sterile distilled water following contact with the germicide

15. The disinfectant that should not be used on lensed instruments due to the potential for loosening the "cement" around the lens is:

    A. glutaraldehyde
    B. isopropyl alcohol
    C. chlorine compounds
    D. phenolic compounds

16. Spillage of blood that occurs during surgery should be:

    A. covered with an impervious drape
    B. sectioned off from traffic
    C. cleaned up at the end of the procedure
    D. cleaned up immediately

17. The purpose of keeping doors to the operating room closed is to:

    A. decrease noise level
    B. maintain negative pressure
    C. maintain positive pressure
    D. maintain proper temperature

18. The purpose of washing the hands prior to the surgical scrub is to:

    A. render them sterile
    B. remove gross soil and transient microorganisms
    C. protect personnel from contracting disease from the patient
    D. remove resident microorganisms

19. When draping a sterile field, the scrubbed person would do all of the following *except*:

    A. drape from the periphery to the operative site
    B. protect the gloved hand with a cuff
    C. drape the patient and all furniture and equipment to be included in the sterile field
    D. hold drapes in a compact position above the waist level

20. When dispensing sterile items to a sterile field, the circulator would:

    A. open the far side of the package last
    B. stand as close to the sterile field as possible

    C. ensure that wrapper tails are properly secured
    D. recap the remaining portion of the sterile saline for dispensing later during the procedure

21. The scrub has completed the sterile setup when notified that the surgeon will be 30 minutes late. He or she would:

    A. remain with the sterile field until further notified
    B. cover the sterile items and take a break
    C. break scrub and get directions from the supervisor
    D. find a comfortable stool and wait for further instruction

22. Bioburden refers to:

    A. an agent that kills microorganisms on inanimate objects
    B. the process of destroying all microorganisms, including spores
    C. inhibition of bacterial growth
    D. the degree of microbial contamination

23. Procedures performed at the end of a surgical case to protect the health care worker who will be handling the surgical instruments in the sterile processing department are known as:

    A. terminal disinfection and sterilization
    B. surgical conscience
    C. strike-through contamination
    D. sanitation

24. Which of the following is not an acceptable method of transporting contaminated instruments down the hall following a surgical procedure?

    A. in a closed case cart
    B. covered in a plastic bag
    C. in an open-mesh bottom tray
    D. any of the above are acceptable methods

25. If the temperature on the steam sterilizer reads 270°F, what should the pressure reading be?

    A. 15 to 17 psi
    B. 20 to 25 psi
    C. 27 psi
    D. 30 to 35 psi

Answers & Rationales

1. **D.** **Rationale:** Antiseptics are chemical agents that are used to inhibit the growth of microorganisms on animate (living) objects.

2. **C.** **Rationale:** Disinfection is the process of destroying microorganisms on inanimate (nonliving) objects.

3. **C.** **Rationale:** Terminal sterilization is the procedure for destroying pathogens at the end of the

procedure to protect the health care worker from exposure to these pathogens.

4. **A.** **Rationale:** Saturated steam under pressure is considered the safest, most practical method for sterilizing fabric, metal, and fluid—anything that is not damaged by heat or moisture.

5. **B.** **Rationale:** The minimal temperature required to kill bacterial spores is 250°F (121°C).

6. D. **Rationale:** The Bowie-Dick test must be run daily in the prevacuum sterilizer to assure complete removal of air. Air and steam cannot occupy the same space at the same time, and sterilization cannot occur if air is present.

7. B. **Rationale:** A gravity displacement sterilizer would require a drying cycle, as there is no vacuum present for the rapid withdrawal of steam, and sterile items would be wet with steam.

8. D. **Rationale:** Ethylene oxide is a toxic gas that requires removal (aeration) prior to use of articles sterilized by this method.

9. A. **Rationale:** Three minutes is the time required to flash (temperature 270°F or 132°C) a small number of instruments.

10. A. **Rationale:** Biological monitors (spore tests) are the most reliable means of monitoring sterilizer effectiveness. Live agent-sensitive spores of nonpathogenic organisms are placed in a test pack, run through the proper cycle, and then tested for viability. *Bacillus stearothermophilus* spores are used to monitor the effectiveness of steam autoclaves, and *Bacillus subtilis* spores are used for ethylene oxide gas sterilizers. Both spores can be **used to monitor** the effectiveness of STERIS® or Sterrad®.

11. D. **Rationale:** When instruments are packaged for sterilization, they must be left open and placed on a rack or "stringer" to ensure that they stay open so that the sterilant can reach all areas of the instruments.

12. B. **Rationale:** When sterile packs are stored, they should be placed behind packs with older dates (stock rotation), away from vents, and in closed cabinets.

13. A. **Rationale:** Critical items are those which, if not properly sterilized, would present a high risk of infection (i.e., those used for dissection of tissue or any time the body's first line of defense is broken).

14. A. **Rationale:** When instruments are disinfected for use, they should be clean to reduce the bioburden, be dry to avoid diluting the solution, have all surfaces exposed to the germicidal agent, and be rinsed thoroughly after removal from the germicide to ensure the removal of toxic residue before being used on a patient.

15. B. **Rationale:** Lensed instruments must never be left to soak in isopropyl alcohol, as that could dissolve the "cement" holding the lens in place.

16. D. **Rationale:** Spillage of blood or body fluids that occurs during surgery should be cleaned up immediately by the circulator wearing proper protection and using a high-powered germicidal agent. This is referred to as concurrent disinfection.

17. C. **Rationale:** Doors to the operating room should remain closed to maintain positive air pressure. Filtered air enters from above the operating table and exits through a vent near the floor, forcing dirty air out.

18. B. **Rationale:** Gross soil and transient organisms are removed by washing the hands prior to the surgical hand scrub. When performed properly, the surgical scrub renders the hands surgically clean.

19. A. **Rationale:** When draping sterile fields, the scrubbed person always protects the gloved hands with a cuff, holds drapes in a compact position above the waist level to avoid contamination by sterile drapes falling below the table level, and drapes all furniture and equipment to be included in the sterile field (from the nearest area to the farthest away to avoid inadvertent contamination). When the patient is draped, the drapes are first placed at the operative site and then extended outward toward the periphery.

20. C. **Rationale:** When dispensing sterile items, the circulator would stand at least 1 foot from the sterile field, open the far side of the package first to avoid reaching over the sterile contents, and secure the wrapper tails to prevent the wrapper edges (nonsterile) from touching sterile areas. Sterile solution bottles are not to be recapped for later use because of possible inadvertent contamination while opening, pouring, and recapping the bottle.

21. A. **Rationale:** Sterile tables are not to be covered because of the difficulty in uncovering them without contamination. To break scrub for further instruction would not be cost-effective. Once prepared, sterile fields cannot be left unguarded. Sitting on stools is not recommended, as gown areas below table level are considered contaminated and the hands should not rest in the "lap."

22. D. **Rationale:** Bioburden refers to the degree of microbial contamination on an object; a disinfectant is an agent that kills microorganisms on inanimate objects; sterilization is the process of destroying all microorganisms including spores; bacteriostasis is the inhibition of bacterial growth.

23. A. **Rationale:** Terminal disinfection and sterilization are the procedures performed after the surgical procedure to protect the health care worker in the sterile processing department who will handle the surgical instruments (this includes placing all instruments used during the case in the washer sterilizer).

24. **C.** **Rationale:** Instruments should be covered for the safe transport to the decontamination area and not in an open tray.

25. **C.** **Rationale:** The addition of 27 pounds per square inch is required to raise the temperature in the chamber to 270°F; 15 to 17 psi is required to raise the temperature to 250°F.

Part II: Deciphering a Surgical Schedule

The following mock surgery schedule will be used to answer several questions pertaining to surgical asepsis. The same schedule, or a similar one, will be used in subsequent chapters to ask questions about the content of the chapter.

Rm# time	Surgeon	Procedure	Anest.	Rm# time	Surgeon	Procedure	Anest.
Rm00				**Rm07**			
OC	Dr. Z	Rt. Knee Arthroscopy	Gen.	7:00	Dr. M	Rhinoplasty	Gen.
OC	Dr. C	Craniotomy	Gen.	TF	Dr. M	Lipoma removal	MAC
OC	Dr. Z	Angioplasty	Gen.				
Rm01				**Rm08**			
7:00	Dr. X	Lobectomy	Gen.	11:00	Dr. E	Bovine Thrombectomy	MAC
TF	Dr. X	Thoracotomy	Gen.				
TF	Dr. X	Tracheostomy	Gen.				
Rm02				**Rm09**			
7:00	Dr. B	Splenectomy	Gen.	8:30	Dr. T	Cholecystectomy	Gen.
TF	Dr. B	Gastrectomy	Gen.	TF	Dr. T	Palatoplasty	Gen.
Rm03				**Rm10**			
7:00	Dr. A	Cystoscopy	MAC	7:00	Dr. K	Nephrectomy	Gen.
TF	Dr. A	Cystoplasty	Gen.	TF	Dr. K	Choledocholithotripsy	MAC
12:30	Dr. F	Pyleogram	MAC	TF	Dr. K	Hepatic resection	Gen.
3:00	Dr. F	Cystocele repair	Gen.				
Rm04				**Rm11**			
7:00	Dr. Y	Carpal tunnel release	Gen.	7:00	Dr. L	Colposcope	Gen.
TF	Dr. Y	Fasciotomy	Gen.	12:00	Dr. L	Mastectomy	Gen.
Rm05				**Rm12**			
7:00	Dr. G	Trans-sphenoidal Adenectomy	Gen.	7:00	Dr. W	Trans-metatarsal amputation	Gen.
TF	Dr. G	Trans-urethral resection of the prostate	Gen.	TF	Dr. W	Osteotomy	Gen.
					Dr. W	Arthroplasty Right Knee	Gen.
TF	Dr. G	Bletharoplasty	Gen.	TF			
Rm06				**Rm13**			
7:00	Dr. R	Lumbar Laminectomy	Gen.	7:00	Dr. O	Hysterectomy	Gen.

The following questions should be answered using the surgery schedule above

1. An implant for use in the knee arthroscopy needed to be processed. What indicator should be used to ensure that there are no living microbes or spores on this?
   A. Chemical indicator
   B. Bowie dick
   C. Biologic indicator
   D. Julian date

2. The splenectomy in Room 2 became more complicated than expected. Many of the instruments in the case have significant bioburden. How should this be handled?
   A. Instruments should be placed directly into the ultrasonic cleaner to remove bioburden
   B. Instruments should be run through the washer sterilizer and then hand washed

    C. Instruments should be disassembled and washed, then placed in the washer sterilizer

    D. Instruments should be rinsed with saline, then run through the washer sterilizer

3. The Surgical Technologist in Room 5 is in a hurry and needs an instrument that is peel packed and stored in the instrument room. When she obtains the instrument, the expiration date shows that the package needs to be reprocessed. What should she do?

    A. Repackage the item and set it aside for reprocessing

    B. Unpackage the instrument and use the flash sterilizer

    C. Use the instrument if the integrity of the package is intact

    D. Wrap the instrument and use the flash sterilizer

4. When the splenectomy experienced complications, there was blood spilled on the OR floor. The circulating nurse needed to decontaminate the area. What type of agent would most likely be used?

    A. Bleach

    B. Glutaraldehyde

    C. Sterile water

    D. Hospital Grade Disinfectant

5. The scrub scheduled to assist in the Cystoscopies in Room 3 has retrieved an item from the Cidex solution. This item has a lumen. What precautions does the scrub need to take?

    A. The item needs to be flushed and rinsed well with sterile 0.5% alcohol solution

    B. The item needs to be rinsed and the lumen flushed with sterile water

    C. The item is safe for patient use after aeration has occurred

    D. The item must be reprocessed in STERIS solution before use

6. The same item must be reprocessed after use. What does the scrub need to remember?

    A. The item should be damp, with water in the lumen before being processed

    B. The item should be cleaned and dried before placing in solution

    C. The item must be processed in a closed unventilated room

    D. The solution can be used indefinitely

7. The scrub tech in Room 11 will need to process an item using Sterrad. How long will this process take?

    A. One hour

    B. 20–30 minutes

    C. 10 hours

    D. 16 hours

8. The Surgical Technologist in Room 11 has set up the scope when the surgery is postponed. The scope has been processed with STERIS. What is important for the ST to remember?

    A. The item processed with STERIS cannot be stored

    B. The item processed with STERIS must be placed into a rigid container for storage until surgery is rescheduled

    C. The item processed with STERIS must be peel packed for storage

    D. The item processed with STERIS must be wrapped in muslin for safe storage

9. The ST who scrubbed in the On Call arthroscopy needs to process the instruments after the surgery. There are several instruments that have multiple parts. How should this be handled?

    A. The instruments should remain assembled throughout the process

    B. The parts should be disassembled, washed by hand and reassembled for processing

    C. The parts should be disassembled and processed

    D. The parts should be separated into multiple trays for processing

10. The Surgical Technologist in Room 4 is finished with cases, and is helping the turn over team process rooms. What must he remember when helping this team?

   A. It is not necessary to wipe down the surgical table after every surgery, new linen, however, must be placed on the table.
   B. You must use a clean mop-head for each room
   C. ORs are terminally cleaned every other day
   D. OR tables should not be moved during the cleaning process

Answers & Rationales

1. **C. Rationale:** The only way to ensure sterility is the use of biologic indicators. The result of this test should be known before an implant is inserted. The use of other monitors will guarantee that the sterilizer has reached the appropriate temperature, humidity, or length of time. This cannot, however, ensure that the item is sterile. It is only through the use of biologic indicators that sterility is confirmed.

2. **C. Rationale:** Instruments with a lot of bioburden must be washed manually before they are processed through the washer sterilizer. Generally, the ST will rinse instruments in sterile water throughout the procedure to reduce the amount of bioburden dried onto the surfaces. However, occasionally, this cannot be done. When the instruments are being prepared for processing, it may be necessary for them to be cleaned manually. STs should never use saline to wash instruments as this may pit the surface.

3. **B. Rationale:** If the instrument is needed immediately, the ST will not have the time to have the instrument reprocessed. The use of flash sterilization should only be utilized when other options are not viable. If flash is used, the instrument should be unwrapped and placed in a special pan or a closed flash sterilization tray.

4. **D. Rationale:** While several of these are commonly used disinfectants, the most commonly used type of disinfectants used during surgery to clean spills are Phenolic compounds or quats, depending on the hospital. While chlorine bleaches are sometimes used for this purpose, their use is discouraged due to the possibility of damage to certain equipment, as well as its corrosive effects. Glutaraldehyde is not routinely used in cleaning of floors or surfaces,

and sterile water has no germicidal properties.

5. **B. Rationale:** Instruments processed with Cidex must be rinsed with sterile water before use as the chemical is toxic to tissues. This rinse must also include a flushing of any lumens to ensure that the chemical residue has been removed. This is done with sterile distilled water prior to the use of the object.

6. **B. Rationale:** Items processed in Cidex must be clean and dry before processing. Any moisture may dilute the solution, causing it to be ineffective. Gross bioburden should always be removed before processing any instrument or equipment. Glutaraldehyde must be used in a well ventilated area, and the expiration date should always be checked before use.

7. **A. Rationale:** The actual processing time for Sterrad is one hour. There is no aeration time needed for items processed with Sterrad.

8. **A. Rationale:** Items processed with STERIS cannot be stored. They are processed for immediate use. Therefore, the ST will need to reprocess the item.

9. **C. Rationale:** Instruments and items with pieces that are detachable should be disassembled before the processing begins. All of the items should be kept together while they are being processed, to avoid losing pieces.

10. **B. Rational:** Mop heads should be changed to new for every room. Tables should be wiped down after every case, and tables should be moved, and rolled through a disinfectant. Terminal cleaning will be performed daily with a rotation schedule for deeper cleaning of walls, vents, ceilings, and other areas.

A patient entering the operating room is entrusting his or her life to the members of the surgical team. Remember, the patient is not Dr. Green's gallbladder; he or she is someone's family member, friend, or loved one. Honor their trust by doing everything possible to meet the needs of the patient and make the surgical experience the best it can be. Each patient brings unique problems to the table, and should always be approached with a personalized plan of care. There are specific needs for different segments of the population, and these needs must be understood by the Surgical Technologist before surgery begins. Patients may be extremely nervous or agitated when they are brought to the surgical suite. The ST must appreciate what the patient is going through in order to give the best possible patient care.

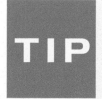

TIP   **How to Answer Surgical Patient Questions**

Understanding the psychology of the surgical patient may not seem important at first. The issues are very complex and impact many aspects of patient care. When faced with a question on surgical patients, the Surgical Technologist must remember that each patient is an individual. This means that while there are distinct patterns in behavior and thought among groups, every person may not re-act the same. Understanding some basic guidelines regarding patient care is essential for the ST. Remember that while each patient is an individual, there are guidelines that should be followed to ensure safety.

Surgery is divided into three distinct periods: preoperative, intraoperative, and postoperative. Certain things occur during each phase of surgery. For example, patients are evaluated during the pre-operative phase of surgery. This will include baseline monitoring, assessments, consents, and other variables which must be evaluated before any patient is brought to the surgical suite. During the intra-operative phase, the patient is induced, positioned prepped, and catheterized. Post operatively, the patient is evaluated, transferred and must recover from the procedure. Each phase has its own dangers that must be known before the next phase may begin. The ST must rely upon knowledge gained from experience and texts to answer these questions.

Example:
If a surgeon needs the results from a tissue specimen during a procedure, how will the specimen be sent?

A. In formalin
B. In a container or on Telfa without solution
C. On a slide as a smear
D. In a culture tube

To answer this question, you need to understand what the reason is for this specimen. Generally, specimens that need to be evaluated immediately should be passed off the field dry. They are immediately sent to the lab for evaluation. When a specimen is placed in formalin, it is usually reserved for a routine analysis, and cultures are generally used to establish infections. Therefore, the best answer to this question would be B.

The Preoperative Patient

I. Patient Needs and Bill of Rights

   A. Physical needs and rights
     1. Capacity for the adequate exchange of oxygen and carbon dioxide
     2. Adequate hydration
     3. Nutrition and the best possible state of health
     4. Adequate elimination of waste
     5. Sleep, rest, and warmth

   B. Spiritual needs
     1. Support for religious beliefs
     2. Respect for the expression of religious beliefs
     3. Visit with clergy
     4. Right to refuse treatment

   C. Emotional needs
     1. Freedom from fear or anxiety: fears include the unknown, loss of self-control, financial loss, disfigurement, pain, death, loss of security, and incompetent personnel
     2. Self-esteem, security, acceptance, and recognition
     3. Stress factors: family concerns, being in a strange environment, employment issues, and financial concerns

D. Social and cultural needs
  1. Respect for patients' differences

E. Helping to meet the patient's psychological needs
  1. Observe patient behaviors.
  2. Listen closely to what the patient says.
  3. Give verbal encouragement to the patient.
  4. Reassure the patient: convey warmth, acceptance, respect, and caring.
  5. Report any observed needs to
     a. Surgeon (concerns relating to surgery)
     b. Anesthesia provider (concerns relating to anesthesia)
     c. Registered nurse (general concerns and/or observations)

F. Patients with special needs
  1. *Pediatric patients:* They are not "small adults." Needs differ based on age (infants, birth to 18 months; toddlers, 1½ to 2½ years; preschoolers, 2½ to 5 years; school-aged children, 6 to 12 years; adolescents, 12 to 18 years). The special needs of the pediatric patient include
     a. Pediatric patients have an increased need for oxygen and food because of increased metabolism. Children under age 2 are generally scheduled for surgery early in the day to decrease their time without nourishment and fluid. Infants may receive formula up to 6 hours before the surgery and clear liquids up to 2 hours before the surgery.
     b. Infants become dehydrated rapidly (especially with vomiting and diarrhea), creating an imbalance of electrolytes. Fluid and blood loss are closely monitored (sponges weighed) and replaced in a careful and exacting manner using special catheters and infusion sets. As little as 30 cc of blood loss may need to be replaced in the neonate.
     c. Body temperature can change rapidly due to their large skin surface in relationship to their small volume. Core body temperature is continuously monitored using a rectal thermometer. Heat loss during surgery is prevented by the use of warm blankets, increased room temperature (80°F for infants and 75°F for a child), the use of heat sources such as a radiant heat lamp, warm solutions (prep, irrigating, and IV), hyperthermia blankets, forced air warming blanket, and/or thermal head coverings.
     d. Because of their narrow airway, infants and children are more prone to respiratory obstruction and must be monitored closely (chest movements should be observed for retraction, and oximetry readings should be taken).
     e. Infants are more susceptible to infection, demanding meticulous surgical aseptic technique on the part of all team members.
     f. Separation from the mother is traumatic for infants over 6 months, toddlers, and preschool children. The mother's presence is encouraged whenever possible. Favorite toys are also important for children from 6 months to school age. Be aware of the age and developmental level and provide age-appropriate emotional support. Provide emotional support to parents.
     g. Anesthesia induction for children is generally performed by inhalation and requires more active assistance by the circulator.
     h. Positioning requires special devices such as rolled gauze for restraint straps, wash cloths for chest rolls, foam rings and pads.
     i. Instruments, suture, and supplies are selected with consideration given to the size of the patient.
  2. *Geriatric patients (over 65 years old)*
     a. Assessment for cognitive function (memory, learning), sensory functions (vision, auditory, tactile), anxiety (self-esteem, fears), mental state (will to live), and physical limitations (stiff joints, malnutrition) is essential.

   b. Special needs

Prevent the loss of heat. Loss of subcutaneous tissue and reduced muscle mass leads to hypothermia.

Care in positioning must be used to avoid pain in joints or skin damage (provide extra padding, move slowly and gently, lift, do not slide).

Skin loses its elasticity and is more prone to shearing forces; there is increased risk for skin breakdown; use hyposensitive tape.

Because of altered circulation, antiembolic measures are used to avoid venostasis and clot formation.

Careful monitoring of vital signs is essential.

Geriatric patients are more prone to infection, pulmonary complications, urinary problems, and drug reactions. Patient may experience sensory deficit, have a slower reaction time, and may become disorientated especially under stress.

   3. *Obese patients (at least 20% overweight)*
      a. Common complications are an overworked heart, hypertension, varicose veins, pulmonary function problems, gallbladder disease, osteoarthritis, diabetes mellitus, and malnutrition.
      b. Special needs

Transporting and lifting: use mechanical devices.

Since obese people are often self-conscious about their weight, avoid unnecessary exposure.

Anesthesia: induction, intubation, and maintenance may be more difficult.

Surgical intervention: more difficult and requires longer instruments and more retraction.

Positioning on the operating table is more difficult and requires more assistance.

Vascular complications: obese patients are more prone to clot formation and require antiembolic measures.

Delayed healing: because of decreased circulation in adipose tissue.

   4. *Patients with diabetes*
      a. Common complications of diabetes mellitus

Dehydration and electrolyte imbalance

Infection

Inadequate circulation

Delayed wound healing

Nervous system disorders

      b. Special needs

Monitor blood sugar levels.

Monitor changes in insulin requirements.

Give intravenous dextrose.

Use antiembolic stockings or devices.

Observe and guard skin integrity.

Use hyposensitive tape to attach dressings.

Air or water mattresses are useful in a pressure area over bony prominences.

SURGERY HINT

Have long instruments and standing stools available in the room when working on an obese patient. Check bed weight limits and have positioning devices ready. Never attempt to position an obese patient without extra assistance.

Allow for extra time during the intubation and for exposure.

5. **Malnutrition**
   a. Problems associated with malnutrition
      Inadequate wound healing
      Alterations in blood clotting
      Increased susceptibility to infection
      Increased risk of morbidity (complications) and
         mortality (death)
   b. Special needs
      Nutritional supplements to counteract negative nitrogen balance (pro-
         vided by proteins) and build up plasma albumin; supplied by oral
         intake, nasogastric tube feedings, gastrostomy tube feedings, or
         intravenous infusion
      Hyperalimentation: total parenteral nutrition (TPN), in which essen-
         tial nutrients are delivered into a vein through central venous can-
         nulation

6. **Immunocompromised patient**
   a. Includes the very young or old, patients with autoimmune diseases,
      transplant recipients, patients with AIDS
   b. Complications of the surgical patient with AIDS
      Overall poor health
      Presence of external and internal lesions
      Swollen, painful lymph nodes
   c. Care of the surgical patient with AIDS
      Careful handling to avoid disturbing lesions
      Use of comfort measures, physical and verbal
      Use of extra personnel when lifting and positioning
      Careful placement of monitoring devices and electrosurgical unit
         (ESU) grounding pad

G. **Patients' rights**
   1. Considerate and respectful care
   2. Complete information regarding surgery
   3. Refuse treatment
   4. Privacy
   5. Confidentiality of records (HIPAA regulations)
   6. Be advised of and refuse to participate in human experimentation
      and/or research
   7. Expect continuity of care before, during, and after
      surgery
   8. Know hospital rules and regulations applicable to conduct

H. **Health and wellness**
   1. Physical health
   2. Nutrition and metabolism
   3. Mental health
   4. Stress: internal/external; physical/psychological
   5. Stress reduction techniques
      a. Relaxation/meditation
      b. Exercise
      c. Biofeedback
      d. Defense mechanisms
   6. Alternative healing methodologies
      a. Massage therapy
      b. Touch therapy
      c. Aroma therapy
      d. Music therapy
      e. Herbal remedies
      f. Acupuncture

II. **Consent for Surgery**

A. **Concepts**
   1. Written medical consent is based on hospital policies
   2. Informed consent is required for each procedure involving surgery or hazardous therapy and must include understandable language.

B. **Types of consent**
   1. General consent: authorizes the physician in charge of the hospital staff to render treatment as he or she deems necessary
   2. Surgical consent: authorizes performance of surgical intervention
   3. Anesthesia administration: the part of the surgical consent that lists the anesthesia provider, risks, and possible alternatives. Some facilities require a separate anesthesia consent
   4. Sterilization consent: some states require spouse's signature
   5. Blanket consent: authorizes any related procedure deemed necessary by the surgeon if unforeseen circumstances are found

C. **Purposes of consent**
   1. Protect the patient from unapproved and unwanted procedures.
   2. Protect the surgeon and health care facility and its personnel from claims of unauthorized procedures.

D. **Contents of consent**
   1. Patient's legal name and signature
   2. Surgeon's name and signature
   3. Procedure to be performed (no abbreviations) in medical terms and lay terms
   4. Signature of witness
   5. Date and time of signatures

E. **Responsibility for consent**
   1. The surgeon is ultimately responsible for obtaining consent and explaining to the patient and/or family member the following:
      a. Nature of proposed procedure, including its necessity
      b. Benefits, risks, and potential complications
      c. Alternative treatment options
   2. Both the anesthesia provider and the circulator are responsible for ensuring that the operative permit/informed consent form is correct, on the chart, and is properly signed and witnessed before bringing the patient into the room and beginning the procedure.

F. **Persons authorized to witness consents are a physician, nurse, or other hospital employee who attest to identification of the patient, voluntary signing, and mental competence of signatory.**

G. **Legal guidelines for consents**
   1. Consent is given freely and without coercion.
   2. Patient is of legal age or is an emancipated minor (married or independently earning a living, or has given birth).
   3. Parent or legal guardian must sign for a minor. (*Note:* A spouse of legal age may sign for emancipated minor.)
   4. If the patient is mentally incompetent, a legal guardian (person or agency) must sign, or in absence of a legal guardian, a court of competent jurisdiction may legalize the procedure.
   5. If the patient is unconscious or intoxicated, a responsible relative or guardian must sign.
   6. Consent must be signed prior to the administration of preoperative sedative medications and/or entry into surgery or area for treatment.
   7. Hospital policy or state law dictates who may sign a consent form: parent, legal guardian or agency, next of kin, administrator, or court order.

8. Consent alternatives in life-threatening circumstances may be by telephone, e-mail, telegram, fax, or by two consulting physicians (not including operating surgeon) or by administrative consent.

III. **The Patient Record**

   A. **Legal document:** may go to court and must be accurate, complete, and objective with no erasures

   B. **If there is an error, strike through with a single line, initial, and date it**

   C. **Confidential:** protected by HIPAA

   D. **Guide to patient's history, current condition, and treatment**

   E. **Documentation verified before surgery**
      1. History and physical
      2. Documentation of treatment
      3. Diagnostic and therapeutic reports, such as blood studies, urinalysis, chest x-ray, and consultation reports
      4. Signed forms: consent forms for surgery, sterilization, disposal of extremity, etc
      5. Preoperative preparation (preoperative checklist)
      6. Special patient concerns, such as allergies
      7. Record of vital signs (baseline for surgery)
      8. Physician's order sheet
      9. Documentation related to Universal Protocol to Prevent Wrong Person, Wrong Site Surgery

   F. **Intraoperative documentation**
      1. Anesthesia records
      2. Intraoperative procedure record
      3. Count sheets for sponges, sharps, and instruments
      4. Surgeon's progress notes
      5. Surgeon's dictated record of operative procedure(s)
      6. Pathology report
      7. Charge slips, if required by the facility
      8. Specimen record book, if required by the facility
      9. Laboratory requisitions
         a. *Pathology:* for organ or tissue
         b. *Cytology:* for smears, fluids, and washings
         c. *Bacteribiology:* for cultures and sensitivity tests (acid-fast, aerobic, anaerobic)

IV. **Preoperative Routine**

   A. **Lab tests**
      1. Complete blood count (CBC)
         Hemoglobin: 12–14 grams; less than 10 indicates anemia
         Hematocrit: percentage of red blood cells: 45%
         Red blood cell count (RBC): 5 million
         White blood cell count (WBC): 5000–10,000; elevated WBC indicates infection
         Differential count: measures the percentage of each type of WBC
      2. Urinalysis (UA): pH = 6, bacterial count over 5000 indicates GU infection, protein or albumin may indicate renal disease, specific gravity denotes concentration of urine, normal specific gravity is 1.001–1.035, and high specific gravity indicates dehydration.
      3. Blood chemistry
      4. Prothrombin time (if on anticoagulant therapy)
      5. Type and cross match for blood (if there is a need for blood replacement)
      6. Drug toxicity/screening

B. Other diagnostic tests
  1. Electrocardiogram (EKG)
  2. Radiology: x-ray, CT scan, MRI

C. Photographs (particularly for plastic surgery)

D. Complete history and physical examination

E. Completed preoperative treatments as ordered (e.g., enema, surgical skin prep, and urinary catheterization)

F. Preoperative assessment by the anesthesia provider and assignment of ASA (Anesthesia Society of America) classification (classes I to VI, with I being best health and lowest risk)

G. Identification of allergies, concerns, or limitations

H. Operative and other special permits

I. Vital signs for baseline

J. NPO (nothing by mouth) at midnight unless otherwise ordered

K. Morning of surgery: removal of prostheses (dentures, wigs, etc.); bladder elimination; bath/shower; clean gown; secure patient possessions; administration of preoperative medication; removal of hairpins, nail polish, and makeup; oral hygiene; and family visit

L. Provide safe and quiet environment.

V. Patient Identification, Transfer, and Transport

A. Transfer and transport the correct patient for the correct surgeon and the correct procedure in the correct location (top priority).
  1. Introduce self to the patient.
  2. Read the patient's identification band. Ask the patient to state the name and ensure information matches
  3. Compare the identification band with the name on the patient's record/chart, computerized patient labels, and name on surgical schedule. *(Note: Basic information included on the patient label is the patient's name, age, hospital number, and physician.)*
  4. Ask the patient to verbally state the name and pertinent information, if possible; report any discrepancy to the nurse.

B. Patient transfer
  1. *To stretcher* (after greeting and identification)
    a. Ensure that the hospital gown is on, prosthesis and jewelry removed, and the bladder is emptied.
    b. Request visitors to leave, screen the patient, cover the patient with a clean cotton sheet/blanket, and avoid unnecessary exposure.
    c. Position the stretcher alongside bed, raise the bed to stretcher level, lock wheels, and assist the patient in moving; use good body mechanics (get help if needed), and give special attention to tubes, catheters, IVs, traction, or other apparatus.
    d. Ensure maximum patient comfort and safety: pillows, arms, and hands fully on stretcher and covered with sheet, restraint strap fastened, side rails up, IV properly positioned above the patient.
  2. *To wheelchair:* align the wheelchair alongside the bed, flip up footrests and lock wheels, assist the patient to don bathrobe and slippers, assist the patient as needed in moving, and cover legs with sheet or cotton blanket.

C. Patient transport to surgery holding area (by stretcher or wheelchair)
  1. Take the patient and record to the OR.
  2. When using a stretcher
    a. *along corridors:* push the stretcher from the head, patient feet first
    b. *into elevator:* pull the stretcher from the head, patient head first into elevator, feet first off elevator

3. A minimum of two persons are needed for the transportation of a patient in a bed or on a special frame, a patient receiving oxygen, a patient in traction, or whenever there are doubts or concerns about patient safety.

4. Avoid unnecessary talking, abrupt movements, banging into walls or furniture; proceed at safe speed. If patient is in traction, do not let the traction weights swing. Do not allow the patient to hold onto the side rails as hands may be inadvertently injured.

5. Never leave the patient alone on a stretcher.

6. Observe the patient for any changes or reactions to medications (difficulty in breathing, coughing, flushed face, perspiration, nausea, or undue anxiety).

7. Carefully observe the intravenous fluid to ensure that it is dripping into the drip chamber and the IV site is not swelling; observe other appliances which may be connected to the patient; carry drainage devices below bed level.

8. Report any untoward reactions or observations to the nurse.

The Intraoperative Patient

I. **Admitting the Patient to Surgery**

   A. **Receiving the patient in the OR**
     1. Patient is identified by the circulator (asks name, checks the name band against the chart and against the name on the surgical schedule).
     2. Convey warmth, respect, and caring.
     3. Check the chart for lab work, signed operative permit, history, physical, and doctor's orders completed
     4. Ask the patient to verbalize what procedure is being performed (including side on multiple sites/levels), when he or she last had something to eat or drink, and any known allergies.
     5. Nurse may take and record vital signs and start an IV if the anesthesia provider is not available.
     6. Ensure that the patient is warm and as comfortable and safe as possible.
     7. The Association of periOperative Registered Nurses (AORN) has developed a "Time Out" protocol to help ensure the correct surgery is being performed on the correct patient and correct site.

   B. **Transfer to the OR table ("bed" in presence of patient)**
     1. Lock wheels, assist the patient as needed, protect modesty, guide and secure tubes, and apply safety strap across thighs, two inches above knees.
     2. Patient may self-transfer with the help of at least two persons, one at the side of the gurney and the other at the side of the operating table, or need a four-person assisted transfer.
     3. Transfer devices include slider board, roller, backboard, or lift sheet.
     4. Use good body mechanics.
     5. Instruct the patient to uncross legs, secure arms at the side on the table, or place on padded armboard (not to exceed 90° abduction to avoid damage to the brachial plexus).

   C. **Preliminary preparation for patient positioning**
     1. *Operating table:* ensure that the table is an appropriate type and configuration for the procedure (orthopedic, urologic, fluoroscopic, etc.).
     2. *Special equipment and table attachments:* check safety (knee) strap, anesthesia screen or IV poles to separate sterile from nonsterile areas, lift sheet, armboard(s), wrist or armstrap, hand table, shoulder roll, shoulder braces, kidney rests, hip restraint, stirrups, metal footboard, headrest, pressure mattress or bean bag (air evacuation mattress), and/or other equipment or padding which may be needed.

D. Activities performed by anesthesia personnel before anesthesia induction
  1. *Assembly of equipment and supplies:* airways, endotracheal tubes, laryngoscope, suction catheters, labeled prefilled medication syringes
  2. *Patient care:* ensure patient warmth and comfort, check vital signs, attach monitoring devices (EKG, pulse oximeter, blood pressure cuff, bispectral index monitor, and temperature monitor), ensure intravenous access (peripheral or central), apply thermoregulatory devices (hyper/ hypothermia blanket, warmed air device), and inform patient of activities

E. *Role of the circulator during anesthesia induction:* correct identification of the patient; provide patient comfort and reassurance; ensure therapeutic environment and close doors leading to corridor; never leave a patient unguarded; never leave anesthesia care provider alone during the induction of and emergence from anesthesia; be ready to perform Sellick's maneuver (cricoid pressure) if needed; and assist with the assessment of blood loss, blood transfusion, and other procedures as requested

II. Positioning the Patient for Surgery

A. Critical factors in positioning patients for surgery
  1. *Type of anesthesia:* patients are anesthetized in the supine position and then repositioned for the surgical intervention as necessary under the direction of the anesthesia provider and the surgeon.
  2. *Incision site:* dorsal recumbent (supine) is chosen whenever possible.
  3. *Surgeon's preference:* when more than one position provides access to operative site
  4. *Safety:* airway access, IV access, security, and physiological and anatomical considerations
  5. *Qualifications for a good position*
    a. Maximum safety for the patient
    b. Correct body alignment
    c. Freedom for respiration
    d. Freedom for circulation
    e. No pressure on nerves or bony prominences, and body surfaces not touching other body surfaces or the metal table
    f. Accessible operative site
    g. No extreme flexion or extension of joints; joint movement should follow the normal range of motion
  6. *Why positioning is so critical for the surgical patient*
    a. An anesthetized patient will be unable to feel and/or verbalize pain (a protective mechanism).
    b. Unnatural or uncomfortable positions would be identified were the patient awake.
    c. Immobility is forced, often for long periods of time, and the patient cannot move to relieve discomfort or pain caused by pressure.
    d. Circulation is impeded during surgery because of the effects of drugs and anesthetics on the vascular system, leading to decreased tissue perfusion especially at pressure areas.
    e. Protective muscular mechanisms are decreased during surgery due to the use of neuromuscular blockers; the patient may experience more soreness after surgery.
  7. *Protect yourself:* use good body mechanics, get help as needed, allow patients to do all they can for themselves, and use lifting and moving devices for the patient who cannot assist you.
  8. Once the surgical procedure is complete, check all skin surfaces for injury and document findings.

SURGERY HINT

Most facilities utilize a "time out" or "moment of silence" to ensure that the patient and procedure are correct. This reduces wrong site surgeries. Follow facility procedure during this routine.

Be prepared for emergency procedures during induction. Malignant hyperthermia, cardiac events, and difficult airways can occur during this phase of surgery. Generally, as a rule of thumb, the Surgical Technologist will maintain the sterile field during emergencies unless otherwise directed.

B. Positions (Figure 8-1)
   1. *Dorsal recumbent (supine) position:* the most common position; the patient lies with his or her back flat on the OR bed.
      a. Head aligned with the body; safety strap 2 inches above knees
      b. Arms secured under the lift sheet with palms down or against the thigh or extended on padded armboards (palms up) at an angle not to exceed 90° to avoid injury to the brachial plexus.
         (*Note:* Arms hanging beside the OR table can cause damage to the ulna nerve; crossing arms across the chest may cause interference with respirations.)
      c. Ankles uncrossed to prevent damage to peroneal and tibial nerves and to avoid circulatory compression
      d. Possible pressure areas: occiput, scapulae, elbows, sacrum, ischial tuberosities, and heels (any bony areas); padding should be provided
      e. Use of this position: surgery on the ventral surface of body
      f. Modifications
         Head hyperextension with head in "donut" or turned toward affected side: for procedures of face and neck (thyroid position) support may be placed under the shoulders for hyperextension
         Pad under affected side to elevate body part: for anterolateral procedures
         Frogleg: supine with knees flexed and thighs externally rotated for Foley catheter placement; a pillow should be placed under each knee for support
         Arm extension: for breast, axillary, upper extremity, or hand procedures
         For cesarean section: right side slightly elevated with a wedge under the right flank to prevent pressure on the vena cava by the pregnant uterus
         For an abdominal/perineal resection: a combination of supine and modified lithotomy may be used
   2. *Trendelenburg position:* supine, knees flexed over a break in the table, head of table tilted downward 45° and padded shoulder braces may be applied over acromion processes; used for procedures in pelvis or lower abdomen to force abdominal contents upward toward the diaphragm, and sometimes for a patient in shock; reduces venostasis in legs and decreases lung volume because of compression on diaphragm. Observe patient's feet to make sure that Mayo stand is not compressing the patient's toes.
   3. *Reverse Trendelenburg position:* supine with table titled head up, feet down, padded footboard, safety strap 2 inches above knees; may be used for upper abdominal surgery to improve visualization by forcing abdominal contents downward, or for surgery of the head and neck to facilitate breathing and decrease venous congestion. For thyroid or neck surgery, a roll may be placed horizontally under the shoulders to hyperextend the head.
   4. *Semi-Fowler position (beach chair):* supine with buttocks at flex in table and knees over lower break, foot of table slightly lowered, knees flexed, and body raised 45° as a backrest with feet on padded footboard; used for cranial (head supported in headrest), shoulder, or breast procedures

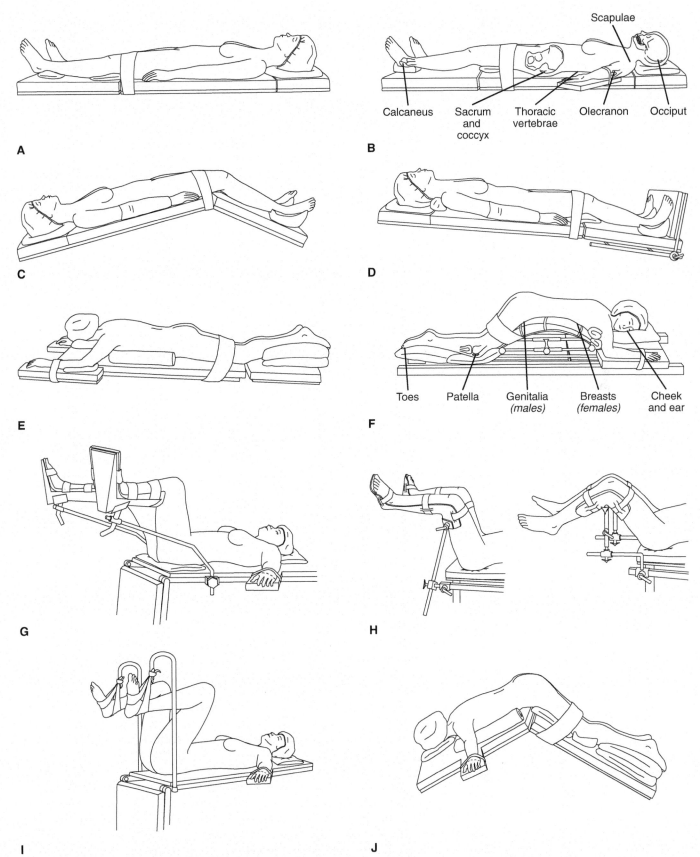

A

B

Scapulae

Calcaneus   Sacrum   Thoracic   Olecranon   Occiput
            and   vertebrae
            coccyx

C

D

E

F

Toes   Patella   Genitalia   Breasts   Cheek
                 (males)   (females) and ear

G

H

I

J

Figure 8-1 Surgical Positions: A. Dorsal recumbent (supine) position; **B.** Potential pressure areas for dorsal recumbent position; **C.** Trendelenburg position; **D.** Reverse Trendelenburg position; **E.** Prone position; **F.** Potential pressure areas for prone position; **G–I.** Lithotomy positions using different types of stirrups; **J.** Kraske (jackknife) position.

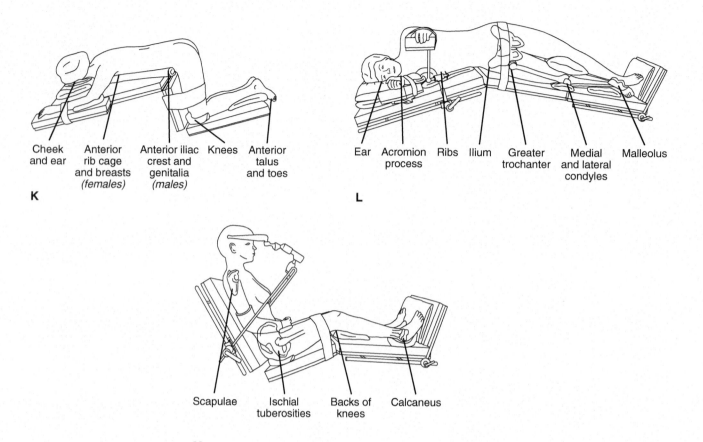

Figure 8-1   (continued) **K.** Potential pressure areas for knee-chest position; **L.** Potential pressure areas for lateral kidney position; **M.** Potential pressure areas for Fowler position.

    5. *Fowler (sitting) position:* ischial tuberosities padded to avoid pressure on sciatic nerve, arms flexed on a pillow, and head in cranial headrest; used for Occipital Craniotomy or posterior cervical procedures. Potential complications include:

       a. Potential for air embolism due to negative venous pressure in head and neck area (Doppler device and Central Venous Pressure line used for monitoring)

       b. Postural hypotension (antiembolitic hose, elastic bandages, or a sequential compression device may be used for prevention)

    6. *Lithotomy position:* supine with patient's buttocks along the break between the body and leg section of table and stirrups secured in holders at equal height and correct height for patient's legs. The most common types of stirrups are candy cane with foot straps, posts with knee crutches, and boot type that extend to the midcalf. Buttocks should not extend over table edge

       a. Legs are raised simultaneously by two persons by grasping the sole of the foot with one hand and cradling the calf of the leg with the other (permission obtained from anesthesia provider before moving patient).

       b. Legs should be padded and should not contact with any metal surface to avoid damage to the peroneal nerves.

       c. Leg section of the table is lowered and the mattress is removed. The buttocks should be even with the edge of the middle section of the bed.

       d. Hands are extended on armboards. Hands and fingers that are tucked at the side can get caught in the break of the table when raising/lowering the leg section. Arms crossed over the chest can compromise respiration.

e. Postoperatively, legs are lowered slowly and simultaneously to avoid a sudden drop in blood pressure.

f. During long procedures, distal pulses, skin color, or evidence of edema should be assessed; vulnerable areas include knees, hips, and back.

g. Used for perineal, vaginal, rectal, or endourologic procedures

7. *Prone position* (turned after anesthesia induction): patient is lying with the abdomen resting on the OR bed.

a. Positioning supervised by anesthesia provider and surgeon

b. A minimum of four persons are required (head, feet, and each side).

c. Patient is logrolled onto chest rolls, lateral bolsters, or frame, with weight borne by the iliac crests and acromion processes to avoid pressure on the sternum and abdomen.

d. Female breasts and male genitals are protected.

e. Arms are placed on angled armboards by lowering arms along the side of the OR bed and rotating upward beside the head, with palms down or placed by the side, palm up, secured with lift sheet.

f. Head is placed on headrest, donut, or pillow and turned to the side.

g. Pillows are placed under the ankles to prevent pressure on the toes, padding is placed under the knees to protect patellae, and a safety belt is applied above the knees.

h. Vulnerable areas include eyes, ears, breasts, genitalia, and toes.

i. Used for procedures on the dorsal side of the body

8. *Modified prone position:* a Relton's, Wilson, Hastings, or Andrews frame may be used in positioning for spinal surgery.

9. *Kraske (jackknife) position:* anesthetized in supine position and turned as with prone position; hips over the center break of table which is flexed about 90°, and table tilted downward so that the hips are elevated above the rest of the body; used for rectal procedures or Pilonidal Cystectomy; a possible concern is venous pooling in head and feet; patient returned slowly to the horizontal position; for rectal procedures, the buttocks may be taped apart

10. *Knee–chest position:* a foot extension added, and the table flexed at the center break, with leg section brought to a right angle with the table; patient kneels on foot extension and entire table is tilted cephalad to elevate the pelvis: may be used for sigmoidoscopy or Culdoscopy and occasionally for Lumbar Lamincectomy with the back of the table flat

11. *Lateral position:* patient is placed on his or her nonoperative side.

a. Named according to the side the patient is lying on (right lateral position for surgery on the left)

b. Used for access to the kidney, unilateral thoracic cavity, hip, or retroperitoneal space

c. Decreases effectiveness of ventilation and circulation

d. A minimum of four people are required to position the patient after anesthesia induction.

e. Lower leg is flexed and upper leg is extended on a pillow.

f. Bean bags or pillows may be used to stabilize the patient.

g. Safety strap is placed across the hips (adhesive tape may be used).

h. Arms are placed on a double armboard with a small roll placed under the axilla resting on the OR bed.

i. Blood pressure is measured using the lower arm.

j. Head is in alignment with the spine and supported on a small pillow.

k. *Pressure points:* ears, acromion process, iliac crest, greater trochanter, lateral knee, and malleolus

   a. *Lateral kidney position:* lateral position with the patient's lower iliac crest over kidney rest on the table; when the kidney rest is raised and the bed is flexed, accessibility to the kidney region is provided; the lower leg is flexed and upper leg extended on a pillow; circulation is compromised by pressure on the abdomen from kidney rest; prior to closing the incision, the kidney rest is lowered to facilitate closure.

    b. *Lateral chest position:* for unilateral transthoracic procedures; bean bags, bolsters, or a second strap (or adhesive) may be placed over the shoulder for stability.

12. *Anterior chest position:* for thoracoabdominal procedures; the patient is supine with pillows under the shoulder and buttocks on the affected side.

13. *Sims' position:* patient is lying on left side, table flat, with the upper leg flexed at the hip and knee; preferred position for administration of enema and anal endoscopic examination

III. Urinary Catheterization

A. Purposes
1. Keep bladder deflated during abdominal or pelvic surgery to avoid injury.
2. Prevent bladder distention during long procedures.
3. Monitor urine output.
4. Sterile specimen collection
5. Management of incontinence

B. Procedure (sterile technique essential); requires a physician's order
1. Position patient (females in "frog leg", males in supine with pillow under knees) and ensure adequate lighting
2. Open sterile catheter set, don sterile gloves using open gloving technique, check integrity and function of balloon and value before inserting by inflating with 10 ml of sterile water for a 5-cc balloon (balloons range from 5 to 30 cc). (*Note:* A straight catheter [Robinson] is used to collect a specimen or empty the bladder. The balloon [Foley] catheter is a retention catheter. A 30-cc balloon is used to provide pressure and hemostasis following prostate surgery. A three-way Foley provides continuous bladder irrigation, in addition to drainage and retention)
3. Clean the perineum with antiseptic from anterior to posterior (not retracing) or use circular motion around the glans penis for males, starting at the urethral meatus
4. Hold labia back (penis erect with slight tension) with nondominant hand and insert lubricated catheter into urethra with the other hand until the flow of urine begins. Then insert an additional inch to avoid damaging the urethra with the balloon.
5. Inflate the balloon (3–5 ml more than required for the balloon to allow for the fluid in the tubing) and connect the catheter to a drainage bag. Saline should not be used to inflate the balloon as it may crystallize.
6. Catheter should be secured with tape to the patient's thigh and the drainage bag placed below patient level, preferably in view of the anesthesia provider.

C. Monitoring urinary output
1. *Amount:* to check kidney function
2. *Color:* blood could indicate damage or injury

IV. Skin Preparation: The skin serves as the body's first line of defense against pathogens by being composed of layers of tightly packed stratified squamous epithelial tissue, oil, and normal flora. Before this protective barrier is broken (surgery), it must be cleansed of the oil and normal flora (remove transient and reduce resident organisms) to avoid transfer of these opportunistic pathogens into deeper body tissue. To ensure proper cleansing of the operative site, the patient showers and puts on a clean gown before coming to surgery. The surgical team prepares the operative site with antiseptic soap (scrub) and/or antiseptic solution (paint) just prior to surgery.

A. **Preliminary procedures**
   1. Mechanical cleansing of the incision site with agents such as isopropyl alcohol, chlorhexidine gluconate, iodine, iodophor, or hexachlorophene is performed to reduce bacterial flora.
   2. Checks for allergies and general skin condition are done prior to the use of any antiseptic.

B. **Hair is removed when ordered by the surgeon; however, the wound infection rate is considerably higher in patients who are shaved preoperatively. Hair removal may be accomplished by**
   1. *Clippers:* electric or battery operated with a detachable head that can be disinfected or is disposable; is the preferred method; use short strokes against the direction of hair growth with the blade flat against the skin.
   2. *Depilatory cream:* perform preliminary skin patch to test for sensitivity, apply thick layer over hair to be removed, wait required time (usually 20 minutes), and wash off; not used around the eyes or genitalia; follow manufacturers' directions.
   3. *Razor:* wear gloves, use a sterile sharp razor, soak hair in lather, hold skin taut, stroke in the direction of hair growth, shave as close to the time of surgery as possible in the preadmit area or holding room, and *only* if ordered. Nicks made in the skin several hours before surgery are considered contaminated and could result in surgical site infection (SSI) or cancellation of the case.
   4. *Other*
      Never remove eyebrows or eyelashes without a specific order.
      Hair from a patient's head is considered patient property and is saved and labeled unless a consent is signed for disposal.
      Hair may need to be removed from skin sites selected for placement of the dispersive electrode for the electrosurgical unit (ESU) and the EKG electrode.

C. **Patient's skin prep (scrub) in the OR**
   1. *Setup:* prep tray with sterile gloves, towels, sponges (not radiopaque), small basins, and antiseptic solution is opened on a separate small table or prep stand
   2. *Antiseptic solutions:* should be a broad-spectrum germicide that is easily applied; remains effective; is nontoxic and not irritating to the skin; remains active in presence of alcohol, organic matter, soap, or detergent; and is nonflammable (for use with LASER or electrosurgery)
      a. *Chlorhexidine gluconate (Hibiclens) may be mixed with 70% alcohol (Hibitane tincture):* effective 4 hours, nontinted or tinted, irritating to the eyes
      b. *Iodine and iodophors:* 1% to 2% solutions of iodine in water or 70% alcohol, which may cause skin burns if not allowed to dry or wiped off with alcohol; some patients are allergic to iodine; leaves a stain on the skin
      c. *Isopropyl alcohol:* not applied to mucous membranes; volatile, effective fat solvent, must not pool under patient if LASER or electrosurgical unit (ESU) is used
      d. *Hexacholorophene:* develops a cumulative effect, is neutralized by alcohol, and is ineffective against gram-negative organisms and fungi; used on patients who have washed with it for several days
      e. Single-use applicators containing an alcohol-based antiseptic which leaves an antimicrobial film are available (Dura Prep®)
   3. *Procedure:* get permission from the anesthesia provider, fold coverings back to expose area to be prepped, don sterile gloves, place absorbent barriers to avoid solution pooling under the patient, and wet a sponge with antiseptic (squeeze out excess); scrub the skin with friction in a

circular motion beginning at the incision site and scrub in ever-widening circles to the periphery; discard the sponge after reaching the periphery and use a clean sponge to repeat the process for a minimum of 5 minutes. (*Note:* Always clean from clean to dirty area and do not retrace.) After scrubbing for 5 minutes, the area is blotted dry with sterile towels, and the antiseptic "paint" is applied in the same manner using sponge sticks.

4. If a question exists regarding the area to be prepped, as in the case of cancer or for a skin graft, ask the physician.

5. *Specific areas*

   a. *Umbilicus:* clean first with a cotton-tipped applicator and discard or fill with antiseptic solution to soften detritus. Prep the umbilicus last or with a separate sponge.

   b. *Stoma (colostomy):* seal off with self-adhering drape or come back to this "dirty" area last.

   c. *Traumatic wounds:* irrigate and cover with sterile gauze, change gloves, and then scrub around them.

   d. *Graft areas:* separate setup for recipient and donor sites, prep donor site first

   e. *Eye:* never shave eyebrows; eyelashes may be trimmed, if ordered by the surgeon, with petrolatum-coated fine scissors; a nonirritating antiseptic is used around the eyes; prep begins at the inner canthus of the eyelid and then outward toward the brow and cheek; the conjunctival sac is flushed with a nontoxic agent (normal saline, ½ strength iodophor solution) with a bulb syringe from the medial to the lateral side. Local anesthetic drops such as tetracaine hydrochloride may be placed in the eye prior to prepping for the awake patient to avoid discomfort.

   f. *Ears, face, and nose:* protect the eyes with sterile plastic sheeting; cotton-tipped applicators are used for the nostril and external ear canal.

   g. *Neck:* scrub from mandible to top of the shoulders, chest to nipple lines, and laterally to the bedline.

   h. *Lateral thorocoabdominal:* remove gown; affected arm held up and scrub is extended from site of incision to axilla, chest, and abdomen from crest of ileum to the neck, axillary area is prepped last due to high microbe count.

   i. *Abdomen:* prep extends from nipple line to pubis and bedline to bedline; used for various abdominal incisions.

   j. *Chest and breast:* arm on affected side is elevated; area scrubbed includes shoulder, upper arm to elbow, axilla, chest wall to bed line, and beyond the sternum. If cancer is suspected, prep the breast gently to avoid dispersal of cancer cells; prep axillary area last due to high microbe count.

   k. *Shoulder:* arm is elevated; area scrubbed includes circumference of arm to below elbow, from base of neck over shoulder, scapula, and chest to midline; prep axillary area last.

   l. *Upper arm:* arm is elevated; area scrubbed includes circumference of arm to wrist, axilla, and over the shoulder to the scapula; prep axillary area last.

   m. *Elbow and forearm:* scrub entire arm from shoulder to hand.

   n. *Hand:* scrub hand and arm to 3 inches above the elbow.

   o. *Rectoperineal:* begin scrub with pubis, genitalia, perineum, and anus; discard sponge and use separate sponge for inner aspect of the thighs.

   p. *Combined abdomen and perineum:* complete rectoperineal prep first with the patient in lithotomy position; obtain a second prep set for the abdominal area.

   q. *Vagina:* after surrounding areas are scrubbed, sterile sponge and sponge forceps are used for vagina and cervix.

r. *Hips:* leg on affected side is elevated; area scrubbed includes abdomen, thigh to knee, buttocks to bed line; groin and pubis area are prepped last due to high microbe count.

s. *Thigh:* affected leg is elevated; area scrubbed includes circumference of thigh and leg to ankle, over hip and buttocks to bed line; groin and pubis are prepped last.

t. *Knee:* circumference of leg from foot to upper thigh is scrubbed.

u. *Ankle and foot:* scrub foot and ankle to just below the knee.

6. *Skin marking:* may be done before prep if marking can not easily be scrubbed off; generally done after prep, with sterile skin marking pen, gentian violet, or methylene blue

V. **Surgical Specimens:** Specimens are a very important part of surgery; they serve as legal evidence and a basis for analysis of the patient's condition. They demand of the surgical team the utmost care in handling.

A. *Definition:* a surgical specimen is a sample of tissue, fluid, organ, or foreign material collected from the patient during surgery.

B. *Surgical specimen protocol*

1. Based on hospital policy dictated by the pathology department

2. Handling of specimen should be kept to a minimum (and never with unprotected hands).

3. Specimens are collected by the surgeon and passed to the scrub.

4. The surgeon may mark the specimen with sutures for orientation or identification purposes.

5. Scrub listens carefully as the surgeon identifies the specimen and repeats the identification for verification.

6. Scrub places specimen in the specimen basin on the back table until the circulator is ready to take it. *(Note:* Specimens are *never* passed off on a sponge, as doing so could result in an incorrect sponge count. Specimens should be passed off field when the surgeon is finished examining it and gives permission.)

7. Scrub identifies the specimen as it is passed to the circulator.

8. The circulator completes the pathology requisition *(Note:* Surgical specimens are kept separate, unless ordered otherwise.)

9. The circulator places the specimen in the appropriate container or holds the container to receive the specimen from the scrub.

10. Specimens should not be allowed to dry out.

11. Formaldehyde (10% formalin) is the solution frequently used for the preservation of permanent specimens.

12. If the outside of the specimen container becomes contaminated, the circulator cleans it with a disinfecting solution.

13. The circulator labels the specimen on the side of the container and takes it, along with the pathology requisition, to the pickup area and records it in the specimen log.

14. Types of specimens

a. **Frozen section (small pieces of tissue for immediate examination by the pathologist):** placed in the specimen container without solution, circulator notifies pathology to pick it up or sends it to them with proper identification label and requisition. A verbal report is given by the pathologist in a matter of minutes.

b. *Embryo/fetus:* regulated by hospital policy

c. *Stones and teeth:* placed in dry containers to avoid dissolution

d. *Body fluids or washings:* left in the syringe or trap (e.g., sterile Luken's trap for bronchial or peritoneal washings) in which they were collected and sent to the lab immediately

e. *Amputated limbs:* placed in a fluid impervious bag and sent to the morgue for refrigeration

     f. *Foreign bodies:* saved for police if involved in a crime (bullet, knife, etc); follow hospital policy for transfer

     g. *Cultures:* aerobic and anaerobic cultures may be taken by the physician (transport media differ and care must be taken to use the proper containers) and passed off the field to circulator immediately for transport to the lab. *(Note:* Culture tubes are replaced in the container in which they came and dropped into the wrapper held by the circulator.)

     h. *Cytology smears:* placed on a slide and sprayed with a fixative

     i. *Breast tissue:* generally sent without fluid or fixative for evaluation of hormone sensitivity.

     j. *Small specimens:* may be sent on telfa to avoid loss

     k. Whenever a doubt exists regarding a specimen name or preparation, ask the surgeon.

15. *Labeling specimen:* label must include the patient's name, identification number, diagnosis, date, time, surgeon, exact specimen title, and precise test required, and must be written on the appropriate requisition and logged in the specimen book. Circulator places label on the side of the container and not the lid to avoid inadvertent switching of lids.

16. *Specimen storage:* depending on hospital policy, specimens are kept at room temperature in the department and generally picked up daily by courier and taken to the lab; fluids, smears, and cultures must be refrigerated or sent to the lab immediately. Some specimens are taken to x-ray for testing before being sent to the lab.

VI. **Thermoregulatory Devices:** Because of the combined effects of cool temperatures in the surgical suite coupled with a high humidity, skimpy clothing, and effects of cold prep solutions, drugs, and anesthetics, patients frequently encounter inadvertent hypothermia, which can lead to very serious complications such as increased blood pressure, tissue hypoxia, increased metabolism, increased oxygen consumption, and increased strain on the cardiovascular and respiratory systems. Hypothermia affects up to 60% of all surgical patients, and the goal for every patient should be the maintenance of a normal core temperature. Intraoperative heat loss occurs through radiation, convection, conduction, and evaporation.

A. **Prevention of inadvertent hypothermia in surgical patients**

1. Use a Bair Hugger® (forced-air skin surface warmer) or ultraviolet or infrared heat lamps to raise the body temperature.
2. Apply warmed blankets and/or thermal drapes upon arrival in OR.
3. Keep the patient covered as much as possible, especially the extremities.
4. Limit time between skin prep and application of drapes.
5. Keep patient dry.
6. Warm irrigation fluids, IV fluids, blood, and prep solutions unless contraindicated.
7. Monitor body temperature.
8. Apply head covering: Special thermal caps and blankets are available, as well as plastic coverings for the head and neck areas.

SURGERY HINT

When receiving multiple (permanent) specimens from the surgeon, the Surgical Technologist may not have the opportunity to pass them off the field immediately. In this situation, isolate each specimen and use a sterile marking pen to detail the information about each specimen until they can be received by the circulator.

    An important reminder: Bilateral surgical specimens must be isolated and sent separately when warranted. Make sure that they are clearly marked as either right or left.

9. Use a reflective or hypo/hyperthermia blanket (or a radiant heat source for an infant). (*Note:* A hyperthermia blanket or heated mattress pad is set at 104°F [40°C] for adults or 100°F [38°C] for infants.)

B. **Indications for use of thermoregulatory devices**
   1. *Infants:* lose heat rapidly due to underdevelopment of thermoregulating mechanism in their bodies and greater surface to volume ratio.
   2. *Debilitated patients:* have lower metabolism and a greater surface-to-volume ratio
   3. *Geriatric patients:* have poor circulation and lose heat rapidly

C. **Induced hypothermia:** artificial lowering of the body temperature below normal limits to reduce metabolic rate, oxygen requirements, anesthesia requirements, and blood loss
   1. Indications (uses)
      a. Organ transplantation
      b. Neurosurgery: to decrease cerebral blood flow and intracranial pressure
      c. Septic shock
      d. Hypertensive crisis or Malignant Hyperthermia
      e. Following cardiac resuscitation
      f. Procedures requiring cardiopulmonary bypass
   2. Methods
      a. *Surface-induced hypothermia:* immerse in ice water, pack body in ice, sponge with alcohol, or use hypothermia blanket
      b. *Internal cooling:* use iced saline slush packs around an organ, and irrigate with cold fluids
      c. *Systemic hypothermia:* blood is cooled through heat-exchanging devices in extracorporeal circulation, as with open heart surgery; may be lowered to 26°C (78.8°F) and then progressively rewarmed to 35°C (95°F)
   3. Complications of hypothermia
      a. May predispose patient to cardiac arrest
      b. Shivering and vasoconstriction poses a problem, as it increases oxygen needs (overcome by muscle relaxants, IV chlorpromazine, or an analgesic such as meperidine).
      c. Rewarming may lead to reactive bleeding or circulatory collapse.

VII. **Vital Signs**

A. **Pulse (heartbeat felt through the walls of arteries)**
   1. *Locations:* temporal, carotid, apical (heard with stethoscope over apex of the heart), brachial, radial, femoral, popliteal, dorsalis pedis
   2. *Rhythm:* abnormal rhythm may be called dysrhythmia or arrhythmia
   3. *Rate:* varies with age (70 beats per minute for adults to 130 beats per minute for infants) and increases with activity, temperature elevation, increased metabolism, or infection. Tachycardia is a rapid heart rate (over 100 beats per minute), and bradycardia is a slow heart rate (below 60 beats per minute).
   4. *Quality (strength):* may be full, bounding, weak, or thready

B. **Respiration**
   1. *Rate:* varies with age (ranges from 12–20 per minute for normal adult to 50 per minute for infant) and increases with increased metabolism, or activity
   2. Rhythm and volume vary
   3. Terms related to respiration
      a. *Eupnea:* normal breathing
      b. *Apnea:* without breathing
      c. *Bradypnea:* slow breathing
      d. *Tachypnea:* rapid breathing

e. *Dyspnea:* difficult breathing

f. *Rales:* rattling or bubbling sounds heard on auscultation (listening with a stethoscope) and caused by mucus in air passages

g. *Rhonchi:* wheezing sounds due to a partial obstruction, heard on auscultation

h. *Kussmaul's respiration:* fast deep, gasping respiration as seen in a diabetic coma

i. *Cheyne-Stokes respiration:* irregular breathing pattern of apnea and hyperpnea (seen in critically ill patients)

j. *Orthopnea:* breathing that is possible only when the patient is sitting or standing

C. Temperature

1. *Measured by a thermometer:* mercury, electronic, or thermistor probe connected to an instrument for readout; skin surface probes or adhesive strips have chemicals which change color to indicate rises in temperature.

2. *Normal:* 98.6°F (37°C)

3. *Febrile or pyrexia:* elevated temperature

D. Blood pressure

1. *Definition:* blood pressure is the amount of pressure exerted against arterial walls when the heart contracts and relaxes.

2. Measured by a sphygmomanometer and stethoscope or other pressure device

   a. *Systolic:* first sound heard while the cuff of the sphygmomanometer is being deflated; pressure exerted against arterial walls when ventricles contract to force blood out of the heart and is the highest number in the blood pressure reading. Normal for the average adult 90 to 130 mm Hg (millimeters of mercury pressure).

   b. *Diastolic:* last sound heard during deflation of the cuff; represents pressure exerted against the walls of arteries when heart is filling (relaxation phase of ventricles); and is the lowest number in the reading. It ranges from 60 to 90 mm Hg for the average adult.

3. Blood pressure is determined by the force of the heart, diameter of the vessels, blood volume, and blood viscosity (thickness).

4. Terms relating to blood pressure

   a. *Hypertension:* high blood pressure

   b. *Hypotension:* low blood pressure

   c. *Pulse pressure:* difference between systolic and diastolic

   d. *Murmurs:* rasping sounds generally made by defective heart valves or septal defect

   e. *Doppler:* a device for measuring blood pressure or pulse which uses ultrasonic high-frequency sound waves to assess the movement of blood through a vessel and provides audible sounds reflected to a probe connected to a monitor

VIII. Emergency Procedures: Regardless of how simple an operation may seem, the patient is always exposed to risks, not only from the hazards of surgery but also from anesthesia. The surgical team must be aware of possible complications and risks, preventive measures, and appropriate action to take in emergencies.

A. Indication of an emergency

1. Difficulty in breathing: dyspnea or choking

2. Disorientation, confusion, or changes in level of consciousness

3. Chest pain or tightness

4. Changes in skin color

5. Changes in vital signs

6. Bleeding

7. Inability to move a body part

B. **Objectives of emergency care**
   1. Preserve life.
   2. Prevent further deterioration.
   3. Restore to a level of optimal wellness.

C. **Priorities in emergency care of a patient**
   1. Establish unresponsiveness (shake, shout) and summon help.
   2. *Open airway:* tilt the head and lift the jaw (head tilt, chin lift). (*Note:* The most common cause for an obstructed airway in the unconscious victim is the tongue falling back to block off the pharynx, a condition that can be corrected by lifting the jaw and tilting the head back.)
   3. *Check for breathing:* look, listen, and feel; if not breathing, ventilate (give two slow breaths initially); use an ambu bag if available, otherwise use mask-to-mouth or mouth-to-mouth resuscitation. (*Note:* If airway is obstructed, use Heimlich maneuver or chest thrusts [back blows or chest thrusts for infants].)
   4. *Check circulation:* feel carotid pulse (brachial for infants); if no pulse, initiate a proper hospital procedure and begin CPR—15 chest compressions over lower third of sternum at a rate of 80–100 compressions per minute, with patient in dorsal position on flat surface, to every two ventilations; continue until the patient is resuscitated or more experienced person arrives. Check for return of pulse and breathing after one minute and every few minutes thereafter.
      (*Note:* With child and infant CPR, the ratio of breaths to compressions is 1:5.)
   5. *Monitor vital signs:* observe for changes, and report; observe for shock.
   6. *Bleeding:* external bleeding is first controlled by direct pressure, elevation, and application of cold.
   7. *Chest injuries:* open wound in the chest is a "sucking" wound and must be closed off to prevent lung collapse.
   8. *Fractures* (pain, swelling, loss of motion, and deformity): splint to immobilize.
   9. Comfort measures and calm reassurance are important.

D. *Shock:* decreased circulating volume; may be due to trauma (burns, fractures, wounds), loss of blood volume, or anaphylactic reaction, or may be cardiogenic or septic
   1. Traumatic shock (neurogenic or vasogenic)
      a. *Signs and symptoms:* apprehension; weakness; cool, clammy skin; dilated pupils; shallow, irregular breathing; rapid, weak pulse; and nausea and vomiting.
      b. *Treatment:* supine position with legs elevated or Trendelenburg (unless dyspneic); prevent the loss of body heat.
   2. *Hypovolemic shock (hemorrhagic):* due to the loss of blood: signs, symptoms, and treatment are similar to that of traumatic shock with the need to reestablish blood volume (IV fluids/blood).
   3. *Septic shock:* due to severe infection; temperature will be elevated; treated additionally with antibiotics.
   4. *Cardiogenic shock:* due to failure of the heart to circulate fluid; heart contraction must be strengthened with adrenergic drugs.
   5. *Anaphylactic shock* (**due to severe allergic reaction**): circulating volume decreased due to the movement of fluids from vascular bed into tissues (causing edema); release of histamines, causing rash and redness of skin (increased peripheral blood) and constricted bronchioles. Treatment of choice is 0.3 to 1.0 cc of epinephrine (vasoconstrictor and bronchodilator) and oxygen. Anti-inflammatory drugs and antihistamines may also be prescribed. (*Note:* Preventive measures include checking for allergies and giving test dose for "first-time" drugs.)

E. *Seizure (convulsion):* caused by epilepsy, high temperature, head injury, or toxic condition (may occur with certain anesthetics)
   1. *Signs and symptoms:* crying out, eyes rolling back, loss of consciousness, muscle twitching and shaking, and frothing at the mouth
   2. *Treatment:* protect patient from injury, reassure, and reorient.

F. *Malignant Hyperthermia:* life-threatening, metabolic crisis triggered by some anesthetic agents in susceptible patients.
   1. *Signs and symptoms:* unexplained tachycardia, tachypnea with elevated expired carbon dioxide levels, muscular rigidity, unexplained rise in temperature (late sign) [*Note:* soda lime (agent used to remove carbon dioxide from the patient during closed-circuit ventilation) turns blue]
   2. *Treatment:* discontinue suspected trigger agent(s); hyperoxygenate and administer drugs (dantrolene sodium [to allow movement of calcium], procainamide [cardiotonic], sodium bicarbonate [buffer], regular insulin and Dextrose 50% [carbohydrate source for cell metabolism], mannitol or furosemide [to flush kidneys of waste products produced by cell metabolism]); cool internally and externally by packing the patient in ice, use of ice water through a nasogastric tube, use of chilled irrigating solutions; correct electrolyte imbalance; monitor urinary output and Central Venous Pressure (CVP); and change soda lime canisters.
   3. *Prevention:* patient history, lab studies, and muscle biopsy. (*Note:* All OR personnel should be aware of the location and inventory of the Malignant Hyperthermia cart and established protocol.)

G. *Aspiration:* gastric contents inhaled into lungs
   1. *Signs and symptoms:* dyspnea and cyanosis
   2. *Treatment:* suctioning of airway, administration of steroids, and antibiotics
   3. *Prevention:* NPO before surgery or gastric lavage (evacuation) by nasogastric tube; cricoid pressure (Selleck's maneuver); careful administration of inhalation anesthesia; and positioning unconscious patient on side with head-down tilt

H. *Laryngospasm:* complete closure of the vocal cords resulting in a totally obstructed airway
   1. *Treatment:* 100% positive-pressure oxygen and administration of neuromuscular blocker (succinylcholine hydrochloride)

I. Toxic reaction to local anesthesia
   1. *Signs and symptoms:* dilated pupils, confusion, muscle spasms, tachycardia, tachypnea, and nausea and vomiting
   2. *Treatment:* Patients must be closely monitored, by an oximeter with ready access to oxygen.

J. *Hemolytic transfusion reaction:* caused by mismatched blood transfusion
   1. *Signs and symptoms:* leads to agglutination (clumping) of RBCs and may result in Disseminated Intravascular Coagulation (DIC), obstruction of vessels and organ necrosis (death), depletion of clotting factors and platelets, and activation of the fibrinolytic system
   2. *Treatment:* stop transfusion, report, send blood back to blood bank, monitor urine output, and administer drug therapy.

K. Cardiac arrest
   1. Clinical manifestations of impending arrest are unstable blood pressure, rapid pulse, respiratory changes, cardiac dysrhythmias, and symptoms of shock.
   2. Roles of the surgical team in cardiac arrest
      a. *Anesthesia provider:* director of resuscitation
      b. *Surgeon:* cardiac compressions, external or internal
      c. *Circulator:* summons help, secures emergency cart, draws up medicines, provides documentation, and starts time clock

      d. *Scrub:* remains sterile, guards the sterile field, keeps track of counts, and assists surgeon(s) as needed

   3. *Emergency supplies and equipment (crash cart):* available at all times with current inventory; contains resuscitation and oxygen equipment, intubation supplies, tracheotomy tray, sterile gloves and dressings, suction machine and catheters, IV infusion solutions and sets, cutdown tray, thoracotomy supplies, EKG monitor and supplies, defibrillator with paddles and supplies, cardiac pacemaker, flow sheets for documentation, CVP manometer, sutures, needles, syringes, and drugs (epinephrine, sodium bicarbonate, calcium chloride, lidocaine hydrochloride, and others)

   4. *Advanced life support:* includes the use of special equipment and techniques to establish and maintain effective ventilation and circulation, and monitor and control dysrhythmias, drug administration, and postresuscitative care

   5. *Defibrillation:* use of electric shock to restore the heart to a normal rhythm

      a. Applied by physician or trained health care provider

      b. External (electrode paddles applied to the chest) or internal (sterile electrode paddles applied directly to the heart) defibrillation may be performed.

      c. External electrode paddles must be kept clean.

      d. Electrode paste, jelly, or special adhesive gauze pads are placed beneath the paddles.

      e. When using the defibrillator, no one touches the metal operating table, patient, paste, or operator (who gives a loud verbal warning before each discharge).

      f. Automated external defibrillators (AEDs) are available and easy to use by trained medical or nonmedical personnel.

IX. Monitoring Equipment in the Operating Room

  A. *Hemodynamic monitoring:* indwelling arterial, venous, and intracardiac catheters measure cardiac output and intracardiac pressures; provide information about the function of the heart and other major organs.

  B. *Central Venous Pressure (CVP):* Catheter (Hickman, Broviac) placed in the subclavian vein to the right atrium

  C. *Arterial blood gases and/or pressure:* intraarterial catheter

  D. *Pulmonary artery pressure:* Swan-Ganz catheter

  E. *Electrocardiogram:* for rhythm and rate on monitor screen

  F. *Arterial blood gases:* pulse oximetry measures arterial hemoglobin oxygen saturation and may be placed on the finger, toe, earlobe, or bridge of the nose. A reading of less than 90% could indicate hypoxia.

  G. *Respiratory tidal volume:* volume of air moved with each respiration. (*Note:* Patients are observed both for the rate and depth of respiration.)

  H. *Body temperature:* electronic measurement with thermistor probes inserted into a body orifice (esophagus, bladder, rectum, nasopharynx) or cutaneous strips

  I. *Urinary output:* indwelling (Foley) catheter with urimeter

  J. *Electroencephalogram (EEG):* scalp electrodes

  K. *Somatosensory evoked potentials:* used to assess spinal cord function during orthopedic or neurosurgery of the spine.

  L. *Bispectral index monitoring system (BIS):* noninvasive method of monitoring depth of general anesthesia level through processed EEG parameters

X. **Death and Dying**

   A. **Perceptions of death and dying**
     1. Religious beliefs
     2. Cultural beliefs
     3. Attitudes of family members
     4. Attitudes of caregivers

   B. **Classifications of death**
     1. Accidental
     2. Terminal
     3. Prolonged
     4. Sudden

   C. **Responses to loss/grief (Kübler-Ross)**
     1. Denial
     2. Anger
     3. Depression
     4. Bargaining
     5. Acceptance

   D. **Quality of life versus quantity of life**
     1. Euthanasia
     2. Right to die
     3. Advance directives
       a. Living will
       b. Durable power of attorney
     4. Do Not Resuscitate (DNR)

   E. **Death of a patient in the operating room**
     1. Notification of perioperative manager
     2. Notification of family and significant others
     3. Notification of chaplain/clergy
     4. Forensic issues and coroner's cases: all forensic evidence is preserved by following the chain of evidence
     5. Preparation of the body for family viewing: viewing should take place in a clean, private area
     6. Postmortem patient care: follow hospital policy and state law

   F. **Coping strategies**
     1. Empathy
     2. Grieving process
     3. Share feelings with others
     4. Verbalize fears
     5. Team effort
     6. Support groups for staff members and bereaved families
     7. Chaplain/clergy

   G. **Organ procurement and transplantation**
     1. Establishment of brain death
     2. Procurement
       a. Living donor: blood-dependent organs
       b. Cadaveric procurement: cornea, bones, skin

The Postoperative Patient

I. **Postanesthesia Care Unit (PACU):** The anesthesia provider and circulator transport the patient to the PACU and give a report to nursing staff.

   A. Patients are covered with warm blankets and moved gently to avoid any sudden decrease in blood pressure.

   B. Patency of airway is monitored; oxygen is given by mask to lessen hypoxia and help flush anesthetics.

C. Level of consciousness, skin condition, and vital signs are checked every 5 to 15 minutes and recorded.

D. Surgical wound, drain, catheters, and dressings are assessed for drainage, and the surgeon is notified of any complications.

E. Medications are given to control pain and nausea. Other postoperative discomforts are thirst, abdominal distension, and urinary retention.

F. Intravenous fluids and urinary output are closely monitored.

G. Bedside equipment includes airway devices, oxygen, suction, emesis basin, bedpan, urinal, and monitoring devices. Emergency equipment such as crash cart, defibrillator, and tracheotomy tray must be immediately available.

H. Common postoperative complications may include hemorrhage, shock, pulmonary embolus, deep-vein thrombosis, and respiratory issues.

I. Following a return to stable vital signs, the patient is transferred back to the nursing unit or the ambulatory unit in preparation for discharge.

II. Discharge Planning

A. Begins early in the treatment process (i.e., before or on admission).

B. Follows institutional discharge policy.

C. Patient evaluation: mental and physical.

D. Critical readiness criteria for discharge: vital signs, respiratory status, reflexes, mental status, surgical consideration, pain, nausea and vomiting, oral intake, voiding, anesthesia considerations, and ambulation

E. Family support system: assist with activities, ensure patient complies with postoperative instructions, monitor the patient's progress toward recovery.

F. Provide written postoperative instructions: to include medications, activity restrictions, diet and elimination, surgical side effects, possible complications and symptoms, treatments, access to post discharge care, follow-up care.

Show What You Know

Directions
Each of the numbered items or incomplete statements in this section is followed by answers or by completions of the statement. Select the ONE lettered answer or completion that is BEST in each case.

1. An expressed concern of the patient that he or she will be paralyzed following spinal anesthesia should be reported to the:
   A. surgeon
   B. anesthesia provider
   C. circulating nurse
   D. OR supervisor

2. One way the surgical technologist could help meet the psychosocial needs of the surgical patient is to:
   A. tell the patient that everything will be just fine
   B. observe the patient's behavior and listen carefully to what the he or she says
   C. report your observations to the patient's family
   D. embrace the patient and tell him or her you know just how he or she feels

3. Obtaining an informed consent for surgery is the ultimate responsibility of the:
   A. anesthesia provider
   B. circulator
   C. OR supervisor
   D. surgeon

4. Persons witnessing the signing of the consent for surgery attest to all of the following *except*:
   A. the person signing the form is the person whose name appears on the form
   B. that the surgeon fully explained the surgery to the patient and family and they understand it
   C. the signature of the patient is given voluntary
   D. the patient is mentally competent to sign the consent

5. The operative permit must be signed:
   A. before the patient enters the hospital
   B. before the preoperative sedative medication is given
   C. after the patient arrives in the holding area
   D. just before surgery is begun

6. In life-threatening circumstances, consent for surgery may be granted by any of the following methods *except:*
   A. telephone conversation with nearest relative
   B. two consulting physicians
   C. signature of the assistant surgeon
   D. telegram or fax consent from nearest relative

7. During a preoperative visit, the anesthesia provider assigned an ASA classification of class V to the patient. This means that:
   A. the patient is a very poor risk for surgery
   B. the patient is in the best of health for surgery
   C. the patient will be unable to pay for the surgery
   D. the patient is a minor

8. Patient identification can best be made by:
   A. comparing the name on the bed with the name on the OR schedule
   B. asking the nurse to identify the patient
   C. comparing the name on the patient's identification band with the name on the OR schedule
   D. asking the patient if he is Mr. Jones

9. When transporting a patient to surgery, you would:
   A. pull the stretcher from the foot when entering an elevator
   B. push the stretcher from the head when traveling through a corridor
   C. have the patient hold onto the side rails
   D. place IV fluids beside the patient on the stretcher

10. The reason for the 90° limit for extension of a patient's arms on a padded armboard is:
    A. avoiding injury to the brachial plexus
    B. avoiding injury to the ulnar nerve
    C. avoiding injury to the peroneal nerve
    D. avoid injury to the sciatic nerve

11. Which of the following positions for surgery might require the use of shoulder braces?
    A. lateral
    B. dorsal recumbent
    C. Kraske (jackknife)
    D. Trendelenburg

12. Permission for turning the anesthetized patient from a dorsal recumbent to a prone position must be obtained from the:
    A. surgeon
    B. anesthesia provider
    C. OR supervisor
    D. circulator

13. The position that permits enhanced visualization during pelvic surgery is:
    A. reverse Trendelenburg
    B. Trendelenburg
    C. lithotomy
    D. Sims

14. Postural hypotension is a threat when the patient is placed in which of the following positions?
    A. Fowler
    B. Trendelenburg
    C. lateral kidney
    D. prone

15. The number of persons required to position a patient in stirrups is:
    A. one
    B. two
    C. three
    D. four

16. For the patient in the prone position, the weight of the body should be borne by the:
    A. iliac crests and acromion processes
    B. ischial spines and coccyx
    C. sternum and pubis
    D. abdomen and chest

17. For a Right Nephrectomy, the patient would be placed in the _____ position.
    A. right lateral kidney
    B. left lateral kidney
    C. Sims
    D. Kraske

18. Which of the following antiseptics could stain the skin?
    A. isopropyl alcohol
    B. chlorhexidine gluconate
    C. hexachlorophene
    D. iodine

19. The skin preparation area for a Carpal Tunnel Release would include:
    A. the foot to 3 inches above the knee
    B. the hand and arm to 3 inches above the elbow
    C. the abdomen from nipple line to pubis
    D. the chest from sternum to bedline and from clavicle to umbilicus

20. The surgical specimen which is examined immediately by the pathologist is a/an:

    A. amputated limb
    B. culture
    C. foreign body
    D. frozen section

21. Which of the following lab values falls within the normal range?

    A. hemoglobin of 6–8 grams
    B. white blood cell count of 15,000
    C. specific gravity of urine 1.055
    D. hematocrit of 45%

22. Induced hypothermia may be accomplished by all of the following *except:*

    A. drugs
    B. packing the body in ice
    C. irrigating with cold fluids
    D. use of cooling blanket

23. Correct hand placement for cardiac compressions during CPR is:

    A. lower third of the sternum
    B. epigastrium
    C. between the scapulae
    D. on the left side of the chest above the heart

24. The symptoms of traumatic shock are:

    A. cool, clammy skin, weak, rapid pulse; dilated pupils
    B. hot, dry skin; fast pulse; constricted pupil
    C. redness, rash, swollen eyes, dyspnea
    D. cool, clammy skin; slow pulse; Kussmaul breathing

25. Should a cardiac arrest occur in the OR, the role of the scrub would be:

    A. perform mouth-to-mouth resuscitation
    B. perform cardiac compression
    C. obtain crash cart
    D. maintain the sterile field and keep track of counts

Answers & Rationales

1. **B.** **Rationale:** Expressed patient concerns regarding anesthesia should be reported to the anesthesia provider, who should address those concerns directly with the patient.

2. **B.** **Rationale:** Surgical Technologists can help meet the psychosocial needs of patients by listening, reassurance, demonstrating concern, and touching. To tell a patient that everything will be just fine or that you know how they feel will block further communication.

3. **D.** **Rationale:** The surgeon is responsible for explaining to the patient the nature of the proposed procedure, the necessity for the operation, the risks, the benefits, and alternative treatment options.

4. **B.** **Rationale:** A witness to the signing of an operative consent form attests to the fact that the patient was signing voluntarily, was mentally competent to sign, and is, indeed, the person whose name appears on the form. A witness may be a physician, nurse, or other staff member.

5. **B.** **Rationale:** The operative permit must be signed before the preoperative sedative medication is given as the medication could alter the patient's cognitive ability. It is not necessary that the permit be signed before the patient enters the hospital.

6. **C.** **Rationale:** In life-threatening circumstances when the next of kin is not available and the patient is unable to sign the operative permit, consent may be given by telephone, fax, e-mail, or telegram by a near relative or by two consulting physicians not performing the surgery.

7. **A.** **Rationale:** ASA classification is assigned by the anesthesia provider on the basis of patient status for surgery. Poor-risk patients are assigned a class V; lower-risk patients are assigned a class I.

8. **C.** **Rationale:** Patient identification is a serious matter for OR personnel and is done by asking the patient to state his or her name, reading the name on the patient's armband, and comparing that name with the name on the patient's record/chart, and the OR schedule.

9. **B.** **Rationale:** When transporting a patient to surgery, you would stand near the head of the patient and push the stretcher feet first through the corridor. This would allow for close observation of the patient and provide better control of the stretcher.

10. A. **Rationale:** When a patient's arm is extended on an arm board during surgery, it is not extended beyond a 90° angle, as this would put stress on the brachial plexus and may lead to damage.

11. D. **Rationale:** Padded shoulder braces should be applied to the OR table for the patient in the Trendelenburg position to protect the person from sliding cephalad. It is important that the pressure/weight be borne by the acromion process.

12. B. **Rationale:** Permission must be obtained from the anesthesia provider to move the patient once anesthesia is initiated, as they are responsible for monitoring the patient's airway and state of homeostasis.

13. B. **Rationale:** During pelvic surgery, visualization is improved by tilting the OR table cephalad (Trendelenburg) to allow abdominal contents to move up toward the diaphragm.

14. A. **Rationale:** The Fowler position may cause a pooling of blood in the lower extremities and lead to hypotension.

15. B. **Rationale:** Two persons are needed to position a patient in stirrups, as both legs should be raised and rotated simultaneously to avoid damage to the hip joint.

16. A. **Rationale:** When placing a patient in the prone position, the weight of the body should be borne by the iliac crests and acromion processes. Pressure on the abdomen and chest would impede respiration and venous return.

17. B. **Rationale:** For a Right Nephrectomy, the patient would be placed in the left lateral kidney position—"lateral" because the kidneys are retroperitoneal, "kidney" because the kidney flex on the table is raised, and "left" because the position is named for the side on which the patient is lying.

18. D. **Rationale:** Iodine leaves a brownish stain on the skin and is not appropriate for plastic surgery.

19. B. **Rationale:** A Carpal (wrist) Tunnel Release would require a skin prep of hand and arm to 3 inches above the elbow.

20. D. **Rationale:** A frozen section is a sample of tissue examined by the pathologist immediately while the patient is still under anesthesia.

21. D. **Rationale:** The normal hematocrit (percentage of red blood cells) is 45%. The normal hemoglobin is 12–14 grams—a hemoglobin less than 10 indicates anemia; the normal white blood cell count is 5000–10,000—an elevated white blood cell count indicates infection; the normal specific gravity of urine is 1.005–1.025—a high specific gravity indicates dehydration.

22. A. **Rationale:** Body temperature may be lowered by external cooling, internal cooling, or by cooling the blood. Drugs are not used to lower temperature.

23. A. **Rationale:** For CPR, the heel of one hand is placed on the lower third of the sternum with other hand locked onto it, elbows kept straight, and compressions done by applying pressure straight down to depress the sternum 1½ to 2 inches for an adult.

24. A. **Rationale:** Symptoms of traumatic shock are: dilated pupils; cool, clammy skin; rapid, thready pulse; anxiety; and rapid, shallow breathing. Hot, dry skin may be noted in patients in anaphylactic shock as well as swollen eyes and dyspnea. Kussmaul breathing is a slow, deep-breathing pattern seen in patients in diabetic coma.

25. D. **Rationale:** The role of the scrub during a cardiac arrest during surgery is to maintain a sterile field, keep track of counts, and assist the surgeon as needed.

Part II: Deciphering a Surgical Schedule

The following mock surgery schedule will be used to answer several questions pertaining to surgical patients. The same schedule, or a similar one, may be used in subsequent chapters to ask questions about the content of the chapter.

Rm.# time	Surgeon	Procedure	Anest.	Rm. # time	Surgeon	Procedure	Anest.
Rm.00				**Rm07**			
OC	Dr. Z	Rt. Knee Arthroscopy	Gen.	7:00	Dr. M	Rhinoplasty	Gen.
OC	Dr. C	Craniotomy	Gen.	TF	Dr. M	LAVH	MAC
OC	Dr.Z	Angioplasty	Gen.				
Rm.01				**Rm08**			
7:00	Dr. X	Lobectomy	Gen.	11:00	Dr. E	Bovine	MAC
TF	Dr. X	Thoracotomy	Gen.			Thrombectomy	
TF	Dr. X	Tracheostomy	Gen.				
Rm02				**Rm09**			
7:00	Dr. B	Splenectomy	Gen.	8:30	Dr. T	Cholecystectomy	Gen.
TF	Dr. B	Gastrectomy	Gen.	TF	Dr. T	Palatoplasty	Gen.
Rm03				**Rm10**			
7:00	Dr. A	Cystoscopy	MAC	7:00	Dr. K	Nephrectomy	Gen.
TF	Dr. A	Cystoplasty	Gen.	TF	Dr. K	Choledocholithot-	MAC
12:30	Dr. F	Pyleogram	MAC	TF		ripsy	
3:00	Dr. F	Cystocele repair	Gen.		Dr. K	Hepatic resection	Gen.
Rm04				**Rm11**			
7:00	Dr. Y	Carpal tunnel release	Gen.	7:00	Dr. L	Colposcope	Gen.
TF	Dr. Y	Fasciotomy	Gen.	12:00	Dr. L	Mastectomy	Gen.
Rm05				**Rm12**			
7:00	Dr. G	Trans-sphenoidal Adenectomy	Gen.	7:00	Dr. W	Trans-metatarsal amputation	Gen.
TF	Dr. G	Trans-urethral resection of the prostate	Gen	TF	Dr. W	Osteotomy	Gen.
TF	Dr. G	STSG	Gen.	TF	Dr. W	Arthrocentesis	Gen.
Rm06				**Rm13**			
7:00	Dr. R	Lumbar Laminectomy	Gen.	7:00	Dr. O	Hysterectomy	Gen.

The following questions should be answered using the surgery schedule above

1. How will the patient in Room 6 be positioned?

    A. Dorsal recumbent
    B. Lateral
    C. Prone
    D. Lithotomy

2. A patient scheduled in Room 5 is morbidly obese. What is a special precaution that should be taken?

    A. Morbidly obese patients are more prone to infections, therefore, prophylactic antibiotics should be given
    B. There should be extra personnel on hand for transporting and positioning
    C. The patient must be prepped before induction
    D. The patient should be positioned before induction

3. The patient in Room 13 is suffering from diabetes. What precautions should be taken?

    A. The room should be heated to prevent hypothermia
    B. Nutritional supplements should be given pre-operatively
    C. Antiembolic stockings may be used postoperatively to aid in circulation
    D. Diabetes patients are prone to respiratory obstructions

4. How will the patient scheduled for the LAVH in Room 7 be positioned?

    A. Lithotomy
    B. Trendelenburg
    C. Dorsal Recumbent
    D. Prone

5. Where will the safety strap be located on the patients in Room 1?

   A. Across the lower legs
   B. 2" above the knee
   C. At the waist
   D. There will not be a safety strap in these surgical procedures

6. How will the Cystoscopy patient be positioned?

   A. Lithotomy
   B. Supine
   C. Trendelenburg
   D. Kraske

7. A Wilson frame will be used in one of the surgeries listed. Which one is the most likely to use this device?

   A. Hepatic Resection
   B. LAVH
   C. Craniotomy
   D. Lumbar Laminectomy

8. The patient who will undergo the Nephrectomy in Room 10 will be placed in a lateral position. How many people are required to position the patient?

   A. 2
   B. 3
   C. 4
   D. 5

9. The surgeon requires the patient in Room 2 to have an indwelling catheter. Why would this be ordered?

   A. For patient comfort postoperatively
   B. For sterile specimen collection
   C. For convenience during rehabilitation
   D. To keep the bladder inflated during the procedure

10. The patient scheduled in Room 5 for a skin graft needs to be prepped. What does the Surgical Technologist need to do?

   A. Use one kit of providone Iodine for the recipient site, and leave the donor site clear
   B. Use a separate setup for each site and prep the donor site first
   C. Use separate setup for each site and prep the recipient site first
   D. Do not prep either site

Answers & Rationales

1. **C.** **Rationale:** Lumbar Laminectomies are performed on the spine with the patient in the prone position. The other positions will not be suitable for most Laminectomies. Occasionally, a spinal surgery will be done with the patient in another position, depending on what the goal of the surgery is.

2. **B.** **Rationale:** A morbidly obese patient presents many obstacles in surgery, one of which is the possibility of injury to staff when positioning and transferring the patient. For this reason, there should always be extra personnel on hand when transferring and positioning the morbidly obese patient.

3. **C.** **Rationale:** Patients with diabetes suffer from many health issues, including decreased circulation to extremities. For this reason, the surgeon may order the use of antiembolic stockings or devices both during the procedure and afterward.

4. **A.** **Rationale:** LAVH stands for Laparoscopic Assisted Vaginal Hysterectomy. This procedure is done with the patient in the lithotomy position.

5. **B.** **Rationale:** The safety strap for a patient in the supine position is 2" above the knees, unless otherwise directed.

6. **A.** **Rationale:** Patients undergoing Cystoscopies are generally placed in a lithotomy position to facilitate the insertion of the Cystoscope. Precautions must be taken whenever lithotomy is used, as it can easily result in patient injury due to improper positioning.

7. **D.** **Rationale:** The Wilson frame is a positioning device sometimes used when a patient is in the prone position. It must be properly positioned on the table before the patient is placed in position.

8. **C.** **Rationale:** There must be four people to properly place a patient in the lateral position. There should be one person at the head (anesthesia), one person at each side, and a fourth at the feet.

9. **B.** **Rationale:** There are several reasons that an indwelling catheter would be placed in a patient. It may be to monitor urine output, to keep the bladder deflated during the procedure, or to collect a sterile specimen. Catheterization is a sterile procedure that needs to be performed carefully to avoid urinary tract infections.

10. **B.** **Rationale:** Donor and recipient sites in skin grafts should be prepped separately with the donor site being prepped first.

PEARSON
myhealthprofessionskit™

Use this address to access the interactive Companion Website created for this book. Simply select "Surgical Technology" from the choice of disciplines. Find this book and click to enter.

The wound is a visible evidence of surgery, the yardstick by which patients often measure both the technical skill of the surgeon and the success of surgery. Wounds represent unique problems. They must be managed correctly to heal properly, and create issues when they do not. Many patient populations, especially those suffering from diabetes, deal with wounds that must be dealt with through surgical interventions. The proper care and management of wounds may mean the difference between healing and further surgeries. Knowing the physiology behind wound healing is instrumental in being able to accurately predict which sutures, drains, and dressings will be used in the procedure.

CHAPTER OUTLINE

How to Answer Questions about Suture

Sutures are always challenging to students and seasoned Surgical Technologists alike. With all of the variations, brands, strands, needle points, and sizes, it is easy to see why. When dealing with sutures, there are several easy tips to select the appropriate type. Remember that there are actually not that many kinds of suture: absorbable or nonabsorbable, natural or synthetic, and single strands or multiple strands. Always choose the size based upon the area of the body to be sutured. You would need a very small suture strand for an ophthalmic case, while you will need a larger stronger suture for abdominal muscles. Remember that sizes are denoted by the number on the packet. The smaller the suture the more 0s there are (example: 5-0 represents 00000: Very small; while 2-0 represents 00: larger diameter) Once you know the approximate size that will be needed, you can then concentrate on the type of suture that will be required. Some basic rules are that you must select suture based on the wound type, you must select the needle based on the tissue type, and you should select length based on the suture line and the size of the wound. Keeping these guidelines in mind should make the selection of suture easier for the Surgical Technologist.

Needle types are also challenging, but, again, several rules apply. Each needle type has a specific type or types of tissue it is commonly used for. Sizes and gauge and curvature all play into which the needle type will be chosen. The needle that is pictured on the package is the actual size of the needle, so if you are in doubt, the packaging should offer a hint.

Example:
Which type of suture needle would be used to repair Liver tissue?

a. Blunt
b. Keith
c. Spatula
d. Cutting

To answer this question, and ones like it, remember that every needle has specific characteristics that will make it most suited to the tissue that it will be used on. Remember the anatomy of the liver, as well as liver tissue. Is it tough and fibrous or friable and delicate? We know that liver tissue is friable, and requires a specific needle type. We also know that cutting needles are most commonly used during skin closures, so they can be eliminated. Keith needles are straight and are not commonly used, but would not be used on liver tissue. Thus, we can eliminate the Keith needle. This leaves blunt and spatula needles. Spatula needles are used primarily in eye cases, not on liver tissue, leaving the blunt needle as the correct answer. Blunt needles are routinely used for friable tissues. Remember, the surgeons preference card should always be consulted for individual preferences, but the Surgical Technologist must be able to anticipate the suture selection for the cases they are assigned.

Definitions

1. *Adhesions:* two surfaces "stick" together that are normally separated
2. *Collagen:* the chief constituent of connective tissue
3. *Contracture:* formation of excessive scar tissue in skin, fascia, muscle, or a joint
4. *Dead Space:* gap left in wound caused by separation of wound edges
5. *Debridement:* removing dead, devitalized tissue from a wound to promote healing
6. *Edema:* swelling; abnormal accumulation of fluid in an area
7. *Granulation tissue:* scar tissue formed by fibrous collagen to fill in the wound
8. *Granuloma:* inflammatory lesion surrounding a foreign substance in a wound
9. *Hematoma:* blood clot
10. *Hemostasis:* controlling bleeding or hemorrhage

11. *Ischemia:* lack of blood supply to an area
12. *Necrosis:* death of tissue
13. *Serosanguinous:* blood tinged

Types of Wounds

A wound is a break in the continuity of tissue.

I. *Traumatic Wounds:* those caused by injury
   A. *Laceration:* irregular tear
   B. *Abrasion:* scraping away of the tissue
   C. *Puncture:* wound made with a piercing object
   D. *Burns:* chemical, thermal, and irradiation
   E. *Decubitus ulcers (pressure sores):* damage to skin or underlying structures due to tissue compression and inadequate blood supply usually over a bony prominence
   F. *Contusion (hematoma):* bruise; skin is not broken (closed wound)
   G. *Avulsion:* tissue torn from its site of attachment
II. **Classifications of Wounds by Severity**
   A. *Open:* the integrity of the skin is destroyed
   B. *Closed:* the skin is intact
   C. *Simple:* no loss of tissue and no foreign body present in the wound
   D. *Complicated:* tissue is lost or destroyed; foreign body present in the wound
   E. *Clean:* no infection, wound edges are approximated
   F. *Contaminated:* an object containing microbes or foreign matter that has penetrated the skin
   G. *Delayed full-thickness injury:* the full effects of the injury may not be seen for several days; tissue necrosis or full-thickness tissue loss; seen in electrocution, lightning strikes, and crushing injuries
III. *Surgical Wound:* cut with a sharp instrument (intentional, incision, excision)
IV. *Chronic Wounds:* pressure sores, ulcers

Wound Healing

I. **Types of Wound Healing (three ways that wounds heal)**
   A. **First intention, primary union (ideal healing)**
      1. Wound edges are approximated (brought together) layer by layer
      2. Clean, incised wounds
      3. Healing occurs from side to side; all layers at the same time; minimal edema
      4. Minimal tissue loss and drainage
      5. Freedom from infection
      6. Minimal scarring; results in a strong union
   B. **Second intention, granulation (indirect union)**
      1. Excessive tissue loss and drainage
      2. Bacterial contamination
      3. Wound left open to heal from the inside out
      4. Granulation tissue forms in the defect between the wound edges from bottom up, and epithelial cells migrate from the wound edges. (*Note:* Granulation is small masses of tissue formed from budding capillaries and collagen during wound healing. Good granulation tissue appears pink and clear and bleeds easily.)

5. Excessive granulation tissue (proud flesh) may extend above the skin margins.
6. Requires longer to heal, leaves a wide irregular scar, and results in weak union or hernia

C. **Third intention (delayed primary closure)**
   1. *Examples:* ruptured appendix, gunshot wound to bowel, or other infected traumatic wound
   2. Wound is debrided (cleansed of debris) and purposely left open to heal by second intention for several days.
   3. Absorbent packing material and/or drains are placed between wound edges to avoid premature closure or trapping of infection deep inside.
   4. Patient is brought back to surgery (secondary closure), after danger of infection period has passed, for wound closure (approximating two surfaces of granulating tissue).

II. **Phases of First Intention Wound Healing**

A. *Phase 1:* Lag phase or inflammatory response phase (days 1 to 5)
   1. *Hemostasis:* bleeding control
      a. Within seconds of injury, blood vessels near injured tissue constrict to help occlude blood flow (whitening of tissue is evident).
      b. Platelets collect to form a plug.
      c. Clot is formed by deposits of fibrin threads made from fibrinogen.
      d. Scab is formed as proteins in the wound dry, making a shield against bacteria.
   2. *Signs of inflammation*
      a. *Redness:* due to dilated capillaries, which bring blood to the area
      b. *Heat:* due to increased blood and metabolic activity in the area
      c. *Swelling (edema):* caused by a leakage of plasma from capillaries, which have become more permeable; swelling may last several days
      d. *Pain:* caused by injury to nerves or pressure from edema
      e. *Loss of function:* due to edema, pain, and pressure on nerves
   3. *Phagocytosis:* white blood cells, by changing their shape, pass through the permeable capillary walls to engulf and digest bacteria. White blood cells and phagocytic debris become the ingredients in pus.
   4. **Wound strength is limited to the wound closure material holding it together.**
   5. **Wound should be observed for swelling and discoloration.**

B. *Phase 2:* Proliferation phase: lasts up to 2 weeks
   1. Fibroblasts (connective tissue cells) multiply rapidly and bridge the wound edges and form collagen (works like tissue glue to give strength to the wound).
   2. Capillary buds sprout to form a network.
   3. Wound should be supported and free from excess stress or pull.

C. *Phase 3:* Maturation, remodeling, or differentiation phase: begins at 2 weeks and lasts for months
   1. Scar begins to fade as the formation of new blood vessels decreases leaving a mature white scar called a cicatrix.
   2. The wound gains in tensile strength as collagen density increases.

III. **Factors That Affect Wound Healing**

A. *Age:* pediatric and geriatric patients are more prone to infection

B. **Compromised circulation caused by atherosclerosis, venous stasis, anemia, diabetes, etc**

C. **Poor nutrition or fluid and electrolyte imbalance; vitamin C is necessary for good scar formation**

D. **Obesity**

E. **Drugs such as anti-inflammatory agents (corticosteroids) and antineoplastic drugs**

   F. Radiotherapy: x-ray or irradiation

   G. Smoking, which reduces functional hemoglobin, constricts blood vessels, and promotes postoperative coughing, which puts pressure on the wound

   H. Preoperative skin shave, with resultant abrasions, permits transient bacteria to enter the wound

   I. Presence of acute or chronic disease: cancer, metabolic disease

   J. Immunocompromised patient

   K. Preoperative stress level

   L. Presence of infection

   M. Allergic reactions

   N. Wounds located near joints or other areas of stress

   O. Contaminated wound

   P. Lengthy surgical procedures

   Q. Presence of foreign bodies in the wound

   R. Wound complications

IV. Intraoperative Techniques to Enhance Wound Healing

   A. Follow sterile technique to avoid introducing bacteria.

   B. Do not leave culture media in the wound for bacteria.
      1. Minimize dead tissue.
         a. Preserve blood supply.
         b. Irrigate to debride blood clots and dead tissue.
         c. Avoid excessive cauterization of tissue.
      2. Hemostasis with minimal accumulation of blood
         a. Careful dissection
         b. Use of drains when oozing is expected
      3. Eliminate dead space by close approximation of tissue.
      4. Minimize foreign material left in the wound, such as the long ends of a suture (excess debris increases the workload of the lymphatic system and provides a culture medium for bacteria).
      5. High-risk (dirty) wounds are left open to heal by granulation.
      6. Inoculum of bacteria present during surgery should be decreased.
         a. Bowel preparation
         b. Use antibiotics prophylactically and therapeutically.
         c. Minimize talking and movement.
         d. Decrease wound exposure time through organization and work efficiency.

   C. Tissue handling
      1. *Manipulation:* gentle, clean, decisive movements; proper instruments; and proper tissue approximation without tissue strangulation (Halstead principles of tissue handling)
      2. *Dissection:* sharp cuts following anatomical lines
      3. *Protect tissue:* keep moist and minimize exposure; use devices such as bowel bag, wound protector ring, and viscera retainer

   D. *Hemostasis:* secure knots, double ligate high-risk vessels, coagulate precisely to avoid damage to surrounding tissue, and tie off proximal vessels first.

   E. Length and direction of incision

Classification of Wounds

I. Class I (clean): Infection rate 1%–5%

   A. Elective procedure under ideal conditions

   B. Primary closure with or without closed wound drainage

C. No break in aseptic technique

D. No inflammation present

E. Examples include Thyroidectomy, Breast Biopsy, Total Hip Arthroplasty

II. **Class II (clean—contaminated): Infection rate 8%–11%**

A. Entry made into a tube leading to the outside (mucous membrane), such as gastrointestinal (GI), genitourinary (GU), or respiratory tract under controlled conditions

B. Minor or no break in aseptic technique

C. No infection present

D. Examples include Hysterectomy and Pneumonectomy

III. **Class III (contaminated): Infection rate 15%–20%**

A. Gross spillage of contamination (e.g., feces)

B. Major break in aseptic technique

C. Acute inflammation present

D. Open traumatic wound less than 4 hours old

E. Examples include gunshot wound to the abdomen, open fracture.

IV. **Class IV (dirty or infected; highest infection rate expected): Infection rate 27%–40%**

A. Bacteria present in wound before surgery

B. Perforated viscera/viscus

C. Infection with pus or drainage

D. Dirty traumatic wound over 4 hours old or with a foreign body

E. Examples include incision and drainage of an abcess.

Wound Management

I. **Surgical Drains, Tubes, and Catheters**

A. **Drains and catheters**

1. Provide an exit for fluids that may exist or be expected (closed vacuum wound drain). Accumulated fluids:

   a. Provide a culture media for bacteria

   b. Cause tissue irritation (bile, urine, pus)

   c. Cause elevation of skin flaps with loss of vascularity and increase wound disruption potential

   d. Cause pressure on adjacent organs

2. Provide access for contrast media for x-ray studies (cholangiogram catheter, ureteral catheter).

3. Provide access for medication and/or irrigation (Port-a-Cath, for medication; Tenckhof for peritoneal dialysis).

4. Remove purulent (pus) or necrotic (dead) material with sump drains.

5. Remove air or secretions from organs or body cavities.

   a. Closed underwater-seal drainage (chest drain)

   b. Foley two-way and three-way catheter (retention catheters for urine)

   c. Salem sump and Levin tube (nasogastric tubes)

   d. Cantor or Miller-Abbott tubes (small intestine)

   e. Red Robinson catheter (temporary drainage of urine from the bladder, irrigation of ducts)

6. Remove blood clots, emboli, or biliary stones (Fogarty catheter).

7. Catheters are made of latex, rubber, silicone, PVC, Teflon; sized according to the French scale; special adaptors are used to connect to tubing.

B. Types of wound drains
   1. *Penrose:* flat cylinder latex drain, which is available in ¼- to 1-inch diameters, usually placed in a separate stab wound, secured with a sterile safety pin, and serves as an avenue for exit of fluid based on positive pressure inside the body. A cigarette drain is a penrose with a gauze inside the lumen.
   2. *Gravity drain:* tube placed in body organ (bile duct, bladder) and connected to a drainage bag positioned below the patient level; secured with a stitch (T-tube for the bile duct; Malecot, Pezzer, and Mushroom for Suprapubic Cystostomy)
   3. *Closed vaccum wound drain:* drain left in tissue where "weeping" is expected, brought out through skin, sutured in place, and connected to a vacuum-type reservoir (examples are Jackson-Pratt or Hemovac).

      (*Note:* Air is removed from the reservoir before the drain tubing is connected.)
   4. *Sump drains:* double or triple lumen tubes used for aspiration (drawing fluid out), irrigation (washing out), or to introduce medication; brought out through a stab wound and connected to suction.

      (*Note:* One lumen is for drainage, one is for escape of air, and one is for irrigation.)

C. Factors for consideration when using drains or catheters.
   1. Patency must be maintained.
   2. Sterility of components must be maintained until drains and/or catheters are connected.
   3. If an air leak exists, a suction drain is ineffective; connections must be secure.
   4. Drain sites are dressed separately from incision sites with a slit sponge or nonadhering dressing.
   5. Drains are secured to the skin with a 0 to 3-0 nonabsorbable suture on a cutting needle. (*Note:* Granulating tissue forms a fibrous wall around a tube, sealing it off. If the tube is pulled out too soon, a leak can occur, often with serious consequences. This may not be the case when tubes such as the Foley catheter or Levin tube are placed in natural orifices [openings].)
   6. Gravity drainage bags must be kept below the level of the patient.
   7. Type and placement of drains are recorded on the intraoperative record and reported to the PACU nurse.

II. Wound Complications

A. Hemorrhage (open or concealed)
   1. *Indications:* drop in blood pressure, weak, fast pulse; apprehension; cyanosis, and cold, clammy skin
   2. *Causes:* inadequate hemostasis during surgery, improper tying of suture
   3. Methods of hemostasis
      a. Direct pressure, pressure dressing, and packings
      b. Tourniquets: pneumatic tourniquet, blood pressure cuff, Esmarch bandage, rubber tubing, and rubber band; used on extremities
      c. Clips and sutures: hemostatic clamps, ligating clips, and ligatures (ties) to occlude vessels
      d. Pledgets, packs, patties

SURGERY HINT

Closed vacuum wound drains such as hemovacs cannot be connected until the tissue closure has been achieved. Always use a heavy instrument to handle trochar points on the drain tubing.

      e. *Thermal methods:* cryosurgery to seal a small bleeding area, electrocautery, electrosurgery, fulguration (tissue destruction by electric sparks generated by a high frequency current), LASER, hemostatic scalpel, and photocoagulation

      f. *Chemicals:* absorbable gelatin (Gelfoam), absorbable collagen (Collostat, Helistat), microfibrillar collagen (Avitene), and oxidized cellulose (Surgicel, Oxycel)

      g. *Drugs:* phenol with alcohol, styptics, epinephrine, silver nitrate, oxytocin, thrombin, fibrinogen, and vitamin K (enables the liver to produce clotting factors)

    4. Hemostasis during dissection
      a. Electrosurgical unit (ESU)
      b. Harmonic Scalpel
      c. Argon-enhanced coagulation
      d. LASER

B. Wound disruptions
    1. *Dehiscence:* wound gapes open (partial or total)
    2. *Evisceration:* abdominal contents (viscera) protrude from the wound; requires immediate surgical intervention
    3. Generally occur 2 to 6 days after surgery
    4. *Signs and symptoms:* profuse serosanguinous (thin, bloody) drainage, wound bulging, patient feels something give way, vomiting, and tachycardia
    5. *Herniation (eventration):* the surface layers remain intact but the deeper layers (fascia) separate, allowing muscles and organs to bulge.

C. Sinus tract formation caused by collection of fluid without an outlet; fluid makes its own way out by forming a passage (fistula) to another hollow organ or to the outside of the body.

D. Hematoma (localized collection of blood); seroma (collection of serum) in a wound

E. Infection (invasion by pathogens); endogenous (caused from microbes within the body) or exogenous (caused from microbes that came from outside the body)
    1. Measures to prevent wound infection
      a. Surgical aseptic technique
      b. Meticulous wound closure and gentle tissue manipulation
      c. Control of airborne and environmental contamination
      d. Removal of endogenous organisms (as with skin prep, bowel prep, and vaginal prep)
      e. Antibiotics (prophylactic and therapeutic)
      f. Use of sterile dressing application
      g. Adequate tissue perfusion
      h. Use of wound drains

F. *Adhesions:* fibrous bands of scar tissue that bind organs together and may result in obstruction of the bowel; tend to occur more frequently when dry sponges and glove powders are introduced into a body cavity.

SURGERY HINT

Many surgical gloves contain powder to facilitate ease of application. This powder, if allowed into the surgical incision, can cause tissue reactions and adhesions. When changing gloves during a procedure, or when removing top gloves after a contamination or dirty phase of the case, have sterile water available to rinse powder off of the gloves.

Adhesions may be surgically managed through LOA, or lysis of adhesions.

There are chemical adhesion barrier films available to cut down on the formation of adhesions after abdominal or pelvic cavity cases.

G. Excessive scar formation
1. *Cicatrix:* scar
2. *Keloids:* excessive scar formation that extends beyond the borders of the scar; may continue to grow over a long period; common among people with dark skin tones; injection of an anti-inflammatory drug into tissue may prevent them along with use of a pressure dressing
3. *Proud flesh:* excessive granulation tissue; may extend above skin margins

III. **Wound-Closure Materials and Techniques**

A. **Terms**
1. *Suture (stitch):* material used to approximate tissue; to "sew" together until healing occurs
2. *Tensile strength:* amount of pull a knotted strand of suture can withstand; usually decreases as diameter decreases
3. *Gauge:* size (diameter) of a strand; ranges from 5 (largest) to 11-0 (smallest)
4. *Monofilament:* one strand
5. *Multifilament:* more than one strand; braided or twisted
6. *Ligature reel (tie):* suture material on a reel used to tie off blood vessels
7. *Instrument tie/tie on a passer:* a strand of suture loaded on an instrument such as a right angle or tonsil adson clamp
8. *Suture ligature (stick tie, transfixion suture):* suture on a noncutting needle used to anchor the suture into the surrounding tissues prior to tying
9. *Free-tie:* strand of suture placed into a surgeon's pronated, cupped hand
10. *Anastomosis:* creation of an opening between two formerly separated structures such as a vessel or intestine; joining two structures by suturing

B. **Specification for suture materials**
1. Sterile
2. Predictable uniform tensile strength
3. Minimum gauge for safety for specific tissue use
4. Provide knot security and support during tissue healing
5. Inert, or cause minimal reaction, as a foreign body in tissue

C. **Choice of suture materials (based on healing potential): Remember that there are several suture companies. Each company has its own brand name for the sutures that it produces.**
1. *Healing characteristics:* absorbable suture is used for rapidly healing tissue (mucous membrane), and nonabsorbable for slow-healing tissue (tendons, fascia).
2. *Incision:* small monofilament suture for good cosmetic results; larger sutures when greater holding power is needed
3. *Infection or drainage:* suture may act as a foreign body harbor microorganisms (multifilament) or lead to granulation or stone formation (e.g., silk).
4. *Characteristics of suture:* knot placement and security and ease in use
5. *Rate of absorption based on*
   a. *Type of tissue:* fast in serous or mucous membranes, slow in tissues such as tendons, ligaments.
   b. *Condition of tissue:* more rapid in infected tissue
   c. *General health of the patient:* slow in debilitated or aged patient, but rapid in undernourished patient
   d. *Type of absorbable suture used:* plain absorbs more rapidly than chromic
6. *Surgeon's choice:* listed on surgeon's preference card
7. *Availability:* hundreds of suture–needle combinations are available for purchase, but all may not be in stock due to the cost of maintaining a large inventory.

> **SURGERY HINT**
>
> Many sutures have "memory." If a suture has memory, do not pass it to the surgeon until it has been straightened. Hold the suture and gently pull on it to remove the curves. Do not pull too hard as the suture may snap.

D. **Absorbable sutures**
   1. **Surgical gut**
      a. Digested by enzymes
      b. Derived from intestinal mucosa of sheep
      c. Packed in alcohol solution (should be rinsed before use in the eyes); must not be soaked in saline: use immediately following removal from the package, unwind carefully to avoid knot formation, and grasp ends and tug gently to straighten; never run gloved fingers down length or jerk to stretch surgical gut.
      d. **Plain surgical gut:** untreated
         Loses tensile strength in 5 to 10 days
         Digested within 70 days
         Used to ligate small superficial vessels, suture subcutaneous and rapidly healing tissues, tie tonsil knots
         Yellow package and suture
         Causes marked tissue reaction
      e. **Chromic surgical gut:** treated with chromium salts to resist absorption
         Used to ligate larger vessels and in urinary and biliary tracts; may be used in infected tissues
         Supports wound about 14 to 21 days; completely absorbed in 90 days
         Brown suture in a beige package
         Causes limited tissue reaction
         Exhibits a marked decrease in knot security and tensile strength when wet; tails must be left long to prevent knot slippage
      f. Collagen (made from flexor tendon of beef) used primarily in ophthalmic surgery
   2. **Synthetic absorbable suture**
      a. Absorbed by hydrolysis
      b. Inert (causes little or no tissue reaction), nonallergenic, nonpyogenic, and available in monofilament or multifilament; packaged dry
      c. **Polydioxanone (PDS and PDS II suture)**
         Monofilament
         Used in slow-healing tissue, when extended wound support is needed, as with elderly patients, or in the presence of infections
         Seventy percent of tensile strength remains after 2 weeks; completely absorbed in 6 months
         Silver package, violet or clear (for ophthalmic use) suture
      d. **Polyglecaprone (Monocryl)**
         Monofilament
         Used in soft tissue, frequently for subcuticular closure
         Fifty percent of tensil strength remains after 1 week
         Peach colored package, clear or violet suture
      e. **Polyglyconate (Maxon suture)**
         Monofilament
         Used in soft tissue except neural, ophthalmic, or cardiovascular tissue
         Seventy percent of tensile strength remains after 2 weeks; absorbed in 6 months
         Green color or clear

      f. **Polyglactin 910 (Vicryl)**

        Uncoated monofilament; dyed violet

        Coated multifilament; dyed violet, or undyed; smooth passage through tissue and precise knot placement; one of the most popular sutures used today

        Fifty percent of strength remains after 2–3 weeks; absorbed within 90 days

        Violet package

      g. **Polyglycolic acid (Dexon)**

        Uncoated multifilament; dyed green in a gold package and undyed

        Coated multifilament (Dexon Plus suture); coated for smooth passage in tissue and good knot security

        Fifty percent of tensile strength remains at 2–3 weeks; absorbed in 90 days

      h. Other synthetic absorbables: Polysorb, Biosyn

  E. **Nonabsorbable suture**

    1. **Natural nonabsorbable suture**

      a. *Surgical silk:* natural fiber from silkworm cocoons; braided; available in black or white suture in light-blue package; loses much strength in 1 year and disappears in 2 years, gives good wound support, and is used dry; not used in the presence of infection or where a stone may form (bile or urinary system); used on serosa of gastrointestinal tract, fascia, and for ligating larger vessels; excellent handling characteristics and average knot holding and tensile strength

      a. *Virgin silk:* for ophthalmic surgery

      b. *Dermal silk:* coated

      b. *Surgical cotton:* natural fiber twisted; weak; is stronger when wet; white sutures in pink box; not commonly used today as suture, but cotton is used as umbilical tape which can be used as a retractor for vessels or ducts

      c. *Surgical stainless steel:* must be compatible with other metals used in the area to avoid electrolytic reaction; Brown and Sharp (B&S) gauge 18–40, with 40 being smallest; most difficult suture to manipulate; inert with highest tensile strength of any suture, but lacks elasticity and knot tying is a problem; used for tendon repairs, bone repair, sternal closure, abdominal wound closure if infection; handling characteristics: keep strands straight to avoid kinking, and use wire scissors (Smith).

    2. **Synthetic nonabsorbable suture**

      a. Has high tensile strength, less tissue reaction than silk, retains strength in tissue, and knots may require additional flat and square ties; multifilament easier to tie than monofilament

      b. Coatings (silicon, PTFE/Teflon, polybutilate) decrease drag through tissue and provide knot security.

      c. Suture is clamped only at the ends, as clamping can weaken the suture.

      d. *Surgical nylon:* monofilament (Ethilon, Dermalon, Monosof), black or green; used in ophthalmic, plastic, microsurgery, tendon repair, skin closure, and retention sutures; one of the most inert suture materials; because of poor knot security requires extra knots and ends must be cut longer

        Uncoated multifilament nylon (Nurolon), braided, black or white, high tensile strength

        Coated multifilament (Surgilon), treated with silicone to enhance passage in tissue, high tensile strength

      e. *Mersilene and Dacron:* braided polyester fiber; pliable; white or green; useful in respiratory and cardiovascular procedures

      f. *Polybutilate (Ethibond):* coated polyester fiber, braided; green or white; in orange packages

g. *Polytetrafluroethylene (Polydek, Tevdek):* Teflon-coated braided polyester; may produce foreign body granuloma; flexible and strong

h. *Silicone (Ti-cron):* Polyester coated with lubricant; white or blue

i. *Polybutester (Novafil suture):* monofilament, more flexible and elastic; clear or blue

j. Polypropylene (Prolene, Surgilene, Dermalene, Surgipro)
Monofilament
Most inert of synthetic materials
Acceptable substitute for steel
Can be used in the presence of infection
Choice for many plastic and cardiovascular procedures because of smooth pull through tissue and inertness; used for abdominal fascia closures, subcuticular pull-out sutures, or for retention sutures
Available in blue and clear

F. **Surgical needles**
1. *Characteristics:* made of steel, strong, rigid, sharp, same diameter as suture, appropriate shape and size for tissue to be sutured, and detectable by x-ray. Three parts of a needle are point, body, and eye.
2. *Needle points:* honed for specific type of tissue
    a. *Cutting:* razor sharp for tough tissue that is hard to penetrate (skin, tendon, sclera)
        i. *Conventional cutting:* three cutting edges (inside curve) allow smooth passage through tissue that heals quickly
        ii. *Reverse cutting:* triangular configuration extends along the body of the needle with a precision point; frequently used on the skin
        iii. *Side cutting:* for ophthalmic surgery; relatively flat on top and bottom and cutting edge on sides
        iv. *Trocar point:* three sharp cutting edges
        v. *Taper cut:* Combination of tapered body with a slight cutting tip
    b. *Taper point:* used for soft, delicate tissue
    c. *Blunt point:* tapered with rounded blunt point for friable tissue (liver, kidney)
3. *Needle shaft* (body)
    a. Heavy gauge for fibrous tissue, and fine gauge for microsurgery
    b. Length determined by depth (bite)
    c. Straight shaft (Keith) may be used for skin; curved shafts (¼-, ⅜-, ½-, ⅝-circle, and half-curved needles) are passed to the surgeon on needle holder; increased curvature needed for deeper tissue penetration.
    d. *Smooth finish:* some coated with plastic or silicone to enhance passage in tissue.
4. **Needle eyes (for attachment of sutures)**
    a. *Eyed needle–closed eye (Mayo, Ferguson, Martin, Keith):* opening may be round, oblong, or square; suture is threaded through 2 to 4 inches and locked into the needle holder; causes more tissue damage than the eyeless needle
    b. *French eye needle (spring or slit eye):* loaded by pulling the suture strand into a v-shaped area above the eye.
    c. *Eyeless needles (atraumatic, swaged):* continuous with the suture, eliminate threading, and minimize tissue trauma
        i. *Single-armed attachment:* one needle
        ii. *Double-armed attachment:* needle on each end of the suture strand; commonly used to anastomose a vessel
        iii. *Permanently swaged attachment:* needle attached and must be removed by cutting with suture scissors
        iv. *Controlled release attachment (pop-off or detach):* needle may be detached from the suture with a quick, sharp pull.

SURGERY HINT

Preloading suture can be a dangerous practice that many facilities frown upon. Preloading can be dangerous, as it allows sharps to be exposed. The Surgical Technologist should be able to quickly load and pass suture as the surgeon requests it, not before. Sutures are preloaded in packs for a right-handed surgeon.

Suture packets should be opened to expose needles during the initial count to ensure that the number of needles in the packet is accurate.

5. Placement of the needle in the needle holder (arming or loading the needle holder).
   a. Select needle holder with appropriate size jaws for needle size.
   b. Select needle holder with the appropriate length for depth in wound.
   c. Determine if surgeon is left-handed or right-handed, and position the needle accordingly.
   d. Set the needle 1–2 mm into the needle holder jaw.
   e. Clamp the needle body at the right angle to the holder, one-third the distance from eye or swag (*never* on swaged area, as it is the weakest area of a swaged needle).
   f. Newer suture packets allow arming the needle without touching it to avoid a needle stick.
   g. Seat needle securely in holder and close needle holder to second ratchet.
   h. Pass with needle point toward the chin of the surgeon while holding on to the end of the suture if it is long or with the suture over the back of your hand if it is short or a "pop-off." Pass a pair of appropriate pick-ups or tissue forceps to the surgeon. If the suture is long, hand the end to the first assistant so that they may "follow" or "run" the suture. The first assistant may want an instrument (hemostat or empty needle holder) to grasp the needle as it is passed through the tissue.
   i. Hospital policy may dictate a "no-touch" technique with sharps. This technique eliminates hand-to-hand passing of sharps by the use of a neutral zone or designated container.

G. Suturing terminology and techniques
   1. *Primary suture line* (refers to the sutures that approximate the wound edges)
      a. *Continuous suture (running stitch):* series of stitches with one strand that provides for a rapid closure, even distribution of tension, and a leakproof suture line; the strand is tied after the first stitch and then tied again after the last stitch is placed.
      b. *Interrupted suture:* each stitch is taken and tied separately; if one strand breaks, the others may hold; in the presence of infection, microbes are less likely to follow the strand; known as the Halstead technique; various techniques are used to insert an interrupted suture, i.e., mattress.
      c. *Buried sutures:* continuous or interrupted sutures beneath the skin
      d. *Purse-string suture:* continuous suture around a lumen which, when tightened, closes the lumen; used for the appendix and in the right atrium and ascending aorta when inserting cannuale for cardiopulmonary bypass
      e. *Subcuticular suture:* short, lateral continuous stitches beneath the epidermis, which is secured at each end of the incision; creates a minimal scar
      f. *Suture patterns*
         Distance between stitches is equal to the width of each stitch.
         Sutures are tied loosely to accommodate for edema.
         Vertical mattress provides precise edge approximation.
         Eversion is achieved by the horizontal mattress stitch.
         Skin suture marks can be avoided by sewing a continuous subcuticular stitch

Skin bites are of equal distance on each side.

Buttons may be used to prevent tissue damage (when using tendon suture).

When a continuous stitch is used, the remaining strand is untwisted after each bite.

A continuous locking stitch prevents slippage and aids hemostasis, but it may strangulate the tissue.

The Connel stitch is a continuous inverting suture which may be used for bowel mucosa (inner layer).

The Limbert stitch is used for bowel serosa (outer layer).

The Halsted stitch is an interrupted horizontal mattress stitch.

The Cushing stitch is a continuous horizontal mattress stitch.

2. *Secondary suture line* (**tension, stay, or retention sutures**): heavy, interrupted, nonabsorbable widely spaced suture placed lateral to the primary suture line and through multiple layers.
   a. Used with abdominal incisions to reinforce the primary suture line in patients that have predisposing factors that may lead to wound disruption.
   b. Bridges, bolsters, or bumpers are used to prevent the heavy suture (nylon, silk, polyester, wire) from cutting into the primary suture line.
3. *Traction suture:* nonabsorbable suture used to stabilize or retract tissue to the side of the operative field for the enhancement of visualization during dissection; used on the sclera, myocardium, or tongue

H. **Packaging and preparation**
   1. *Suture packet:* with or without swaged needle; comes in a double wrap
      a. May have one or more suture needles
         Opened only as needed; are not resterilized
         Color-coded labels with needle silhouette
         Designed for easy dispensing
         Observe for expiration dates on sutures
      b. Standard length suture (54 inches for absorbable and 60 inches for nonabsorbable) may be cut in half, third, or quarter lengths. Precut lengths (18, 24, and 30 inch strands) are also available.
      c. Ligating reel (54-inch suture, color-coded with size identification by the number of holes in the radiopaque reel; included in counts, and used in place of free ties to ligate bleeders).
      d. The surgical assistant helps with the placement and cutting of ligatures by holding the hemostatic clamp (attached to the vessel) with the point exposed. After the surgeon ties the first knot, the clamp is removed. Once the knots are secured, the suture is cut, leaving a 6-mm (¼-inch) tail if it is monofilament and a short 3-mm (1/8-inch) tail if it is multifilament.
   2. *Overwrap:* outside wrapper for an easy transfer to the sterile field; circulator peels back edges for scrub to take with a clamp or flips it onto the sterile field
   3. *Box:* contains one to three dozen packets, color coded, contains all printed suture information

I. **Surgical staples: Come in reusable and preloaded disposable staple guns and appliers**
   1. *Uses:* biopsy, ligate, divide, resect, close skin or fascia, and anastomosis
   2. Advantages
      a. *Speed:* decreases operating time and increases efficiency
      b. *Accelerates wound healing:* reduced blood loss, trauma, edema, tissue reaction, and necrosis; provides even surface and leakproof closure; and nutrients can pass the B-shaped staple line into edges of tissue
      c. Reduces chance of needle sticks

3. Disadvantages of staples
   a. *Cost:* expensive and once opened cannot be used for another patient
   b. Special instruction and practice with use of each type of stapler is essential to avoid error.
   c. Must be placed precisely
   d. Stainless steel staples may interfere with CT or MRI procedures.
4. Stapling instruments
   a. *Skin stapler:* each squeeze of the trigger fires a single staple to approximate skin edges; preloaded with staples of varying widths which are removed in 5 to 7 days with a special extractor.

      (*Note:* Assistance is needed in placing skin staples; while surgeon everts and approximates skin with forceps, assistant fires staple gun with a single squeeze of the handle.)
   b. *Linear stapler (Thoracoabdominal [TA]):* two rows of staples are placed simultaneously; for transection of internal tissues; available in different sizes and colors to accommodate tissue thickness
   c. *Linear cutter (Gastrointestinal anastomosis [GIA]):* two double-staggered rows of staples with a cutting bar; places staples on both sides of the cut line.
   d. *Intraluminal stapler (ILS, end to end anastomosis [EEA]):* for anastomosis of the gastrointestinal tract; a circular knife within the head of the circular stapler trims tissue
   e. *Ligating and dividing staplers (LDS):* ligates, divides, and staples tissue; useful for omentum and mesentery
   f. *Ligating clips:* used on vessels, nerves, and ducts
      Available in various sizes; color-coded clips available in presterilized disposable packets for use with non-disposable clip appliers
      Disposable clip appliers are available preloaded and in different lengths.
      Made of stainless steel, titanium, or tantalum

J. **Endoscopic suturing**
   1. Suturing through a trocar cannula during endoscopy can be performed through the extracorporeal (outside the body) method; the knot is tied outside the body and slid in place with a knot pusher.
   2. Preknotted endo-loops may be introduced with plastic delivery devices.
   3. Intracorporeal knot tying is performed completely with the abdomen.

K. **Tissue repair materials**
   1. Tissue adhesive
      a. *Biological adhesive*
         Fibrin glue made from fibrinogen and thrombin; hemostatic
         Autologous or homologous plasma is used to produce fibrinogen.
         Pooled-donor plasma is used commercially to prepare fibrin glue in Europe.
      b. *Synthetic adhesives:* polymethylmethacrylate, a synthetic glue (bone cement) used in fixation of fractures or joint replacement to stabilize prosthetic devices in bone

---

SURGERY HINT

Stapling devices may become clogged with staples that did not discharge or with tissue. Have a small basin of fluid available to swish the tip in before re-loading the device. Do not use this fluid as irrigation.

Always check clips appliers before using as some may not hold staples well. These should be set aside and tagged after the case for repair. Never hand a surgeon a clip applier that is malfunctioning as it can damage tissue.

Hemoclip appliers may be non-disposable. If so, the appliers are color coated to match the boats, or trays, of clips.

Generally, the trays are considered a countable item.

Cyanoacrylate, used for skin closure; Dermabond is applied with an applicator and dries in 2 ½ minutes. It remains on the wound 5–10 days and should not be used in the presence of infection.

2. Biological materials

Fascia lata: strips of fascia from beef (heterogenous graft), patient's thigh (autogenous graft), or from cadavers (allograft), used to strengthen defects in fascia

3. Synthetic meshes (used to reinforce or bridge tissue deficiencies)

   a. Easily cut to the desired size
   b. Easily sutured or stapled
   c. Pliable, inert, porous, and allow fibrous tissue to grow through openings
   d. Types

      Polyester fiber mesh (Mersilene mesh)
      Polyglactin 910 mesh (Vicryl mesh)
      Polypropylene (Prolene mesh, Marlex mesh)
      Polytetrafluoroethylene (PTEF, Gore-Tex soft tissue patch)
      Ingrowth mesh (Surgisis)
      Stainless steel mesh

L. **Skin closure devices**

1. *Skin staples:* in disposable applier, easy to use, reduce tissue trauma and operating time
2. *Skin clips:* form more scar tissue than other methods; Michelle Clips are rarely used.
3. *Wound zipper:* commercially prepared nylon zipper used when frequent reentry of a wound is necessary
4. *Skin closure strips:* adhesive-backed strips placed at intervals across an incision to approximate skin edges (Steri-strip, Proxistrip); a skin tackifier (benzoin or mastisol) may be used to increase adhesiveness.

IV. Wound Dressings

A. **Purposes of wound dressings**

1. Protect from microbial contamination and injury.
2. Absorb drainage and secretions.
3. Support or compress to control bleeding, eliminate dead space, and decrease edema.
4. Immobilize when movement might interfere with healing (e.g., joints).
5. Apply medication (e.g., infected wound).
6. Cover the wound aesthetically.
7. Provide a healthy environment.
   a. Wick away excessive exudate (e.g., urine, bile) to prevent skin maceration (skin soft due to wetting).
   b. Provide moist environment for rapid epithelization.
8. Wound debridement (e.g., decubitus ulcer)

B. **Types of dressings**

1. *Primary:* placed directly on the wound to preserve a moist environment and wick away exudate (drainage) from the wound
2. *Secondary:* placed over the primary dressing to absorb drainage and secretions
3. *One-layered dressing:* used to cover a small incision with minimal drainage, consists of a transparent film with adhesive backing (Op-Site, Bioclusive); liquid collodion may be applied to form a seal over the wound
4. *Three-layer dressing:* used when drainage is expected. The inner contact layer is one of three types:

   Nonocclusive: permeable, nonadherent dressings which wick away exudate and allow exposure of the wound to air (Telfa, Adaptic)

Occlusive: a nonpermeable dressing made of tightly woven gauze with petrolatum to seal a wound (e.g., following removal of a chest tube) or to prevent the loss of fluid (e.g., burns). (Vaseline gauze, Xeroform gauze).

Semiocclusive: semipermeable hydroactive materials such as hydrogels (Tegasorb, Exuderm) and hydrocolloids (Nu-Gel, Aqua-Gel); may be used on a decubitus ulcer or burn.

The intermediate layer is placed over the inner layer to absorb any drainage (4 × 4 gauze sponges, ABD pad, combine pad). The outer layer is used to secure the contact and absorbent layers and includes
a. Paper, silk, or adhesive tape
b. Rolled gauze (Kerlix, Kling)
c. Rolled cotton sheeting (Webril)
d. Elastic bandage (Ace, Coban)
e. Seamless tubular cotton (Stockinette)
f. Tubular gauze on a digit
g. Montgomery straps—used when wound requires frequent inspection or dressing change, used in pairs

5. *Nonadhering:* prevents primary dressing from sticking to the wound, skin staples, or sutures and allows exudate to flow into dressing
6. *Rigid dressing:* used to support and immobilize limb (splint, cast)
7. *Pressure dressing:* dressings which provide compression and increase bulk to prevent swelling.
8. *Stent dressing:* long suture ends are tied over a dressing to hold it in place.

C. **Application of dressings**
1. Opened by the circulator *after* the final sponge count is complete to avoid potential errors in counting.
2. Scrub person cleans around incision with damp sponge
3. A separate dressing is used for the drain (slit dressing).
4. Applied before drapes are removed or protect the site with a sterile towel until drapes are removed
5. Benzoin (Mastisol) may be applied to enhance the adhesiveness of the skin.
6. Tape is applied by circulator. Care should be taken to select appropriate tape. Be aware of tape allergies.
7. Elastic bandages, pressure dressing, stockinette, casts, and splints are generally applied by the surgeon or first assistant.
8. Bandages used on extremities should be applied from distal to proximal, and compress without obstructing, with each spiral covering about one-third of the previous spiral.

Show What You Know

Directions

Each of the numbered items or incomplete statements in this section is followed by answers or by completions of the statement. Select the ONE lettered answer or completion that is BEST in each case.

1. A patient is brought into the emergency room with the following injuries: a large bruise on the thigh, an irregular cut on the forehead, and skin scraped off the arm. The wounds would be described as:

   A. incise wound of thigh, abrasion of forehead, burns of the arm
   B. avulsion of thigh, contused forehead, abrasion of arm
   C. contused wound of thigh, laceration of forehead, abrasion of arm
   D. abrasion of thigh, puncture wound to forehead, lacerated arm

2. You are assigned to scrub on a gunshot wound of the abdomen with a perforated bowel and will expect the surgeon to:

   A. clean up the wound and approximate wound edges for primary intention healing
   B. irrigate and suction in preparation for second intention healing
   C. suture individual layers of tissue after debridement of the wound
   D. clean up the wound, pack the wound to keep wound edges apart, and bring the patient back at a later date for delayed closure

3. Control of bleeding is called:

   A. homeostasis
   B. granulation
   C. inflammatory process
   D. Hemostasis

4. During which phase of wound healing is the strength of the wound limited to the suture holding it together?

   A. granulation
   B. lag phase (inflammatory)
   C. epithelization (proliferation)
   D. remolding (maturation)

5. All of the following factors delay wound healing *except:*

   A. smoking
   B. steroid or cancer drugs
   C. emotional stress
   D. good circulation

6. Which of the following intraoperative techniques would *not* promote wound healing?

   A. inoculum of bacteria into the wound
   B. preservation of blood supply

   C. elimination of dead space
   D. irrigation to debride the wound

7. Based on the potential for infection, which one of the following described wounds would be classified as a class I?

   A. removal of the appendix with no major spill
   B. inguinal hernia repair without break in technique
   C. compound fracture
   D. gunshot wound to the abdomen

8. A collection of fluid in tissue would result in all of the following *except:*

   A. hemostasis
   B. a culture medium for bacteria
   C. pressure on adjacent organs
   D. elevation of skin flap with the loss of vascularity and predisposition to wound disruption

9. For which of the following wound drains would a sterile safety pin be needed?

   A. sump drain
   B. closed wound suction drain
   C. Penrose drain
   D. gravity drain

10. Inadvertent removal of which one of the following drains during the first 48 hours after placement would cause the *least* concern?

    A. T tube (gravity drain)
    B. wound sump drain
    C. closed-wound suction drain
    D. nasogastric tube

11. Which of the following signs would you expect if the patient is hemorrhaging?

    A. slow pulse
    B. hypertension
    C. cool, moist skin
    D. flushed face

12. Which of the following methods of hemostasis is thermal?

    A. absorbable gelatin (Gelfoam)
    B. thrombin
    C. Esmarch bandage
    D. electrocautery

13. When fibrous bands of scar tissue bind organs together, the condition is:

    A. adhesions
    B. cicatrix

C. evisceration

D. sinus tract

14. A suture at the secondary suture line is a:

A. stick tie

B. ligature

C. traction suture

D. retention suture

15. Of the following sutures, which will be absorbed quickest?

A. surgical gut

B. polyglycolic acid (Dexon)

C. polypropylene (Prolene)

D. polydioxanone (PDS)

16. Which suture is contraindicated both in the presence of infection and in the urinary or biliary tract?

A. chromic gut

B. polypropylene (Prolene)

C. polydioxanone (PDS)

D. silk

17. Which suture gauge would be more appropriate for ophthalmic surgery?

A. 7

B. 0

C. 4–0

D. 8–0

18. The needle point most appropriate for suturing liver, pancreas, or spleen is:

A. taper

B. blunt

C. cutting

D. trocars

19. Which of the following statements best describes the placement of the needle holder on the needle?

A. one-fourth of the distance from the point

B. on the swaged section

C. in the center of the needle

D. one-third the distance from the eye or swage

20. The stitch which provides the most rapid closure, even distribution of tension, and a leakproof suture line is:

A. interrupted

B. continuous

C. purse string

D. buried

21. The purpose of a secondary suture line is to:

A. reinforce the primary suture line

B. provide traction to immobilize tissue

C. secure the wound drain

D. suture around a lumen to occlude a vessel

22. With which of the following staplers would the surgeon need assistance in application?

A. ligating clip

B. linear stapler

C. intraluminal stapler

D. skin stapler

23. The dressing that should be placed nearest the wound is:

A. primary dressing

B. secondary dressing

C. pressure dressing

D. rigid dressing

24. Dressing sponges are opened by the circulator:

A. before the surgical procedure begins

B. before the counts are taken

C. after the final count is taken

D. anytime the scrub calls for them

25. After the blood around the wound is wiped away with a damp sponge, the dressings are applied by the:

A. circulator as soon as the drapes are removed

B. circulator before the drapes are removed

C. scrub before the drapes are removed

D. physician after the drapes are removed

Answers & Rationales

1. **C.** **Rationale:** A bruise is a contused wound, a cut with irregular edges is a lacerated wound, and a scraped wound is an abrasion.

2. **D.** **Rationale:** A gunshot wound of the abdomen would result in gross contamination from bowel contents and would require thorough irrigation and packing wound edges apart to permit granulation to begin. The patient would be brought to surgery at a later date for delayed closure—third intention healing.

3. **D.** **Rationale:** *hemo:* blood; *stasis:* control.

4. **B.** **Rationale:** The inflammatory phase, also known as the lag phase, is the first few days, when the strength of the wound is limited to the strength of the sutures holding it together. Epithelization (up to 2 weeks) is the proliferative phase when collagen is being formed and stitches are removed. Wound strength is returned during the remolding or maturation phase.

5. **D.** **Rationale:** Wound healing is delayed by poor circulation, smoking (constricts blood vessels and reduces functional hemoglobin), and emotional stress (lowers body defenses).

6. **A.** **Rationale:** Wound healing is promoted by a good blood supply, elimination of dead space, irrigation to debride wounds, and avoiding inoculum of bacteria in the wound.

7. **B.** **Rationale:** A class I wound is an elective procedure done under ideal conditions with primary closure, and with no major breaks in sterile technique; an inguinal hernia repair would belong to this class. A compound fracture would be class III, with greater chance of infection due to protruding bone. A major spill from the appendix and a gunshot wound to the abdomen would constitute class IV, with the greatest chance of infection.

8. **A.** **Rationale:** Fluid collecting in tissue provides a culture medium for bacteria, puts pressure against adjacent organs, and causes elevation of skin flap, which results in the loss of vascularity and predisposes to wound disruption. It would not provide hemostasis.

9. **C.** **Rationale:** A Penrose drain is a flat cylinder latex drain, generally placed in a stab wound and secured with a safety pin. It serves as an avenue for fluid to exit the body.

10. **D.** **Rationale:** Granulating tissue forms around tubes placed in stab wounds to wall them off. If they are pulled out within 48 hours, a leak can result with serious consequences. Tubes placed in natural orifices, such as a nasogastric tube, would not cause granulation.

11. **C.** **Rationale:** Signs and symptoms associated with hemorrhaging are rapid, weak pulse, rapid, shallow respiration, and cyanosis, which results from decreased circulating volume with resulting hypoxia. Cool, moist skin results from circulatory collapse, which accompanies a decreased blood volume.

12. **D.** **Rationale:** Thermal methods of hemostasis include electrocautery, electrosurgical unit, laser, fulguration, hemostatic scalpel, photocoagulation, and cryosurgery. The Esmarch bandage provides hemostasis by pressure, absorbable gelatin is a chemical, and thrombin is a drug.

13. **A.** **Rationale:** Adhesions are fibrous bands of tissue, resulting from trauma or irritation to tissue, which bind organs together and often require surgery for lysis.

14. **D.** **Rationale:** A retention/tension/through and through suture creates the secondary suture line.

15. **A.** **Rationale:** Surgical gut suture is made of animal protein and therefore is more rapidly absorbed by the body and also causes the most tissue reaction.

16. **D.** **Rationale:** Silk suture is a braided nonabsorbable suture which is not used in the presence of infection because it provides a wicking action and is contraindicated in biliary and urinary tract surgery because it serves as a nucleus for stone formation.

17. **D.** **Rationale:** Ophthalmic surgery requires a very fine suture from 5–0 to 11–0.

18. **B.** **Rationale:** A blunt-point needle is used on friable tissue, such as liver, pancreas, or spleen.

19. **D.** **Rationale:** The needle holder is clamped one-third the distance from the eye or swage of the needle to allow for entry of the point of the needle into tissue with sufficient space for grasping with a needle holder to pull it through.

20. **B.** **Rationale:** The continuous suture is a series of stitches with one strand (running stitch) that provides for rapid closure, even distribution of tension, and a leakproof suture line.

21. **A.** **Rationale:** The secondary suture line (tension, stay, or retention suture) is a heavy, nonabsorbable suture, used with some abdominal closures in patients with low healing potential to prevent wound disruption. It is passed through multiple layers of tissue, widely spaced, to reinforce the primary suture line.

22. **D.** **Rationale:** When placing skin staples, two hands are needed to hold wound edges together, thereby requiring an assistant to position and fire the staple gun.

23. **A.** **Rationale:** When dressing a wound, the primary dressing should be placed next to the incision to wick away the exudate, which if held next to the skin would lead to tissue irritation and maceration.

24. **C.** **Rationale:** Radiopaque sponges are never used to dress the wound. Dressing sponges are not opened until the final sponge count is taken, to avoid an incorrect count.

25. **C.** **Rationale:** Following the placement of the final stitch or staple, the scrub cleans the blood from around the wound with a damp sponge, places dressings on the wound, and holds them with one hand while removing drapes with other hand. The circulator or physician secures the dressing with tape or another type of bandage.

Part II: Deciphering a Surgical Schedule

The following mock surgery schedule will be used to answer several questions pertaining to wound management. The same schedule, or a similar one, may be used in subsequent chapters to ask questions about the content of the chapter.

Rm# time	Surgeon	Procedure	Anest.	Rm# time	Surgeon	Procedure	Anest.
Rm00				**Rm07**			
OC	Dr. Z	Rt. Knee Arthroscopy	Gen.	7:00	Dr. M	Rhinoplasty	Gen.
OC	Dr. C	Craniotomy	Gen.	TF	Dr. M	Lipoma removal	MAC
OC	Dr. Z	Angioplasty	Gen.				
Rm01				**Rm08**			
7:00	Dr. X	Lobectomy	Gen.	11:00	Dr. E	Bovine Thrombectomy	MAC
TF	Dr. X	Thoracotomy	Gen.				
TF	Dr. X	Tracheostomy	Gen.				
Rm02				**Rm09**			
7:00	Dr. B	Splenectomy	Gen.	8:30	Dr. T	Cholecystectomy	Gen.
TF	Dr. B	Gastrectomy	Gen.	TF	Dr. T	STSG	
Rm03				**Rm10**			
7:00	Dr. A	Cystoscopy	Gen.	7:00	Dr. K	Nephrectomy	Gen.
TF	Dr. A	Cystoplasty	MAC	TF	Dr. K	Open Appendectomy	MAC
12:30	Dr. F	Pyleogram	Gen.	TF	Dr. K	Hepatic resection	Gen.
3:00	Dr. F	Cystocele repair MAC					
Rm04				**Rm11**			
7:00	Dr. Y	Carpal tunnel release	Gen.	7:00	Dr. L	Colposcope	Gen.
TF	Dr. Y	Fasciotomy	Gen.	12:00	Dr. L	Mastectomy	Gen.
Rm05				**Rm12**			
7:00	Dr. G	Trans-sphenoidal Adenectomy	Gen.	7:00	Dr. W	Trans-metatarsal amputation	Gen.
TF	Dr. G	Trans-urethral resection of the prostate	Gen	TF	Dr. W	Osteotomy	Gen.
TF	Dr. G	Bletharoplasty	Gen.	TF	Dr. W	Arthrocentesis	Gen.
Rm06				**Rm13**			
7:00	Dr. R	Lumbar Laminectomy	Gen.	7:00	Dr. O	Hysterectomy	Gen.

The following questions should be answered using the surgery schedule above

1. What type of suture line will be used to close the appendix stump during the open appendectomy in Room 10?

   A. Continuous
   B. Interrupted
   C. Mattress
   D. Purse String

2. What size suture will be most appropriate for the Bovine Thrombectomy in Room 8?

   A. 5–0
   B. 2
   C. 1–0
   D. 11–0

3. The Surgical Technologist in Room 5 has a packet of suture that is yellow. What type of suture is in this packet?

   A. Nylon
   B. Silk
   C. Gut
   D. Polyglactin 910

4. The ST in Room 9 needs a Vicryl suture. What color packet will he get?

   A. Yellow
   B. Green
   C. Peach
   D. Violet

5. The surgeon in Room 2 needs a stapler that can cut and staple a straight line simultaneously. Which stapling device should the ST get?

   A. EEA
   B. TA
   C. LDS
   D. Wound zipper

6. The surgeon in Room 6 will be placing interrupted stitches rapidly. What type of needle attachment will he most likely request?

   A. Pop-offs
   B. Swaged
   C. French eye
   D. Double armed

7. The surgery in Room 1 will require closure of the sternum. What type of suture material will be most likely used?

   A. Surgical Cotton
   B. Stainless steel
   C. Surgical Gut
   D. Polyglecaprone (Monocryl)

8. The surgeon in Room 7 has asked the Surgical Technologist for a stick tie. What is he requesting?

   A. A tie on an instrument
   B. A non-cutting needle with attached suture
   C. A Mayo needle
   D. A ligature reel

9. The patient having his Appendix removed in Room 10 has been in intense pain. Once the surgeon gets to the cecum, she discovers that the appendix has burst. What classification would this wound be?

   A. Class I
   B. Class II
   C. Class III
   D. Class IV

10. Dr. T in Room 9 has asked for Xeroform dressing for the STSG. What type of dressing is this?

    A. Non-occlusive
    B. Semi-occlusive
    C. Occlusive
    D. Non-adhering

Answers & Rationales

1. **D.** **Rationale:** The suture line most commonly used to close a lumen, like an appendix stump, is the purse string suture line. This will then be inverted, and another suture line will be placed on the tissue.

2. **A.** **Rationale:** 5–0 is the only appropriate choice in the Thrombectomy. The other options are either too large or too small.

3. **C.** **Rationale:** colored packets make it easier to quickly identify suture materials. Generally the companies that produce suture use these color codes for the suture that they produce. Yellow is the color that denotes surgical gut.

4. **D.** **Rationale:** Violet or purple suture packets denote Polygalactin 910, also called Vicryl or Polysorb.

5. **C.** **Rationale:** The LDS is a Ligating and Dividing Stapler. It cuts and staples in one device. While the EEA also staples and cuts, it is reserved for end-to-end anastomosis, involving the gastrointestinal tract, and cuts in a circle.

6. **A.** **Rationale:** When surgeons are doing a large closure using interrupted stitches, they may want to use pop-offs or control release suture.

This allows the surgeon to move quickly, without having to cut before moving to the next stitch.

7. **B.** **Rationale:** Stainless steel is used to close the sternum in most cases. The Surgical Technologist must handle this with extreme care, as stainless steel may be sharp, especially after being cut. Extra precautions should be taken to prevent punctures of gloves and barriers.

8. **B.** **Rationale:** Stick ties are generally used to anchor tissue or other structures. It is generally a non-cutting needle with attached suture. It may also be called a suture ligature or a transfixion suture.

9. **C.** **Rationale:** A ruptured appendix would be classified as a class III wound, or contaminated. This will increase the risk of infection to 15%–20%.

10. **C.** **Rationale:** Xeroform is an occlusive dressing that is primarily woven gauze infused with petroleum. It is used to seal wounds.

Instrumentation, Equipment, and Case Preparation

Surgery is performed by a team, and each member is a vital link in a chain encircling the patient. Any missing link in the chain can break the protective barrier, causing serious consequences to the patient. Each specialist on the team understands his or her role and is familiar with the roles of every other team member, providing a vigilant system of checks and balances. It is essential that each team member pay close attention to detail, exercise self-control, keep lines of communication open, economize time and motion, be knowledgeable of the scheduled procedure, be prepared both physically and emotionally, and perform consistently under stress. The Surgical Technologist must know all of the instrumentation, equipment, and preparation that go into a case in order to properly function in their role.

CHAPTER OUTLINE

How to Answer Questions on Instrumentation

Instrumentation like suture may be confusing to some students and Surgical Technologists. There are so many different instruments in existence today that learning them all can be a daunting undertaking. As with suture, there are some basic rules that will make it easier to prepare for cases. Always match the instrument to the case, or section of anatomy it is going to be used on. Make sure that the instrument is the correct size; neither too small nor too large for the task. There are specialized instruments that will be used in each surgical case that the Surgical Technologist should familiarize himself with prior to the beginning of the case. Above all, if there is a doubt about an instrument, NEVER hand a crushing or traumatic instrument to a surgeon if it has not been requested. This could irreparably damage the structure that is being worked on.

When faced with a question about instrumentation, attempt to visualize the procedure that is being discussed. What type of tissue is being worked on or repaired? What will the visualization be? Is it being performed laparoscopically or under microscopic visualization? All of these variables must be determined to properly plan the instrumentation for a case. Once these variables have been established, determine which surgical specialty is involved. Is there a specialized instrument that should be identified? You should also determine if the instrument is traumatic or atraumatic. Is it grasping or crushing? Is it a forcep or a clamp? All of these will help you determine the correct answer to the question posed.

Example:
Which instrument is most likely to be used during a bowel resection?

a. Babcock
b. Davidson
c. Herrick
d. Cooley

To answer this question, first identify the type of procedure that is being performed. The bowel resection is a general surgical procedure. This means that you can eliminate instruments that are from other surgical specialties. Eliminating the Cooley, Herrick, and Davidson leaves the Babcock as the correct answer.

Instrumentation

I. Classification of Instruments (based on function)

    A. Cutting/dissecting (used to incise, excise, or separate tissue)

        1. *Scalpels:* #3, #4, and #7 handles: The #3 and #4 handles come in long and angled sizes.

            a. Disposable blades are applied and removed with a needle holder.

            b. Blades #20, #21, and # 23 fit scalpel handle #4.

            c. Blades #10, #11, #12, and #15 fit handles #3 and #7.

            d. Scalpel used for making the skin incision is often considered contaminated and is isolated after the use.

            e. Scalpel may be passed to the surgeon a "no touch" technique is used; scapel is placed in the neutral zone and retrieved by the surgeon to avoid injury

        2. *Scissors:* may be straight or curved; sharpness must be maintained; cutting edges are aligned; used for a designed purpose

            a. *Tissue scissors:* sharpest at tip; usually curved or angled; common names are Mayo (for tough tissue), Metzenbaum (for delicate tissue), episiotomy, Iris, Stevens, and Potts-Smtih (cardiovascular scissors)

            b. *Suture scissors:* blunt points for cutting sutures (straight Mayo, metzenbaum scissors)

            c. *Wire scissors:* short, heavy blade for cutting wire (Smith)

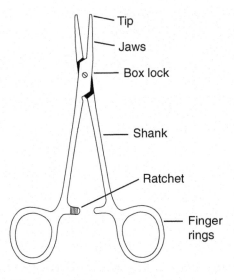

Figure 10-1

3. *Bone cutters:* chisels, osteotomes, gouges, rasps, files, rongeurs, nitrogen, battery, or electric-powered drills, saws, and reamers
4. *Other sharp dissectors:* biopsy forceps, punches, currettes, and snares

B. Grasping and holding (used for manipulation and fine tissue traction)
   1. *Tissue forceps*
      a. *Smooth tips:* for delicate tissue, may be bayonet (angled) or straight, short or long, delicate or heavy; used as pincers (Adson)
      b. *Toothed forceps:* single, double, or multiple teeth for a firm hold on tough tissue; concentrates forces on a small amount of tissue for a maximum holding and minimal tissue destruction (Brown)
   2. *Allis forceps:* contains teeth for gentle but secure hold on tissue without tissue damage
   3. *Babcock forceps:* fenestrated (window) round tip for grasping delicate tubes, ovaries, or intestinal tissue
   4. *Stone forceps* (Randall): for grasping stones
   5. *Tenaculum forceps* (Lahey, Schroeder, Jacobs): sharp tips provide firm grasp
   6. *Bone holders:* hold bone in position (Lane, Lowman)

C. Clamping and occluding (used to apply pressure to prevent leaking of contents)
   1. *Parts of a clamp* (Figure 10-1)
      a. Tip
      b. Jaw (from box lock to tip)
      c. Box lock (hinge joint)
      d. Shank (from box lock to finger rings)
      e. Ratchet (locks instrument)
      f. Finger rings (ringed handles)
   2. *Hemostatic forceps:* used to occlude blood vessels; Hemostat: straight or curved; Halsted, Crile, Lahey, Kelly, Rochester Pean, Mixter (right angle), and tonsil (Schnidt)

SURGERY HINT

Always use caution when handing sharp instruments such as penetrating towel clamps or gelpis. The sharp prongs can easily snag gloves or drapes creating contamination or injury to both the staff and the patient.

When retracting, take care not to move the retractor or change the pressure of the retractor. If it is necessary to move the retractor, or to let go of the retractor, ask if it is OK to let go. Never let go of retraction unless it is announced or expected.

Always hand self-retaining retractors in the closed position and in the proper orientation for use.

Again, be aware of sharp prongs and always practice safe handling.

3. *Crushing clamps:* for crushing tissue or vessels; jaws may be straight, curved, or angled; serrations may be horizontal, diagonal, or longitudinal (Kocher, Oschner intestinal clamps)
4. *Noncrushing vascular and intestinal clamps:* for temporary occlusion; jaws with opposing rows of finely serrated teeth; shape of jaws varies; multi-ratcheted (Statinsky, DeBakey, Cooley: vascular)

D. **Exposing and retracting (used to enhance visualization during dissection)**
   1. *Handheld retractor (manual):* narrow or wide; depth of blades varies; may be dull, sharp, have hooks, or be malleable (bendable) (Rake, Deaver, Harrington, Richardson, vein, Senn, U.S. Army)
   2. *Self-retaining retractors:* advantage of fixed position to free assistant for other tasks (Balfour, Bookwalter, Weitlaner, Gelpi, and Finochetti rib retractor). (*Note:* Moist lap pads may be used to protect tissue from contact with metal.)

E. **Suturing or stapling**
   1. *Needle holder:* short, sturdy jaws for grasping a needle (Webster, Castroviejo, Heaney)
   2. *Staples:* various types; disposable or reusable

F. **Viewing (used for examining interior of the body)**
   1. *Speculum:* used to hold open a canal (vaginal, ear, nasal)
   2. *Endoscopes:* hollow or lensed; pass into a body orifice or through a small incision

G. **Suctioning and aspirating**
   1. *Suction:* tube with suction tip, connected to a vacuum or suction source; used for removing irrigation, blood, or body fluids
   2. *Suction tips:* Poole abdominal tip, Ferguson-Frazier tip, Yankauer tonsil tip, aspirating tube (through an endoscope).

H. **Probing: wirelike, may be malleable, used to explore ducts or a fistula, may be used with a guide (grooved director) (Bowman lacrimal probes)**

I. **Dilating: used to enlarge an orifice or duct (Bakes common duct dilators, Hanks, Hegar, or Pratt cervical dilators)**

J. **Accessory instruments include mallet and screwdriver**

II. **Care and Handling of Instruments**

A. **Check function and integrity: check scissors, forceps, and clamps for alignment, imperfections, cleanliness, and working conditions; set aside if defective**

B. **Sort instruments by classification, keep them in their proper place, and handle gently.**

C. **Protect sharp edges, blades, and tips.**

When suctioning the plume from the ESU, keeps the tip of the suction ¼ inch away from the tip of the bovie, ensure that you do not block the operative field.

SURGERY HINT

Keeping the instruments organized on the back table and Mayo take practice, but is essential for a seamless count. Following the protocol of always replacing instruments in their original space will help the ST remain organized.

For students and new STs, identification of new instruments can be challenging. Before the beginning of the case, read the count sheet, identify instruments that are unfamiliar, and write the name of the instrument(s) on the back table using a sterile marker.

Many facilities require a standard setup for certain cases. Others will allow techs to set up using individual preferences. Check with the facility to ensure compliance.

D. Use instruments only for their designed purpose.

E. Pass instruments decisively and firmly to the palm of the physician's extended hand. (*Note:* Ratcheted instruments are closed before passing.)

F. Keep instruments free of gross soil during surgery: wipe blood and debris from instruments promptly with sponge moistened with sterile water; keep suction tip flushed, and keep electrosurgical tip clean.

G. Close ratcheted instruments on the first ratchet.

H. Keep instruments organized and accessible for the final count.

I. Ensure that all instruments are removed before drapes are discarded.

J. In preparation for terminal sterilization, disassemble instruments with movable parts, open hinged instruments, separate instruments of dissimilar metals, flush cold distilled water through hollow instruments, and rinse blood and debris from other instruments.

K. Instrument cleaning methods (manually or by presoaking)
   1. Microsurgical and ophthalmic instruments are *not* processed through a washer–sterilizer.
   2. Instruments are *not* cleaned in scrub sinks or sinks in a substerile room.
   3. Cover instruments or place in case cart and take to the decontamination area. (*Note:* Personnel must wear protective gloves, aprons, and face shields while cleaning instruments.)
   4. Never scrub surfaces with abrasive agents or leave to soak in saline; saline rusts and pits instruments.
   5. Rinse instruments in distilled or deionized water.
   6. Load instruments into sterilizer trays with racks and run through washer–sterilizer/washer–decontaminator or put in basin with 2% trisodium phosphate solution and steam sterilize for 45 minutes at 250°F (121°C) (rarely done).
   7. Lensed instruments may be immersed in high-level disinfectant after manual cleaning, or processed through an automatic cleaning and disinfecting machine.
   8. *Ultrasonic cleaning:* high-frequency sound waves generate tiny bubbles that dislodge, dissolve, or disperse debris from serrations, box locks, and crevices of instruments (by cavitation).
      a. Instruments are cleaned and terminally sterilized before processing through the ultrasonic cleaner and should be open and disassembled; cutting edges should be protected, dissimilar metals separated, and plated instruments not included.
      b. Instruments are rinsed thoroughly and dried promptly after removing from ultrasonic cleaner.

L. Lubricate instruments after cleaning according to the manufacturer's guidelines.
   1. Place in water-soluble lubricant bath.
   2. Avoid the use of mineral oil, machine oils, and silicone (impermeable to many sterilizing methods).

M. **Inspect and test instruments.**
1. Hinged instruments for flexibility
2. Jaws and teeth for proper alignment
3. Serrations for perfect mesh
4. Forceps for alignment
5. Ratchet teeth (interlocking part between finger rings) for holding power; check for chipping from plated surfaces
6. Tension between shanks
7. Needle holder for needle security
8. Scissors tip for sharpness
9. Microsurgical instruments under magnifying glass for alignment, burrs, nicks, and sharpness of cutting edges
10. Remove all damaged instruments from circulation.

N. **Package and sterilize instruments.**
1. Rigid containers (metal or heavy plastic) used with increasing frequency; filters changed after every use
2. Wrapped trays with perforated bottoms; absorbent towel or foam in bottom to absorb condensate; double wrapped in linen or paper
3. **Prepackaged instruments:** single instrument or small set may be double wrapped in linen or paper or sealed in a paper-plastic pouch (peel pack)
4. **Assembling instrument sets:** use checklist; count and record dry instruments; arrange in definite pattern with heavy instruments on the bottom of the tray; open hinges and box locks; remove detachable parts; separate dissimilar metals; evenly distribute weight; place in rigid container or double wrap; add internal and external chemical indicator and label for intended use. (*Note:* Opened position of ring-handled instruments must be maintained [an instrument holder' pins or rack is useful for this purpose].)
5. Steam sterilize
   a. Gravity displacement sterilizer 30 minutes at a minimum temperature of 250°F (121°C)—rarely used
   b. Prevacuum sterilizer 3–4 minutes at minimum temperature of 270°F (132°C)

III. **Powered Surgical Instruments**

A. *Uses:* precision drilling, cutting, shaping, and beveling bone; taking skin grafts; and abrading skin

B. *Advantages:* increased speed, decreased fatigue, and decreased blood loss

C. *Disadvantages:* dispersal of fine mist of blood or bone; may be hazardous

D. *Accessories:* drill bits, burrs, cutting blades, reamer, or abrader

E. *Power sources*
1. *Air powered:* uses medical-grade compressed air or dry nitrogen (cylinder or piped in)
   a. Set and monitored by pressure gauges on the regulator while the instrument is running and/or as determined by manufacturer's instructions
   b. Instrument assembled, turned on, and psi (pounds per square inch) pressure set at manufacturer's recommendation; minimum cylinder pressure of 500 psi
   c. Small, lightweight, free of vibration, easy to handle, and pinpoint accuracy at high speed, with minimal heating of bone
2. *Electric powered (saws, drills, dermatomes, nerve stimulators)*
   a. Battery powered: cordless, rechargeable battery in handpiece
   b. Alternating current: keep power switch off when plugging cords into electrical outlets, and avoid accidental activation by disconnecting power source or moving foot pedal when not in use.
   c. Because of heat generated from electrical instruments, cooling is provided by the assistant dripping sterile saline from a bulb syringe onto

area, which also serves to wash away particles; care must be taken to avoid touching blade; protection from splash is provided by masks, goggles, shields, and impervious gowns.

F. Handling powered instruments
   1. Set power instruments and attachments on a separate small table or basin stand.
   2. Handle and store air hoses or power cords with care.
   3. Assemble carefully, ensure proper setting, test before use, and keep trigger or handles in safety position when changing attachments or not actively in use

G. Cleaning and sterilizing powered instruments
   1. Decontaminate and clean immediately after use; wipe off organic debris between uses, disassemble, keep cord or air hose attached, wipe with detergent, and dry.
   2. Do not immerse motor or hoses in liquid.
   3. Lubricate as recommended by the manufacturer.
   4. Wrap for sterilization; disassemble, protect sharp edges, and loosely coil hose or cords.
   5. Sterilize (disassembled with hoses coiled and delicate parts protected) as recommended by the manufacturer.

Equipment

I. Electrosurgery (routine surgical technique in cutting and coagulating body tissue with a high-frequency current)

A. *Electrosurgical unit (ESU):* current flows from a generator to an active electrode, through tissue, and back to the generator through the inactive electrode
   1. Generator must be properly grounded.
      a. *Coagulating current:* coagulates tissue and seals the ends of small vessels to control bleeding
      b. *Cutting current:* cuts tissue
      c. *Controls:* start with the lowest setting and increase as necessary based on surgeon's request; may be operated by foot pedal or hand-controlled switch; circulator verbally confirms power setting.
   2. *Active electrode:* directs current to operative site from the generator (electrosurgical pencil)
      a. *Tips:* blade, loop, ball, and needle (extension available for coagulating/cutting deep in a wound)
      b. *Handles:* pencil-shaped, tissue forceps, or suction tube, either disposable or reusable
      c. *Conductor cord:* connected to generator (scrub passes cord off to circulator for attachment; keep free from kinks or stress, do not wrap around metal instruments); kept clean, visible, and dry.
      d. Electrode kept in container when not in use to avoid fire or patient burns in the event of inadvertent activation
      e. Tips must be kept free of charred tissue, which absorbs heat and decreases effectiveness. Use the scratch pad to remove eschar
   3. *Inactive dispersive electrode:* grounding pad
      a. Provides return of current to the generator
      b. Fastened firmly to the grounding connection on the generator
      c. Placed on surgically positioned patient on a clean, dry skin surface, over a large muscle mass, and as close to the operative site as possible. Areas to be avoided: scar, bony prominence, hairy surface, or pressure points; placement should be noted in the operative record along with the condition of the skin before application and upon the removal of pad.

4. *Bipolar versus monopolar unit*
   a. *Bipolar unit:* dispersive electrode is incorporated into the forceps used by surgeon; provides precise control and does not require the use of a grounding pad current flows from tip to tip of the forceps.
   b. *Monopolar unit:* current flows from active electrode, through patient, to inactive dispersive (grounding pad) electrode, and back to the generator.
5. *Safety factors:* more patient injuries result from the ESU than from any other electrical device in surgery.
   a. Precaution taken around mouth, head, or pleural cavity when high concentrations of oxygen or nitrous oxide are used.
   b. EKG electrodes are placed as far away from the operative site as possible.
   c. Flammable prep solutions such as alcohols or tinctures should not be allowed to pool under the patient and should be allowed to dry completely before applying the drapes.
   d. Other electrical equipment is connected to a separate source of current unless an isolated power system is used.
   e. Ensure that the correct generator receptacle is used for connecting bipolar versus monopolar electrode.
   f. Pacemaker or internal defibrillator may malfunction when using the ESU; careful monitoring of the patient is essential.
   g. Jewelry and other metallic objects can cause alternate ground site burns on the patient and should be removed.
   h. Dry sponges on the operative field may lead to fire.
   i. Repeated requests to increase current may indicate a problem and merit investigation.
   j. Active electrode should be kept in holder when not in use.

II. **Endoscopy (introduction of a scope inside the body for purpose of diagnosis, biopsy, or surgery)**

   A. *Parts of an endoscope*
      1. *Viewing sheath (scope):* rigid or flexible tubelike supporting structure through which the lighting source and various accessories are introduced
      2. *Light source:* fiber-optic light bundle attached to a light source; for the illumination of the body cavity
      3. *Power source:* fiber-optic light projector. (*Note:* Power source for fiber optics should be on the lowest setting; the unit should be turned off when connecting the cable to the light source, and the intensity is increased or decreased gradually; allow light bulb to fully cool before shutting off the main power switch.)
   B. *Accessories:* **suction tube, snare, biopsy forceps, grasping forceps, electrosurgical tip, sponge carrier, ligature carrier, suturing device, and irrigation equipment**
      1. *Operating microscope (optical system):* can be connected to the endoscope
      2. *LASER surgery:* LASER beam focused through endoscopes; argon and Nd:YAG can pass through fiber-optic scopes, and carbon dioxide (CO_2) lasers can be directed through a rigid endoscope or arm of an operating microscope; plume cleared by smoke-evacuation suction device; dulled, ebonized, or reflective instruments decrease reflection and scatter of the beam; appropriate backstops are used to protect the nontargeted tissue.
      3. *Ultrasonography:* ultrasound transducer provides visualization of the heart, liver, pancreas, spleen, and kidneys.
      4. *Cameras:* video cameras with recorder/player/audio equipment can be adapted to endoscopes and transmit images to a closed-circuit television screen; procedural documentation can be obtained by recording images using high-resolution pictures, videotape, CD-ROM, or DVD.

C. *Hazards of endoscopes*
1. *Perforation:* more probable from rigid scopes
2. *Bleeding:* at biopsy or dissection site
3. *Electrical hazards:* improperly grounded electrical equipment: bipolar active electrodes are preferable; if monopolar is used, an inactive dispersive electrode must be in place; only solid-state generators should be used, to avoid any variance in voltage.

D. *Types of endoscopic procedures*
1. *Surgically clean endoscopic procedures:* endoscopes (laryngoscope, gastroscope, cystoscope, colonoscope, for examination or treatment) are introduced into a natural orifice; scopes are terminally sterilized or high-level disinfected after use.
2. *Sterile endoscopic procedures:* trocar is used to establish a passageway directly into a sterile body cavity for the introduction of endoscopes for various surgical procedures (laparoscopy, thoracocopy, mediastinoscopy, arthroscopy, nephroscopy, etc.).

E. *Care and handling of endoscopes*
1. Thoroughly clean immediately after each procedure, terminally sterilize or high-level disinfect, and dry before storing.
2. Avoid kinking fiber-optic light cables and test before each use by holding up to light and looking with a magnifying glass focused on the opposite end for dark spots, which indicate broken fibers.
3. Handle gently: delicate and expensive equipment, especially scopes and cameras.

F. *Sterilization:* **disassemble, encase in a tray, and sterilize according to manufacturer's recommendations (STERIS unit used most frequently).**

G. *High-level disinfection: not frequently used*
1. Clean in nonresidue liquid-detergent solution, rinse, dry, and immerse in 2% solution of activated glutaraldehyde with parts disassembled. A 20–30-minute soak is recommended.
2. **Time:** 10 minutes at temperature of 68°F to 86°F to kill vegetative bacteria, fungi, HBV, and HIV viruses (45 minutes to be tuberculocidal and 10 hours to be sporicidal).
3. Scopes are removed from solution with sterile gloves.
4. Rinse all parts thoroughly in sterile distilled water before use on patient tissues.

H. *Storage:* **terminally sterilize or disinfect, dry, and store unwrapped in soft material. Flexible endoscopes are stored vertically; store light carriers with the scope.**

I. *Considerations for patient safety*
1. Ensure proper disinfection/sterilization of the equipment.
2. Hydrogen gas and methane gas present in the colon are flushed out with carbon dioxide before electrosurgery is used in the area.
3. Endoscopes, accessories, and related equipment are tested at all stages of handling: prior to use, during the procedure, immediately after use, prior to cleaning, after rinsing and drying, and prior to disinfection or sterilization.
4. Ensure dissipation of heat generated from the projection lamp.
5. Observe the patient after procedure for complications.
6. Ensure proper grounding when a monopolar active electrode is used.

J. Critical factors with laparoscopic surgery
1. *Preparation:* gather equipment and supplies, verify that all equipment is in working order
   a. Video tower: monitor, light source, CO_2 insufflator, camera unit, data storage
   b. Instrumentation: telescope, light cord, CO_2 tubing, ESU cord, laparoscopic instruments, and supplies vary with each procedure.

2. *Pneumoperitoneum:* insufflation of the abdomen with CO_2
   a. Need Verres needle (closed laparoscopic approach) or Hasson cannula (open approach using a small incision for the introduction of the first trocar) with CO_2 tubing
   b. Patient must be relaxed to avoid increased abdominal pressure.
   c. Intraabdominal pressure must be at least 10 mm Hg but not exceed 15 mm Hg.
   d. If pressure is being lost, check for the following:
      Leakage; may need converter, reducing sleeve, or blocker
      Open stopcock
      CO_2 tubing for kinking
      Incision too large; may need to be sutured using a 5/8 inch curved needle
3. *Cords:* connect to sterile field securely.
   a. Ensure that the correct end is passed off the field to the correct side of the table.
   b. Include CO_2 tubing, fiber-optic light cord, camera cord, suction-irrigation tubing, electrosurgery, LASER, etc., as necessary.
4. *Trocars/cannula*
   a. *Primary trocar:* first one inserted (infraumbilical); others inserted under telescope visualization
   b. *Secondary or working trocar:* used to pass laparoscopic instruments
5. *Telescope:* optical portion of scope: handle with extreme care
   a. Defog by placing in warm saline for 15 to 20 seconds and blotting gently or use defogging solution (FRED); if in the abdomen, gently touch the end of the scope against viscera or flush with irrigating solution.
   b. Ensure that fiber-optic light is turned on and the intensity is increased gradually.
   c. *Never* place lighted scope on drapes, as the intense light may ignite them; have the circulator decrease the light intensity as soon as surgeon is finished (allow unit to cool before turning off or disconnecting).
6. *Camera:* handle gently and connect to scope eyepiece.
   a. White balance on 4 × 4 ray-tec sponge once attached to the telescope and full light intensity is achieved.
   b. Camera person must maintain proper orientation as to position inside the abdomen; pull back to watch all instruments entering (especially trocars, scissors, and aspirating tips).
   c. Camera may be held in place by a robotic arm.
   d. Obstructed view from abdominal contents may be managed by adjusting the patient's position to shift abdominal organs.
7. *Electrosurgery:* bipolar with footpedal and adapter in position
8. *Techniques of endoscopic surgery*
   a. Place instruments in surgeon's hands as they will be needed to avoid the surgeon having to take his or her eyes from the field, guide working tip to the cannula portal for ease of insertion.
   b. Call the name of the instrument being placed in the surgeon's hand, especially scissors and aspirating needles, to avoid inadvertent injury.
   c. Test endoclip applicator; should be empty when going through the scope and loaded under direct vision.

K. **Advantages of laparoscopic surgery**
   1. More efficient
   2. Decrease postoperative pain and complications with earlier return to activities of daily living
   3. Adaptable to CO_2, argon, and KTP (potassium titanyl phosphate) LASERs to decrease risk of bleeding, infection, and shock

4. Data storage provides a permanent record, better assisting, and a more interested staff.

5. Decrease adhesions, especially with gentle tissue handling, hemostasis, and nonreactive suture

    L. Disadvantages of laparoscopic surgery

      1. Requires hand–eye coordination

      2. High cost of equipment purchase and maintenance

      3. Additional training of personnel

III. Microsurgery

    A. *Advantages:* better visualization for dissection and repair of fine structures, safer dissection with less trauma, and superior lighting

    B. *Operating microscope (compound binocular instrument which uses light waves for illumination)*

      1. *Optical lens system:* magnifying power and resolving power (ability to discern details)

      2. *Components:* objective lens (closest to the object) oculars/eyepieces

      3. *Magnification:* enlarging power of the objective lens multiplied by the ocular lens. A zoom lens, operated by foot control, permits the surgeon to change magnification without removing hands from the operative field.

      4. *Focus:* changed manually or by foot-controlled motor; adjusted by the surgeon

      5. *Illumination system*

        a. *Paraxial illuminators:* light tubes with halogen bulbs and focusing lenses

        b. *Coaxial illuminators:* fiber optic; illuminates same area as objective field; requires wound irrigation with a cool solution to protect against radiant heat

      6. *Mounting systems:* stability is essential

        a. *Floor mount:* base can be locked into position; arms should be folded close to the column and attachments locked in place before moving.

        b. Ceiling mount

        c. Wall mount

      7. *Care of microscopes*

        a. Damp dust before use (except lens) using clean cloth saturated with detergent-disinfectant; clean wheels.

        b. Clean lens according to manufacturer's recommendations.

        c. Circulator prepares the microscope; avoid dropping and fingerprinting lenses; avoid dropping observation tubes; have extra bulbs and fuses available and know how to change them; check electrical connections and knobs for security; conveniently position foot controls.

        d. Properly store microscope and accessories to protect lenses, viewing tubes, and cords and apply dust cover.

      8. *Accessories*

        a. *Assistant's binoculars:* can be attached

        b. *Broadfield viewing lens:* for overall view or grasping a needle

        c. *Cameras:* may be attached to beam splitter, allows for connection to a monitor or data storage (pictures, video, CD-ROM, DVD)

        d. *LASER microadapter:* for directing a LASER beam through operating microscopes

        e. *Remote foot controls:* for focus, zoom, or tilt

        f. *Armrest and chair:* support for surgeon's hand is mandatory

        g. *Microscope drape:* disposable transparent drape is applied by scrub (gloved hands protected by a cuff) and secured by circulator

      9. *Microinstrumentation:* instruments have a dull finish, are angled to prevent obstruction of the surgical view, and have handles with springs that are held like a pencil; includes knives, scissors, and saws (cutting); spatulas and retractors (exposure), forceps, clamps, special needle holder, and

---

SURGERY HINT

The scrub tech should ensure that the surgeon does not need to look away from the field when working under the microscope. Make sure that instruments are passed correctly so that attention from the surgery is not interrupted. If using patties during a neurosurgical procedure, either place them at the periphery of the field or place them on the back of the hand and pass bayonets for the surgeon. Some surgeons prefer to have the cottonoid already loaded on the bayonet while under the scope.

---

microsurgical air-powered drills and saws with fingertip or foot control; microsuture sizes range from 8-0 to 11-0; sponges are nonfibrous or lint-free patties (compressed cellulose).

10. *General considerations for microsurgery*
   a. Patient must be safely and comfortably positioned, the table locked, and the operative site immobilized.
   b. *Anesthesia:* if local, the patient is instructed to lie still; if general, planning is necessary for the placement of team members and microscope.
   c. *Scrub's duties:* care in handling delicate instruments, especially tips; place instruments on Mayo stand in order of use (room is generally darkened); place instruments in the surgeon's hand in a position for use and guide hand toward operative field; keep instruments clean by gently wiping with lint-free gauze; keep hands out of operative line of sight; and be alert and observant.

IV. **Pneumatic Tourniquet**
   A. *Use:* decreases blood loss during surgery of the extremities on or below the knee or elbow
   B. *Function:* similar to blood pressure cuff; inflated with compressed gas, ambient air, or from a piped-in system
   C. *Special considerations*
      1. Tourniquet cuff, tubing, connectors, contact closures, and ties are inspected prior to use.
      2. Select an appropriate-sized tourniquet cuff for the size of the extremity.
      3. Apply wrinkle-free padding to the extremity prior to cuff application; should be positioned at the point of maximum circumference of the limb.
      4. Apply tourniquet cuff prior to skin prep (or during draping if using a sterile cuff).
      5. Avoid collection of fluid or prep/scrub solutions beneath the cuff.
      6. With extremity elevated, an Esmarch bandage may be applied—distal to proximal—to exsanguinate blood prior to cuff inflation. The Esmarch is removed after cuff inflation; not used on patients with compromised circulation, such as diabetics.
      7. Tourniquet inflation pressure depends on the patient's age, systolic blood pressure, width of tourniquet cuff, and circumference of the limb (50 to 75 mm Hg above systolic pressure for an upper extremity and 100 to 150 mm Hg above systolic pressure for lower extremity).
      8. Inflation time should be kept to a minimum and the surgeon notified at intervals starting at 1 hour then every 15 minutes; generally doesn't exceed 1 1/2 hours.
      9. Documentation includes location of cuff, name of person applying cuff, cuff pressure, time of inflation and deflation, skin integrity after cuff is removed, and identification number of the tourniquet.

10. *Cleaning:* reusable cuffs should be cleaned and stored after each patient use.

V. **Other Equipment**

   A. *Harmonic Scalpel:* uses ultrasonic energy friction to cut and coagulate tissue simultaneously; because of the lower temperature used, there is less surrounding tissue damage and less vaporized tissue plume than with the ESU; no electricity passes through the patient, therefore no grounding pad is needed

   B. *Argon-enhanced coagulator:* uses argon gas in a portable tank attached to a specialized electrosurgical pencil, uses argon to carry the electrical current from the active electrode to the tissue, patient must be grounded since monopolar electricity is used

   C. *Dermatome:* used in taking split-thickness skin grafts (STSGs); there are three basic types: knife (Ferris-Smith, Humbly, Weck), drum (Reese, Padgett), motor driven (Brown air, Zimmer); electricity or compressed nitrogen or air may be used as the power source; mineral oil is used to prepare the donor site, and a wooden tongue blade may be used to hold the skin taut; the thickness of the graft is controlled by adjusting the depth of the cut on the dermatome head; the width of the graft is determined by the width of the opening on the dermatome head

   D. *Fiber-optic headlight:* allows the wearer to focus a small diameter intense light beam in the surgical field; the electrical light source is usually mounted on a small portable cart

   E. *Cavitron Ultrasonic Suction Aspirator (CUSA):* uses a sharp, hollow vibrating tip to emulsify abnormal tissue; irrigation is delivered through the handpiece and then aspirated back into the unit along with the tissue fragments.

   F. *Autologous blood retrieval system (cell saver):* a blood salvaging device that suctions blood directly from the wound, anticoagulates and filters it, and permits reinfusing the blood intravenously; contraindications to its use include blood contaminated by GI contents, infection, cancer, or the use of certain antibiotics and hemostatic agents

   G. *Nerve stimulator:* used to identify nerves to avoid damage as in parotid gland surgery or excision of an acoustic neuroma to avoid the facial nerve. The nerve integrity monitor (NIM) uses electrodes placed in the muscles to monitor the nerve location.

   H. *Cryotherapy unit:* uses an extremely cold probe to freeze diseased tissue without damage to surrounding tissue; liquid nitrogen, CO_2 gas, or Freon may be used to create the low temperatures ($-50°C$ or more); used to remove cataracts, treat retinal detachments, remove brain tumors and liver tumors, and treat prostatic cancer and cervical dysplasia and skin cancer

   I. *Irrigation/aspiration unit:* uses a power device to pulse saline solution into a wound to cleanse and debride it; may be powered by nitrogen, or battery; surgical team must be protected from the splatter by a shield placed on the handpiece and face shields

   J. *Sequential compression devices:* used to prevent venous stasis in the lower limbs or to prevent edema in the upper limbs following an axillary lymph node dissection; consist of inflatable vinyl or fabric wraps that alternately compress and relax by the use of a motorized pump attached to each wrap by tubing

   K. *Loupes:* special glasses used for magnification

   L. *Doppler:* uses ultrasonic waves to monitor the movement of blood through arteries; measurement is changed into an audible signal.

Process of Surgery

I. Preliminary Preparation

    A. Before the first operation of the day

        1. Perform handwashing.

        2. Remove unnecessary equipment and tables from the room.

        3. Damp dust all horizontal surfaces, overhead lights, and mounted equipment.

II. Before Each Operation

    A. Prepare operating table; clean sheet, lift sheet, safety strap, armboard, and other equipment as needed; check functioning.

    B. Position OR table, lights, and furniture.

    C. Connect and check suction and electrosurgical generator.

    D. Line linen hamper, waste containers, and kick buckets with impervious, anti-static bags.

    E. Gather instruments, supplies, and equipment based on surgeon's preference card.

    F. Gather positioning devices.

    G. Check the function of basic and specialty equipment.

    H. Remove and report any defective equipment or furniture.

    I. Open sterile supplies.

        1. Check chemical sterility indicators.

        2. Utilize aseptic technique.

        3. Open near the time of the scheduled procedure.

        4. Leave a wide margin of safety between sterile and nonsterile areas.

        5. Do not reach over sterile areas.

III. Duties of Scrub before the Surgeon Arrives

    A. Remove jewelry, secure mask and protective eyewear, open gown and gloves (double glove), perform surgical scrub, and don sterile gown and gloves.

    B. Apply sterile drapes to Mayo stand and basin stand as appropriate.

    C. Arrange drapes; prep, basins, gowns, and gloves for surgical team; arrange instruments and accessory items on the back table.

    D. Count sponges, needles, sharps (blades and electrosurgical tips), instruments, and other items which could be retained in the surgical wound with circulator.

    E. Sponges counted include

        1. *Gauze sponges (x-ray detectible 4×4s) may be called Ray-tecs:* for swabbing superficial tissue. Usually come in packs of 10

        2. *Tapes, lap pads, and lap packs:* for swabbing deep tissue, absorbing fluid, or for walling off viscera and keeping it moist and warm. Usually come in packs of 5

        3. *Peanut sponges/Kitner dissectors:* attached to a clamp and used for blunt dissection. Rosebuds are used for pediatric patients. Usually come in packs of 5

        4. *Cottonoid (patties):* compressed rayon or cotton; moistened and used on delicate tissue (nerve, brain, and mucous membrane). Usually come in packs of 10

        5. *Pledgets:* buttress under sutures in friable tissue or to reinforce a vascular graft

    F. Arrange instruments and accessory items on Mayo stand; apply scalpel blades with a needle holder; prepare sutures in sequence of use; fill and label syringes as needed; attach appropriate size needles, and label all drugs; prepare irrigation fluids. Syringes used for irrigation include ear/infant (bulb without a barrel) and Asepto/Dakins (bulb with barrel).

SURGERY HINT

When setting up the back table, orient the layout to the patient position on the bed. Keep sharps and softs closest to where you will stand. Make sure that the instruments are accessible while retracting. Keep it small and compact for ease of use and organization. Work efficiently and keep the movement of supplies to a minimum. Place extra towels and drapes out of the way

     G. Follow functional organizational patterns. Work rapidly without compromise of the sterile field.

IV. Duties of Scrub after the Surgeon Arrives

     A. Gown and glove surgeon and assistant(s) and provide wet cloth for the removal of glove powder.

     B. Assist with prepping and draping as directed

     C. Position Mayo stand over the patient; connect suction, electrosurgical cords, and other tubing or cords to the sterile field; apply sterile light handles; and place sponges on field.

     D. Pass skin knife (in basin if using "no touch" technique), clamps, suture, ESU, and instruments as needed based on observation, anticipation, and verbal requests.

     E. Keep the field organized and free of debris, replace bloody sponges as needed, and transfer bloody ones to kick bucket.

     F. Take special care in handling specimens, sponges, needles, and scalpels.

     G. Monitor sterile technique.
       1. If contaminated, step back from the sterile field, and secure or request the needed sterile item (glove, sleeve), and make adjustments. May require assistance of the circulator.
       2. If a needle contaminates a glove, discard the needle from the sterile field (but it must be accounted for), have circulator remove the glove, and change the glove (open method).
       3. Items falling below table level are discarded.
       4. Contact with the sterile field is kept to a minimum.
       5. Leave a wide margin of safety when passing close to an unsterile field or area.
       6. Do not turn your back to the sterile field and pass other sterile team members back to back or front to front.
       7. Keep the sterile field dry to avoid strikethrough.
       8. Keep talking to a minimum; avoid coughing or sneezing over the sterile field.

     H. During the closure, count sponges, sharps, and instruments beginning with items on the field, Mayo stand, and back table. Count all items in one category before proceeding to the next category.

     I. Keep the surgeon supplied with sutures and other items as needed.

     J. With a damp sponge, clean around the incision site and prepare the dressing.

     K. Keep the Mayo stand and instrument table sterile until the patient leaves the room.

V. Postoperative Routine

     A. Check drapes and floor for instruments.

     B. Break down the sterile field after the patient leaves the room.

     C. Dispose of sharps in a puncture-proof container according to the policy.

     D. Dispose of single-use items in an impervious bag.

E. Remove trash and linen from the OR.

F. Deposit OR records in the correct location.

G. Log in specimens and leave them at the proper location.

H. Complete terminal disinfection and sterilization of instruments.

I. Clean contaminated furniture and floor.

J. Restock cabinets.

K. Prepare the room for the next operation.

VI. Duties of Circulator

A. Fasten gown backs of sterile team members.

B. Open sterile supplies as needed, pour solutions, and present medications.

C. Count sponges, sharps, and instruments with scrub and record.

D. Greet and identify the patient, check chart, position the patient safely and appropriately, assist the anesthesia provider as needed, and apply warm blankets as needed.

E. During the induction of general anesthesia, stay in the room and near the patient; ensure a quiet environment.

F. After the patient is anesthetized and after receiving permission from the anesthesia provider, assist with repositioning the patient, and apply grounding pad; expose to appropriate area for skin preparation; turn on spotlights; perform skin preparation according to surgeon's preference and hospital policy.

G. Tie gown backs of surgeon and assistant(s) and observe for breaks in technique during draping; assist scrub in moving instrument table and Mayo stand into position; secure standing stools (platforms) as needed; position kick buckets and splash basins; connect suction and active and inactive electrodes; activate electrosurgical unit; and verbalize settings on the generator to the surgeon.

H. Stay in the room during surgery and monitor the sterile field; keep discarded sponges separated by using forceps or gloved hand; obtain IV fluids, blood, or additional supplies and equipment as needed; assist in monitoring blood loss; and keep control desk informed of changes in the patient, marked delays, cancellations, etc.

I. Prepare specimens for transport.

J. Complete perioperative documentation.

K. Be alert to breaks in technique.

L. During closure, count sponges, sharps, and instruments with scrub, report to surgeon, and document on count sheet and/or OR record.

M. Call for the next patient; send for the patient's bed, etc.

N. After the operation is completed:
1. Untie gown backs (if reusable).
2. Assist with securing dressings and drains.
3. Cleanse the patient of body fluids, blood, or residual prep solution.
4. Cover the patient with a clean gown and warm blanket.
5. Assist with the patient transfer and transport to **Post Anesthesia Care Unit (PACU)** and give report to the PACU nurse.

Sponge, Sharp, and Instrument Counts

A sponge, needle, or instrument inadvertently left in a wound can cause serious complications or death, can result in further surgery, and can be an object of litigation. Institutional policies regarding counts must be understood and rigidly followed to protect the patient, the institution, and the staff. Instruments are counted initially in the sterile processing area, and a count sheet is signed by the individual preparing the set.

1. In the OR, initial counts are taken preferably after all items are on the back table but before preparation of the Mayo stand.

2. Subsequent counts are taken:
   a. When additional items are added to the sterile field
   b. Before the closure of a hollow organ
   c. After the closure of any body cavity
   d. At the time of permanent relief of scrub and/or circulator
   e. At the closure of subcutaneous layer and skin

3. Items are counted audibly with the scrub and circulator concurrently viewing each item as it is separated.

4. Counted items are x-ray detectable and are kept in the OR until the patient is transferred out.

5. If initial sponge or needle count is incorrect, remove the entire package from the room, document, get a new pack, and start again.

6. Procedure for incorrect counts at the end of the procedure
   a. Inform the surgeon immediately.
   b. Repeat the entire count.
   c. Search for the missing item.
   d. Notify the person in charge.
   e. Have x-rays taken of the surgical site or cavity to locate items.
   f. Document all actions and findings.

7. Safety measures in the count procedure.
   a. Keep various sizes of sponges together.
   b. Keep small items (e.g., cottonoids and peanuts) on the field after use until the final count is completed.
   c. Replace Ray-tec 4 × 4 sponges with laparotomy sponges when the abdominal or thoracic cavity is entered.
   d. Account for all parts of broken needles or instruments.
   e. Place used needles in the appropriate numerical space in needle box, holder, or magnetic pad.
   f. Do not allow sponges or instruments to be removed from the room until the final count is completed.
   g. Open dressing sponges (non-x-ray detectable) only *after* the final count is complete.
   h. Pass needles to the surgeon on an exchange basis.
   i. Do not give the surgeon an x-ray detectable sponge to wipe powder from gloves.
   j. Do not add or remove sponges from the operative field while counting.
   k. Count from the field, Mayo, back table, and off the field.
   l. Never leave needles, blades, electrosurgical tips, safety pins, or other loose sharps on the Mayo stand.
   m. The number of needles must be verified as each suture pack is opened.
   n. Keep a mental count of sponges in the incision, needles on the field, etc. Be alert at all times.

SURGERY HINT

If the surgeon is packing the abdominal cavity with moist laps, keep a count of the number of laps that he or she places in the cavity. Let the circulator know the number of laps in the cavity, and alert the circulator as they are removed. Some surgeons will want the laps "tagged" before placement. Use instruments that are least likely to be needed during the procedure to attach to the lap loops.

Show What You Know

Directions: Each of the numbered items or incomplete statements in this section is followed by answers or by completions of the statement. Select the ONE lettered answer or completion that is BEST in each case.

1. Which one of the following scalpel handles would be needed for a #20 blade?

   A. #3
   B. #4
   C. #7
   D. a and c

2. Which of the following instruments would be used to cut bone?

   A. rongeurs
   B. Allis forceps
   C. # 4 scalpel handle with #10 blade
   D. tenaculum

3. Any of the following instruments could be used for hemostasis *except:*

   A. Babcock
   B. Crile
   C. Kelly
   D. Schnidt

4. Which one of the following is a manual retractor?

   A. Gelpi
   B. Harrington
   C. Finochetti
   D. Weitlaner

5. Which one of the following instruments would *not* be used for suction?

   A. Ferguson-Frazier
   B. Yankauer
   C. Poole
   D. Richardson

6. Instruments should be closed:

   A. when placed on the instrument table (back table)
   B. when placed in the autoclave
   C. when passed to the surgeon
   D. when washed in the ultrasonic cleaner

7. When the box locks on instruments are stiff and difficult to open, they are placed in:

   A. sterile saline
   B. mineral oil
   C. a water-soluble lubricant bath
   D. the washer–sterilizer

8. When assembling instrument sets, you will need the:

   A. surgeon's preference card
   B. surgical schedule
   C. patient's chart
   D. instrument checklist

9. The most effective and efficient method for sterilizing wrapped instrument sets is a/an:

   A. prevacuum sterilizer
   B. flash autoclave
   C. ultrasonic cleaner
   D. peracetic acid sterilizer

10. To counteract the heat produced by an electric-powered instrument, the scrub will:

    A. disconnect the instrument when not in use
    B. drip sterile saline from a bulb syringe onto the blade of the instrument while it is in action
    C. place the instrument in ice water when not in use
    D. cool it with a solution of alcohol while it is in action

11. The most commonly used electrical instrument in surgery is a/an:

    A. drill
    B. microscope
    C. pneumatic tourniquet
    D. electrosurgery unit

12. The grounding pad which connects the patient to the electrosurgical generator is called a/an:

    A. active electrode
    B. inactive dispersive electrode
    C. bipolar electrode
    D. monitor

13. The power source for fiber optics should:

    A. be turned on at the time the cable is connected
    B. always be at the highest setting
    C. be rapidly increased in intensity
    D. be turned off before the power cord is disconnected from the wall outlet

14. Which of the following endoscopic procedures would be a sterile procedure?

    A. laparoscopy
    B. gastroscopy
    C. laryngoscopy
    D. colonoscopy

15. Which of the following instruments is a stone forcep?

    A. Adson-Brown
    B. Lahey, Jacobs

C. Randall

D. Potts

16. Which of the following types of equipment would require sterile draping by the scrub?

A. electrosurgical unit

B. bronchoscope

C. video tower

D. microscope

17. A device applied while an extremity is elevated for the purpose of exsanguinating blood prior to inflation of a pneumatic tourniquet cuff is a/an:

A. Esmarch bandage

B. ace bandage

C. sterile Kerlix bandage

D. Elastoplast bandage

18. Scalpel blades are applied with:

A. gloved hands

B. Kocher

C. needle holder

D. thumb forceps

19. All of the following are safety measures for the sponge, sharp, and instrument count *except:*

A. if a sponge pack contains an incorrect number of sponges, repeat the count and make the necessary adjustments on the count sheet

B. counts are performed before the closure of a hollow organ such as the uterus or stomach

C. specimens going to pathology should not be placed on a counted sponge

D. needles should be handed to the surgeon on an exchange basis

20. Following anesthesia induction, permission for changing the patient's position must be obtained from the:

A. surgeon

B. anesthesia provider

C. circulator

D. surgical assistant

21. Subsequent counts are taken for all of the following *except:*

A. before the closure of a body cavity

B. after the closure of any body cavity

C. at the time of permanent relief of scrub and/or circulator

D. after the dressing sponges are opened

Match the following sponges with their use.

---

22. blunt dissection of tissue

23. swabbing delicate (brain) structures

24. walling off viscera

25. swabbing superficial tissue

a. cottonoid patties

b. lap pads

c. peanut sponges

d. 4 × 4 sponges

Answers & Rationales

1. **B.** **Rationale:** A #4 scalpel handle takes a #20, #21, or #23 blade. A #7 scalpel handle and a #3 scalpel handle take #10, #11, #12, and #15 blades.

2. **A.** **Rationale:** Rongeurs are used for cutting bits of bone. A #4 scalpel handle does not take a #10 blade.

3. **A.** **Rationale:** Hemostasis is provided by such clamps as mosquito, Halsted, Crile, Kelly, Schnidt; a Babcock is a grasping instrument for delicate tissues.

4. **B.** **Rationale:** A Harrington (Sweetheart) retractor is a manual (handheld) retractor designed to retract the liver. The Gelpi, Finochetti, and Weitlaner are self-retaining retractors.

5. **D.** **Rationale:** A Richardson is a manual retractor used to retract deep wounds. The Poole is used for abdominal suction, the Yankauer is used for oral suction, and the Ferguson-Frazier is used for smaller areas or more delicate suctioning.

6. **C.** **Rationale:** Instruments passed to a physician should be closed and placed firmly into the

palm of an extended hand in a functional position. Instruments are always opened for cleaning and sterilization. Instruments on the back table are usually left open to speed the cleanup process at the end of the procedure.

7. **C.** **Rationale:** Stiffness of box locks is corrected by placing or soaking in a water-soluble lubricant bath such as instrument milk. Oil is impermeable to steam, and saline would promote rusting.

8. **D.** **Rationale:** An instrument checklist is used in counting and assembling sets, as well as for count procedures before surgery begins and before wound closure.

9. **A.** **Rationale:** Steam sterilization is the method of choice for any non–heat-sensitive items. The prevacuum sterilizer uses a shorter timed sterilization process. The flash autoclave is used sparingly for unwrapped items. The ultrasonic cleaner does not sterilize. Paracetic acid cannot be used for wrapped items.

10. **B.** **Rationale:** Electric-powered instruments such as saws and drills generate a great deal of heat, which is damaging to tissue. Cooling is provided by dripping sterile saline from a bulb syringe onto the blade or drill point during sawing or drilling.

11. **D.** **Rationale:** The electrosurgery unit (ESU) is the most commonly used electric instrument in surgery and is designed both for coagulating bleeders and cutting tissue.

12. **B.** **Rationale:** The inactive dispersive electrode, commonly referred to as the grounding pad, returns current to the ESU generator. The active electrode directs the current to the operative site.

13. **D.** **Rationale:** The power source for fiber optics should be on the lowest setting and turned off when the power cord is connected or disconnected to the wall outlet; and intensity should be increased and decreased gradually to prevent the damage to fiber-optic bundles.

14. **A.** **Rationale:** Endoscopic procedures that are performed through a natural body orifice, such as the GI tract, respiratory tract, or GU tract, are surgically clean procedures due to insertion into mucous membrane which opens to the outside of the body. When an incision is made to introduce a scope, such as a laparoscope, all items must be sterile and sterile technique must be used.

15. **C.** **Rationale:** Randall is a stone forcep; Adson-Brown are tissue forceps; Lahey and Jacobs are tenaculi; Potts are cardiovascular scissors.

16. **D.** **Rationale:** A microscope may be mounted on the base, ceiling, or wall for stability. Since it cannot be sterilized, it is covered by a plastic transparent drape. The scrub, protecting gloved hands with a cuff, places the drape over the microscope, and the circulator grasps it from beneath and helps secure it.

17. **A.** **Rationale:** An Esmarch bandage is a latex-rubber rolled bandage, applied to a raised extremity following application of a pneumatic tourniquet to exsanguinate blood before the inflation of the pneumatic cuff. It is applied by wrapping in a spiral fashion from distal to proximal, overlapping each spiral by one-third. It is removed immediately after the tourniquet is inflated.

18. **C.** **Rationale:** A scalpel blade is applied with a needle holder, holding the cutting edge down and away from eyes; it is locked into the groove of the handle.

19. **A.** **Rationale:** If the initial sponge or needle count is incorrect, remove the entire package from the room, document the event, and get a new package and start again.

20. **B.** **Rationale:** The anesthesia provider must be consulted prior to changing the position of an anesthetized patient, as well as before beginning the skin prep and/or beginning surgery.

21. **D.** **Rationale:** All sponges, sharps, and instruments are counted prior to the beginning of surgery, and subsequent counts are taken when additional items are added to the sterile field, before closure of a deep incision or body cavity, after closure of a body cavity, at the time of permanent relief of scrub or circulator, and at the closure of the subcutaneous layer/skin and before opening dressing sponges.

22. **C.** **Rationale:** Peanut sponges are secured on a clamp, such as a Kelly, and used for blunt dissection of tissue.

23. **A.** **Rationale:** Cottonoid patties, compressed cotton or rayon, are moistened and used to swab delicate tissue such as nerve, spinal cord, or brain tissue.

24. **B.** **Rationale:** Lap packs, pads, and tapes are moistened and used to wall off viscera.

25. **D.** **Rationale:** 4 × 4 gauze sponges, often referred to as Raytex, are used for swabbing superficial tissue.

Part II: Deciphering a Surgical Schedule

The following mock surgery schedule will be used to answer several questions pertaining to instrumentation, equipment, and case preparation. The same schedule, or a similar one, may be used in subsequent chapters to ask questions about the content of the chapter.

Rm.# time	Surgeon	Procedure	Anest.	Rm. # time	Surgeon	Procedure	Anest.
Rm.00				**Rm07**			
OC	Dr. Z	Rt. Knee Arthroscopy	Gen. Gen.	7:00	Dr. M	Rhinoplasty	Gen.
OC	Dr. C	Craniotomy	Gen.	TF	Dr. M	Lipoma removal	MAC
OC	Dr.Z	Angioplasty					
Rm.01				**Rm08**			
7:00	Dr. X	Lobectomy	Gen.	11:00	Dr. E	Bovine Thrombectomy	MAC
TF	Dr. X	Thoracotomy	Gen.				
TF	Dr. X	Tracheostomy	Gen.				
Rm02				**Rm09**			
7:00	Dr. B	Splenectomy	Gen.	8:30	Dr. T	Cholecystectomy	Gen.
TF	Dr. B	Gastrectomy	Gen.	TF	Dr. T	Palatoplasty	Gen.
Rm03				**Rm10**			
7:00	Dr. A	Cystoscopy	MAC	7:00	Dr. K	Nephrectomy	Gen.
TF	Dr. A	Cystoplasty	Gen.	TF	Dr. K	Choledocholithotripsy	MAC
12:30	Dr. F	Pyleogram	MAC	TF	Dr. K	Hepatic resection	Gen.
3:00	Dr. F	Cystocele repair	Gen.				
Rm04				**Rm11**			
7:00	Dr. Y	Carpal tunnel release	Gen.	7:00	Dr. L	Colposcope	Gen.
TF	Dr. Y	Left Hip Arthroplasty	Gen.	12:00	Dr. L	Mastectomy	Gen.
Rm05				**Rm12**			
7:00	Dr. G	Trans-sphenoidal Adenectomy	Gen.	7:00	Dr. W	Trans-metatarsal amputation	Gen.
TF	Dr. G	Trans-urethral resection of the prostate	Gen	TF	Dr. W	Osteotomy	Gen.
TF	Dr. G	Bletharoplasty	Gen.	TF	Dr. W	Arthroplasty Right Knee	Gen.
Rm06				**Rm13**			
7:00	Dr. R	Lumbar Laminectomy	Gen.	7:00	Dr. O	Hysterectomy	Gen.

The following questions should be answered using the surgery schedule above

1. Mark is the Surgical Technologist who is assigned to Room 8. When he pulls his instrument set, what is one of the instruments he is likely to see in it?

   A. Potts Smith Scissors
   B. Lane bone holding clamp
   C. Harrington retractor
   D. Lambotte Osteotomes

2. Which of the following instruments may be found in Room 13?

   A. Pratt dilatators
   B. Heaney needle drivers

    C. Castroviejo needle driver

    D. Rongeur

3. Which surgery on the schedule may require the use of a CUSA?

    A. The on call craniotomy to remove a brain tumor

    B. The lumbar laminectomy to free a compressed spinal nerve

    C. The trans-metatarsal amputation from infection

    D. The bovine Thrombectomy to remove a clot

4. Which instrument is likely to be found in Room 1?

    A. Duval

    B. O'Sullivan–O'Connor

    C. Tenaculum

    D. Verees needle

5. Mark has a missing raytec sponge. The room has been searched, but it has not been found. What should happen at this point?

    A. Notify the person in charge, have x-rays taken, and document the incident

    B. The patient must be given prophylactic antibiotics, and the incident must be reported to the next of kin

    C. The surgeon must initiate a report that is sent to the insurance company to cover the cost of x-rays

    D. No action should be taken. The sponge is not likely in the cavity.

6. The Scrub Tech in Room 13 will need a large self-retaining retractor. What should she look for?

    A. Richardson

    B. O'Sullivan–O'Connor

    C. Harrington

    D. Davidson

7. Which surgical procedure will most likely use Cottonoids?

    A. Hysterectomy

    B. Osteotomy

    C. Lobectomy

    D. Craniotomy

8. Wendy is a Surgical Technologist working in a circulating role in Room 3. What is the duty she will be expected to perform?

    A. Surgical scrub

    B. Assist with dressings and drains

    C. Retract tissue for visualization

    D. Run the anesthesia machine

9. Which of the following instruments might be found in Room 12?

    A. Lane

    B. Haney clamp

    C. Maryland dissector

    D. Finochetto

10. Dave is scheduled to perform the right knee replacement scheduled in Room 12. He is looking for an orthopedic tray. Which room may have orthopedic instruments that he can use?

    A. Room 1

    B. Room 11

    C. Room 5

    D. Room 4

Answers & Rationales

1. A. **Rationale:** A bovine Thrombectomy is a peripheral vascular procedure which will require vascular instruments. The only vascular instrument on the list is a potts-Smith scissor. The Lambotte and Lane are orthopedic instruments, and a Harrington retractor would be much too large for the procedure.

2. B. **Rationale:** Heaney needle drivers are used in GYN surgical procedures in place of regular needle drivers. They possess a curved jaw that helps the surgeon with the anatomical structures she must reach. The other instruments would not be found on a GYN set. Castroviejo needle drivers are used for an extremely fine suture or micro surgery, and Rongeurs are used on bone.

3. A. **Rationale:** The CUSA is used to break up abnormal tissue and aspirate it along with irrigation, away from the site. The CUSA would not be used in the other cases listed.

4. A. **Rationale:** Duval is a lung forcep that is used to grasp lung tissue. It would be used in either the Lobectomy or the Thoracotomy. O'Sullivan O'Connor and Tenaculum are both GYN instruments, and the Verees needle is used in laparoscopic surgery to achieve pneumoperitoneum.

5. A. **Rationale:** When a sponge or other item is missing, and the team is unable to locate it, the next steps are to notify the person in charge, obtain an X-ray, and document the incident in the record. The sponge or other item may have been disposed of, or the beginning count may have been wrong; however, this cannot be assumed. It must be handled with the correct protocol.

6. B. **Rationale:** The O'Sullivan–O'Connor is a self-retaining retractor used in GYN surgical procedures. Richardson, Harrington, and Davidson retractors are all manual retractors used in other surgical procedures.

7. D. **Rationale:** Cottonoids are used in neurosurgical procedures.

8. B. **Rationale:** The circulator may be asked to assist in the placing of surgical dressings and drains. The other duties will be performed by the Surgical Technologist in the Scrub role.

9. A. **Rationale:** The Lane is a bone holding forcep that may be included in orthopedic instrument sets. The Finochetto is a rib spreader that may be used in Thoracic surgeries, the Haney is used in GYN, and the Maryland dissector is a laparoscopic dissector.

10. D. **Rationale:** The only room that may have an orthopedic set would be Room 4. The other rooms are dedicated to different procedures that would not use these trays.

PEARSON
myhealthprofessionskit™

Use this address to access the interactive Companion Website created for this book. Simply select "Surgical Technology" from the choice of disciplines. Find this book and click to enter.

11 Professional Aspects

A profession, as defined by Webster's Dictionary, is a principal calling, vocation, or employment requiring specialized knowledge and often long and intensive academic preparation. The profession of Surgical Technology requires the practitioner not only to develop a strong knowledge base and skills set, but also to embrace the behaviors and attitudes attributed to any true profession. This chapter identifies the areas of affective behaviors and knowledge related to the practice of Surgical Technology and the professional Surgical Technologist. Even Surgical Technologists with a broad knowledge base must remember that skill is only part of the job. Dependability, teamwork, and critical thinking skills are among the attributes that are necessary for success in the field.

CHAPTER OUTLINE

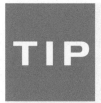

Some of the most important questions associated with this subject deal with communication and procedural management. The Surgical Technologist must be able to communicate effectively in all situations, including emergencies. It is also imperative for the ST to be aware of the different agencies that play an important part in the Operating Room environment. When answering questions dealing with the professional aspects of the job, you should always use both common sense and critical thinking skills.

Example:
A Surgical Technologist, faced with an emergency situation during a routine procedure, should be able to exhibit this behavior.

a. Empathy
b. Autonomy
c. Self-direction
d. Adaptability

While all of these behaviors are affective in nature, as well as being important to STs, one behavior fits the proposed scenario better than the others. While empathy is an absolute need in the ST, this situation would not be an example where empathy is highlighted. Autonomy is also a desired affective trait for STs, but again does not present the best answer in this scenario. The only affective trait that would be the BEST possible answer in this scenario is the trait of adaptability. When a case goes south, the ST must be able to quickly and seamlessly adapt to the changing procedure.

I. **Information Management**

   A. **Formats**

      1. Electronic
         a. World Wide Web
         b. Computers
         c. DVD/CD-ROM/videotape
         d. Teleconferences
      2. Verbal
         a. Educational lectures/audioconferences
         b. Inservices
      3. Written
         a. Periodicals
         b. Books
         c. Industry resources/guides

   B. **Uses**

      1. Documentation
      2. Information storage
      3. Maintain currency in a knowledge base
      4. Research

II. **Credentialing**

   A. *Individual*

      1. *Types:* At this time, the requirement for Surgical Technologists varies from state to state. Some states REQUIRE the ST to be certified in order to work. Other states do not require certification, but strongly recommend it. For the Surgical Technologist, certification is a logical step to professional status, and is becoming a necessity.
         a. *Certification:* voluntary demonstration of competency; least restrictive type of credentialing

      b. *Registration:* state requirement for practice; may be based on minimum standards or testing

      c. *Licensure:* state requirement for education, practice, minimum competency, and enforcement; most restrictive type of credential

  2. *Continuing education:*

      a. May be required for the renewal of credential

      b. Goal is to assist in maintaining a current knowledge base

B. *Institutional accreditation:* recognition of maintaining standards

  1. *Educational programs:* in Surgical Technology, accreditation assures compliance with **Commission on Accreditation of Allied Health Education Programs (CAAHEP)** standards and guidelines for education

  2. *Health care facilities:* through **Joint Commission on Accreditation of Healthcare Organizations (JCAHO). Now called the Joint Commission.**

C. *Professional organizations*

  1. Directly related to the profession of Surgical Technology

      a. *Association of Surgical Technologists (AST):* professional membership organization

      b. *Accreditation Review Committee on Education in Surgical Technology and Surgical Assisting (ARC-STSA):* addresses standards for Surgical Technology educational programs

      c. *Commission on Accreditation of Allied Health Education Programs (CAAHEP):* accreditation body for Surgical Technology education programs.

      d. *National Board of Surgical Technology and Surgical Assisting (NBSTSA):* formerly Liaison Council on Certification for the Surgical Technologist (LCC-ST) certification body for the profession of Surgical Technology

  2. Associated with the profession

      a. *American College of Surgeons (ACS):* professional organization for surgeons

      b. *American Hospital Association (AHA):* organization related to the administration of hospitals, health systems, health services, and integrated delivery networks

      c. *American Medical Association (AMA):* professional organization for physicians

      d. *American National Standards Institute (ANSI):* administers and coordinates voluntary standardization and conformity assessment systems

      e. *American Society of Anesthesiologists (ASA):* professional organization for anesthesiologists and anesthesia care providers

      f. *American Society of PeriAnesthesia Nurses (ASPAN):* professional organization for nurses in the pre-, post-, and ambulatory surgery roles

      g. *Association for the Advancement of Medical Instrumentation (AAMI):* developer of medical device standards

      h. *Association of Operating Department Practitioners (AODP):* professional organization for allied health practitioners in Great Britain

      i. *Association of periOperative Registered Nurses (AORN):* professional organization for registered nurses in the perioperative role

      j. *Centers for Disease Control and Prevention (CDC):* monitors disease outbreaks, health topics, and emergency preparedness

      k. *Emergency Care Research Institute (ECRI):* research/consulting agency for the health care technology assessment and cost-effectiveness

      l. *Food and Drug Administration (FDA):* regulates medications and medical devices used in the health care setting

      m. *Joint Commission on Accreditation of Healthcare Organizations (JCAHO) or Joint Commission:* sets standards for quality in health care

n. *National Fire Protection Association (NFPA):* establishes regulations related to fire safety

o. *National Institute for Occupational Safety and Health (NIOSH):* prevention of work-related illness and injuries

p. *Occupational Safety and Health Administration (OSHA):* monitors the workplace environment for safety

q. *World Health Organization (WHO):* United Nations-based organization that monitors worldwide health issues

III. Teamwork

A. Group dynamics

1. *Total Quality Management (TQM)*

2. *Group dynamics:* five stages in order of occurrence

a. *Forming:* members become oriented to the tasks and group members to one another; discussion centers on defining the task, how to approach it, and concerns; members rely on the group leader for guidance and direction.

b. *Storming:* group members organize for work and conflict may result; members bend and mold their feelings, ideas, attitudes, and beliefs to suit the group organization; conflict results over leadership, structure, power, and authority; group members must move from a "testing and proving" mentality to a problem-solving mentality; group members need to develop good listening skills.

c. *Norming:* group trust and cohesion with active acknowledgment of all members' contributions; community building and solving of group issues; positive data flow between group members, sharing feelings and ideas, soliciting and giving feedback to one another, and exploring actions related to the task; creativity is high, and interactions are characterized by openness and sharing of information on both a personal and task level; the group is effective.

d. *Performing:* people work easily in independent subgroups or as a total unit; roles and authorities dynamically adjust to the changing needs of the group and individuals; the group is productive; members are highly task- and people-oriented; there is a sense of unity, group identity, high group morale, and group loyalty; the task function becomes genuine problem solving, leading toward optimal solutions and optimum group development.

e. *Adjourning:* the termination of tasks and disengagement of the group; a planned conclusion usually includes recognition for participation and achievement and an opportunity for members to say personal goodbyes.

3. *Conflict management*

a. Negotiation

b. Bargaining

c. Consensus through collaboration

4. *Cooperative behaviors*

a. Open communication

b. Focus on issues and not personalities

5. *Networking:* sharing thoughts and ideas with peers, fellow professionals, interested individuals

B. Communication

1. Components

a. The message

b. The meaning

2. Types

a. Verbal

b. Nonverbal

i. Body language

    ii. Eye contact

    iii. Space and territory

  3. Effective communication techniques

   a. Active listening

   b. Responding to cues

   c. Clarifying

   d. Using open-ended sentences

   e. Showing acceptance

  4. Ineffective communication

   a. Giving false reassurance

   b. Speaking for others

   c. Being defensive

   d. Being judgmental

   e. Blocking communication

C. Leadership

 1. Types

  a. Formal

  b. Informal

 2. Styles

  a. *Autocratic:* unilateral leadership; the group follows orders directed by the leader; bureaucratic leadership is similar to this style and assigns duties to groups or team members.

  b. *Democratic:* the leader makes decisions by consulting the team while still maintaining control of the group; the team decides how the task will be tackled and who will perform which task.

  c. *Laissez-faire:* the leader has little control or involvement with the group; the group is self-motivated and directed.

D. Motivation

 1. Maslow's Hierarchy of Needs (in order from simple to complex)

  a. *Physiological needs:* "survival" needs: oxygen, water, basic nutrition, a pain-free and temperature-regulated environment

  b. *Safety needs:* the desire to be free from physical danger and deprivation of the basic physiological needs the need for self-preservation; personal and environmental safety

  c. *Love and belonging:* social affiliation, including a sense of security involving those who will care for them and the sense that caregivers will provide compassionate care while maintaining the patient's sense of dignity

  d. *Self-esteem:* a need for both a positive self-concept and respect of both self and others

  e. *Self-actualization:* the need to maximize one's potential, whatever it may be; includes the concepts of self-fulfillment, self-purpose, and self-worth

 2. Erickson's developmental stages

  a. **Trust versus Mistrust:** birth to 1 year

  b. **Autonomy versus Shame and Doubt:** 1–3 years

  c. **Initiative versus Guilt:** 4–6 years

  d. **Industry versus Inferiority:** 6–12 years

  e. **Identity versus Role Confusion:** 12–18 years

  f. **Intimacy versus Isolation:** 18–30 years

  g. **Generativity versus Stagnation:** 30–65 years

  h. **Ego Integrity versus Despair:** 65 years+

 3. American Hospital Association (AHA) Patient Bill of Rights: The patient has the right to:

  a. Considerate and respectful care

  b. Information concerning diagnosis, treatment, and prognosis

c. Make decisions about the plan of care
d. Have an advance directive
e. Every consideration of privacy
f. Expect that all communications and records pertaining to his or her care will be treated as confidential
g. Review the records pertaining to his or her medical care and to have the information explained or interpreted as necessary, except when restricted by law
h. Expect that a hospital will make reasonable response to the request of a patient for appropriate and medically indicated care and services
i. Ask and be informed of the existence of business relationships among the hospital, educational institutions, other health care providers, or payers that may influence the patient's treatment and care
j. Consent to or decline to participate in proposed research studies or human experimentation
k. Expect reasonable continuity of care when appropriate and be informed by physicians and other caregivers of available and realistic patient care options when hospital care is no longer appropriate
l. Be informed of hospital policies and practices that relate to patient care, treatment, and responsibilities

4. Association of Surgical Technologists (AST) Code of Ethics
a. To maintain the highest standards of professional conduct and patient care
b. To hold in confidence, with respect to patient's beliefs, all personal matters
c. To respect and protect the patient's legal and moral right to quality patient care
d. To not knowingly cause injury or any injustice to those entrusted to our care
e. To work with fellow technologists and other professional health groups to promote harmony and unity for better patient care
f. To always follow the principles of asepsis
g. To maintain a high degree of efficiency through continuing education
h. To maintain and practice Surgical Technology willingly, with pride and dignity
i. To report any unethical conduct or practice to the proper authority
j. To adhere to the code of ethics at all times in relationship to all members of the health care team

5. Precepting
a. Adult learning principles: adults
   i. Are autonomous and self-directed
   ii. Need to connect learning to life experiences and knowledge to learning
   iii. Are goal-oriented
   iv. Are practical, focusing on the aspects of a lesson they view as most beneficial to them in their work
   v. Need to be shown respect

E. **Affective behaviors related to the Surgical Technologist**
1. *Adaptability:* able to adjust to rapidly changing situations
2. *Anticipation:* the "surgical eye and ear"; listening and observing events to prepare items to meet the patient and surgeon's needs before they are requested
3. *Autonomy:* responsibility for one's own actions and decisions
4. *Commitment:* doing whatever it takes to meet the needs of the patient
5. *Critical thinking:* ability to assess, plan, implement, and evaluate situations and decisions on an ongoing basis

6. *Discrimination:* acquiring professional behaviors
7. *Empathy:* giving quality care without becoming "emotionally" attached to the patient
8. *Flexibility:* prepared to meet the individual needs of each patient
9. *Internalization:* delivering the same quality care to others as you would desire for yourself
10. *Motivation:* independent, quality skills, and behaviors
11. *Nonjudgmental:* impartial and accepting of patient's culture, religion, beliefs, and decisions
12. *Prioritization:* assessment and decision-making based on principles
13. *Self-direction:* work independently; assess personal and professional needs and continuing education
14. *Self-monitoring:* assessment of one's own practice and skills
15. *Surgical conscience:* delivering the highest quality care based on standards of practice
16. *Positive work ethic:* stamina and endurance; participating in long cases without relief; working as a team member

IV. **Critical Thinking**

A. **Process**
1. Assessment
   a. Subjective information—interpretations
   b. Objective information—the facts
2. Planning—based on assessment and knowledge
3. Implementation
4. Evaluation
5. Predicted outcomes

B. **Procedural management**
1. Anticipated
   a. Surgeon's preference
   b. Routines
2. Unanticipated
   a. Changes in planned intervention
   b. Emergency situations
      i. Hemorrhage
      ii. Malignant Hyperthermia
      iii. Cardiac arrest
      iv. Fire

V. **Employability Skills**

A. **Qualities**
1. *Positive work ethic:* works within their scope of practice while making positive contributions to the team
2. *Ambition:* drive and determination to deliver quality care
3. *Positive communication skills:* ability to use verbal and nonverbal communication skills with various team members and the patient
4. *Motivation:* desire to be a contributing team member
5. *Integrity:* strong sense of professional "right and wrong"
6. *Dedication:* desire to deliver the highest quality of care
7. *Flexibility:* ability to adjust to changes in job demands
8. *Adaptability:* broad knowledge base and ability to manage unanticipated situations
9. *Attendance:* dependability and timeliness
10. *Appearance:* following policies for attire
11. *Commitment:* desire to give the best care possible
12. *Competencies:* strong and continually increasing knowledge and skills base

B. Job search
  1. *Cover letter:* accompanies a resume or curriculum vitae; gives brief description of employment position desired
  2. *Resume:* provides candidate information, including name, address, and contact information, education history, work experience, and professional topics; may also include reference contact information
  3. *Application:* employer's document requiring standard candidate information
  4. *Interview:* one-on-one meeting between an employer and potential candidates

C. **Resignation: formal, written notification of employee's termination of employment with an institution**

Show What You Know

Directions
Each of the numbered items or incomplete statements in this section is followed by answers or by completions of the statement. Select the ONE lettered answer or completion that is BEST in each case.

1. Ineffective communication techniques include all of the following *except:*
   A. speaking for others
   B. being judgmental
   C. using open-ended sentences
   D. blocking communication

2. Which of the following is a voluntary demonstration of competency in a professional area?
   A. registration
   B. certification
   C. accreditation
   D. licensure

3. Critical thinking skills require the Surgical Technologist to develop and implement plans of care based on knowledge and experience. Place the steps of critical thinking skills in order.
   1. evaluate   A. 1, 2, 3, 4
   2. plan   B.   2, 4, 3, 1
   3. assess C.   3, 2, 1, 4
   4. implement D. 3, 2, 4, 1

4. Being impartial and accepting of a patient's culture, religion, beliefs, and decisions is an affective behavior called:
   A. discrimination
   B. being nonjudgmental
   C. internalization
   D. autonomy

5. Which professional organization accredits the education of the profession of Surgical Technology?
   A. Joint Commission on Accreditation of Healthcare Organizations (JCAHO)
   B. Commission on Accreditation of Allied Health Education Programs (CAAHEP)
   C. American National Standards Institute (ANSI)
   D. National Institute of Occupational Safety and Health (NIOSH)

6. Nonverbal communication consists of all of the following *except:*
   A. eye contact
   B. body language
   C. space and territory
   D. all of the above are true; there are no exceptions listed.

7. Development of the "surgical eye" and the "surgical ear" helps the Surgical Technologist develop which affective behavior?
   A. empathy
   B. motivation
   C. surgical conscience
   D. anticipation

8. Which of the following credential is the most restrictive type of professional credentialing?
   A. registration
   B. certification
   C. accreditation
   D. licensure

9. Place the five stages of group dynamics in order.
   1. performing   A. 4, 5, 2, 3, 1
   2. storming   B. 5, 2, 4, 1, 3
   3. adjourning   C. 2, 4, 5, 1, 3
   4. norming   D. 3, 4, 2, 5, 1
   5. forming

10. Which organization regulates medications and medical devices used in the health care setting?
    A. Federal Food and Drug Administration (FDA)
    B. Occupational Safety and Health Administration (OSHA)
    C. American National Standards Institute (ANSI)
    D. Centers for Disease Control and Prevention (CDC)

11. In Erickson's developmental stages, the 12- to 18-year-old adolescent patient is addressing which major psychological issues?
    A. trust versus mistrust
    B. identity versus role confusion
    C. intimacy versus isolation
    D. ego integrity versus despair

12. Which credential attests to the quality of an educational program in Surgical Technology?
    A. registration
    B. certification
    C. accreditation
    D. licensure

13. The type of leadership characterized by team decision making is called _____ leadership.
    A. autocratic
    B. bureaucratic

C. laissez-faire

D. democratic

14. In Erickson's developmental stages, the elderly patient over 65 is addressing which major psychological issues?

A. initiative versus guilt

B. generativity versus stagnation

C. ego integrity versus despair

D. autonomy versus shame and doubt

15. Place the five stages of Maslow's hierarchy in order from simple to complex.

1. love and belonging   A. 4, 2, 1, 5, 3
2. safety needs   B. 5, 3, 4, 1, 2
3. self-actualization   C. 2, 4, 3, 1, 5
4. physiological needs   D. 3, 4, 2, 5, 1
5. self-esteem

16. The AST Code of Ethics includes all of the following *except:*

A. maintaining the highest standards of professional conduct and patient care

B. always following the principles of asepsis

C. respecting and protecting the patient's legal and moral right to quality patient care

D. all of the above are true; there are no exceptions listed.

17. When considering the principles of adult learning, which of the following is false?

A. adult learners are autonomous and self-directed.

B. adult learners do not connect learning to life experiences and knowledge to learning.

C. adult learners are goal-oriented.

D. adult learners need to be shown respect

18. When considering employment qualities, the desire to give the best care possible is called:

A. commitment

B. flexibility

C. competency

D. ambition

Answers & Rationales

1. **C.** **Rationale:** Ineffective communication techniques include speaking for others, being judgmental, and blocking communication. Using open-ended sentences is an effective communication technique to gather or clarify information.

2. **B.** **Rationale:** Certification is a voluntary demonstration of competency in a professional area and is the least restrictive type of credentialing. Registration is more restrictive and licensure is the most restrictive. Accreditation addresses adherence to standards of education or practice.

3. **D.** **Rationale:** The steps of critical thinking skills, in order, are assess, plan, implement, and evaluate.

4. **B.** **Rationale:** Being impartial and accepting of a patient's culture, religion, beliefs, and decisions is an affective behavior called being nonjudgmental. Discrimination involves acquiring professional behaviors, internalization involves delivering the same quality care to others as you would desire for yourself, and autonomy involves being responsibility for one's own actions and decisions.

5. **B.** **Rationale:** CAAHEP accredits the education of the profession of Surgical Technology. JCAHO accredits hospitals and other health care settings, ANSI administers and coordinates voluntary standardization and conformity of assessment systems, and NIOSH is a government agency that addresses the issues of the prevention of work-related illness and injuries.

6. **D.** **Rationale:** Nonverbal communication consists of all of the following: eye contact, body language, and space and territory. There are no exceptions listed.

7. **D.** **Rationale:** Development of the "surgical eye" and the "surgical ear" helps the Surgical Technologist develop anticipation, the skill of preparing items for the team's use before they are needed. Empathy involves giving care without becoming emotionally attached to the patient; motivation involves the delivery of quality skills and behaviors; and the surgical conscience is delivering the highest quality care based on standards of practice.

8. **D.** **Rationale:** Licensure is the most restrictive type of professional credentialing of those listed.

9. B.   **Rationale:** The five stages of group dynamics, in order, are forming, storming, norming, performing, and adjourning.

10. A.   **Rationale:** The Federal Food and Drug Administration (FDA) regulates medications and medical devices used in the health care setting. The Occupational Safety and Health Administration (OSHA) monitors the workplace environment for safety, the American National Standards Institute (ANSI) administers and coordinates voluntary standardization and conformity assessment systems, and the Centers for Disease Control and Prevention (CDC) monitors disease outbreaks, health topics, and emergency preparedness.

11. B.   **Rationale:** In Erickson's developmental stages, the 12- to 18-year-old adolescent patient is addressing identity versus role confusion, a stage that addresses body image and self-discovery. Trust versus mistrust occurs in 0- to 1-year-olds; intimacy versus isolation occurs in 18- to 30-year-olds; and ego integrity versus despair occurs in individuals 65 years old and older.

12. C.   **Rationale:** Accreditation attests to the quality of an educational program in Surgical Technology.

13. D.   **Rationale:** In the democratic leadership style, the leader makes decisions by consulting the team while still maintaining control of the group and the team decides how the task will be tackled and who will perform which task. Autocratic leadership styles dictate tasks to the group, and laissez-faire leadership gives the group no direction. Bureaucratic leadership assigns duties to groups or team members and is similar to the autocratic leadership style.

14. C.   **Rationale:** In Erickson's developmental stages, the 65-year-old and above elderly patient is addressing ego integrity versus despair, a stage that addresses a review of life accomplishments and a sense of contribution. Initiative versus guilt occurs in 4- to 6-year-olds; generativity versus stagnation occurs in 30- to 65-year-olds; and autonomy versus shame and doubt occurs in 1- to 3-year-olds.

15. A.   **Rationale:** The five stages of Maslow's hierarchy, in order from simple to complex, are physiological needs, safety needs, love and belonging, self-esteem, and self-actualization.

16. D.   **Rationale:** The AST Code of Ethics includes maintaining the highest standards of professional conduct and patient care, always following the principles of asepsis, and respecting and protecting the patient's legal and moral right to quality patient care. There are no exceptions listed.

17. B.   **Rationale:** When considering the principles of adult learning, adult learners are autonomous and self-directed, they are goal-oriented, and they need to be shown respect. Adult learners do connect learning to life experiences and knowledge to learning.

18. A.   **Rationale:** The desire to give the best care possible is called commitment. Flexibility is the ability to adjust to changes in job demands, competency refers to a strong and continually increasing knowledge and skills base, and ambition involves the drive and determination to deliver quality care.

PEARSON
myhealthprofessionskit™

Use this address to access the interactive Companion Website created for this book. Simply select "Surgical Technology" from the choice of disciplines. Find this book and click to enter.

General Surgery

Surgery is a branch of medicine that treats diseases, injuries, and deformities by manual or operative methods. Surgery has evolved over time to allow for many different specialties. This chapter provides an overview of indications for surgery, abdominal incisions, and procedures related to hernias, breast surgery, the gastrointestinal tract, and the biliary system, spleen, and pancreas, all of which fall under the heading of general surgery. These surgeries tend to utilize the same or similar instrumentation, and have grown to include laparoscopic and bariatric surgeries. All Surgical Technologists should have an intimate knowledge of general surgery and the procedures that are performed, as this is the cornerstone for other specialties. Without this basic knowledge base, the ST will struggle in other specialty areas.

CHAPTER OUTLINE

TIP

Answering questions dealing with general surgery requires basic knowledge of anatomy and physiology, positioning, and other subjects. Remembering anatomy is the key to answering questions involving positioning, prepping, and draping, as well as gauging which sutures are most likely to be used during the case. Knowledge of medical terminology is also key when dealing with procedures, as they are couched in these terms. Remember that the surgery will not be "removal of the gallbladder" but will be a cholecystectomy. Knowing the basic incisions is also important in being able to anticipate draping and prepping. The most likely incision will give you a large amount of information that is necessary for the procedure.

Example #1:
During a cholecystectomy, which anatomical structure will be ligated?

a. The common bile duct
b. The hepatic duct
c. The cystic duct
d. The hepatic vein

To answer this question, first identify the relevant anatomy including using medical terminology. A cholecystectomy is the removal of the gallbladder. The gallbladder is a small sac connected to the liver. The purpose of the gallbladder is to store bile that is created by the liver, to be used in the digestive process. When the gallbladder is surgically removed, it must be freed from the liver, and several anatomical structures must be ligated and divided. One of these is the cystic duct. The hepatic duct conducts bile from the liver into the common bile duct, which then enters the duodenum. The hepatic vein is necessary for liver circulation. Therefore, the correct answer would be C.

Example # 2:
Which incision is most likely to be used in an open cholecystectomy?

a. Left subcostal
b. Right subcostal
c. mcBurneys
d. Left Paramedian

Again, anatomy must be used to answer this question. You must know the location of the gallbladder in order to anticipate the incision site. Once you know that the anatomical structure to be removed is located in the upper right quadrant, this will immediately rule out the left side incisions, leaving only the right subcostal and mcBurneys. Since mcBurneys is not an incision used to remove the gallbladder, this leaves the right subcostal incision as being the most likely one used in this scenario. While there are several incisions that may be used during a cholecystectomy, none of the others were an option for this particular question.

I. **Indications for Surgery**

    A. **Patient indications (Table 12-1)**
        1. Diagnosis
        2. Trauma
        3. Metabolic diseases
        4. Inflammation/infection
        5. Congenital defects
        6. Neoplasms
        7. Obstruction
        8. Reconstruction
        9. Other

TABLE 12-1   Patient Indications for Surgery

Diagnosis	Pathological specimens are obtained for study by such procedures as direct visualization through a flexible or rigid lighted instrument—a scope (endoscopy), biopsy (removal of tissue for pathological analysis), or exploratory laparotomy (opening into the abdomen to determine the cause of a problem not evident by other methods)
Trauma	Injury caused by burns or accidents; includes surgical procedures such as repair of injured organs or tissues such as fractured bones or a ruptured spleen, removal of foreign bodies, debridement of burns, or reimplantation of limbs
Metabolic diseases	Removal of tissues or organs that are malfunctioning, such as a Splenectomy for thrombocytopenia (bleeding problem due to a clotting deficiency) or the removal of thyroid tissue that is overproducing thyroid hormones
Inflammation/Infection	Some infections such as appendicitis, cholecystitis, or abscesses do not respond to medical treatment and are treated by surgery
Congenital defects	Birth defects that require or are aided by surgical correction, which includes such procedures as Herniorrhaphy for indirect inguinal hernia or Pyloroplasty for pyloric stenosis
Neoplasms	Surgical procedures are performed to remove both benign and malignant neoplasms. Cancer treatment may also be supplemented by radiation therapy and/or chemotherapy
Obstruction	Tubes, vessels, or ducts in the body can become obstructed by stones, growths, blood clots, twisting (volvulus), or intussusception (telescoping in on itself)
Reconstruction	Body parts may be replaced, supplemented, or reduced to make them more functional or attractive. Degenerative disease of a joint may be corrected by Joint Arthroplasty, or a breast enlarged by Augmentation Mammoplasty

B. Surgical indications
   1. *Diagnosis:* determination of the nature of a cause of a disease
   2. *Prophylaxis:* disease prevention
   3. *Restoration:* to return to as normal as possible
   4. *Palliation:* giving relief but not curing

II. **Surgical Incisions of the Abdominal Wall (Figure 12-1)**
   A. **Midline**
      1. Incision made between the two rectus abdominis muscles, down the linea alba, and curving around the umbilicus
      2. Offers good exposure to any part of the abdomen
      3. Can easily be extended
      4. High incidence of dehiscence/evisceration
      5. Retention sutures (secondary suture line), extending through all layers, may be used to provide wound support
      6. Uses: Exploratory Laparotomy, Gastrectomy, Colectomy, during trauma surgery, and many other procedures
   B. **Paramedian**
      1. Vertical incision approximately 4 cm lateral to midline on either side, either above or below the umbilicus
      2. Following incision in skin and subcutaneous tissue, the rectus sheath is split vertically and the muscles retracted laterally

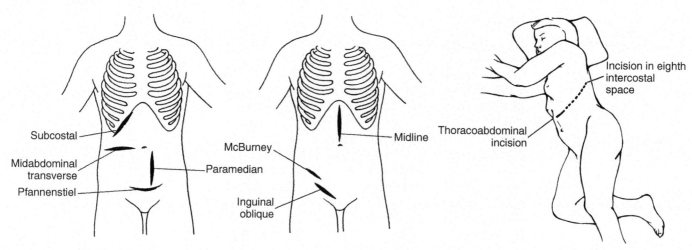

FIGURE 12-1

3. Incision into peritoneum is done midline
4. Right upper paramedian used for biliary/pancreas procedures; left upper paramedian used for Gastrostomy; left lower paramedian used for sigmoid procedures

C. **Subcostal (Kocher)**
   1. Oblique incision that follows the margin of the rib—right or left; the eighth intercostal nerve is cut
   2. Can be extended across the midline
   3. Good cosmetic incision
   4. Produces less tension on wound edges than with a vertical incision
   5. Right subcostal for biliary/pancreas procedures; left subcostal for procedures of the spleen

D. **McBurney**
   1. Oblique; muscle-splitting
   2. Right lower quadrant of the abdomen over McBurney's point (just below the umbilicus and 4 cm medial to the anterior iliac spine)
   3. Fibers of the external oblique, internal oblique, and transversalis muscles are split and retracted and the peritoneum is entered
   4. Limited exposure
   5. Common use: Appendectomy

E. **Inguinal lower oblique**
   1. Follows the fold at the groin or just superior to the groin on either side
   2. Provides access to the inguinal canal, internal and external inguinal rings
   3. Used for Inguinal Herniorrhaphy, Femoral Herniorrhaphy, and Orchiopexy for cryptorchidism

F. **Pfannenstiel**
   1. Curved transverse incision along the lower abdominal fold, 1½ inches above the symphysis pubis (bikini incision)
   2. Skin, subcutaneous tissue, and fascia (rectus sheaths) are incised; the rectus muscle is separated in midline; peritoneum is entered through a vertical midline incision
   3. Provides strong closure; has a low incidence of disruption
   4. Used for pelvic gynecological procedures such as Cesarean Section, Abdominal Hysterectomy, or Suprapubic Prostatectomy

G. **Midabdominal transverse (horizontal flank) incision**
   1. Begins at the center midline point between the xiphoid and umbilicus and extends laterally to the lumbar region between the ribs and the iliac crest

2. Incision is carried through skin, subcutaneous tissue, anterior sheath, and rectus sheath; underlying muscles are split in the direction of their fibers; posterior sheath and peritoneum are divided

3. Used to provide approach for retroperitoneal organs, such as the kidney, adrenal gland, proximal ureter, lumbar sympathetic nerves, and inferior vena cava

H. Thoracoabdominal incision

1. Patient will be in the lateral or a modified supine position

2. Begins midway between xyphoid and umbilicus and extends across the seventh or eighth rib interspace to the midscapula line (transverse incision)

3. Rectus and oblique abdominal muscles are divided down to the peritoneum and pleura; the costal cartilage and diaphragm are divided

4. Used for procedures involving the lower esophagus, upper stomach, or hiatal hernia

I. Transverse

1. Incision made at a 90-degree angle to midline

2. Examples include extension of the midline incision when greater exposure is needed

3. Common use: Liver resection or transplant

III. Basic Laparotomy: An Incision through the Abdominal Wall to Enter the Abdominal Cavity

A. Tissue layers

1. Skin
2. Subcutaneous/adipose
3. Anterior fascia/linea alba
4. Muscle
5. Posterior fascia
6. Peritoneum

B. Patient preparation

1. Preoperative
   a. NPO
   b. Foley catheter
   c. NG tube
2. Anesthesia
   a. General
   b. Spinal
   c. Epidural/Caudal: intra- and postop pain management
3. Positioning and aides
   a. Supine (dorsal recumbent)
   b. Arm boards
   c. Safety strap
   d. Pillow/padding
4. Skin preparation
   a. Shave/clip, as ordered
   b. Antimicrobial scrub/solution
   c. One-step skin prep
5. Draping
   a. Wound towels
   b. Fenestrated sheet
6. Procedural preparation
   a. Instruments
      i. *Cutting/Dissecting* —skin knife, deep knife, Metzenbaum scissors, Mayo scissors
      ii. *Forceps* —toothed utility, dressing forceps
      iii. *Hemostatic* —hemostats, Kellys/Peans

     iv. *Retracting* —Kelly/Richardsons

     v. *Accessory* —suction tips, towels clips

    b. Supplies

     i. Sponges (radiopaque 4×4s or Ray-tecs, laparotomy sponges, dissectors)

     ii. Electrosurgical unit active and inactive electrodes

     iii. Suction tubing and tip—Yankauer and Poole

     iv. Light handles

     v. Sutures

     vi. Medications/Irrigation solutions

    c. Equipment

     i. Electrosurgical unit (ESU)

     ii. Suction

     iii. Hypothermia unit

   7. Procedure

    a. Midline incision is made through skin and subcutaneous tissue with "skin knife" and forceps or sponge; vessels are clamped and ligated or cauterized

    b. Fascia is incised with "clean" knife or electrosurgical pencil; muscles are retracted or transected

    c. Peritoneum is grasped with forceps and incised with deep knife and Metzenbaum scissors (*Note:* Once the peritoneum is opened, loose radiopaque 4×4 sponges are removed from the field—if used, these sponges and dissectors are commonly secured on an instrument before use in the surgical incision)

    d. Abdomen is explored; moist laps are used to pack viscera aside; retractors are placed for visualization

    e. Surgical intervention is performed based on findings

    f. Wound is irrigated (saline or saline with a broad-spectrum antibiotic added); a drain is placed as indicated

    g. Incision is closed; fascia with suture (absorbable or nonabsorbable) and skin (staples, suture, or suture placed subcuticularly and wound closure strips)

    h. Incision cleaned and dressing applied

   8. Postoperative complications (Table 12-2)

    a. Postoperative/Paralytic ileus

    b. Atelectasis

    c. Wound dehiscence or evisceration

    d. Wound infection

    e. Urinary retention

IV. Minimally Invasive Surgery (MIS)/Laparoscopic Procedures

 A. Definition: operative interventions performed via portals placed within several small incisions in the abdominal wall: uses include diagnosis, tissue/organ sampling, tissue/organ repair, and tissue/organ removal

 B. Advantages

  1. Direct observation of anatomy under magnification with projection onto a monitor

  2. Less tissue trauma

  3. Shorter hospital stay—commonly done as an ambulatory procedure

  4. More rapid return to optimum level of wellness and activities of daily living

 C. Disadvantages

  1. Cost

  2. Procedure length—may be longer based on learning curve to acquire skills and overall technical skills of surgeon and team

  3. May need to convert to an open procedure

TABLE 12-2   Postoperative Complications

Condition	Definition	Prevention/Treatment
Postoperative/Paralytic ileus	Absence of peristalsis with abdominal distention	Use of a nasogastric tube for decompression; NPO (nothing by mouth) until bowel sounds return
Atelectasis	Collapse of lung tissue due to inadequate respiration, secondary to shallow breathing	Encouraged to take deep breaths, cough, and turn frequently
Wound dehiscence/evisceration	Partial/complete disruption of the incision line	Due to excessive stress on the suture line during the early phases of healing; support incision during straining/coughing/sneezing
Wound infection	Formation of pus at the surgical site	Maintain aseptic technique and sterile field; use irrigation with or without antibiotics
Urinary retention	Inability to micturate (void)	Urinary output should be closely monitored and record first voiding

D. **Specialty instrumentation**
   1. Telescope, light cord, and camera
   2. Insufflation tubing and Verres needle
   3. Trocars/cannulas—diameter corresponding to instrumentation
   4. Endoscopic instrumentation: can include graspers, dissectors, scissors, suturing devices, and retractors

E. **Specialty equipment**
   1. Video tower/boom (may use a primary and "slave" monitor)
      a. Monitor
      b. CO_2 insufflator
      c. Fiberoptic light source
      d. Camera generator
      e. Image storage—photography or VCR

F. **Anesthesia:** general

G. **Position:** supine—Trendelenburg/reverse Trendelenburg positions used to enhance visualization by using gravity to displace intestine (*Note:* Footboard may be used for reverse Trendelenburg position to prevent the patient from sliding and skin shear from occurring)

H. **Procedure**
   1. Access
      a. *Open Laparoscopy* —small peri-umbilical incision made and dissected down through peritoneum; trocar/cannula placed under direct visualization of underlying tissues; traction sutures placed into fascia layer—sutures secured to Hasson device on the cannula
      b. *Closed Laparoscopy* —peri-umbilical skin incision (½ inch) and insertion of Verres needle; primary trocar/cannula inserted blindly through tissues
      c. *Working portals* —two to three other small incisions may be used for introduction of telescope and applicable instrumentation; secondary trocars are inserted under visualization of the telescope and using transillumination of the abdominal wall
      d. Carbon dioxide (CO_2) is used to insufflate the peritoneal cavity to an intraabdominal pressure of 12 to 15 mm Hg (creation of a pneumoperitoneum)
   2. **Closure:** Fascia (open laparoscopic approach or w/large trocar usage) and subcutaneous tissue are commonly closed with suture
   3. Dressings consist of adhesive bandages or bio-occlusive

SURGERY HINT

If the ST is in charge of the camera during a laparoscopic procedure, he or she must remember to keep the camera view on the operative instrument tips. Follow trocars as they enter peritoneum, and always orient the image to the center of the screen. Remember, the camera angles are essentially backward, meaning that if the scope needs to focus cephalad, the ST should move the scope physically caudally, to accommodate the view.

4. **Surgical contraindications:** extensive adhesions, obesity, malignant disease, large stones, pregnancy, abdominal sepsis/peritonitis

5. Surgical hazards: perforation of organ with the trocar, persistent bleeding from the biopsy site, and injury to a major vessel

6. Postoperatively, patients may experience moderate abdominal and shoulder pain (due to CO_2 under the diaphragm)

V. Hernia Repair/Herniorrhaphy

    A. **Definition:** a protrusion of a tissue or organ through a weakness in the abdominal wall due to a congenital or acquired defect in the supporting fascia layer. It can result in an obstruction of abdominal viscera. Predisposing factors to acquired hernias include straining at work, chronic cough, straining to void, straining at stools, ascites (collection of fluid in the abdomen), or obesity.

    B. **Hesselbach's triangle:** formed by the rectus abdominus muscle, inguinal ligament, and deep epigastric vein and artery; most common site for hernia formation

    C. **Inguinal canal:** contains the spermatic cord in men and round ligament of the uterus in women and runs parallel to the groin area

    D. **Types of hernias**
       1. Indirect/Direct
       2. Congenital/Acquired
       3. Reducible: contents of hernia sac can be returned to the abdominal cavity
       4. Incarcerated: unnatural confinement of the contents of a hernia sac
       5. Strangulated: impairment of the blood supply to the contents of a hernia sac

    E. **Specifics**
       1. *Direct inguinal hernia*
          a. Protrusion of peritoneal sac with abdominal viscera into the inguinal canal resulting from a defect in the transversalis fascia
          b. More common in men
          c. Typically acquired
          d. Layers of tissue in the abdominal wall in this area are Scarpa's fascia (the membrane below the subcutaneous tissue), external and internal oblique muscles and aponeuroses, internal oblique, transversalis fascia (major supporting structure), and peritoneum
          e. Inguinal (Poupart's) ligament is formed by the lower border of the external oblique muscles and extends from the iliac crest to the pubic tubercle
          f. Surgical hazards of inguinal hernia repair include damage to spermatic cord, testicular artery or vein, and femoral artery or vein
          g. Postoperative complications include: scrotal hematoma, acute urinary retention
       2. *Indirect inguinal hernia*
          a. Definition—protrusion of peritoneal sac with abdominal viscera into the inguinal canal resulting from a defect in the internal inguinal ring; hernia sac commonly follows the spermatic cord
          b. Most common type of hernia
          c. Repair—similar to direct inguinal hernia

3. *Femoral hernia:* protrusion of peritoneum and viscera through the femoral ring just below the inguinal (Poupart's) ligament due to a defect in the transversalis fascia; more common in women
4. *Ventral hernia:* found on the anterior abdominal wall
5. *Epigastric hernia:* defect found above the level of the umbilicus
6. *Incisional hernia:* defect found within a previous surgical incision
7. *Diaphragmatic hernia/hiatal hernia:* defect in the diaphragm at the area of passage of the esophagus into the abdominal cavity
8. *Spigelian hernia:* located between different muscle layers of the abdominal wall and may be called interparietal, interstitial, or intramuscular; difficult to diagnose—ultrasonic or computerized tomography (CT) scanning may be necessary; may be associated with an intestinal obstruction

F. Hernia repair
1. *Open—Inguinal/Femoral hernia*
   a. Instruments: basic laparotomy set, self-retaining retractor and Penrose drain
   b. Surgical prep includes abdomen, anterior thighs, and scrotum
   c. Anesthesia: general, spinal, or local anesthesia may be used
   d. Incision is made parallel to the inguinal ligament through subcutaneous tissue (vessels clamped and ligated); the external oblique fascia is opened and retracted
   e. Spermatic cord is retracted with a moistened Penrose drain
   f. Hernia sac (peritoneal tissue) is freed from the cord, transfixed, doubly ligated, and divided or pushed back into the peritoneal cavity
   g. Transversalis fascia is repaired using primary suturing or placement of mesh (may or may not be sutured into place)
   h. Scarpa's fascia closed with suture
   i. Skin is closed and dressing is applied
2. *Laparoscopic—Inguinal hernia repair*
   a. Instruments: telescope and light cord, trocars/cannula, endoscopic dissectors, endoscopic stapler/tacker
   b. Balloon dissection of the pre-peritoneal space with placement of a synthetic mesh which is stapled over the fascia defect; may also be approached through the peritoneum

VI. Breast Surgery
A. Anatomy: located on the chest between the sternum and axillary line; breasts receive their blood supply from branches of the internal mammary artery, lateral branches of the intercostal arteries, and a branch of the axillary artery; consist of breast and tail of Spence; lymph drains to the axillary nodes and internal mammary chain

B. Diagnostic measures: mammography, thermography, ultrasonography, fine-needle aspiration, CT, magnetic resonance imaging (MRI), and breast biopsy with or without needle localization, and sentinel node biopsy

C. Psychosocial issues to be considered: body image issues for both male (enlargement, especially during adolescence) and female patients (equated with femininity and sexuality)

D. Patient position: supine with operative side near the edge of the table, pad under operative side or slight Fowler's with a lateral tilt and arm on affected

---

SURGERY HINT

To reduce waste, do not open mesh patches until the surgeon asks for a specific patch. Have the mesh in the room and ready to be opened, but wait until a final size and type of mesh has been decided upon.

side extended on a padded armboard, not to exceed 90-degrees abduction to avoid injury to the brachial plexus

E. **Skin preparation:** from umbilicus to the base of the neck, from bed line to beyond the sternum on unaffected side, including the axilla and possibly upper arm on the operative side

F. **Instrumentation:** breast biopsy set or major instrument set, depending on procedure; Geiger counter (sentinel node biopsy)

G. **Anesthesia:** general; biopsy may be done under local

H. **Concepts of breast surgery**
   1. **Incisions:** inframammary, infra-areola, supra-areola, radial, transverse elliptical, or axillary
   2. Breast tissue is approximated with absorbable suture on a cutting needle, and skin is closed with fine suture or staples
   3. Irradiation or chemotherapy may be done if more than one lymph node is involved
   4. Closed-wound drain used for more significant tissue removal—left in place and anchored to the skin with a nonabsorbable suture
   5. Skin graft may be necessary to cover areas of skin deficit following radical surgery

I. **Surgical procedures of the breast for neoplasm**
   1. *Breast biopsy:* small amount of tissue is removed for pathologic examination
   2. *Needle biopsy:* tissue is obtained with disposable cutting needle or Vim-Silverman needle
   3. *Excisional biopsy/lumpectomy:* removal of the entire mass, including nonaffected tissue margins
   4. *Simple mastectomy:* removal of a breast without lymph node dissection; generally done as a palliative measure for extensive benign disease or for gynecomastia
   5. *Sentinel node biopsy:* removal of radioactive axillary nodes following injection of Lymphazurin at the suspected tumor site
   6. *Axillary node dissection/sentinel node biopsy:* removal of unilateral lymph nodes that drain breast tissue; may perform sentinel node biopsy—injection of radioisotope and dye which is absorbed by the first (sentinel) node draining the tumor area; this node is located with a Geiger counter and removed and examined for metastasis.
   7. *Modified radical mastectomy with axillary node dissection*
      a. Incision: oblique elliptical with lateral extension toward the axilla
      b. Bleeding points are controlled with hemostats and electrocautery
      c. The knife blade may need to be changed frequently due to the tough nature of fibrous breast tissue
      d. Axillary contents are dissected using Mixters and blunt dissection
      e. Wound is irrigated and a closed vacuum drain placed in the wound and secured with a nonabsorbable suture on a cutting needle
      f. Skin flaps are approximated and closed with staples or an interrupted nonabsorbable suture
      g. Dressing is bulky and commonly includes compression of the surgical site

J. **Surgical hazards associated with radical breast surgery include pneumothorax, injury to axillary blood vessels, long thoracic or lateral thoracic nerve, or brachial plexus**

K. **Prognosis is good if no or limited metastasis to lymph nodes or other organs**

L. **Surgical procedures of the breast for infection**
   1. *Incision and drainage of abscess:* cultures are taken: abscess is generally caused by staphylococci or streptococci

VII. **Gastrointestinal Surgery**

   A. **Pathophysiology**

      1. **Esophagus**

         a. GERD—GastroEsophageal Reflux Disease

         b. Esophageal varices

         c. Zenker's diverticulum

         d. Esophageal stenosis

      2. **Stomach**

         a. PUD—Peptic Ulcer Disease

         b. Pyloric stenosis

      3. **Small intestine/large intestine**

         a. Obstruction

         b. Neoplasms

         c. Diverticulum

         d. Intussusception

         e. Strangulation/infarct/necrosis

      4. **Rectum/anus**

         a. Hemorrhoids

         b. Fissure/fistula

         c. Polyps

         d. Hirschsprung's disease

   B. **Diagnostic interventions**

      1. EGD—esophagogastroduodenoscopy

      2. Colonoscopy

   C. **General considerations**

      1. Bowel preparation preoperatively

         a. Mechanical

            i. Enema/bowel evacuation agents

            ii. NPO/clear liquid diet

         b. Chemical

            i. Antibiotics

      2. Patient is placed in supine position

      3. General anesthesia is usually administered

      4. Abdominal prep, basic draping, and midline incision are routine

      5. "Bowel technique" (isolation of items contacting inner lining of GI tract) is implemented

      6. Bowel serosa is approximated with nonabsorbable interrupted suture; bowel mucosa is approximated with absorbable suture using a continuous running stitch

      7. The mesenteric defect is closed with absorbable suture using a continuous running stitch to prevent bowel entrapment and obstruction

   D. **Specialty instruments**

      1. Intestinal instruments

         a. Crushing (kockers/oschners)

         b. Occluding clamps (Glassman, Payr, Allen, or Doyen shod)

      2. Intestinal staplers

         a. Linear/TA (thoracoabdominal)

         b. Linear cutter/GIA (gastrointestinal anastamosis)

         c. End-to-end stapler/EEA (end-to-end anastamosis)

         d. Mesenteric/omental stapler/LDS (ligate, divide, staple)

   E. **Surgical procedures**

      1. **Esophagus**

         a. *Nissen fundoplication:* surgical procedure for correction of the treatment of GERD (GastroEsophageal Reflux Disease)/hiatal hernia

            i. **Repair of hiatal or diaphragmatic hernia:** repair of a defect in the diaphragm where the esophagus normally passes through that permits the stomach to slide into the chest cavity and may result in esophagitis, with bleeding and discomfort in both the chest and back

ii. Fundus of the stomach is anchored against the diaphragm and the proximal stomach is wrapped around the gastroesophageal junction.

iii. **Position:** supine

iv. **Incision:** midline, subcostal, or transabdominal

v. **Specialty instruments:** long instruments are essential

vi. May be performed laparoscopically

b. *Esophagogastrectomy/Partial esophagectomy*

i. Removal of diseased portion of the esophagus and stomach for relief of strictures in the lower esophagus (caused by trauma, infection, corrosion, or tumors) or management of esophageal varices or varicose (tortuous, dilated) veins; may be secondary to cirrhosis of the liver and result in hemorrhage; may initially be treated by the following:

• Insertion of tube with inflated balloon (Sengstaken-Blakemore) to control bleeding by pressure

• **Sclerotherapy:** caustic agent is injected into varices to cause clotting and hardening using a flexible gastroscope

ii. Lower end of the esophagus is removed and anastamosis of distal segment to proximal stomach using EEA (end-to-end) stapler or hand sewn

iii. **Incisions:** thoracoabdominal

iv. **Specialty instrumentation:** thoracotomy and abdominal instruments—rib spreader, Deaver, Harrington (with moist packs), Allen clamps or staples

v. **Supplies:** intestinal suture 2-0 chromic, 3-0 silk, and chest tubes and water seal drainage

c. *Excision of Esophageal (Zenker's) Diverticulum*

i. **Diverticulum:** a weakening in the wall of a canal that balloons out to form a blind pouch

ii. Occurs in the cervical portion of the esophagus, collects small amounts of food, and causes a feeling of fullness in the neck

iii. **Position:** semi-Fowler

iv. **Specialty instruments:** neck dissection instruments; stapler, esophageal dilator

v. **Incision:** inner border of sternocleidomastoid muscle from hyoid bone to clavicle

vi. **Procedure:** sac of diverticulum is freed, ligated or stapled, and wound is closed

2. **Stomach**

a. *Vagotomy:* resection of a portion of the vagus nerve to interrupt parasympathetic stimulation, thereby reducing gastric acid secretions; requires a high abdominal incision and long instruments, Penrose drain, nerve/vagotomy hooks, and ligating clips

b. *Pyloroplasty:* drainage procedure for the stomach following a Vagotomy or a widening procedure for acquired pyloric stenosis; pylorus is opened longitudinally and sutured side-to-side

c. *Gastrostomy:* palliative procedure to prevent malnutrition and starvation in a patient with an obstructed esophagus or mechanical swallowing problems

i. Left paramedian or midline incision

ii. Purse string suture is placed while stomach is held with Babcock or Allis forceps, #15 blade is used to make the incision within the purse string; a catheter is inserted, and the suture tightened around it. A stomach flap may be formed around the catheter; may be performed percutaneously (PEG—Percutaneous Endoscopic Gastrostomy Tube Placement)

      iii. **Gastrojejunostomy (Roux-en-Y Gastroenterostomy):** permanent communication between the wall of the stomach and proximal jejunum without the removal of a section; done to bypass a pyloric obstruction

      iv. **Gastrectomy:** removal of a diseased portion of the stomach (ulcer or tumor)

- *Billroth I (Gastroduodenostomy):* duodenum is anastomosed to the remaining stomach leaving one continuous tract
- *Billroth II (Gastrojejunostomy):* following the removal of the diseased portion of the stomach, the duodenal stump is closed and a loop of the jejunum is anastomosed to the remaining stomach, creating a larger opening
- *Total Gastrectomy:* complete removal of the stomach; performed for palliative or curative treatment for a malignant lesion. A loop of the jejunum is anastomosed to the distal esophagus.

      v. **Biliopancreatic Diversion (BPD):** gastric bypass

- Resection of part of the stomach; division of the duodenum from jejunum; gastrojejunostomy and anastamosis of the duodenal limb to the distal ileum

3. **Small intestine/large intestine**
   a. *Appendectomy*
      i. Removal of the appendix from the cecum for acute inflammation
     ii. **Incision:** right McBurney incision
    iii. **Specialty instruments:** laparotomy instruments, babcocks
    iv. **Procedure**
   - Cultures of peritoneal fluid taken if murky/cloudy
   - Poole suction may be needed if fluid present
   - Babcock used to grasp the appendix; mesoappendix is dissected from the wall of the appendix and ligated
   - Base of appendix ligated and divided
   - Appendix and contaminated instruments are isolated
   - Protective gauze sponges are placed around the cecum during division
   - Wound is closed in layers

     v. **Ruptured appendix**—drain may be placed: closed vacuum in cavity, penrose in subcutaneous tissue
    vi. Procedure may also be performed laparoscopically

   b. *Excision of Meckel's Diverticulum*
      i. Unobliterated congenital duct in the distal ileum which may ulcerate, bleed, or perforate
     ii. Procedure resembles that of an Appendectomy or may involve resection of ileum—bowel resection and anastamosis

   c. *Small Bowel Resection:* removal of diseased portion of intestine through an abdominal incision with an end-to-end anastomosis of remaining portions; done for tumors and for gangrenous portions caused by strangulation, adhesions, herniation, volvulus (twisting), or intussusception (telescoping of the bowel).

   d. *Ileostomy:* surgical creation of an opening in the ileum to the body surface to reduce activity in the colon; done for colitis or as a diversion when the large intestine has been removed

   e. *Colostomy:* surgical creation of an opening in the colon to the surface of the body
      i. *Purposes:* treat an obstruction caused by a malignant lesion, advanced inflammation or trauma (such as colitis, diverticulitis, or ruptured diverticulum) to decompress and give the bowel a rest
     ii. *First-stage Loop Colostomy:* loop of colon is freed from the mesentery and brought through a small incision made on the left side of the abdominal wall and secured with a loop ostomy bridge;

the abdomen is closed and the loop of bowel is dressed with petro-latum gauze

    iii. *Second-stage Loop Colostomy:* after 48 hours, the colon is opened with an electrosurgical blade (a painless procedure for the patient), and an ostomy appliance is attached. (*Note:* This avoids exposure of peritoneal structures to intestinal bacteria.)

    iv. *Transverse Colostomy:* loop colostomy

    v. *Closure of a Colostomy:* reestablishment of intestinal continuity; incision is made around colostomy to free it from the skin margins; end-to-end anastomosis is performed and wound is closed

f. *Anterior Resection of Sigmoid Colon:* removal of the lower sigmoid colon and rectum with an end-to-end anastomosis of the sigmoid colon to the rectum; an end-to-end anastomosis is performed, either by suturing in layers or using EEA (end-to-end anastomosis) staplers, which may be introduced through the abdomen or transanally

g. *Abdominoperineal Resection/Miles Resection (Proctocolectomy)*

    i. *Position of patient:* supine and later placed in lithotomy or modified lithotomy; two surgical teams may operate concurrently

    ii. *Specialty instruments:* laparotomy sets (one for abdominal approach, one for rectal approach), intestinal instruments

    iii. *Procedure:*

        midline incision is made;

        bowel is mobilized;

        blood supply is isolated and ligated with care to avoid damage to left colic artery (which will supply the colostomy);

        rectum is freed with care to avoid presacral nerve injury, resulting in sexual and bladder dysfunction;

        proximal colon is exteriorized as a colostomy (end or single-barrel);

        ostomy appliance is attached;

        wound is closed;

        patient is changed to the lithotomy position, and the team changes gowns and gloves and uses a "new" set of instruments;

        perineal area is prepped and draped;

        anus is closed with a purse string suture to prevent contamination;

        incision is made around rectum into the hollow sacrum;

        distal segment (rectum and anus) is removed;

        incision is closed. (*Note:* This procedure may be done by one or two teams with the patient in a modified lithotomy position.)

4. Rectum/Anus

  a. *Hemorrhoidectomy:* removal of varicose veins of the rectum

    i. *Position:* lithotomy or jackknife (Kraske); the buttocks are retracted with wide adhesive tape attached to the OR table

    ii. *Specialty instruments:* minor set plus rectal instruments (penningtons, rectal retractors, anoscope/sigmoidoscope)

    iii. *Supplies:* base of hemorrhoid may be sutured (absorbable) or cauterized (ESU)

    iv. *Anesthesia:* general or spinal

    v. *Dressing:* gauze packing commonly left in the anal canal and a dressing with T-binder applied

---

SURGERY HINT

When dealing with bowel, have the extra gown and gloves ready for the change from "dirty" to "clean". Remember which instruments have been utilized during the "dirty" part of the surgery, as they will need to be incorporated into the count at the end of the case. Be careful of sharps used during this part, as they are also considered contaminated, and need to be separated from the "clean" instruments and sharps. Having a second needle board for these is a good idea, if allowed by the facility.

   b. *Excision of anal fissure/fistula:* benign lesion/tract of anal wall
   c. *Pilonidal Cystectomy:* "nest of hair" cyst of congenital origin on the posterior surface of the lower sacrum in the intergluteal fold
      i. *Position:* jackknife (Kraske) position
      ii. *Procedure:* sinus tract is identified with probe and/or dye (methylene blue);
         elliptical incision is made down to fascia, and the cyst is removed en bloc;
         wound is left open to heal by granulation, packed, and pressure dressing is applied
   d. *Polypectomy:* removal of polyp (benign tumor that grows on a stalk and may occur on any mucous membrane); potentially malignant. Polyps of the colon are generally removed through a colonoscope by electrocoagulation.
   e. *Anoplasty:* surgical restoration or formation of an anus; performed on infants with an imperforate anus or congenital absence of an anus
   f. *Pediatric colorectal resection:* resection of a diseased portion of colon and rectum with an end-to-end anastomosis of the colon to the lower rectum; performed on children with Hirschsprung's disease—congenital aganglionic megacolon: a section of the colon or rectum lacks ganglion cells in the muscle layer, thereby resulting in an inability of the segment to relax and permit the passage of feces and leading to constipation, megacolon, and other problems

VIII. **Surgery of the Biliary Tract, Liver, Pancreas, and Spleen**
   A. **Hepatobiliary system (liver, gallbladder, and biliary ductal system) surgery**
      1. *Biliary tract*
         a. Bile flows from the liver through right and left hepatic ducts (one from each lobe)
         b. Join to form the common hepatic duct (CHD)
         c. Becomes the common bile duct (CBD) at the level where the CHD joins the cystic duct (from gallbladder)
         d. The CBD joins the pancreatic duct (duct of Wirsung) and enters the duodenum at the ampulla of Vater—controlled by the sphincter of Oddi
      2. *Biliary pathology*
         a. *Cholelithiasis:* gallstones
         b. *Choledocholithiasis:* gallstones in the common bile duct
         c. *Biliary atresia:* congenital absence of the bile duct, leading to obstructive jaundice
         d. *Cholecysitis:* inflammation of the gallbladder
      3. *Hazards of biliary surgery*
         a. Hemorrhage
         b. Injury to the extrahepatic duct system
      4. *Preoperative preparation and diagnosis*
         a. Liver function tests: fat and protein metabolism; coagulation properties, bilirubin
         b. Radiographic studies: ultrasound, CT, radioisotope scanning, MRI
         c. Endoscopic Retrograde Cholangiopancreatography (ERCP)
      5. *Specialty instrumentation*
         a. Harrington retractor
         b. Mayo common duct scoops
         c. Oschner gallbladder aspirating trocar
         d. Randall stone forceps
         e. Bakes common duct dilators
         f. Potts scissors
      6. *Anesthesia:* general
      7. *Position of patient:* supine with reverse Trendelenburg and table tilted to the left. (*Note:* If a cholangiogram is to be done, an operating table with x-ray cassettes or C-Arm/fluoroscopy is used.)

8. *Procedures*
   a. *Laparoscopic Cholecystectomy*
      i. Trocar/cannulas are placed—telescope, working portal, two-grapsing/retracting portals
      ii. cystic duct, cystic artery, and cystic vein are ligated with hemo-clips and divided
      iii. gallbladder is isolated and freed and removed via largest incision
   b. *Open Cholecystectomy:* surgical removal of the gallbladder
      i. Incision: right subcostal (Kocher), right paramedian, or transverse
      ii. Liver retracted with Harrington retractor
      iii. Cystic duct, cystic artery, and cystic vein are ligated with hemo-clips and divided
      iv. Gallbladder is isolated and freed and removed
      v. Wound drain may be used
      vi. Gallbladder bed may be closed with chromic or other absorbable suture
   c. *Common Bile Duct (CBD) exploration*
      i. Duct opened with #7 Knife handle with #11 blade, incision extended with Potts scissors
      ii. Stone forceps, scoops, dilators, stone baskets, and balloon-tipped catheters may be used to remove stones—choledochoscope may be used to assist visualization
      iii. T-tube may be left in the common bile duct to provide a stent, duct closed with absorbable suture, tube secured to the skin with a nonabsorbable suture and connected to a gravity drainage device
   d. *Operative Cholangiogram*
      i. Imaging—fluoroscopy commonly used; C-arm/image intensifier but can use flat plate x-rays
      ii. Contrast media injected via cholangiogram catheter placed in cystic duct—diatrizoate sodium (Hypaque or Renografin) commonly used for contrast media. (*Note:* Care is taken to ensure that all air has been removed from the syringe and tubing, as bubbles may appear as stones on the x-ray; the sterile field is protected with a sterile drape before the x-ray machine is brought over the field or the C-arm is covered with a sterile drape.)
   e. *Cholecystostomy:* drainage of the gallbladder through the abdominal wall with a mushroom/Pezzar catheter attached to gravity drainage device
   f. *Choledochostomy:* drainage of the common bile duct through the abdominal wall with a T-tube inserted in the CBD
   g. *Common bile duct exploration:* dilation and examination of the CBD and placement of a stent drain (T-tube)
   h. *Choledochojejunostomy/Choledochoduodenostomy:* bypass procedure in which an end-to-side anastomosis of the CBD to the jejunum/duodenum is done to relieve obstruction in the distal end of the CBD.
   i. *Cholecystojejunostomy/Cholecystoduodenostomy:* bypass procedure in which a side-to-side anastomosis of the gallbladder to the jejunum/duodenum is done to relieve obstruction in the CBD.
   j. *Liver biopsy:* a biopsy needle (Silverman, Tru-Cut) is passed into the liver, activated, and removed. A small sample of liver tissue is obtained for pathological examination. If done percutaneously, the patient is then placed on the right side to enhance hemostasis by pressure on the needle insertion site.
   k. *Hepatic resection:* lobectomy or segmental resections done to remove cysts, tumors, or severely traumatized areas
      i. Hemorrhage is a major concern since the liver is friable.
         • Hemostatic methods may include microfibrillar collagen (Avitene), oxidized cellulose (Gelfoam); flaps of tissue sutured

with a blunt needle to the bleeding area for tamponade; argon-enhanced coagulator
- May use CUSA to reduce blood loss during dissection
- Drain is placed in the wound and brought out through a stab wound

l. *Portosystemic shunts:* to treat hemorrhaging esophageal varices, generally secondary to cirrhosis of the liver; surgical treatment by decompressing the portal vein and shunting blood away from the liver
  i. *Portocaval shunt:* anastomosis between the portal vein and the inferior vena cava (IVC)
  ii. *Mesocaval shunt:* superior mesenteric vein (SMV) is anastomosed to the vena cava, or a graft is used to create a shunt between the IVC and the SMV
  iii. *Splenorenal shunt:* anastomosis of the splenic vein to the left renal vein

m. *Liver transplant:* replacing a diseased liver with a donor liver

B. Pancreatic surgery
  1. *Pathophysiology:* inflammation, cysts, and tumors
  2. *Procedures*
     a. *Pancreaticojejunostomy (Roux-en-Y):* anastomosis of a loop of the jejunum to the pancreatic duct; a drainage procedure done for chronic alcoholic pancreatitis and pseudocysts of the pancreas. (*Note:* A Roux-en-Y is any Y-shaped anastomosis involving the small intestine, with the distal end of the divided intestine implanted into another organ and the proximal end into the small intestine below the anastomosis site to provide for drainage without reflux.)
     b. *Pancreaticoduodenectomy (Whipple procedure):* surgical removal of the duodenum, head of the pancreas, distal stomach, and lower half of the CBD with the following anastomoses: Choledochojejunostomy, Pancreaticojejunostomy, and Gastrojejunostomy; a radical procedure done for carcinoma of the head of the pancreas or ampulla of Vater
        i. **Instrumentation:** general laparotomy and gastrointestinal instruments
        ii. **Incision:** long midline or upper transverse
        iii. Wound generally closed with a long-term absorbable or nonabsorbable suture
     c. *Pancreatectomy:* removal of segment/all of the pancreas for malignancy; hormonal, enzyme, or organ replacement necessary

C. Splenic surgery
  1. *Pathophysiology*
     a. **Hypersplenism** (overactive destruction of blood cells)
     b. Enlargement of the spleen (seen in Hodgkin's Disease)
     c. Severe organ trauma
     d. Tumors or cysts
  2. *Specialty instrumentation:* angled pedicle clamps, long instruments
  3. *Incision:* left subcostal or upper midline
  4. *Procedures*
     a. *Splenorrhaphy:* repair of a splenic laceration
        i. Topical hemostatic agents or argon-enhanced coagulation used for hemostasis with small lacerations
        ii. Splenic artery may be ligated
        iii. Lacerated section may be wrapped in a synthetic mesh or omental pouch
        iv. Closed vacuum drainage may be placed in wound
     b. *Splenectomy:* surgical removal of the spleen; hemorrhage is the major hazard
     c. *Laparoscopic Splenectomy:* minimally invasive approach; organ may be removed using a morcellator

Show What You Know

Directions
Each of the numbered items or incomplete statements in this section is followed by answers or by completions of the statement. Select the ONE lettered answer or completion that is BEST in each case.

1. The incision for an Exploratory Laparotomy would be the:

   A. McBurney
   B. Pfannenstiel
   C. periumbilical
   D. midline

2. A vertical incision 4 cm lateral to the midline of the abdomen is a/an _____ incision.

   A. McBurney
   B. paramedian
   C. subcostal
   D. inguinal lower oblique

3. Which of the following anatomical structures could best be approached through a thoracoabdominal incision?

   A. esophagus
   B. duodenum
   C. appendix
   D. sigmoid colon

4. The suture most appropriate for closure of the intestinal mucosa is:

   A. 4-0 silk
   B. 0 silk
   C. 3-0 chromic
   D. 1 chromic

5. The tube used to drain bile from the common bile duct following exploration is a:

   A. Sengstaken-Blakemore tube
   B. T-tube
   C. Foley catheter
   D. Pezzar Catheter

6. For a Pilonidal Cystectomy, the patient will be placed in the _____ position.

   A. supine (dorsal recumbent)
   B. jackknife (Kraske)
   C. Fowler (sitting)
   D. lateral (kidney)

7. Femoral hernias occur:

   A. within Hesselbach's triangle
   B. at the esophageal hiatus
   C. in the periumbilical region
   D. below Poupart's ligament

8. Which of the following surgical procedures would require the use of an image intensifier (C-arm)?

   A. Operative Cholangiogram
   B. Direct Inguinal Herniorrhaphy
   C. Modified Radical Mastectomy
   D. Colon Resection

9. The surgical incision for a Splenectomy could be:

   A. left subcostal
   B. right subcostal
   C. left inguinal oblique
   D. Pfannenstiel

10. What is the term used to describe male breast enlargement?

    A. volvulus
    B. diverticulum
    C. gynecomastia
    D. ptosis

11. Relief of symptoms without curing a disease is referred to as a/an _____ procedure.

    A. diagnostic
    B. palliative
    C. interventive
    D. prophylactic

12. The divisions of the small intestines in order beginning at the pyloric sphincter are:

    A. ileum, jejunum, duodenum
    B. jejunum, duodenum, ileum
    C. duodenum, ileum, jejunum
    D. duodenum, jejunum, ileum

13. Hernias that significantly reduce the blood supply to the hernia contents are said to be _____ hernias.

    A. incarcerated
    B. strangulated
    C. direct
    D. ventral

14. The surgical incision commonly used for Open Choleystectomy is the _____ incision.

    A. inguinal lower oblique
    B. right subcostal
    C. right lower paramedian
    D. midabdominal transverse

15. The surgical incision that is commonly used for pelvic gynecological procedures and has a low incidence of dehiscence is the _____ incision.

    A. midline
    B. thoracoabdominal
    C. McBurney
    D. Pfannenstiel

16. The abdominal incision commonly used for trauma surgery because it provides quick access to the peritoneal cavity and the ability to extend it easily if necessary is the _____ incision.

    A. subcostal
    B. midabdominal transverse
    C. midline
    D. inguinal lower oblique

17. When setting up the Mayo stand for an Exploratory Laparotomy, which of the following instruments would NOT be placed there?

    A. curved Metzenbaum scissors
    B. Kelly/Richardson retractor
    C. hemostatic clamps/forceps
    D. #3 knife handle with a #11 blade

18. The abdominal cavity is filled with which gas to create pneumoperitoneum during minimally invasive surgery (laparoscopy)?

    A. nitrous oxide
    B. oxygen
    C. carbon monoxide
    D. carbon dioxide

19. What specialty supply is used when performing minimally invasive surgery (laparoscopy) using the open method?

    A. Hasson device
    B. Verres needle
    C. disposable Poole suction
    D. 1×3 cottonoids/patties

20. A hernia that forms due to a defect in the internal inguinal ring is referred to as a _____ hernia.

    A. indirect inguinal
    B. direct inguinal
    C. Spigelian
    D. ventral

21. A hernia whose contents cannot be "pushed back" into the abdominal cavity is referred to as a/an _____ hernia.

    A. direct
    B. indirect
    C. incarcerated
    D. ventral

22. The inguinal canal contains the:

    A. round ligament in the man
    B. spermatic cord in the woman
    C. vas deferens in the woman
    D. round ligament in the woman

23. Following Modified Radical Mastectomy, the breast incision would be drained using a:

    A. closed wound drain attached to vacuum drainage
    B. foley catheter attached to gravity drainage
    C. penrose drain attached to vacuum drainage
    D. T-tube attached to gravity drainage

24. A sentinel node biopsy is performed to:

    A. remove breast tissue in a female patient that is suspected of being cancerous
    B. remove enlargened breast tissue in the male patient
    C. remove all inguinal lymph nodes
    D. remove the first lymph node that drains an area of suspected cancer

25. Breast infections are commonly caused by which microbe?

    A. *Staphylococcus aureus*
    B. *Clostridium perfringens*
    C. *Bacillus subtilis*
    D. *Escherichia coli*

26. All of the following are parts of the stomach *except*:

    A. body
    B. antrum
    C. fundus
    D. calyx

27. A "twisting" of the bowel causing obstruction is called a/an:

    A. intussusception
    B. volvulus
    C. dehiscence
    D. adhesion

28. The ligament of Treitz is found between which two structures?

    A. stomach and duodenum
    B. duodenum and jejunum
    C. jejunum and ileum
    D. ileum and cecum

29. Surgical enlargement of the passage between the prepylorus of the stomach and the duodenum is called a:

    A. Cardiomyotomy
    B. Pyloroplasty
    C. Billroth I
    D. Billroth II

30. The telescoping of proximal intestine into the lumen of distal intestine is called a/an:

    A. volvulus
    B. intussusception

C. dehiscence

D. jejuno-ileopexy

31. The surgical procedure performed in conjunction with a Total Colectomy is a/an:

A. Colostomy

B. Cecostomy

C. Ileostomy

D. Jejunostomy

32. All of the following statements refer to pilonidal cyst surgery *except*:

A. performed with a paramedian incision

B. the wound frequently heals by granulation

C. probes are required on the setup

D. methylene blue may be used to outline the walls of the cyst

33. Fine dissecting scissors used during abdominal surgery are:

A. Mayo

B. Potts

C. Metzenbaum

D. Tenotomy

34. The scissors used to open the common bile duct during duct exploration are called:

A. Metzenbaum

B. Potts

C. Mayo

D. Tenotomy

35. The agent used to outline the ducts and associated structures during an intraoperative cholangiogram is:

A. Curare

B. Renografin

C. Coumadin

D. cocaine

36. The liver performs all of the following functions *except*:

A. synthesis of plasma proteins

B. aids in the absorption of vitamin K

C. synthesis of lipoproteins

D. synthesis of insulin

37. The most common type of hernia is the:

A. direct inguinal

B. indirect inguinal

C. umbilical

D. femoral

38. A Meckel's diverticulum is found in the:

A. jejunum

B. ileum

C. ascending colon

D. descending colon

39. The ampulla of Vater is the area in the duodenum where the _____ duct and the _____ duct come together.

A. cystic duct; common bile duct

B. cystic duct; hepatic duct

C. cystic duct; pancreatic duct

D. common bile duct; pancreatic duct

40. The colon walls are made up of axial strips of muscle called the _____ and outpouches of the wall called _____.

A. epiploic appendices; haustras

B. haustras; teniae coli

C. teniae coli; haustras

D. teniae coli; epiploic appendices

41. Upon completion of a colon anastamosis, the defect in the _____ must be closed to prevent postoperative obstruction.

A. lesser omentum

B. greater omentum

C. fascia

D. mesentery

42. The instrument most commonly used to grasp the appendix during an Appendectomy is a/an:

A. kelly

B. kocker

C. babcock

D. allis

43. What medication would NOT be used during hernia repair?

A. protamine sulfate

B. cefazolin

C. lidocaine hydrochloride

D. bupivicaine hydrochloride

44. Instrumentation and supplies for a Vagotomy would include all of the following *except*:

A. ligating clips

B. nerve hook

C. Penrose drain

D. Potts scissors

45. The cyst and sinus tract which is removed from between the intergluteal folds is called:

A. hemorrhoidal cyst

B. pilonidal cyst

C. anal cyst

D. sacral cyst and sinus

46. The hepatic duct system which is anatomically correct is the:

A. cystic duct flows into the common hepatic duct

B. right hepatic duct flows into the pancreas

C. cystic duct flows into the pancreas

D. common hepatic duct flows into the common bile duct

47. The organ that synthesizes cholesterol is the:
    A. liver
    B. spleen
    C. pancreas
    D. gallbladder

48. An anastamosis made between the gallbladder and the duodenum is called:
    A. cholecystoduodenostomy
    B. cholecystoduodenectomy
    C. choledochoduodenostomy
    D. choledochoduodenotomy

Questions 49–53 are based on the following case scenario:

Mr. Robertson, aged 82, enters the hospital, complaining of right upper quadrant pain with nausea and vomiting. He is jaundiced (yellow skin). He is scheduled for exploratory surgery.

49. Preoperative testing for Mr. Robertson would include all of the following *except:*
    A. chest X-ray (CXR)
    B. type and crossmatch
    C. SMA-12
    D. CBC with differential

50. The test that would help decide if Mr. Robertson has cholecystitis would be:
    A. EKG
    B. CBC with differential

C. SGOT/SGPT
D. PT/PTT

51. What medication would be used during an intraoperative evaluation of Mr. Robertson's common bile duct?
    A. heparin sodium
    B. aerosporin
    C. diatrizoate sodium
    D. salicylic acid

52. Intraoperatively the surgeon decides to perform a Cholecystostomy. The drain placed into Mr. Robertson's infected gallbladder would be a:
    A. Foley
    B. Pezzar
    C. T-tube
    D. Jackson-Pratt

53. The retractor used to lift the liver edge during this procedure would be a:
    A. Kelly-Richardson
    B. Balfour
    C. Army-Navy
    D. Harrington/Sweetheart

Instrument Identification

54.

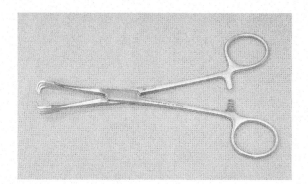

A. Lahey tenaculum
B. Jacobs tenaculum
C. Backhaus clamp
D. Allis forcep

55.

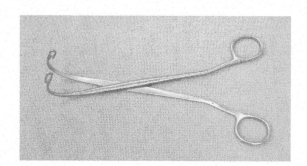

A. Oschner forcep
B. Randall forcep
C. Pean forcep
D. Pennington forcep

56.

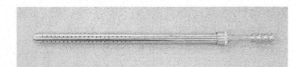

A. Yankauer suction tip
B. Poole suction tip
C. Frazier suction tip
D. Oschner gallbladder trocar

57.

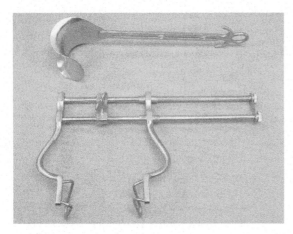

A. Balfour retractor
B. Cushing retractor
C. Sims retractor
D. Weitlaner retractor

58.

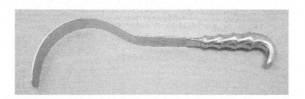

A. Harrington retractor
B. Senn retractor
C. Ribbon/Malleable retractor
D. Deaver retractor

59.

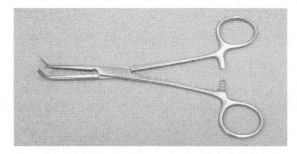

A. Allis forcep
B. Pennington clamp
C. Mixter clamp
D. Heaney Ballentine forcep

Anatomy Review

Gastrointestinal and Biliary Systems

For questions 60–88, label the figures below.

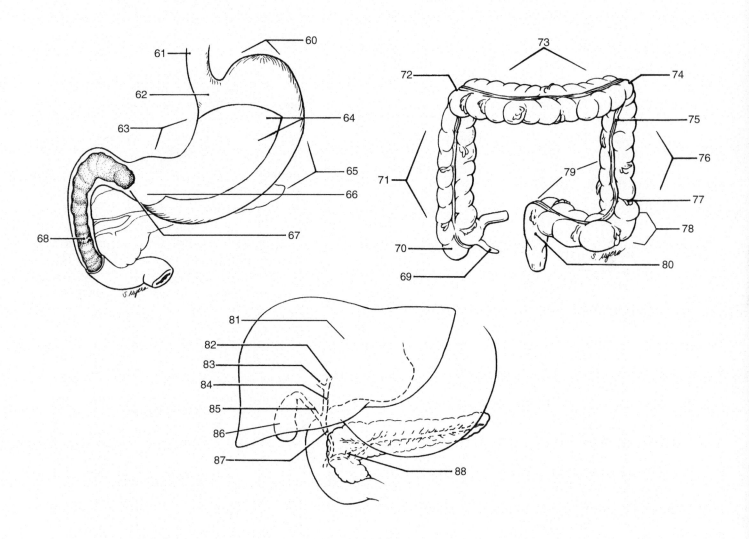

A. ampulla of Vater
B. antrum
C. appendix
D. ascending colon
E. body
F. cardia
G. cecum
H. common bile duct
I. common hepatic duct
J. cystic duct
K. descending colon
L. epiploic appendage
M. esophagus
N. fundus
O. gallbladder

P. greater curvature
Q. haustras
R. hepatic flexure
S. left hepatic duct
T. lesser curvature
U. liver
V. pancreatic duct
W. pylorus
X. rectum
Y. right hepatic duct
Z. sigmoid colon
AA. splenic flexure
BB. teniae coli
CC. transverse colon

Answers & Rationales

1. **D.** **Rationale:** The longitudinal midline is the incision most frequently used for an Exploratory Laparotomy since it is the simplest to perform, offers good exposure, can easily be extended, and contains avascular tough connective tissue.

2. **B.** **Rationale:** The paramedian incision runs parallel to the midline of the abdomen.

3. **B.** **Rationale:** The esophagus extends through the mediastinum and can best be approached through a chest or thoracoabdominal incision. The appendix and duodenum are located in the abdominal cavity and the sigmoid extends into the pelvic cavity.

4. **C.** **Rationale:** 3-0 chromic is the suture of choice (in a continuous stitch) when closing the mucosa of the GI tract. The serosal layer is closed by interrupted stitches of 3-0 silk. The extensive use of staples is rapidly replacing sutures in anastomoses.

5. **B.** **Rationale:** Following exploration of the CBD, the "T" portion of the T-tube is placed in the CBD with the long end brought out through an opening in the CBD and the abdominal wall and is connected to a drainage bag for gravity drainage. The function of the T-tube is to assure patency of the CBD following the trauma of surgery.

6. **B.** **Rationale:** Pilonidal cysts occur on the posterior surface of the sacrum and would require that the patient be placed in a prone or jackknife position for surgical access.

7. **D.** **Rationale:** Femoral hernias are more common in women and occur in the femoral ring where the femoral artery exits the torso, which is below the inguinal (Poupart's) ligament.

8. **A.** **Rationale:** An Operative Cholangiogram is an x-ray of the bile duct and requires contrast media and x-ray equipment.

9. **A.** **Rationale:** The most common incision for Splenectomy is the left subcostal incision.

10. **C.** **Rationale:** *Gynecomastia* is the term used to describe male breast enlargement.

11. **B.** **Rationale:** *Palliative* is the term used to describe a procedure that provides relief of symptoms without curing a disease.

12. **D.** **Rationale:** The small intestines begin at the pyloric sphincter of the stomach and include (in order) the duodenum, jejunum, and ileum.

13. **B.** **Rationale:** The ring of a strangulated hernia compromises the blood supply to the tissues trapped in the hernia sac.

14. **B.** **Rationale:** The right subcostal incision is commonly used because the gallbladder is located under the liver in the right upper quadrant.

15. **D.** **Rationale:** The Pfannenstiel incision is commonly used for pelvic gynecological procedures, and it has a low incidence of dehiscence because the fascia layer is split side-to-side, while the muscle is split and peritoneum is entered using a vertical incision.

16. **C.** **Rationale:** The incision commonly used for trauma surgery is the midline incision because it is easily extended if necessary.

17. **D.** **Rationale:** The #3 knife handle with a #11 blade is not commonly used to perform an Exploratory Laparotomy. The #11 blade is used as the skin knife for minimally invasive (laparoscopy) procedures or to incise a duct or tubular structure.

18. **D.** **Rationale:** During minimally invasive surgery (laparoscopy), pneumoperitoneum is created using CO_2.

19. **A.** **Rationale:** The Hasson device is used, when performing minimally invasive surgery (laparoscopy) using the open method, to secure the cannula to the fascia and create a seal in the peritoneal incision, permitting a pneumoperitoneum to be created.

20. **A.** **Rationale:** An indirect inguinal hernia forms due to a defect in the internal inguinal ring.

21. **C.** **Rationale:** A hernia whose contents cannot be pushed back into the abdominal cavity is referred to as an incarcerated hernia.

22. **D.** **Rationale:** The inguinal canal contains the round ligament in the woman. The remaining structures are all found in the inguinal canal in the man.

23. **A.** **Rationale:** Following Modified Radical Mastectomy, the breast incision would be drained using a closed wound drain attached to vacuum drainage. This system prevents seroma formation and minimizes the potential for postoperative wound infection.

24. **D.** **Rationale:** A sentinel node biopsy is performed to remove the first lymph node that drains an area of suspected cancer. This procedure is done to assist in tumor staging.

25. A. **Rationale:** Breast infections are commonly caused by *Staphylococcus aureus*, a common microbe that is part of the normal flora of the skin.

26. D. **Rationale:** Parts of the stomach include the fundus, body, and antrum/pylorus. The calyx is found in the kidney.

27. B. **Rationale:** A "twisting" of the bowel causing obstruction is called a volvulus.

28. B. **Rationale:** The ligament of Treitz is found at the point where the duodenum ends and the jejunum begins.

29. B. **Rationale:** Surgical enlargement of the passage between the prepylorus of the stomach and the duodenum is called a Pyloroplasty.

30. B. **Rationale:** The telescoping of proximal intestine into the lumen of distal intestine is called an intussusception.

31. C. **Rationale:** The surgical procedure performed in conjunction with a Total Colectomy is an Ileostomy.

32. A. **Rationale:** A paramedian incision is not used when performing pilonidal cyst surgery.

33. C. **Rationale:** Metzenbaum scissors are fine dissecting scissors used during abdominal surgery.

34. B. **Rationale:** Potts scissors are used to extend the incision into the common bile duct during duct exploration.

35. B. **Rationale:** Renografin (diatrizoate sodium) is the agent used to outline the ducts and associated structures during an Intraoperative Cholangiogram.

36. D. **Rationale:** The liver does not synthesize insulin; the pancreas does.

37. B. **Rationale:** The indirect inguinal hernia is the most common type of hernia.

38. B. **Rationale:** A Meckel's diverticulum is found in the ileum.

39. D. **Rationale:** The ampulla of Vater is the area where the common bile duct and pancreatic duct come together.

40. C. **Rationale:** The colon walls are made up of axial strips of muscle called the teniae coli and outpouches of the wall called haustras.

41. D. **Rationale:** Upon completion of a colon anastamosis, the defect in the mesentery must be closed to prevent postoperative obstruction.

42. C. **Rationale:** The Babcock is used to grasp the appendix during Appendectomy.

43. A. **Rationale:** Protamine sulfate is not used during hernia repair.

44. D. **Rationale:** Potts scissors are not used during a Vagotomy.

45. B. **Rationale:** A pilonidal cyst is a cyst and sinus tract removed from between the intergluteal folds.

46. D. **Rationale:** The common hepatic duct flows into the common bile duct.

47. A. **Rationale:** The liver synthesizes cholesterol.

48. A. **Rationale:** Cholecystoduodenostomy is an anastamosis made between the gallbladder and the duodenum.

49. B. **Rationale:** Mr. Robertson should not have significant blood loss during gallbladder surgery to need a blood transfusion, so a type and crossmatch is not usually necessary.

50. B. **Rationale:** The CBC (complete blood count) with differential should indicate the presence of infection if Mr. Robertson had cholecystitis.

51. C. **Rationale:** The medication used during an intraoperative evaluation of Mr. Robertson's common bile duct (intraoperative cholangiogram) is diatrizoate sodium (Hypaque), a contrast media.

52. B. **Rationale:** The Pezzar catheter is placed into Mr. Robertson's infected gallbladder.

53. D. **Rationale:** The Harrington/Sweetheart retractor is designed to lift the edge of the liver with minimal injury.

54. A. **Rationale:** Lahey Tenaculum

55. B. **Rationale:** Randall forcep

56. B. **Rationale:** Poole suction tip

57. A. **Rationale:** Balfour retractor

58. D. **Rationale:** Deaver retractor

59. C. **Rationale:** Mixter clamp

60. (N) fundus

61. (M) esophagus

62. (F) cardia

63. (T) lesser curvature

64. (E) body

65. (P) greater curvature

66. (B) antrum

67. (W) pylorus

68. (A) ampulla of Vater

69. (C) appendix

70. (G) cecum

71. **(D)** ascending colon
72. **(R)** hepatic flexure
73. **(CC)** transverse colon
74. **(AA)** splenic flexure
75. **(BB)** teniae coli
76. **(K)** descending colon
77. **(L)** epiploic appendage
78. **(Q)** haustras
79. **(Z)** sigmoid colon

80. **(X)** rectum
81. **(U)** liver
82. **(S)** left hepatic duct
83. **(Y)** right hepatic duct
84. **(I)** common hepatic duct
85. **(J)** cystic duct
86. **(O)** gallbladder
87. **(H)** common bile duct
88. **(V)** pancreatic duct

Part II: Deciphering a Surgical Schedule

The following mock surgery schedule will be used to answer several questions pertaining to general surgery. The same schedule, or a similar one, will be used in subsequent chapters to ask questions about the content of the chapter.

Rm# time	Surgeon	Procedure	Anest.	Rm# time	Surgeon	Procedure	Anest.
Rm00				**Rm07**			
OC	Dr. Z	Rt. Knee Arthroscopy	Gen.	7:00	Dr. M	Laparoscopic appendectomy	Gen.
OC	Dr. C	Craniotomy	Gen.	TF	Dr. M	Lipoma removal	MAC
OC	Dr.Z	Angioplasty	Gen.				
Rm01				**Rm08**			
7:00	Dr. X	Hemorrhoidectomy	Gen.	11:00	Dr. E	Bovine Thrombectomy	MAC
TF	Dr. X	Colostomy	Gen.				
TF	Dr. X	Bowel resection	Gen.				
Rm02				**Rm09**			
7:00	Dr. B	Splenectomy	Gen.	8:30	Dr. T	Laparoscopic Cholecystectomy	Gen.
TF	Dr. B	Gastrectomy	Gen.	TF	Dr. T	Choledochojejunos-tomy	Gen.
Rm03				**Rm10**			
7:00	Dr. A	Cystoscopy	MAC	7:00	Dr. K	Right Nephrectomy	Gen.
TF	Dr. A	Cystoplasty	Gen.	TF	Dr. K	Choledocholithotripsy	MAC
12:30	Dr. F	Pyleogram	MAC	TF	Dr. K	Hepatic Wedge resection	Gen.
3:00	Dr. F	Cystocele repair	Gen.				
Rm04				**Rm11**			
7:00	Dr. Y	Laparoscopic appendectomy	Gen.	7:00	Dr. L	Colposcope	Gen.
TF	Dr. Y	Whipple	Gen.	12:00	Dr. L	Mastectomy	Gen.
Rm05				**Rm12**			
7:00	Dr. G	Trans-sphenoidal Adenectomy	Gen.	7:00	Dr. W	Trans-metatarsal amputation	Gen.
TF	Dr. G	Trans-urethral resection of the prostate	Gen	TF	Dr. W	Osteotomy	Gen.
TF	Dr. G	Bletharoplasty	Gen.	TF	Dr. W	Arthrocentesis	Gen.
Rm06				**Rm13**			
7:00	Dr. R	Lumbar Laminectomy	Gen.	7:00	Dr. O	Hysterectomy	Gen.

The following questions should be answered using the surgery schedule above

1. During the laparoscopic Cholecystectomy being performed in Room 9, the surgeon announces that he needs to do a CBD exploration. What does the ST need to have available for this added portion of the procedure?

   A. An extra 5 mm trochar
   B. A 10 mL syringe with contrast media
   C. An 11 blade on a 15 handle
   D. An endocatch

2. During the Whipple procedure in Room 4, which section of the gastrointestinal tract is NOT involved?

   A. Distal stomach
   B. Duodenum
   C. Pancreas
   D. Gallbladder

3. All of the following are likely incisions to perform a wedge resection of the Liver, *except:*

   A. Midline
   B. Paramedian
   C. Transverse
   D. Subcostal

4. During the common bile duct exploration that was added in question 1, what does the ST need to remember?

   A. The 5mm trochar will be placed above the camera
   B. Bubbles must be removed from the syringe holding the contrast media
   C. The 11 blade must be a new sterile blade, not the one used for initial skin incisions
   D. The endocatch bag must be closed prior to insertion

5. A patient in Room 9 is scheduled for a choledochojejunostomy. What is the goal of this intervention?

   A. To re-establish the flow of bile by creating a connection between the jejunum and the CBD
   B. To re-establish the flow of bile by connecting the hepatic duct and the jejunum
   C. To create an opening from the common bile duct to the outside of the body
   D. To bypass the hepatic duct and create a passage from the cystic duct to the jejunum

6. Which incision would most commonly be used during an OPEN cholecystectomy?

   A. Midline
   B. Pfannenstiel
   C. Subcostal
   D. McBurneys

7. The Surgical Technologist scrubbed in for the Hepatic Wedge Resection scheduled in Room 9 should have suture on which type of needle?

   A. Blunt
   B. Reverse Cutting
   C. Spatula
   D. Taper

8. In question 1, the surgeon decides to do a CBD exploration. He asks the Surgical Technologist for traction sutures. What are they going to be used for?

   A. To close the duct after it has been cleared of stones
   B. To hold open the duct during the exploration

C. To aid in the closure

D. To retract tissue for better visualization of the cystic duct

9. A patient in Room 4 is scheduled for a laparoscopic appendectomy. What position will the patient most likely be in?

A. Reverse trendelenburg

B. Fowlers

C. Trendelenburg

D. Supine

10. The scheduled gastrectomy in Room 2 is most likely being performed due to:

A. Obesity

B. Hiatal hernia

C. Extreme malabsorptive syndrome

D. Malignancy

Answers & Rationales

1. **B.** **Rationale:** Common bile duct explorations are commonly performed after a cholecystectomy to check for the presence of stones in the tract. Generally, this will be done by injecting a radiopaque dye into the CBD to visualize any stones present. An endocatch would not be used during this portion of the procedure, but may be used during the actual removal of the gallbladder. There is no need to place another trochar for this procedure, and there is no need for an 11 blade.

2. **D.** **Rationale:** Generally, the gallbladder will be left intact unless there are stones present. Generally, the structures removed during a Whipple procedure include the head of the pancreas, the distal portion of the stomach, the duodenum, a portion of the jejunum, and part of the common bile duct.

3. **C.** **Rationale:** The least likely incision for this procedure would be the transverse.

4. **B.** **Rationale:** Under fluoroscopy, air bubbles will look like stones. Therefore, it is important for the Surgical Technologist to make sure that all of the air in the syringe has been removed prior to handing it to the surgeon.

5. **A.** **Rationale:** In this procedure, the patient may have an obstruction preventing bile from entering the small intestine. To correct this, the surgeon will create an anastomosis between the common bile duct and the jejunum.

6. **C.** **Rationale:** A Subcostal incision is the most commonly used incision to access the gallbladder. The Pfannenstiel incision is made near the pubis, generally in abdominal hysterectomies. The McBurneys incision is commonly used for open appendectomies, and a transverse incision would be much larger than necessary.

7. **A.** **Rationale:** Blunt needles are used on friable tissue like the liver.

8. **B.** **Rationale:** Traction sutures are generally placed to hold a structure open. In this case, the structure being explored is the common bile duct. The suture will not be used in closing incisions or the duct itself.

9. **C.** **Rationale:** The surgeon will most likely request the trendelenburg position to help in visualization of internal structures.

10. **D.** **Rationale:** Generally a gastrectomy is performed for malignant cancers.

Obstetrics and Gynecological Surgery

O bstetrics and gynecology are combined specialties for some physicians. Gynecology is the branch of medicine and surgery that deals with women who have diseases of the reproductive system. Gynecological surgeries encompass many aspects of the system from benign ovarian cysts to complete removal of reproductive organs due to malignancies. Obstetrics comes from the Latin word that means "midwife." It deals with the management of pregnancy, labor and delivery, and postpartum care and offers the challenge of delivering care to more than one patient concurrently. Most Surgical Technologists associated with Obstetric surgeries involve cesarean sections.

CHAPTER OUTLINE

When the Surgical Technologist is faced with gynecological surgeries, there are major issues that should be uppermost in the mind. First, the separation between what is considered "clean" and "dirty" has to be clear. Understanding that separate drapes and instrumentation will be required for cases involving a sterile cavity and an unsterile orifice is required for these cases. Separate gowns and gloves may also be necessary when moving between these areas. Second, STs must know the anatomical structures that will be dealt with during these surgeries, as well as the specialty instruments that are utilized during these procedures. With this information in hand, the ST should have little difficulty in answering these questions.

Example:
All of the following ligaments are ligated and divided during an Vaginal Hysterectomy EXCEPT

A. Cardinal ligament
B. Round ligament
C. Uterosacral ligament
D. Suspensory ligament

To answer this question, the ST must know the relevant anatomy. First, there is no indication that the fallopian tubes or ovaries are to be removed. This would be denoted with bi-lateral salpingo-oopherectomy. Therefore, we should proceed with the understanding that these structures will be preserved. The Round, Uterosacral, and Cardinal ligaments are routinely ligated and divided during this procedure. The only ligament that could be preserved is the Suspensory ligament. Therefore, the only appropriate response to this question would be D. This brings into focus the differences between vaginal procedures and abdominal procedures. In abdominal procedures, the Suspensory ligament may be ligated at the proximal end, leaving the distal end preserved.

I. Obstetrics

A. Terminology

1. *Antepartum:* before delivery
2. *Cesarean Section:* incision through the abdominal and uterine wall for delivery of a fetus
3. *Effacement:* flattening and thinning of the cervix
4. *Engagement:* widest part of the fetus in the narrowest part of the mother's pelvis
5. *Episiotomy:* incision in the perineum to facilitate delivery of the fetus and avoid laceration
6. *Gestation:* length of pregnancy (9 months/3 trimesters/10 lunar months)
7. *Lightening:* descent of the fetus into the pelvis; usually occurs about 2 weeks before delivery
8. *Lochia:* vaginal discharge after delivery
9. *Multiparous:* condition of a woman who has given birth to more than one child
10. *Neonate:* newborn
11. *Obstetrics:* branch of medicine that deals with care during the periods of pregnancy, delivery, and postpartum
12. *Postpartum:* after delivery
13. *Preeclampsia:* toxemia of late pregnancy characterized by hypertension, edema, and proteinuria
14. *Presentation:* presenting part of the fetus in birth canal (cephalic, breech, shoulder)
15. *Primigravida:* first pregnancy

16. *Primiparous:* a condition of a woman who has borne one child (500 g or 20-week gestation minimum)
17. *Quickening:* first movement of the fetus felt by the mother
18. *Station:* presenting part of the fetus in relation to mother's ischial spines, expressed in centimeters (−5 to −1 above, +1 to +5 below the ischial spines)

B. Pregnancy
   1. *Fertilization:* uniting of sperm (male gamete) and egg (female gamete)
      a. Occurs at the time of ovulation (release of the egg from the ovary); about the fourteenth day of the ovarian cycle
      b. Usually takes place in the fallopian tube (salpinx) to form a zygote (fertilized egg)
      c. Moves to uterus by peristaltic waves
      d. Usually implants in the fundus (upper portion) of the uterus within 10 days
   2. *Placenta*
      a. Develops from the chorion (an outer membrane of the zygote)
      b. Anchors itself to the uterine wall (made ready by progesterone) through chorionic villi, which serve as a bridge for exchange of nutrients and waste products between the fetus and the mother
      c. Provides nutrition of the fetus
      d. Secretes the hormone HCG (human chorionic gonadotropin), which may be detected in urine as early as 10 days following conception and is used as a pregnancy test
   3. *Amnion*
      a. Developed from an outer layer of the zygote
      b. A sac that contains amniotic fluid that serves as a shock absorber for the developing fetus
   4. *Changes occurring during pregnancy*
      a. Uterus and breasts enlarge
      b. Linea alba (white line) becomes linea nigra (dark line)
      c. Cervix becomes soft and bluish
      d. Brownish pigmentation (chloasma) of the face may occur
      e. Ovulation and menstrual flow commonly cease (amenorrhea)
      f. Urinary frequency, nausea, vomiting, and general fatigue may occur
      g. Pregnancy may be confirmed by human chorionic gonadotropin (HCG) levels, ultrasound, or fetal heart tones (FHT)

C. Signs of labor
   1. *False labor (Braxton Hicks contractions):* felt in the abdomen, with no cervical dilation; irregular, stopped by walking
   2. *True labor:* contractions are regular and increasing in frequency; discomfort is felt both in the abdomen and back and cervix dilates; contractions are intensified by walking; membranes may rupture; and the mucus plug may be lost
   3. *Induced labor:* artificially brought on by the IV administration of oxytocin (Pitocin)

D. Stages of labor
   1. *First stage:* begins with first regular contractions and extends to 10 cm dilation and effacement of the cervix
      a. May begin with ruptured membranes (sudden gush of amniotic fluid from the vagina)
      b. May last 6 to 18 hours for primipara or 4 to 6 hours for a multipara
      c. Fetal heart tone (FHT) monitored (*Note:* FHT decreases during contraction.)
      d. Vaginal bleeding observed
      e. Patient's vital signs are monitored

f. Contractions are monitored for frequency (beginning of one contraction to the beginning of next), intensity, and duration

g. Report to nurse if FHT exceeds 160 per minute or falls below 100, mother's blood pressure goes above 140/90, or contractions are closer than 2 minutes apart or last longer than 90 seconds

h. Patient may have a family member to assist if trained in child-birth classes

i. Patient lies on left side to take pressure off inferior vena cava

j. Saline enema or skin prep may be ordered

2. *Second stage:* from complete cervical dilation and effacement to delivery of the infant

a. If membranes have not ruptured, an amniotomy may be performed by the physician

b. May last 2 hours for a primipara or 30 minutes for a multipara

c. Continue observations as in the first stage; also observe for bulging of perineum, crowning (head of infant appearing), or the mother beginning to push

d. Problems to be reported: prolapsed cord, excessive bleeding, elevated blood pressure, or severe headache

e. Presenting part of infant is a crucial factor; generally cephalic; if feet or buttocks are first (breech), forceps may be needed to turn the fetus

f. Preparations made for delivery: patient placed in the lithotomy position, perineal prep done, drapes applied, and episiotomy performed

g. Anesthesia may be epidural, continuous caudal, pudendal block, spinal, or natural childbirth (without anesthesia)

h. Care of the infant includes positioning on its side with head lower, suctioning to remove mucus or amniotic fluid, maintaining warmth, matching identification bracelets for mother and infant, hand/foot printing, and having oxygen readily available

i. Apgar scoring of infant: assessment of neonate on the basis of heart rate, respiratory rate, muscle tone, color, and reflex irritability, taken at 1 minute and 5 minutes after delivery; 9 to 10 is excellent, 4 to 6 is fair, and 0 is nonviable

3. *Third stage:* from expulsion of infant to expulsion of the placenta

a. Generally lasts about 3 minutes

b. Critical stage; bleeding may occur

c. Cord blood is drawn for tests

d. Episiotomy is sutured; the patient is made comfortable

e. Mother is allowed to see the infant

4. *Fourth stage:* recovery phase (1 hour)

a. Mother is allowed to rest in a dimly lit room with warm blanket

b. Mother is monitored: blood pressure, pulse, respiration, and vaginal bleeding

c. Fundus of the uterus is massaged to express blood clots and stimulate contractions to control bleeding

d. Mother may be given medication (oxytocin or Ergotrate) to stimulate uterine contractions

e. Uterine atony with hemorrhage is the most common postpartum complication

E. Complications of pregnancy

1. **Toxemia (eclampsia):** pregnancy-induced hypertension accompanied by edema, albuminuria, and sometimes convulsions

2. **Ectopic (out of place) pregnancy:** when zygote implants outside the uterine cavity; most common site is the fallopian tube; if not detected early, the tube may rupture and result in bleeding that requires emergency surgery

3. Incompetent cervix: spontaneous abortion occurring during the second trimester; prevented surgically by cerclage (placement of a purse-string mersilene suture around the cervix)
4. Placenta previa: painless bleeding during the second trimester or at the onset of labor due to positioning of the placenta near or over the cervical opening; an indication for C-section
5. Abruptio placenta: painful bleeding caused by the premature separation of the placenta from the uterine wall; leads to rapid demise of the infant and hemorrhage of the mother; emergency C-section indicated
6. Hyperemesis gravidarum: excessive vomiting during pregnancy
7. Gestational diabetes: elevated blood sugar in mother and development of a large fetus

F. **Abortion**
1. Spontaneous or planned intervention resulting in expulsion of the products of conception; may result from incompetent cervical os, blighted ovum, or other reasons
2. Types
   a. *Incomplete abortion:* patient bleeding but entire contents of conception not discharged
   b. *Missed abortion:* nonviable fetus that is not aborted
   c. *Therapeutic abortion:* artificially induced abortion for nonviable or abnormal fetus or for the welfare of the mother; generally performed during the first trimester of pregnancy by a process of cervical dilatation and vacuum extraction of the products of conception

G. **Complications of labor**
1. *Abnormal fetal positions:* transverse lie, breech, and shoulder, presentations indications for a C-section
2. *Dystocia:* difficult labor; contractions fail to expel the fetus; may be an indication for a C-section
3. *Cephalopelvic disproportion (CPD):* head of the infant too large to pass through the pelvis of the mother; indication for a C-section
4. *Retained placenta:* causes bleeding and is generally treated with dilation and curettage (D&C)
5. *Vaginal lacerations:* tears occurring when labor is too rapid and no episiotomy is performed
   a. *First degree:* tear into mucous membrane of vagina and skin of the perineum
   b. *Second degree:* tear into muscles of the perineum
   c. *Third degree:* tear that extends into the external anal sphincter and requires perineorrhaphy
   d. *Fourth degree:* tear that extends into the rectum and requires perineorrhaphy
6. *Ruptured uterus:* may occur during labor of a patient with previous C-section(s) (VBAC—Vaginal Birth After Cesarean) or other uterine surgery
7. *Amniotic fluid embolism:* clotting disorder that occurs when amniotic fluid destroys fibrinogen
8. *Prolapsed cord:* cord precedes fetus down the birth canal and is compressed between the head of the fetus and the pelvic bone of the mother, blocking circulation to the fetus; an indication for emergency C-Section
9. *Inversion of the uterus:* during the third stage of labor, the uterus may prolapse inside out
10. *Multiple pregnancies:* twins, triplets, etc. may lead to labor complications

H. **Complications of the postpartum period**
1. *Infection:* may result from early rupture of membranes or exposure to infectious organisms

2. *Subinvolution of the uterus:* uterus does not go back into normal position in the pelvis.
3. *Hemorrhage due to uterine atony or retained placenta:* most common complication in the fourth stage of labor.
4. *Vulvar hematoma from the trauma of labor.*
5. *Enlargement of the breasts:* managed by compression and ice packs.
6. *Cystitis:* bladder infection; may result from catheterization.
7. *Puerperal psychosis:* mental depression following delivery.
8. *Thrombophlebitis and pulmonary embolism:* generally prevented by early ambulation.

I. Cesarean section
1. *Indications*
   a. *Maternal:* carcinoma of the cervix, dystocias including "failure to progress," eclampsia, herpes infection of the genitalia, previous C-section
   b. *Fetal:* decelerations/fetal distress, meconium staining
   c. *Maternal/fetal:* CPD
   d. *Other:* abruptio placenta, placenta previa, prolapsed cord
2. *Position of the patient:* supine, right side may be elevated to prevent compression of the aorta and vena cava by the enlarged uterus
3. *Anesthesia:* spinal or epidural; if general, anesthesia is not begun until the patient is prepped, draped, and the team is ready to limit the amount of anesthetic agents passed to the fetus
4. *Draping:* towels with cuff and C-section drape (with impervious pockets to catch amniotic fluid); may include incise drape
5. *Incision:* lower midline or Pfannenstiel
6. *Specialty instruments and supplies:*
   a. *Setup for infant:* bulb syringe, warm blankets, isolette or warmed infant table, oxygen, and resuscitation equipment
   b. *Mayo stand setup:* scalpels, clamps, lap sponges, bladder retractor, bulb syringe, suction, ESU, Lister bandage scissors, and Pennington or other uterine clamps for the uterus
7. *Procedure*
   a. Incision is made to expose uterus
   b. Bladder is retracted/separated from anterior uterine wall
   c. Uterus is opened with knife—small "nick" incision (amniotic fluid suctioned) and extended with blunt-tipped bandage scissors
   d. Assistant presses firmly on upper abdomen (simulates a contraction) while the surgeon grasps infant's head and rotates it upward; the surgeon delivers the head and suctions the airway with a bulb syringe before delivering the body; the body is delivered, cord double-clamped with cord clamp and/or Kelly/Peans and divided with bandage scissors; the neonate is passed to the neonatal team (*Note:* Neonatologist, pediatrician, nurse specialist, respiratory therapist, or others care for the infant.)
   e. Surgeon delivers placenta and passes it to the scrub person. (*Note:* Cord blood is drawn for laboratory testing before the placenta is prepared for pathologic examination or storage.)
   f. Care should be taken when suctioning inside the uterus to prevent wound contamination from the cervix
   g. Uterus is closed (one or two layers) with continuous stitch of 0 or 1 absorbable suture on a taper needle while first count is taken
   h. Bladder flap may be reperitonealized with absorbable suture
   i. Peritoneum and/or fascia are closed while second count is taken
   j. Subcutaneous tissue may be closed with interrupted stitches of absorbable suture
   k. Final count taken as skin is closed

l. Wound is cleaned and dressed; perineal pad is applied (*Note:* Uterus may be massaged and clots evacuated before perineal pads are placed)

II. Gynecology

A. Terminology

1. *Carcinoma in situ:* cancer in the endothelial layer that is not invasive
2. *Chocolate cyst:* benign cyst of the ovary that contains dark syrupy contents from old blood; ovarian endometriosis
3. *Cystocele:* herniation of the bladder into the vagina
4. *Dermoid cyst:* sac filled with hair and sebaceous material found in the ovary of young females
5. *Dysfunctional uterine bleeding (DUB):* menstruation that occurs at irregular intervals or postmenopausal bleeding
6. *Dysmenorrhea:* painful or difficult menstruation
7. *Endometriosis:* occurrence of endometrial tissues outside the uterus which slough off during normal menses and cause pain and pelvic congestion
8. *Enterocele:* herniation of the intestine into the cul-de-sac of Douglas
9. *Fornices:* regions in the vaginal vault created by the projections of the cervix into the proximal vagina. The posterior fornix is in close contact with the cul-de-sac (pouch of Douglas); the site for a Colpotomy, Culdocentesis, and culdoscope insertion
10. *Leiomyoma uteri/fibroid:* benign tumor arising from the muscle layer of the uterus
11. *Menometrorrhagia:* excessive uterine bleeding occurring both during menses and at irregular intervals
12. *Pelvic diaphragm:* levator ani and coccygeal muscles with fascial coverings; separates pelvic cavity from perineum and provides support to the abdominal pelvic viscera
13. *Pelvic Inflammatory Disease (PID):* inflammation of the uterus, fallopian tubes, ovaries, and related structures due to infection
14. *Rectocele:* herniation of the rectum into the vagina
15. *Stress incontinence:* leakage of urine when intraabdominal pressure is increased, as with a cough or sneeze
16. *Uterine descensus/uterine prolapse/procidentia:* laxity of the ligaments that suspend the uterus in the pelvic cavity resulting in the uterus "falling" into or out through the vagina; first degree may be treated with a pessary, while second and third degrees may be treated by a Hysterectomy (usually vaginal)

B. Patient preparation for gynecological surgery

1. *Enema:* because of the close proximity of the sigmoid colon and rectum to the uterus, tubes, and ovaries, it is essential that decompression precede pelvic surgery to avoid inadvertent injury and to decrease the chance of postoperative constipation
2. *Urinary catheterization:* a deflated bladder is less likely to be injured during perineal or pelvic surgery. Swelling which may accompany pelvic or perineal surgery makes micturition (voiding) more difficult. A Foley catheter may be left in place until swelling subsides because of the potential for urinary retention
   a. Foley catheter may be inserted prior to the patient's arrival in surgery or inserted just prior to surgery in the OR
   b. "Straight cath": catheterization (red Robinson or metal catheter drains the bladder and is then removed); may be done in the OR immediately prior to a D&C
3. *Deep vein thrombosis (DVT) prophylaxis:* antiembolic stockings with or without sequential compression devices (compression boots), early ambulation, prophylactic anticoagulation, or other measures may be

implemented to lessen the chance of postoperative thrombus formation (*Note:* Surgery in the pelvis can lead to swelling, with resultant pressure on the venous return, which causes stagnation of blood and clot formation.)

4. *Antiseptic douche:* may be ordered prior to surgery to decrease microbial flora in the vagina prior to a Hysterectomy. The vagina is also cleansed with an antiseptic solution in the OR.

C. Diagnostic procedures
   1. *Examination under Anesthesia (EUA):* bimanual examination is frequently done prior to vaginal or abdominal surgery for assessment of the uterus, tubes, or ovaries
   2. *Papanicolaou (Pap) smear:* study of cells taken from the cervix
   3. *Schiller's Test:* staining the cervix or vaginal vault with an iodine (Lugol's) solution to differentiate normal from abnormal tissue
   4. *Biopsy of the cervix:* cervical tissue specimens may be obtained with Gaylor biopsy forceps, scalpel (cold knife conization or cone biopsy), LASER, or LEEP (loop electrosurgical excision procedure)
   5. *Curettage:* scrapings from the uterine cavity for pathological analysis. Usually accompanied by dilation of the cervix
   6. *Colposcopy:* use of colposcope to identify abnormal vaginal epithelium following removal of mucus with acetic acid solution
   7. *Culdocentesis:* aspiration of fluid from the cul-de-sac through the posterior vaginal fornix to determine the presence of blood or pus
   8. *Chromopertubation:* dye (methylene blue or indigo carmine) is introduced into the uterine cavity and fallopian tube through an IV tubing or syringe attached to a uterine manipulator/injector to determine patency of fallopian tubes
   9. *Hystero-salpingography:* x-ray study of the uterus and fallopian tubes following instillation of a radiopaque agent to evaluate infertility

D. Equipment
   1. *Laparoscope with accessories:* see minimally invasive surgery, Chapter 10; bipolar forceps; tubal occlusion devices (silastic rings, clips)
   2. *Pelviscope:* not as frequently used
   3. *Hysteroscope with accessories*
      a. Introduced vaginally
      b. Distention provided by dextran, glucose, glycine, or Hyskon solution—fluid monitoring/control system may be used
      c. Video camera connected to a monitor
      d. Uses: endometrial ablation (resectoscope or balloon therapy); removal of polyps, intrauterine adhesions, and submucous fibroids; or to locate lost intrauterine device (IUD)
   4. Culdoscopy and accessories
      a. used occasionally to investigate cervical/vaginal tissues

E. Abdominal gynecological surgery
   1. *Patient positioning:* supine with slight Trendelenburg for improved visualization of the pelvic organs
   2. *Special instruments and supplies:* abdominal instrument set (to include long instruments, Heaney clamps and needle holders, and Rochester-Pean and Rochester-Oschner forceps), self-retaining retractors (Balfour, O'Sullivan-O'Connor, Martin), and absorbable suture 2-0 to 1
   3. *Incision:* Pfannenstiel or low midline
   4. *Anesthesia:* general, epidural, or spinal may be used
   5. *Skin preparation:* vaginal and abdominal
      a. Place patient in frog-leg position and perform vaginal prep.
      b. Insert Foley catheter and connect to the gravity drainage.
      c. Straighten legs and apply a safety strap.

d. With separate set, perform abdominal prep beginning at the incision site; extend from nipple line to pubis and from bed line to bed line on either side.

6. *Special considerations*
   a. Check sterilization permits if required by hospital policy.
   b. Have moist laps available for packing back abdominal viscera.
   c. Have moist sponges on a forcep for blunt dissection.
   d. Have basin available to receive instruments coming in contact with the vagina; isolate basin/instruments following closure of the vagina cuff.
   e. Counts are taken at closure of vaginal vault, peritoneum, and skin (observe for sponge which may be placed in the vagina).
   f. Perineal pad is placed following Abdominal Hysterectomy.

F. **Abdominal gynecological procedures**
   1. *Oophorectomy:* surgical removal of the ovary; indications include a malignant condition or ovarian cyst (follicular, corpus luteum, dermoid, or chocolate cyst); cyst may be evacuated using a needle aspiration tip and 30-cc syringe; the aspirated fluid is sent for cytology; surgeon attempts to leave some ovarian remnant—estrogen production ceases with bilateral removal—"surgical menopause"
   2. *Salpingo-Oophorectomy:* removal of the tube and ovary when pathology involves both tubes and ovary damage from PID (pelvic inflammatory disease), endometriosis, cysts, or carcinoma. May be designated by initials BSO: Bi-Lateral Salpingo-oopherectomy. If not bilateral, make sure that the correct side is identified.
   3. *Tubal ligation:* interruption in the continuity of the fallopian tubes for sterilization purposes
      a. Presurgical counseling is recommended for the patient
      b. Performed on the first or second postpartum day for a vaginal delivery patient or in conjunction with a Cesarean Section
      c. **Mini-laparotomy**: small transverse incision is made above the pubic hairline down to peritoneum; the tubes are grasped with a babcock, and a section of the tubes is ligated and removed
   4. *Tubal sterilization:* interruption in the continuity of the fallopian tubes for sterilization purposes via laparoscopy; coagulation, and division— bipolar ESU forceps, application of occlusion devices—silastic rings, clips
   5. *Microtubal re-anastamosis/tuboplasty:* reconstruction of fallopian tubes under microscopic assistance for infertility related to previous tubal sterilization
   6. *In-vitro fertilization and embryo transfer:* eggs (oocytes) are retrieved from the ovary through a laparoscope and implanted in the uterine cavity following fertilization
   7. *Myomectomy:* surgical removal of uterine fibroid(s) in premenopausal women wishing to preserve fertility
   8. *Abdominal hysterectomy*
      a. **Indications:** pain associated with pelvic congestion, PID, previous pelvic surgery, endometriosis, fibroids, dysfunctional or postmenopausal bleeding, or malignancy
      b. It also accomplishes sterilization; may be combined with BSO (Bilateral Salpingo-Oophorectomy)
      c. A Supracervical Hysterectomy involves removal of the uterine body with the cervix left in place
      d. **Procedure**
         i. Peritoneal cavity is entered, and viscera is retracted with warm saline packs and self-retaining retractor.
         ii. Round ligaments are clamped with heavy crushing, toothed clamp—Heaney, Masterson, Oschner, or other; ligated, divided— sutured with 0 or 1 absorbable suture, and tagged with hemostats.

     iii. Broad ligaments are excised after identification and protection of the ureters and bladder reflected from the cervix.

     iv. Uterine ligaments are ligated and divided.

     v. Ovarian ligaments are ligated and divided.

     vi. Uterosacral and cardinal ligaments are ligated and divided.

     vii. Vaginal cuff is incised and cut with Jorgensen angled scissors, and the specimen is removed.

     viii. Hemostasis is secured; the vaginal cuff is closed with a continuous stitch or stapled (a drain may be left in place).

     ix. Stumps of uterosacral and round ligaments are sutured to the vaginal cuff.

     x. Contaminated (contact with vagina) instruments are isolated.

     xi. Pelvic cavity is irrigated and counts taken.

     xii. Abdominal wound is closed.

9. *Vesicourethral suspension (Marshall-Marchetti-Kranz procedure):* the periurethral tissues are sutured to the periosteum of the pubic symphysis to reposition the vesico-urethral angle; performed to correct urinary stress incontinence; one hand is placed in the vagina, lifting the urethra upward to assist with suture placement—gloved hand is contaminated.
    a. *Position:* modified lithotomy or frog-legged
    b. *Skin prep:* vaginal and abdominal
    c. *Drapes:* vaginal plus transverse abdominal sheet
    d. *Incision:* Pfannenstiel
    e. *Instruments:* laparotomy set

10. *Wertheim procedure:* Radical Hysterectomy (removal of uterus, tubes, and ovaries, and upper one-third of vagina) and Pelvic Lymphadenectomy. Ureteral catheters are generally inserted prior to surgery as landmarks to avoid damage to them.

11. *Pelvic exenteration:* radical procedure done when metastasis has occurred
    a. *Anterior exenteration:* Wertheim procedure plus Cystectomy (removal of the bladder) with Ileal Conduit; new bladder is formed from a portion of the ileum, intestinal continuity is re-established, and ureters are anastomosed to the ileal conduit with one end of the new bladder pouch brought through the abdominal wall for escape of urine
    b. *Posterior exenteration:* done when metastasis to the rectum has occurred; procedure includes Wertheim procedure plus Abdominoperineal Resection

12. *Laparoscopy:* endoscopic visualization of the peritoneal cavity following insufflation with CO_2
    a. *Indications:* diagnosis of endometriosis, ectopic pregnancy, pelvic mass, and causes of infertility; treatment and surgery for a variety of conditions and/or a sterilization procedure
    b. *Equipment needed:* D&C instrument set plus a laparoscopy set
    c. *Procedure*
       i. Patient is in modified lithotomy position.
       ii. Cervical dilation is performed, and a uterine manipulator is attached to the cervix for manipulation of the uterus.

SURGERY HINT

During an abdominal hysterectomy, the Surgical Technologist should have enough hemostats or other clamps available to clamp off both sides of the uterus as the surgeon frees each side.

Instruments that contact the vaginal vault are to be considered contaminated, and isolated from the other instruments on the field.

---

iii. Chromopertubation: dye may be injected into the tubes through the manipulator to determine tubal patency (observed through the scope for presence in the pelvic cavity).

iv. Small incision is made in umbilical margin; skin is elevated.

v. Verres needle is inserted through the incision into peritoneal cavity, checked by aspiration with 10-ml syringe, connected by plastic tubing to CO_2 insufflator, and 2 to 3 liters of gas is delivered with close monitoring of intraabdominal pressure (approx. 15 mm Hg).

vi. Needle is withdrawn, and trocar and cannula are inserted; trocar is withdrawn, and tubing is attached to cannula.

vii. Telescope is inserted through the cannula and connected to fiber optic light cord; examination begins; defogging may be accomplished by touching the lens to a loop of the intestines or use of chemical agent.

viii. Patient is placed in Trendelenburg position to enhance visualization.

ix. Second/third trocar/cannula may be inserted under direct visualization/transillumination of the abdominal wall.

x. Various procedures may then be performed, including coagulation of tubes for sterilization.

xi. Telescope is withdrawn and CO_2 is allowed to escape from the cannula.

xii. Skin is closed with clips, staples, or a subcuticular stitch, followed by application of an adhesive bandage.

G. **Vaginal and vulvar surgery**
1. *Patient position:* lithotomy
2. *Special equipment*
   a. Stirrups (knee-crutch, string/candy cane, boot/Allen)
   b. Sitting stool for physician
   c. Cryosurgical, electrosurgical unit, or LASER equipment
   d. Vacuum apparatus
3. *Anesthesia:* general, sometimes spinal or caudal
4. *Supplies*
   a. Foley catheter with gravity drainage
   b. Radiopaque sponges on forceps or opened lengthwise for placement around surgeon(s) fingers for blunt dissection
   c. Vaginal packing
   d. Telfa (for endometrial scrapings)
   e. Perineal pad/belt
5. *Special instruments:* D&C set
   a. *Retractors:* vaginal speculum, weighted (Auvard) speculum, and Heaney retractor
   b. *Uterine sound or probe:* measure depth of uterus
   c. *Tenaculum:* single-toothed, doubled-toothed, Jacobs, vulsellum/Lahey; grasp and hold cervix
   d. *Dilators:* Hegar, Hanks, Pratt; dilate cervix (may use lubricating jelly)

SURGERY HINT

Many surgeons will work directly off of the back table. In these cases, have the dilators ready for use from smallest to largest. If handing to the surgeon, always hand smallest to largest.

Place a small sterile glove on the end of the weighted speculum to catch fluids.

Always have lubricating jelly available

---

     e. *Curettes*
       i. Endocervical—Kevorkian
       ii. Endometrial—sharp (Sims) and blunt (Thomas); various sizes
       iii. Use: scrape uterine tissue
     f. *Sponge forceps*
     g. **Uterine dressing forceps (Bozeman)**

6. *Concepts*
     a. Instruments are commonly passed from back table (no Mayo stand)

7. *Skin preparations*
     a. Begin skin prep at pubic symphysis and extend downward over the labia
     b. Cleanse inner thighs
     c. Cleanse labia minora and vestibule (clitoris, urethral meatus, vaginal introitus)
     d. Sponge on forceps is used to cleanse the vaginal vault
     e. Perineum and anus cleaned last and each sponge is discarded after touching the anus. (*Note:* From menarche to menopause, the normal body flora of the vagina are lactobacilli, which produce lactic acid to maintain an acid pH. Microflora in the vagina are a protection against certain bacteria, fluctuate with hormonal variation, and are opportunistic pathogens in a wound.)
     f. Bladder is drained with the use of metal catheter, red Robinson catheter, or a retention catheter (Foley) connected to a gravity drainage

8. *Draping*
     a. Drape sheet/under the buttocks drape
     b. Towels may be placed over thighs
     c. Other drapes
       i. Leggings and abdominal sheet
       ii. Perineal sheet with leggings attached
       iii. Leggings and fenestrated sheet (lithotomy)

9. *Procedures*
     a. *Notes*
       i. If both abdominal and vaginal procedures are indicated, a combined procedure may be performed with the "clean" abdominal procedure done first.
       ii. If one procedure is diagnostic and the other is therapeutic, the diagnostic procedure will be performed first (such as a D&C and an Abdominal Hysterectomy).
     b. *Vulvectomy:* surgical removal of the labia majora and labia minora for carcinoma in situ of the vulva
     c. *Radical Vulvectomy with Lymphadenectomy:* en bloc excision of the labia majora and minora, clitoris, mons pubis, terminal portions of the urethra, vagina, large section of skin from the abdomen and groin, superficial and deep inguinal lymph nodes, portions of the round ligament, and saphenous veins along with the lesion
       i. Skin prep includes abdomen as well as wide perineal area.
       ii. Two closed-wound drainage systems are needed.
     d. *Dilatation and curettage (D&C)*
       i. *Indications:* diagnostic for endometrial carcinoma or an infertility study; therapeutic for incomplete abortion, therapeutic abortion, abnormal uterine bleeding, or primary dysmenorrhea
       ii. *Complication:* uterine perforation
       iii. *Procedure*
         • Bladder is emptied, and vagina is retracted with Auvard or bivalve speculum (Graves or Pederson)
         • Cervix is grasped with a tenaculum.
         • Uterine depth is probed.

- Endocervix is curetted.
- Cervix is gradually dilated.
- Endometrium is curetted.
- Curettings are placed on Telfa for specimen.

    iv. *Alternative procedure:* suction curettage, or vacuum aspiration of uterine contents

- **Uses:** early termination of pregnancy, missed or incomplete abortions
- **Equipment:** D&C instrument set plus placenta forceps, sterile cannula, aspirator tubing, vacuum aspirator unit, and oxytocic drugs
- Specimen (products of conception) is removed from the suction bottle and sent for pathologic examination

    v. *Endometrial treatment:* thermal balloon therapy—balloon inflated within the uterine cavity; superheated to destroy uterine lining; treatment for menorrhagia

e. *Anterior/Posterior Colporrhaphy:* removal of a strip of the anterior vagina with reconstruction for a cystocele and posterior vagina for rectocele to prevent a protrusion of the bladder and rectum into the vagina
  i. Suprapubic cystostomy catheter or Foley catheter placed in urethra may be inserted for bladder drainage.
  ii. Incision is made in the vaginal wall with knife and curved scissors, tissue forceps, Allis forceps, and gauze sponges.
  iii. Interrupted stitches are made with 2-0 absorbable suture on a cutting needle.
  iv. Vaginal gauze packing and self-retaining urethral catheter are left in place.

f. *Vesico-vaginal, urethro-vaginal, or recto-vaginal fistula repair:* fistulae are identified through the vaginal approach and dissected, and the fistula tract is closed with absorbable suture

g. *Cauterization:* removal of a chronic infected area of cervix with the use of a LASER or electrosurgery unit

h. *Conization:* removal of tissue (in the shape of a cone) from the cervix with the use of a knife (cold knife cone biopsy), LEEP (loop endocervical electrocautery procedure), or LASER for inflammation or premalignant lesions of the cervix when fertility is to be preserved
  i. Acetic acid may be used to cleanse the cervix.
  ii. Lugol's solution may be used to identify areas of pathology.
  iii. Specimen is marked with suture to provide orientation.
  iv. Pitressin/saline solution may be injected or sutures used prior to excision to aid hemostasis.

i. *Cervical Cerclage/Shirodkar procedure:* placement of a heavy suture tape (mersilene) around the cervix just under the vaginal mucosa, during the twelfth to fourteenth week of pregnancy, to prevent spontaneous abortion resulting from cervical dilation due to an incompetent cervical os

j. *Cesium rod insertion:* applicators are inserted in the OR, and the patient is taken to the radiation department for insertion of radioactive element; Foley catheter inserted and balloon inflated with radiopaque medium; for treatment of cervical and endometrial malignancy

k. *Marsupialization of a Bartholin's Cyst or Abscess:* incision in the vaginal outlet (outside the ring of the hymen) into Bartholin's duct for drainage; may be incised and drained, excised, or exteriorized by removal of anterior wall of the cyst and suturing the cut edges to nearby skin. Equipment needed includes syringe and 15-gauge 31/2-inch needle; two culture tubes, drain, and iodoform or plain gauze packing

SURGERY HINT

Vaginal hysterectomies can be challenging for the ST. The small area available for the surgeon and Tech to work makes contaminations more likely than in abdominal surgeries. Handing instrumentation while retracting may be impossible, so the ST needs to have the instrumentation oriented so that the surgeon can easily access necessary items.

l. *Perineorrhaphy:* surgical repair of lacerations of the area between the vagina and rectum accompanying childbirth

m. *Vaginal Hysterectomy*
   i. **Indications:** benign disease of the uterus; not greatly enlarged; poor pelvic muscular support, carcinoma in situ, and uterine prolapse
   ii. **Advantages** of this procedure are that it leaves no visible scar and is a shorter procedure with less recovery time
   iii. **Draping:** towels, leggings, fenestrated sheet, and sheet for surgeon's lap (when the surgeon is seated and holds a lap instrument tray)
   iv. **Equipment, instruments, and supplies:** electrosurgical unit, suction, stirrups, vaginal hysterectomy tray, Foley catheter drainage unit; gauze packing, vaginal cream, perineal pad
   v. **Procedure**
      • Vasoconstrictor agent may be injected into the cervical mucosa to facilitate dissection and decrease bleeding
      • Incision made around the cervical mucosa with bladder reflected to expose the peritoneum
      • Uterosacral ligaments are ligated and divided
      • Cardinal ligaments and uterine arteries are ligated and divided
      • Uterus is delivered
      • Cul-de-sac and vaginal vault are closed with uterosacral and round ligament stumps attached

n. *Laparoscopic-assisted vaginal hysterectomy (LAVH)*
   i. Uterus is separated from ligaments, adenexa (adjunct parts), blood, and nerve supply through minimallyinvasive technique.
   ii. Cervical mucosa is incised, and uterus is removed through vaginal incision.
   iii. Vaginal vault is closed.
   iv. Pelvis is re-examined for bleeding via the laparoscope.

o. *Hysteroscopy:* endoscopic visualization of the uterine cavity and tubal orifices
   i. *Indications:* abnormal uterine bleeding, displaced intrauterine device (IUD), chronic pregnancy loss, and infertility
   ii. *Contraindications:* acute infection, cervical malignancy, and pregnancy
   iii. *Complications:* bleeding, perforation, fluid retention, and infection
   iv. *Procedure*
      • Done under local or general anesthesia
      • Patient in lithotomy position
      • Cervix is dilated and hysteroscope is introduced
      • The uterine cavity is distended with solution for irrigation under pressure
      • Resection of endometrial/myometrial tissue may be performed

Show What You Know

Directions
Each of the numbered items or incomplete statements in this section is followed by answers or by completions of the statement. Select the ONE lettered answer or completion that is BEST in each case.

1. The branch of medicine that deals with perinatal care is:
   A. obstetrics
   B. gynecology
   C. neonatology
   D. perinatology

2. A woman who is pregnant for the first time is:
   A. primiparous
   B. primigravida
   C. multiparous
   D. multigravida

3. All of the following are indications for a Cesarean section *except*:
   A. cephalopelvic disproportion
   B. eclampsia
   C. ectopic pregnancy
   D. abruptio placenta

4. The position of choice for the patient with a prolapsed umbilical cord is:
   A. supine
   B. turned onto the patient's on left side
   C. prone
   D. Kraske

5. The clamps most desirable for approximating uterine wound edges for closure during a Cesarean section are:
   A. Pennington
   B. Allis
   C. Adson
   D. hemostat

6. Excessive uterine bleeding occurring both during menses and at irregular intervals is:
   A. menopause
   B. menometrorrhagia
   C. dysmenorrhea
   D. endometriosis

7. A simple diagnostic procedure to differentiate normal from abnormal cervical or vaginal tissue by a staining technique is:
   A. culdocentesis
   B. hysteroscopy
   C. Papanicolaou (Pap smear)
   D. Schiller's test

8. The removal of a fibroid tumor from the uterus is a/an:
   A. Oophorectomy
   B. Fibroidectomy
   C. Myomectomy
   D. Hysterectomy

9. A Radical Hysterectomy with Pelvic Lymphadenectomy is a/an:
   A. Anterior Exenteration
   B. Le Fort operation
   C. Cerclage
   D. Wertheim operation

10. During minimally invasive/laparoscopic pelvic surgery, the peritoneal cavity is insufflated with:
    A. oxygen
    B. nitrous oxide
    C. Hyskon solution
    D. carbon dioxide

11. Stirrups would not be required for which of the following procedures:
    A. Laparoscopic Tubal Ligation
    B. Excision of Bartholin's cyst
    C. Abdominal Hysterectomy
    D. Shirodkar Procedure

12. A basin for contaminated instruments must be provided for which of the following procedures?
    A. Vaginal Hysterectomy
    B. Abdominal Hysterectomy
    C. Anterior and Posterior Colporrhaphy
    D. Vesicovaginal Fistula Repair

13. A self-retaining retractor useful for the Pfannestiel incision is:
    A. Auvard speculum
    B. O'Sullivan-O'Connor
    C. Heaney retractor
    D. Weitlaner

14. You are scheduled to scrub on a D&C and Abdominal Hysterectomy. You will:
    A. set up one table and be prepared to do the D&C first
    B. set up two tables and be prepared to do the Abdominal Hysterectomy first

C. set up one table and be prepared to do the Abdominal Hysterectomy first

D. set up two tables and be prepared first for the D&C, followed by the Abdominal Hysterectomy

15. Ureteral catheters will probably be inserted to provide a landmark to prevent accidental injury during which of the following procedures?

A. Cesarean Section
B. Vaginal Hysterectomy
C. Ovarian Cystectomy
D. Radical Hysterectomy with Pelvic Lymphadenectomy

16. A procedure done on young women who evidence benign tumors of the muscle layer of the uterus but who wish to preserve their fertility is a:

A. Supracervical hysterectomy
B. Oophorectomy
C. Myomectomy
D. Hymenectomy

17. Which of the following self-retaining retractors is used for pelvic surgery?

A. Weitlander
B. O'Sullivan-O'Connor
C. Senn
D. Army-Navy

18. All of the following are uterine ligaments except:

A. broad
B. round
C. perineal
D. uterosacral

19. A Foley catheter is placed into the presurgical Hysterectomy patient to:

A. record accurate intake and output
B. distend the bladder during surgery
C. avoid injury to the bladder
D. maintain a dry perineum postoperatively

20. What would an Anterior and Posterior repair accomplish?

A. repair of a cystocele and rectocele
B. repair of a vesicovaginal fistula
C. repair of a vesicourethral fistula
D. removal of precancerous tissue from the external os of the cervix

21. To confirm the diagnosis of ruptured ectopic pregnancy, it is sometimes necessary to perform a:

A. Cystoscopy
B. Culdocentesis
C. Colonoscopy
D. Pelvectomy

22. An Abdominal Vesicourethral Suspension is known as a:

A. Le Fort
B. Wertheim
C. Marshall-Marchetti Kranz
D. Shirodkar

23. The procedure where only the uterus body is removed is called a/an:

A. Abdominal Hysterectomy
B. Panhysterectomy
C. Supracervical Hysterectomy
D. Vaginal Hysterectomy

24. Indications for Cesarean section include all of the following except:

A. malpresentation
B. toxemia
C. fetal distress
D. endometriosis

25. CPD stands for:

A. cephalopelvic disproportion
B. cephaloperineal disproportion
C. cephaloperineal distortion
D. cephalopelvic distortion

26. Which of the following statements concerning Cesarean sections is not true?

A. Metzenbaum scissors are used to cut the uterus and the umbilical cord
B. delivery forceps may be needed to assist in the removal of the baby's head from the uterus
C. the cervix is open; therefore, care should be taken when suctioning inside the uterus to prevent wound contamination
D. a small bulb syringe is used to aspirate the baby's mouth and nose prior to delivery of the shoulders and body

27. Types of dilators used to dilate or open the cervix include all of the following except:

A. Hanks
B. Pratt
C. Somer
D. Hegar

28. Fallopian tube patency is verified through a procedure called:

A. chromoperitonealization
B. chromopertubation
C. chromointubation
D. chromosomalization

29. The procedure which includes removal of the terminal portions of vulvar orifices and tissues of

the vulva, inguinal lymph nodes, and associated structures is:

A. Vulvectomy
B. Radical Vulvectomy
C. Vulvoplasty
D. Vulvopexy

30. The procedure which is performed postconceptually for the closure of the internal cervical os is the:

A. Shirodkar procedure
B. Marshall Marchetti procedure
C. LASER conization procedure
D. LEEP procedure

31. Cervical conization or biopsy is performed for all of the following *except:*

A. chronic cervicitis
B. cervical incompetence
C. cervical dysplasia
D. carcinoma in situ of the cervix

32. The procedure commonly performed for the treatment of uterine descensus or prolapse is:

A. Vaginal Hysterectomy
B. Total Abdominal Hysterectomy
C. Total Abdominal Hysterectomy, Bilateral Salpingectomy
D. Supracervical Vaginal Hysterectomy

33. Instruments used to grasp the vaginal mucosa during Anterior/Posterior Repair include:

A. hemostatic clamps—criles
B. Allis clamps
C. Oschners
D. Babcocks

34. What does "D&C" stand for?

A. dilation and currettage
B. dilation and conization
C. debridement and conization
D. debridement and curettage

35. The finger-like projections that trap and direct the ova after its maturation and release are called the:

A. endometrium
B. cervical os
C. fimbria
D. vestibule

36. The organ where an "ectopic" pregnancy usually occurs is the:

A. ovary
B. fallopian tube
C. uterus
D. cervix

Questions 37–43 are based on the following scenario.

Ms. Peterson, aged 42, goes to the gynecologist, complaining of pelvic pain. Upon office examination, the physician palpated a pelvic mass on the right adnexa. Ultrasound showed that the mass appears to contain fluid. She is scheduled for surgery.

37. Which procedure would the patient most likely be scheduled for?

A. Hysterectomy
B. Culdoscopy
C. D&C
D. Diagnostic Laparoscopy

38. What equipment would you assemble as you prepared the room for the procedure?

A. video cart with monitor
B. operative microscope
C. vacuum currettage machine
D. Harmonic Scalpel

39. What supplies would you gather in preparation for this procedure?

A. Telfa
B. transverse laparotomy sheet
C. CO_2 insufflation tubing
D. Pitressin injection

40. The mass is found to be a simple ovarian cyst. The surgeon decides to perform an I&D (incision and drainage). What supply/instrument would you have ready?

A. the harmonic scalpel handpiece with cutting blade
B. a Ponsky bag
C. a needle aspiration tip with 30-cc syringe
D. the TA roticulating stapler with absorbable staples

41. The specimen from this procedure would be sent:

A. to Pathology in 10% Formalin solution for permanent section
B. to Cytology without any solution for examination of the cells
C. to Pathology in 10% Formalin solution for frozen section
D. to Cytology in 10% Formalin solution for ERL/PRL levels

42. At the end of the procedure, skin closure is achieved using a subcuticular stitch. What wound closure material would most likely be utilized for this?

A. 5-0 Monocryl on an SH needle
B. 3-0 Vicryl on a PS-2 needle
C. 0 nylon on a TP-1 needle
D. 2-0 plain on a CT-1 needle

43. Which of the following dressing materials would NOT be used for this procedure?

A. Xeroform gauze
B. benzoin/steristrips
C. bio-occlusive dressing
D. adhesive bandages

Instrument Identification

44.

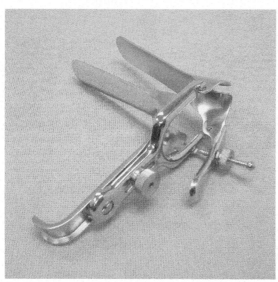

A. Auvard weighted speculum
B. Pederson speculum
C. Jacob tenaculum
D. Sims vaginal retractor

45.

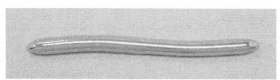

A. Hegar dilator
B. Hank dilator
C. Goodell dilator
D. Pratt dilator

46.

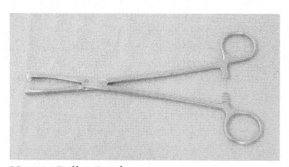

A. Heaney Ballentine forceps
B. Lahey tenaculum

C. Jacobs tenaculum
D. single-toothed Tenaculum

47.

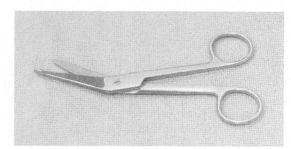

A. bandage scissor
B. Jorgenson scissor
C. Potts scissor
D. tenotomy scissor

48.

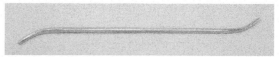

A. Hegar dilator
B. Hank dilator
C. Goodell dilator
D. Pratt dilator

49.

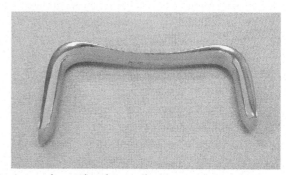

A. Auvard weighted speculum
B. Pederson speculum
C. Jacob tenaculum
D. Sims vaginal retractor

Anatomy Review

Female Reproductive System

50–68.

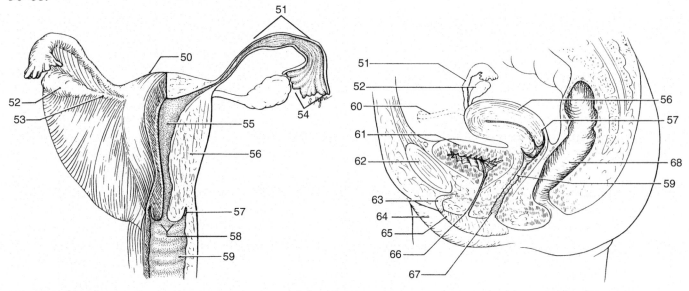

A. bladder
B. cervix
C. clitoris
D. fallopian tube
E. fimbria
F. fornix
G. introitus

H. labia majora
I. labia minora
J. myometrium
K. ovarian ligament
L. ovary
M. pubic symphysis
N. rectum

O. round ligament
P. urethral meatus
Q. uterine cavity
R. uterus
S. vagina

Answers & Rationales

1. **A.** **Rationale:** Obstetrics is the branch of medicine that deals with perinatal care. There is no field of medicine called Perinatology. Neonatology deals with the newborn. Gynecology deals with the study of diseases of the female reproductive tract.

2. **B.** **Rationale:** A woman who is pregnant for the first time is a primigravida. A primiparous woman is one who has borne one child weighing at least 500 g or after 20 weeks of gestation.

3. **C.** **Rationale:** Ectopic pregnancy is not an indication for a C-section (opening into the abdominal and uterine cavity to remove a fetus). With an ectopic pregnancy, one would not go to term but would require surgery during the first or second trimester.

4. **B.** **Rationale:** If a prolapsed umbilical cord is observed, the patient is asked to get into a lateral position with the left side down or is placed in a severe Trendelenburg to allow gravity to relieve pressure on the cord. The

cord should also be kept moist, the nurse and physician notified, and FHTs taken to determine the status of the fetus.

5. **A.** **Rationale:** Pennington clamps are useful in bringing the edges of the uterus together for suturing.

6. **B.** **Rationale:** Menometrorrhagia is heavy vaginal bleeding occurring both during menses and at irregular intervals.

7. **D.** **Rationale:** The Schiller's test is the use of an iodine (Lugol's) solution to stain the cervix and vagina. Staining that is smooth and regular is expected in normal tissue. Irregular staining indicates disease.

8. **C.** **Rationale:** A Myomectomy is the removal of a muscle tumor from the uterus and is used in younger women wishing to preserve fertility.

9. **D.** **Rationale:** A Wertheim operation, developed by Dr. Wertheim for cancer, is the removal of the uterus, tubes, ovaries, upper vagina, and pelvic lymph nodes.

10. D. **Rationale:** Carbon dioxide is the source for pneumoperitoneum necessary during laparoscopic surgery. Hyskon is a solution used to distend the uterus during a Hysteroscopy.

11. C. **Rationale:** Stirrups would not be required when positioning a patient for an Abdominal Hysterectomy. The lithotomy position is used for the remaining procedures.

12. B. **Rationale:** A basin for contaminated instruments is needed during an Abdominal Hysterectomy when the uterus is separated from the vagina.

13. B. **Rationale:** The O'Sullivan-O'Connor retractor is a self-retaining retractor designed for the Pfannenstiel incision.

14. D. **Rationale:** When both a diagnostic and a therapeutic procedure are scheduled for the same patient, the diagnostic procedure is done first. The vagina is considered a "dirty" area and the instruments and setup used for vaginal surgery could not then be used for the abdominal cavity.

15. D. **Rationale:** When radical pelvic surgery is done, ureteral catheters are placed before surgery to serve as a landmark to avoid injury to the ureters.

16. C. **Rationale:** A Myomectomy removes benign fibroids of the uterus. A woman may then become pregnant after healing has taken place.

17. B. **Rationale:** The O'Sullivan-O'Connor retractor is a self-retaining retractor commonly used in pelvic procedures.

18. C. **Rationale:** The broad, round, and uterosacral ligaments are all uterine ligaments.

19. C. **Rationale:** A Foley catheter is used to compress the bladder during pelvic surgery to avoid injury. After surgery, the Foley catheter will be used to monitor urinary output.

20. A. **Rationale:** An Anterior and Posterior Repair is performed for the treatment of a cystocele and rectocele.

21. B. **Rationale:** Culdocentesis is performed to confirm the diagnosis of ruptured ectopic pregnancy.

22. C. **Rationale:** Marshall-Marchetti Kranz is the name for an abdominal vesicourethral suspension.

23. C. **Rationale:** In a Supracervical Hysterectomy, only the uterine body is removed. The cervix is left in place.

24. D. **Rationale:** Endometriosis is not an indication for Cesarean section.

25. A. **Rationale:** CPD stands for cephalopelvic disproportion.

26. A. **Rationale:** Bandage scissors are commonly used to cut the uterus and the umbilical cord during Cesarean section.

27. C. **Rationale:** Hanks, Hegar, and Goodell dilators are used to dilate or open the cervix.

28. B. **Rationale:** Fallopian tube patency is verified through a procedure called chromopertubation.

29. B. **Rationale:** The procedure which includes removal of the terminal portions of vulvar orifices and tissues of the vulva, inguinal lymph nodes, and associated structures is called Radical Vulvectomy.

30. A. **Rationale:** The procedure which is performed post-conceptually for closure of the internal cervical os is the Shirodkar procedure.

31. B. **Rationale:** Cervical conization is performed for the diagnoses of chronic cervicitis, cervical dysplasia, or carcinoma in situ of the cervix.

32. A. **Rationale:** The procedure commonly performed for the treatment of uterine descensus or prolapse is Vaginal Hysterectomy.

33. B. **Rationale:** Allis clamps are used to grasp the vaginal mucosa during anterior/posterior repair.

34. A. **Rationale:** D&C stand for dilation and currettage.

35. C. **Rationale:** The finger-like projections that trap and direct the ova after its maturation and release are called the fimbria.

36. B. **Rationale:** The fallopian tube is the organ where an "ectopic" pregnancy usually occurs.

37. D. **Rationale:** Diagnostic Laparoscopy allows for examination of a mass to determine if it is benign or not. Open Laparotomy can be performed later, if indicated.

38. A. **Rationale:** The video cart and monitor are used for every laparoscopic procedure.

39. C. **Rationale:** CO_2 tubing is used on every laparoscopy to insufflate the abdominal cavity and create the pneumoperitoneum.

40. C. **Rationale:** A needle aspiration tip and 30-cc syringe would be used. The needle will pierce the cyst wall, and the syringe will be used to draw out fluid for analysis.

41. B. **Rationale:** The specimen from this procedure would be sent to Cytology without any solution for examination of the cells.

42. B. **Rationale:** Subcuticular skin closure is achieved using an absorbable suture with a cutting needle.

43. A. **Rationale:** Xeroform gauze would NOT commonly be used as a dressing material for this procedure.

44. B. **Rationale:** Pederson speculum

45. A. **Rationale:** Hegar dilator

46. C. **Rationale:** Jacobs Tenaculum

47. A. **Rationale:** Bandage scissor

48. D. **Rationale:** Pratt dilator

49. **D.** **Rationale:** Sims vaginal retractor
50. **(R)** uterus
51. **(D)** fallopian tube
52. **(L)** ovary
53. **(K)** ovarian ligament
54. **(E)** fimbria
55. **(Q)** uterine cavity
56. **(J)** myometrium
57. **(F)** fornix
58. **(B)** cervix

59. **(S)** vagina
60. **(O)** round ligament
61. **(A)** bladder
62. **(M)** pubic symphysis
63. **(C)** clitoris
64. **(H)** labia majora
65. **(I)** labia minora
66. **(P)** urethral meatus
67. **(G)** introitus
68. **(N)** rectum

Part II: Deciphering a Surgical Schedule

The following mock surgery schedule will be used to answer several questions pertaining to GYN Surgery. The same schedule, or a similar one, will be used in subsequent chapters to ask questions about the content of the chapter.

Rm# time	Surgeon	Procedure	Anest.	Rm# time	Surgeon	Procedure	Anest.
Rm00				**Rm07**			
OC	Dr. Z	Rt. Knee Arthroscopy	Gen.	7:00	Dr. M	LAVH	Gen.
OC	Dr. C	Craniotomy	Gen.	TF	Dr. M	TAH-BSO	MAC
OC	Dr.Z	Angioplasty	Gen.				
Rm01				**Rm08**			
7:00	Dr. X	Anterior-Posterior repair	Gen.	11:00	Dr. E	Bovine Thrombectomy	MAC
TF	Dr. X	Cerclage	Gen.				
TF	Dr. X	Bowel resection	Gen.				
	Dr. X						
Rm02				**Rm09**			
7:00	Dr. B	Splenectomy	Gen.	8:30	Dr. T	Cholecystectomy	Gen.
TF	Dr. B	Gastrectomy	Gen.	TF	Dr. T	Palatoplasty	Gen.
Rm03				**Rm10**			
7:00	Dr. A	Cystoscopy	MAC	7:00	Dr. K	TVH	Gen.
TF	Dr. A	Cystoplasty	Gen.	TF	Dr. K	Myomectomy	MAC
12:30	Dr. F	Pyleogram	MAC	TF	Dr. K	EUA	Gen.
3:00	Dr. F	Cystocele repair	Gen.				
Rm04				**Rm11**			
7:00	Dr. Y	Carpal tunnel release	Gen.	7:00	Dr. L	Colposcope	Gen.
TF	Dr. Y	Whipple	Gen.	12:00	Dr. L	Mastectomy	Gen.
Rm05				**Rm12**			
7:00	Dr. G	D&C	Gen.	7:00	Dr. W	Trans-metatarsal amputation	Gen.
TF	Dr. G	Marsupialization of Bartholin's Cyst	Gen	TF	Dr. W	Osteotomy	Gen.
TF	Dr. G	Laparoscopic tubal ligation	Gen.	TF	Dr. W	Arthrocentesis	Gen.
Rm06				**Rm13**			
7:00	Dr. R	Lumbar Laminectomy	Gen.	7:00	Dr. O	Hysterectomy	Gen.

The following questions should be answered using the surgery schedule above

1. During the setup for the D&C scheduled in Room 5, the Surgical Technologist must arrange the dilators in which way:

   A. From largest to smallest
   B. Smallest to largest
   C. No necessary order
   D. For use before the uterine sound

2. Which of the following scissors is most likely going to be found in Room 13?

   A. Jorgenson
   B. Reynolds
   C. Potts-smith
   D. Jamison

3. The patient in Room 10 is undergoing a TVH. What position is she likely to be in?

   A. Supine
   B. Kraske
   C. Lithotomy
   D. Fowlers

4. When positioning the patient undergoing EUA in Room 10, what is an important patient safety precaution?

   A. Slowly raising each leg separately into the stirrup, starting with the right leg
   B. Raising both legs together quickly to minimize bradycardia
   C. Raising both legs together slowly
   D. Make sure that the left leg is slightly lower than the right to reduce pressure on the vena cava

5. The patient in Room 5 is undergoing laparoscopic tubal ligation. All of the following are likely methods EXCEPT

   A. Coagulation with a Kleppinger
   B. Placement of a fallope ring
   C. Ligating the tubes with chromic gut
   D. Placement of filshie clips

6. For the patient undergoing Marsupialization of a Bartholin's cyst in Room 5, how will the "pouch" be created?

   A. Cyst wall lining is turned out and sutured to vaginal mucosa
   B. Vaginal mucosa is incised and a pouch is created
   C. Pouch is created by suturing mesh to the vaginal wall
   D. Mucosa is excised from an unaffected area a sutured to the affected area to create a pouch

7. A Cerclage is scheduled in Room 1. What is this procedure for?

   A. To prevent spontaneous abortion due to an incompetent cervix
   B. To prevent pregnancy
   C. To irrigate and debride infected cervical tissue
   D. To remove begnin growths from the cervix

8. A patient is scheduled for a Myomectomy in Room 10. The surgeon is having difficulty grasping the Myoma for removal. What instrument should the Surgical Technologist have on hand for the surgeon?

   A. A Babcock
   B. A penetrating towel clamp
   C. A Kelley clamp
   D. DeBakey forceps

9. In the TVH scheduled for Room 10, what draping order should be followed if possible?

   A. Under buttocks drape, towels, leggings, operative sheet
   B. Towels, leggings, under buttocks drape, operative drape
   C. Leggings, operative drape, under buttocks drape, towels
   D. Under buttocks drape, leggings, towels, operative drape

10. Which instrument is LEAST likely to be found on the D&C set opened in Room 5?

    A. Tenaculum
    B. Randall stone forceps
    C. Jorgensen Scissors
    D. Uterine sound

Answers & Rationales

1. **B. Rationale:** When organizing the cervical dilators, the Surgical Technologist should always organize them from smallest to largest. The order that they will be used in is from the smallest diameter to progressively larger diameters; therefore, they should be placed in this order.

2. **A. Rationale:** Jorgensen scissors are the most likely to be found in a Hysterectomy set. Potts smith scissors are vascular scissors, Jamison's are tenotomy scissors also found in vascular cases, and Reynolds is another type of tenotomy scissor not commonly used in GYN surgical procedures.

3. **C. Rationale:** The only position used for vaginal surgical procedures is lithotomy.

4. **C. Rationale:** In positioning the patient for lithotomy, both legs must be raised slowly at the same time. This requires two people to be working in unison for patient safety. The legs must remain at the same height.

5. **C. Rationale:** Using chromic gut was a common sterilization method in open tubal ligation. Most surgeons prefer to do this surgery laparoscopically utilizing any of the remaining methods mentioned.

6. **A. Rationale:** Generally, if Marsupialization is chosen, the standard procedure for attaining a "pouch" is to use the emptied cyst walls to create the opening.

7. **A. Rationale:** Sometimes referred to Shirodkars Procedure, this intervention uses a synthetic tape which is wrapped around the internal os of the cervix to remove the possibility of spontaneous abortion due to incompetent cervix.

8. **B. Rationale:** The Kelley clamp, Babcock, and DeBakey forceps are atraumatic and will give the surgeon no way to grasp to Myoma. Generally, one to two penetrating towel clamps are used to pierce the Myoma, allowing for a good grip on the structure. Depending on the size of the Myoma, the surgeon may need to remove in portions instead of intact. Generally, these portions will be sent to pathology as one unit. If there are multiple myomas that the surgeon wishes sent separately, the ST should ensure that these pieces do not get mixed in with other specimens.

9. **A. Rationale:** Generally, when draping for vaginal procedures, the under buttocks drape will be placed first. The Surgical Technologist must be cognizant of the potential for contamination to gloves and gown during this draping sequence. As a rule, the ST should be double-gloved to ensure that, should a contamination occur, the procedure will not be delayed.

10. **C. Rationale:** Dilation and Curettage should not require the use of tissue scissors. Occasionally, a set will include these scissors, but the procedure requires the use of both the Tenaculum and uterine sound. Generally, the set will include Randall Stone forceps to remove POC (product of conception).

Use this address to access the interactive Companion Website created for this book. Simply select "Surgical Technology" from the choice of disciplines. Find this book and click to enter.

14 Genitourinary Surgery

Urology is a branch of medicine and surgery that deals with problems related to the extraction and excretion of waste products from the bloodstream of men and women of all ages; problems related to the male reproductive organs; and endocrine problems related to the adrenal glands, testes, and prostate. The Surgical Technologist must understand the anatomy and physiology of the genitourinary system in order to assist in these procedures. Cystoscopies, procedures for incontinence, kidney stones, and kidney procedures are included in this branch.

CHAPTER OUTLINE

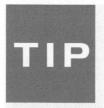

Genitourinary procedures incorporate both the urinary system and the male reproductive system. The specialty may include Cystoscopies, kidney surgeries, or procedures involving the prostate. With such a wide range of procedures, this specialty may be particularly difficult to master. While some of the procedures are relatively straightforward, such a Cystoscopy, they may be extremely complex, such as the removal of the prostate or kidney. Because there is such a wide range of knowledge necessary for proficiency, the Surgical Technologist must have a broad base of understanding in order to work well in this specialty. Answering questions involving this aspect of surgery require knowledge of anatomy, physiology, medical terminology, as well as the procedures and specialty instrumentation.

Example:
When performing a TURP, which irrigation fluid will most likely be used?

a. Normal Saline
b. 3% Sorbitol
c. Sterile water
d. 5% Dextran

To answer this question first think about what is involved with the TURP. This is a trans-urethral resection of the prostate gland. We know that there is fluid that must be used in this procedure. The question is which fluid is the most likely. When doing procedures with fluids, the rule of thumb is that you do not want fluids that carry a current. Since we know that saline is conducive, we definitely would not use that solution. Sterile water is a hemolytic as it is not isotonic, so we would not use this either. That leaves Sorbitol or Dextran. Since Dextran is a volume expander, that leaves the 3% Sorbitol as the answer to this question.

I. Terminology

    A. *Albuminuria:* presence of albumin in urine

    B. *Cysitis:* inflammation of the bladder

    C. *Electrolytic solution:* solution capable of conducting electricity, such as saline

    D. *Glomerulonephritis:* inflammation of the kidneys at the level of the glomerulus (tuft of capillaries that brings blood to the nephron)

    E. *Hemolytic solution:* solution such as distilled water, which causes hemolysis of red blood cells; a hypotonic solution that enters cells, resulting in swelling and rupture

    F. *Lithotomy:* the incision into a duct or organ for the removal of a stone

    G. *Lithotripsy:* crushing of a stone

    H. *Nephrolithiasis:* condition of kidney stones

    I. *Pheochromocytoma:* tumor of the adrenal medulla

    J. *Phimosis:* tight foreskin (prepuce) for which a circumcision is performed

    K. *Uremia:* accumulation of urine products in the blood due to kidney failure

    L. *Urinary incontinence:* inability to control urination

    M. *Vesicoureteral reflux:* backflow of urine from the bladder into the ureters; causes recurrent pyelonephritis (inflammation of the kidney pelvis)

    N. *Wilms' tumor:* malignant kidney tumor in children

II. Surgery of the Bladder, Urethra, and Male Reproductive Organs

    A. Diagnostic tests and procedures

        1. *KUB:* flat-plate abdominal x-ray to visualize kidneys, ureters, and bladder

        2. *Cystoscopy:* visualization of the urethra, bladder, and ureteral orifices through a lighted telescope (30 and 70 degrees used most frequently)

3. *Cystogram:* x-ray visualization of the bladder with the use of contrast media
4. *Urethrogram:* x-ray visualization of the urethra with the use of contrast media
5. *Cystometrogram:* test to measure voiding pressure of the bladder
6. *Serum prostatic-specific antigens (PSA), acid phosphatase, bone scans, CT scan, MRI scan, biopsy, and histologic grading of malignancies:* tests for detecting prostatic cancer
7. *Imaging systems (part of the urologic table):* x-rays, fluoroscopy, tomography, and image intensification
8. *Retrograde Pyelogram:* x-ray visualization of the ureters and kidneys following injection of contrast media through a ureteral catheter
9. *Intravenous urogram (IVU), previously called intravenous pyelogram (IVP):* x-ray visualization of the ureters and kidneys following intravenous dye injection

B. **Equipment, supplies, and instruments**
   1. *Urologic table:* provides an x-ray unit, drainage system, knee supports, hydraulic or electric controls to adjust height and tilt, attachments for irrigating solutions, light source and electrosurgical units
   2. *Endoscopic and ancillary equipment*
      a. Sheath, obturator, telescope, and resectoscope
      b. Fiber-optic light source and cord
      c. Electrodes: cutting loop for TUR (transurethral resection)
      d. Electrosurgical generator for transurethral resection and fulguration (destruction of tissue by high-frequency electricity)
      e. LASERS: Holmium:YAG and argon are adaptable for most cystoscopes
   3. *Irrigating equipment*
      a. Continuous irrigation is essential during Cystoscopy for visualization and washing out blood, stone fragments, or bits of tissue
      b. Sterile, disposable, closed irrigation system
      c. Disposable tandem sets are used to connect several bottles of fluid to allow for changing containers without interrupting the flow
      d. Solution containers are hung 2½ feet above the table; tubing filled with fluid before connecting to the scope
      e. Fluid must be sterile, nonhemolytic, and nonelectrolytic for TUR (saline is never used with an electrosurgical unit); nonelectrolytic, non-hemolytic solutions come premixed; 1.5% glycine, sorbitol, or urogate (uromatic) are more commonly used for TUR; the urologist, by use of a stopcock, controls inflow and outflow
   4. *Evacuators:* attached to the endoscope for aspiration of fragments, clots, or resected tissue
      a. *Ellik:* double bowl-shaped glass evacuator used to irrigate debris (prostatic chips, calculi) from the bladder via a scope sheath
      b. *Toomey:* syringe with a wide opening at the hub; a metal adapter permits use with a catheter
   5. *Ureteral and urethral catheters*
      a. *Ureteral catheters:* sterile, disposable, graduated; used for performing retrograde pyelogram, placed to serve as a landmark during radical pelvic procedures, or to bypass an obstruction; various types of tips available—common are whistle, olive, and cone-tipped
      b. *Self-retaining stents:* placed in ureter with a guidewire; used to maintain ureteral patency; J-stents or pigtail stents
      c. *Urethral catheters*
         i. *uses:* function as a stent or drainage tube, or are used in diagnostic studies
         ii. *Types:* non-retention (red Robinson) and retention/indwelling (Foley)
         iii. *Sizes:* 12 to 30 French (3 French = 1 mm diameter)
         iv. *Foley:* most commonly used self-retaining catheter

6. *Suture:* absorbable suture, such as 2-0 chromic or monocryl, is used on the urinary tract; silk and some other nonabsorbable suture may cause stone formation

7. *Instruments:* Otis bougies, Otis and van Buren urethral sounds, urethral catheter guide, and Mason-Judd bladder retractor

C. Surgical procedures

1. Bladder procedures

   a. *Cystoscopy:* endoscopic examination of the urethra, bladder, and ureteral orifices

      i. **Indications:** hematuria, urinary retention, recurrent cystitis, urinary incontinence, urinary tract infection, tumors, fistulas, stones, to obtain biopsy specimen, treat lesions, or in follow-up examinations of operative or endoscopic procedures

      ii. Patient positioned on urologic table in slight reverse Trendelenburg with legs in padded knee crutch stirrups; anesthesia may be regional, general, or topical

      iii. **Prep:** entire pubic area with antimicrobial soap

      iv. **Draping:** leggings and a disposable fenestrated sheet with sterile screen material to be placed over the drain on the table (*Note:* A disposable urologic drape with rectal sheath is used during a TUR of the prostate)

      v. Topical anesthetic for urethral meatus

      vi. **Procedure:** light cord, electrosurgical unit, and irrigation fluids (2000 to 3000 ml of distilled water) connected to cystoscope sheath

      vii. In the presence of urethral strictures, dilation with sounds or filiform and followers may precede introduction of the scope

      viii. **Scope:** lubricated with water-soluble lubricant and introduced into the urethra; obturator is withdrawn, telescope (0°, 30°, or 70°) inserted into sheath, and bladder is filled with fluid

      ix. Other instruments may be introduced, such as
         • A lithotrite or LASER fiber to crush a stone (lithopaxy)
         • Electrode/resectoscope for fulguration of bladder tumors
         • Catheters for retrograde ureteral catheterization or pyelography

      x. Renografin or Hypaque injected for x-ray

   b. *Cystotomy:* opening into the bladder to relieve obstruction or as an adjunct to another procedure; may be performed percutaneously or as a suprapubic incision; also called Cystostomy or Vesicostomy

   c. *Cystectomy:* removal of the urinary bladder for the treatment of a malignancy: a urinary diversion procedure performed prior to Cystectomy may be one of the following:

      i. *Ileal Conduit:* isolated segment of ileum is removed; continuity of bowel is reestablished; distal end of the segment is sutured to stoma site on the skin of abdomen, and ureters anastomosed to the proximal segment; a stoma appliance is worn to collect urine, or the stoma is formed to be continent and catheterized as needed.

      ii. *Cutaneous Ureterostomy:* distal end of the ureters is brought through the abdominal wall to create an opening to divert urine outside; a stoma appliance is attached

   d. *Bladder neck suspension* for female urinary incontinence; there are numerous procedures, including:

      i. *Marshall-Marchetti-Krantz operation:* done by the gynecologist or urologist; through a suprapubic extraperitoneal incision, the bladder neck is suspended by placement of sutures through the anterior vaginal wall on either side of the urethra and bringing them out through the periosteum on the posterior surface of the pubic symphysis

ii. *RAZ or Stamey procedure (endoscopic suspension):* through short suprapubic incisions (right and left of midline) and a vaginal incision, a Stamey needle with a heavy suture or polyester mesh is used to suspend the bladder neck to the anterior rectus sheath; cystoscopy is performed intraoperatively to guide correct needle passage

e. *Ureteroneocystostomy:* surgical procedure for reimplantation of ureters into bladder to treat vesicoureteral reflux

f. *Periurethral/transurethral injection of collagen:* injection of collagen (Contigen) into the urethral mucosa to treat urinary incontinence in both men and women

2. Urethral, penile, and scrotal procedures

a. *Urethral dilatation:* for strictures following infection and trauma; need balloon dilators, woven filiform and followers, and bougies or metal sounds

b. *Urethrotomy:* an Otis urethrotome is used to cut into a urethral stricture (strictures may also be treated with LASER)

c. *Urethroplasty:* re-establishment of the continuity of the urethra following trauma

d. *Urethral Meatotomy:* incision into the external urethral meatus to enlarge the opening or relieve stenosis or stricture

e. *Circumcision:* excision of the prepuce (foreskin) of the glans penis, done for phimosis or balanoposthitis (inflammation of the glans penis)

f. *Hypospadias repair:* plastic surgery procedure to change the urethral meatus from the ventral surface of the penis to its normal position at the tip of the penis. The extent of the procedure depends on the degree of hypospadias; may require more than one operation. Chordee (ventral curvature of the penis caused by fibrous bands extending from the hypospadiac urethral meatus) is released along with hypospadias repair.

g. *Epispadias repair:* plastic surgery procedure designed to move the urethral meatus from the dorsal surface of the penis to its normal position. When this congenital anomaly occurs, circumcision is delayed in order that the prepuce can be used to create the urethral extension.

h. *LASER ablation of condylomas:* Use of the LASER to destroy diseased tissues of the penis, perineum, and anal area. (*Note:* LASER plume may contain live virus particles, so the Surgical Technologist must take precautions when scrubbed in on condyloma cases.)

i. *Penectomy:* surgical removal of penis for otherwise incurable diseases; may be partial or total

j. *Penile implant:* device placed within the penile shaft to treat organic sexual impotence due to diseases such as diabetes mellitus, priapism, or neurolysis during pelvic surgery; serves as a stent to enable vaginal penetration

   i. *Noninflatable, semirigid:* inserted in the corpus cavernous

   ii. *Inflatable prosthesis:* reservoir is placed in prevesicle space, inflatable silicone rods in the corpus cavernosus, and a pump in the scrotum

k. *Hydrocelectomy:* removal of the sac of fluid from the tunica vaginalis in the scrotum; incision is made in the scrotum for the adult male, but an inguinal incision is used for a congenital hydrocele and accompanied by a hernia repair

l. *Vasectomy:* excision of a section of the vas deferens through a scrotal incision as an elective sterilization procedure. (*Note:* Sterilization permit must be signed and on the chart.)

m. *Vasovasostomy:* microscopic surgery reconnecting the vas deferens for sterilization reversal

n. *Spermatocelectomy:* surgical removal of a spermatocele (intrascrotal cystic mass) through a scrotal incision

o. *Varicocelectomy:* because of venous backflow of blood around the testes, varicose veins develop which interfere with spermatogenesis; usually found on the left side due to anatomy of the spermatic vein; performed through an incision in the upper portion of the scrotum or inguinal canal, the varicose veins are ligated and excised

p. *Orchidectomy:* surgical removal of testes or testis
   i. Bilateral Orchidectomy is done to control metastatic cancer of the prostate gland.
   ii. Unilateral Orchidectomy is indicated for testicular cancer, trauma, or infection.
   iii. Scrotal incision is used for benign conditions, and inguinal approach is used for malignant conditions.

q. *Orchiopexy:* through an inguinal incision, the testis is transplanted to a scrotal pocket and anchored in a normal anatomical position for the treatment of the congenital condition known as cryptorchidism (hidden or undescended testicle).

r. **Testicular detorsion:** through a scrotal incision, the spermatic cord is untwisted and anchored to prevent future twisting (torsion); common to fixate ("pex") both sides.

3. **Prostatic surgery**
   a. *Needle biopsy:* transperineal or transrectal approach is used to obtain a biopsy from the prostate with tru-cut or Vim-Silverman needle when cancer is suspected.

   b. ***Transurethral resection of the prostate (TURP):*** by means of a resectoscope passed through the urethra; a cutting loop electrode is used to resect tissue and coagulate bleeders, enlarging the prostatic urethra, which has become constricted from benign prostatic hypertrophy (BPH); a TURP is the most commonly performed surgical procedure for BPH; a size 22fr to 24fr three-way Foley catheter with a 30-cc balloon is inserted, inflated, and pulled gently to apply traction to the bladder neck to help control bleeding; the third lumen is used for irrigation.

   c. *Transrectal seed implantation:* the percutaneous implantation of radioactive seeds into the prostate gland.

   d. *Open prostate procedures—types*
      i. *Suprapubic prostatectomy:* through a suprapubic incision, the bladder is incised, drained, and a finger inserted to enucleate the prostate gland through the bladder neck
         • Bilateral Vasectomy may precede the Suprapubic Prostatectomy to decrease the potential for postoperative epididymitis.
         • This approach is used for benign conditions and allows access for correction of bladder problems.
      ii. *Perineal prostatectomy:* with the patient in an exaggerated lithotomy position and under general anesthesia, the prostate is enucleated through a half-circle incision made in the perineum.
      iii. *Retropubic prostatectomy:* removal of the prostate gland by an incision behind the pubic symphysis
      iv. *Radical retropubic prostatectomy:* following limited lymph node dissection with no evidence of spread of cancer, the prostate and periprostatic tissue are widely dissected from the bladder, and the bladder neck is reconstructed; this procedure carries a higher incidence of impotence.

   e. *Open prostate surgery—procedure*
      i. *Position:* supine and Trendelenburg with a bolster under the pelvis
      ii. *Anesthesia:* general
      iii. *Drape:* towel under the scrotum, towels around the incision site, sterile lap sheet, another towel over the penis; a urologic incise drape may be used

      iv. *Instruments:* basic lap set and retractors—Mason-Judd (suprapubic) and Dennis-Brown (perineal)

      v. *Supplies:* closed vacuum drains; water-soluble lubricant; 30-cc syringe; Foley catheters with 5- and 30-cc balloons

      vi. *Procedure*
- Pfannenstiel incision
- Rectus abdominis muscle is retracted to expose the space of Retzius anteriorly.
- Prostatic capsule is incised and gland is enucleated.
- Care is taken to preserve neurovascular bundle that abuts the prostate to decrease the chance of postoperative impotence.
- Absorbable suture is used to close the prostate capsule.
- Foley catheters (suprapubic and transurethral) are inserted and connected to drain and provide continuous irrigation.
- Drain is placed in the space of Retzius and brought out through stab wound.

III. Surgery of the Kidneys and Adrenal Glands

A. Major surgical pathology

1. *Acute renal failure and end-stage renal disease:* results in uremia (urine products in the blood) and hypertension; treated medically with renal dialysis—procedure for removing urine products from the blood of a patient in renal failure

    a. *Hemodialysis:* use of an artificial kidney machine with a semipermeable membrane (acts as nephrons) through which blood is dialyzed (cleansed of urea and other impurities). (*Note:* Venous access for hemodialysis will be discussed with vascular surgery.)

    b. *Peritoneal dialysis:* intermittent or continuous dialysis of the peritoneal cavity through a Tenckhoff silicone catheter placed through a paramedian incision and anchored to subcutaneous tissue; the dialysate is instilled into the peritoneal cavity to draw solutes from the body

2. *Renal calculi (stones):* cause pain, obstruction, and infection; surgically managed by removal (lithotomy) or crushing (lithotripsy)

3. *Tumors and cysts:* excision

B. Diagnostic procedures

1. Serum electrolytes, blood sugar, BUN (blood urea nitrogen)
2. Urinalysis and urine cultures
3. Blood chemistry profiles
4. EKG and chest x-ray
5. CT scans, KUB, and urinary flow studies
6. IVP (intravenous pyelogram), IVU (intravenous urogram)
7. Renal arteriography for renal hypertension

C. Special features

1. *Hemorrhage:* possible from large vessels (e.g., renal artery)
2. *Fistulae:* forms when closure of the urinary tract is not watertight; absorbable suture is used on the GU tract
3. *Infection:* combated with antibiotics, irrigation, and drainage systems
4. *Catheters and drains:* must be kept patent
5. Intake and output measurements

D. Special instruments, equipment, and supplies

1. Instruments: routine laparotomy set, kidney instruments (pedicle clamps, DeBakey forceps, set of Randall stone forceps), and rib instruments (Finochietto rib retractors, periosteotome, rib raspatories, Bethune rib cutter, double-action rongeurs, Bailey rib approximator, Langenbeck periosteal elevator)
2. Supplies: red Robinson catheter (8 to 10 French), Asepto syringe, closed wound drainage system, and vessel loops
3. Nephroscope and accessories

4. Suction, electrosurgical unit, hemoclip appliers, and dissectors
5. **Hypothermia measures:** saline slush and ice slush perfusion of cold solutions through renal arteries or surface cooling coils may be used to prolong the safe period of renal ischemia during long procedures
6. Patient x-rays should be in the room
7. If the patient is repositioned for a second incision, an additional instrument set, prep, and drape will be required (as in the case of Nephroureterectomy)

E. **Intraoperative preparation**
1. *Anesthesia:* general
2. *Positioning:* based on the surgical approach used:
   a. *Lateral:* for kidney/adrenal gland; pillows, kidney bar/rests, vacuum (beanbag) positioner, Mayo or elevated armboard for independent arm, axillary roll
   b. *Supine:* for distal ureter/bladder
3. *Incisions*
   a. *Flank or lumbar:* most frequently used; may include the removal of eleventh or twelfth rib; begins at posterior axillary line and follows the twelfth rib and downward between the iliac crest and thorax; patient is in the lateral kidney position
   b. *Transabdominal transperitoneal:* provides an excellent approach to the renal pedicle; used for renal neoplasms; the patient is in supine position with bolsters beneath the flank and lower thorax
4. *Skin preparation*
   a. *Lateral:* begin at twelfth rib and extend from the axilla to 2 inches below the iliac crest and to the bedline on either side
   b. *Supine:* standard lower abdominal prepping; may prep and drape out penis in males
5. *Draping:* folded towels and transverse fenestrated sheet
6. *Surgical procedures*
   a. *Adrenalectomy*
      i. *Indications:* primary tumor such as pheochromocytoma (usually unilateral) or endocrine-dependent tumors such as breast or prostate malignancy (usually, a bilateral Adrenalectomy performed)
      ii. *Position*
         • *Unilateral Adrenalectomy:* lateral position
         • *Bilateral Adrenalectomy:* prone position for a posterior approach or supine position for an anterior approach
      iii. *Instrumentation:* major lap tray, long instruments, kidney tray, and vascular and GI instruments available
   b. *Nephrostomy:* opening into the kidney with tube left in place that exits the skin; used to drain a kidney during healing, or as a temporary urinary diversion; secured to skin and connected to a drainage collection device
   c. *Pyeloplasty:* surgical revision of narrowing, due to stenosis or anatomic obstruction, to increase the size of the outlet from the renal pelvis into the ureter
   d. *Lithotripsy:* crushing of stone, the urinary stone is fragmented
      i. *Electrohydraulic and Holmium YAG LASER lithotripsy:* accomplished with an electrohydraulic lithotriptor Holmium LASER that creates hydraulic shock waves to fragment the stones; fragments may be removed with Randall stone forceps (open procedure) or irrigation

ii. *LASER lithotripsy:* laser beam is directed through a flexible scope to fragment a stone

iii. *Extracorporeal shock wave lithotripsy (ESWL):* noninvasive procedure; anesthetized patient is lifted into water bath, stones are visualized by fluoroscopy, and high-voltage sparks are discharged to generate shock waves to crush the stones

e. *Nephrolithotomy:* removal of a stone from the kidney through an open flank incision

f. *Pyelolithotomy:* removal of a staghorn calculus (stone which completely fills the renal pelvis) from the kidney pelvis through an open incision

g. *Heminephrectomy:* removal of a portion of the kidney
   i. Local hypothermia is essential.
   ii. Absorbable suture on urologic needle for the kidney.
   iii. Gerota's (peri-renal) fat/fascia is sutured over excised portion.
   iv. Renal capsule is reapproximated with a continuous absorbable suture.

h. *Radical nephrectomy:* excision of a kidney, perirenal fat, adrenal gland, Gerota's capsule, and nearby periaortic lymph nodes; indicated for certain renal neoplasms, such as Wilms' tumor

i. *Kidney transplant*
   i. **Living donor**
      • Adjacent operating rooms are used for donor and recipient.
      • Donor must be in good health.
      • Performed for a patient with end-stage renal disease
      • Transplanted into recipient's iliac fossa
      • Renal vein is anastomosed to the side of the recipient's iliac vein with a 5-0 or 6-0 double-armed vascular suture.
      • Renal artery is anastomosed to the recipient's iliac artery.
      • Vessels are irrigated with heparin sodium solution to prevent blood from clotting in the lumen.
      • Ureter is anastomosed through a submucosal tunnel into the bladder.
   ii. **Cadaveric donor**
      • Should be free of infection and cancer, and normotensive (normal blood pressure) until short time before death
      • Permission to harvest the donor kidney is obtained, kidney is removed through a laparotomy incision, and renal perfusion is maintained
      • Equipment and setup are the same as for a Nephrectomy
      • Kidneys, renal vessels, and ureters are carefully dissected
      • Donor organs are transported in a hypothermic pulsatile perfusion machine
      • Artificial life support systems are terminated

j. *Nephrectomy:* removal of a kidney
   i. *Indications:* hydronephrosis (Nephroureterectomy), pyelonephritis, renal atrophy, trauma, tumors, or renal artery stenosis
   ii. *Preparation:* general anesthesia and lateral kidney position; prep and drape for flank incision
   iii. *Procedure*
      • Flank incision through skin, fat, and fascia
      • External oblique, internal oblique, and transversalis muscles are incised.
      • Ribs are resected as needed.
      • Lumbosacral ligaments are cut with a scalpel or heavy scissors.
      • Gerota's fascia is incised with Metzenbaum scissors to expose kidney and perirenal fat.

- Ureter is identified, freed, clamped twice, then divided and ligated with heavy, nonabsorbable suture material.
- Kidney pedicle is isolated, clamped twice, then divided and ligated with heavy, nonabsorbable suture material; kidney is passed off as a specimen.
- Renal fossa is explored, hemostasis is secured, fossa is irrigated, and drain is inserted and brought out through a stab wound.
- Fascia and muscles are closed in layers with an interrupted absorbable suture.
- Skin is approximated with staples or interrupted sutures.
- Drain is secured to the skin with nonabsorbable suture, and the dressing is applied.

iv. *Surgical hazards and complications*
- Clamp slipping off the pedicle with resultant hemorrhage
- Injury to the aorta or inferior vena cava with hemorrhage
- Damage to the spleen (left nephrectomy)
- Accidental entry into the pleural space with lung collapse (left nephrectomy)
- Damage to the duodenum (right nephrectomy)

v. **Postoperative management**
- Careful monitoring of intake and output
- Observe for hemorrhage: dressings and vital signs
- Pulmonary complications may occur: turning, coughing, and deep-breathing exercises are helpful

Show What You Know

Directions
Each of the numbered items or incomplete statements in this section is followed by answers or by completions of the statement. Select the ONE lettered answer or completion that is BEST in each case.

1. Which of the following solutions is electrolytic and would not be used with a fulguration or transurethral resection of the prostate?

   A. normal saline
   B. sterile distilled water
   C. glycine
   D. Sorbitol

2. Inability to control urination is:

   A. uremia
   B. cystitis
   C. urinary continence
   D. urinary incontinence

3. X-ray visualization of the kidneys, ureters, and bladder following an intravenous injection of dye is a diagnostic test called:

   A. retrograde pyelogram
   B. intravenous urogram
   C. KUB
   D. cystometrogram

4. The most commonly used self-retaining urethral catheter is a:

   A. Pezzer
   B. Malecot
   C. Robinson
   D. Foley

5. During an open pelvic procedure, the surgeon asks for the bladder stitch. Of the following sutures on your field, which one would you give the surgeon?

   A. 2-0 chromic
   B. 3-0 silk
   C. 4-0 Prolene
   D. #1 Vicryl

6. Which of the following instruments could be used to dilate a male urethra?

   A. Hegar dilator
   B. van Buren sound
   C. lithotrite
   D. Urethrotome

7. Which of the following is a urinary diversion procedure?

   A. Pyelolithotomy
   B. Ileal Conduit
   C. Lithopaxy
   D. Retrograde Pyelogram

8. Vesicourethral suspension, such as the Stamey procedure and the Marshall-Marchetti-Krantz procedure, is performed to correct:

   A. hypospadias
   B. spermatocele
   C. cryptorchidism
   D. female urinary incontinence

9. The most common surgical management for BPH (benign prostatic hypertrophy) is:

   A. TURP (Transurethral Resection of the Prostate)
   B. Suprapubic Prostatectomy
   C. Retropubic Prostatectomy
   D. Perineal Prostatectomy

10. Possible complications of a Nephrectomy include all of the following *except:*

    A. hemorrhage
    B. impotence
    C. accidental entry into the pleural space
    D. damage to the spleen or duodenum

11. The most common incision for a Unilateral Nephrectomy is:

    A. transabdominal transperitoneal
    B. transthoracic transdiaphragmatic
    C. Pfannenstiel
    D. flank or lumbar

12. Rib instruments should be available for which of the following procedures?

    A. Ureteroneocystostomy
    B. Varicocelectomy
    C. Extracorporal Shock-Wave Lithotripsy
    D. Adrenalectomy

13. Which of the following procedures is designed to remove waste products of urine from the blood of a patient with end-stage renal disease?

    A. peritoneal dialysis
    B. nephroscopy
    C. nephrolithotripsy
    D. pyeloplasty

14. A special sterilization permit would be needed for which of the following procedures?

    A. Hydrocelectomy
    B. Vasectomy
    C. Bilateral Adrenalectomy
    D. Ileal Conduit

15. The syringe used for evacuation of bladder debris, such as prostatic chips or stone fragments, is a/an:

    A. Iglesias
    B. Ellik
    C. van Buren
    D. luer-lock syringe

16. Common tips found on ureteral catheters include all of the following *except:*

    A. spiral
    B. olive
    C. dovetail
    D. whistle

17. Clinical indications for performing Cystoscopy include all of the following *except:*

    A. urinary tract infection, indicated by WBCs in urine upon urinalysis
    B. glomerulonephritis, indicated by a urine specific gravity of 1.020
    C. hematuria, indicated by the presence of RBCs in urine upon urinalysis
    D. acute urinary retention, indicated by voiding 100 cc's of urine in 24 hours

18. Circumcision involves removal of what structure?

    A. glans penis
    B. prepuce
    C. corona
    D. vas deferens

19. Methods for urinary tract calculus removal include which of the following?

    A. Extracorporeal shock wave lithotripsy (ESWL)
    B. Nephrectomy
    C. Varicocelectomy
    D. Ureteral Diversion

20. The instrument(s) used to bypass severe strictures of the urethra is called:

    A. Mason-Judd
    B. Bougies
    C. filiforms and followers
    D. toomeys

21. Common urinary drainage catheters found in the OR would include:

    A. a 34fr, 2-way, 5-cc latex Foley catheter
    B. a 26fr, 3-way, 50-cc silicone Foley catheter
    C. a 22fr, 2-way, 30-cc latex Foley catheter
    D. a 20fr, 4-way, 30-cc red rubber indwelling catheter

22. The three common positions for genito-urinary procedures include all of the following *except:*

    A. supine
    B. modified dorsal recumbent with knees bent (frog-legged)

    C. jackknife
    D. lithotomy

23. During Nephrectomy, instrumentation commonly used would include:

    A. a nephroscope
    B. pedicle clamps
    C. Army-Navy retractors
    D. Potts scissors

24. The procedure of choice to treat irreparable hydronephrosis is:

    A. Ileal Conduit
    B. Hydrocelectomy
    C. Ureteroneocystostomy
    D. Nephroureterectomy

25. The most common telescopes used for cystoscopy include:

    A. 20- and 30-degree scopes
    B. 15- and 30-degree scopes
    C. 15- and 70-degree scopes
    D. 30- and 70-degree scopes\

26. Ureterolithotomy is performed with all of the following instruments *except:*

    A. Potts scissors
    B. #11 blade on a #7 handle
    C. Randall forceps
    D. #10 blade on a #4 handle

27. An Ileal Conduit involves:

    A. implanting the ureters into the sigmoid colon
    B. implanting the ureters into an isolated segment of ileum
    C. reimplanting the ureters into the bladder
    D. implanting the ureters into a connected segment of the ileum

28. The procedure for urinary stress incontinence during which cystoscopy is performed is the _____ procedure.

    A. Stamey procedure
    B. Marshall-Marchetti Kranz procedure
    C. Van Buren procedure
    D. Mason-Judd procedure

29. Suture used to close the ureter would include:

    A. 0 silk
    B. 3-0 nylon
    C. 4-0 silk
    D. 4-0 dexon

30. The tissue of choice used to replace the urinary bladder following Cystectomy is the:

    A. the ileum
    B. the sigmoid
    C. the colon
    D. the jejunum

31. Which plastic surgery procedure is performed to change the urethral meatus from the ventral surface of the penis to its normal position at the tip of the penis?

    A. Hypospadius Repair
    B. Varicocelectomy
    C. Hydrocelectomy
    D. Epispadius Repair

32. Which of the following procedures treats cryptorchidism?

    A. Nephrectomy
    B. Hydrocelectomy
    C. Orchiopexy
    D. Vasectomy

33. Which incision is used to perform Transurethral Resection of the Prostate (TURP)?

    A. midline
    B. Pfannensteil
    C. McBurney
    D. No incision is used; it is performed through the urethra.

34. Positioning aides used during Nephrectomy would include all of the following *except:*

    A. axillary roll
    B. kidney rests
    C. pillows between the legs
    D. stirrups

35. The procedure performed for the treatment of Wilm's tumor is:

    A. Orchiectomy
    B. Radical Nephrectomy

    C. Marshall-Marchetti-Kranz Procedure
    D. Ureteroneocystostomy

36. The term for the surgical crushing of a stone is:

    A. lithopexy
    B. lithotripsy
    C. lithotomy
    D. lithiasis

37. Which organ or structure cannot be seen on a KUB?

    A. bladder
    B. ureter
    C. urethra
    D. kidney

Questions 38 and 39 relate to the following scenario:

Mr. Tovar, aged 64, is scheduled for a kidney transplant to treat his chronic renal failure due to diabetes.

38. During kidney transplantation, the renal artery and vein are anastamosed to the:

    A. iliac artery and iliac vein
    B. femoral artery and saphenous vein
    C. radial artery and basilic vein
    D. aorta and vena cava

39. During kidney transplantation, the blood vessels are irrigated with _____ solution to prevent blood from clotting in the lumen.

    A. cephazolin
    B. pitressin
    C. heparin sodium
    D. bupivicaine hydrochloride

Instrument Identification

40.

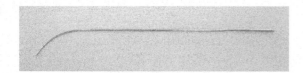

    A. van Buren sound
    B. Aufricht retractor
    C. Hegar dilator
    D. Bougie

Anatomy Review

Genitourinary System

41–56.

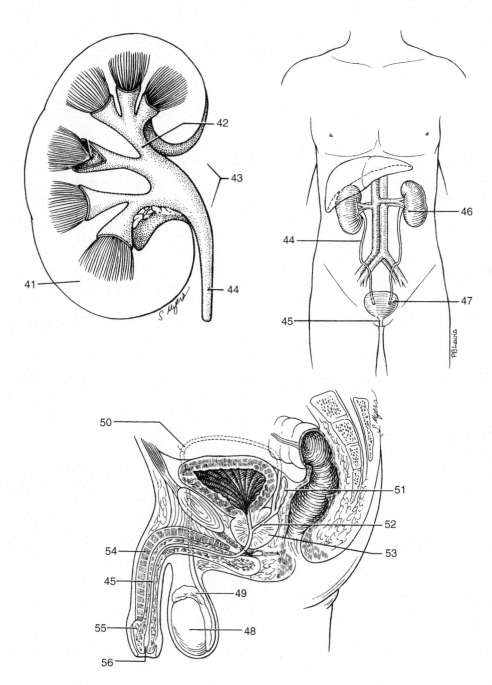

A. bladder
B. calyx
C. corpus cavernosum
D. corpus spongiosum
E. ductus deferens or vas deferens
F. ejaculatory duct
G. epididymis
H. kidney

I. prostate
J. renal cortex
K. renal pelvis
L. seminal vesicle
M. testis
N. ureter
O. urethra
P. urethral meatus

Answers & Rationales

1. **A.** **Rationale:** Normal saline is an electrolytic solution and should not be used with a TURP or fulguration. Sterile distilled water is a hemolytic solution and would not be used during a TURP. Glycine and sorbitol can be used.

2. **D.** **Rationale:** Urinary incontinence is the inability to control urination.

3. **B.** **Rationale:** Intravenous urogram is the x-ray visualization of the kidneys, ureters, and bladder following injection of a contrast media into the vein.

4. **D.** **Rationale:** The Foley catheter is the most frequently used self-retaining urethral catheter. The Pezzer and Malecot may also be left in place but would need to be secured with a suture. The Robinson is a red rubber catheter and is not left in place.

5. **A.** **Rationale:** A 2-0 chromic suture may be used as a bladder stitch. #1 is too large for the bladder, and a nonabsorbable suture may serve as a focus for stone formation.

6. **B.** **Rationale:** Van Buren sounds are designed to dilate the male urethra. Hegar dilators are designed for the cervix. A lithotrite is used to crush stones, and urethrotome is used to "cut" urethral strictures.

7. **B.** **Rationale:** Ileal conduit is the only procedure listed that involves diverting urine.

8. **D.** **Rationale:** Female urinary incontinence is due to a prolapse of the bladder or urethra into a weakened vaginal wall and may be suspended by various methods, including the Marshall-Marchetti-Kranz procedure and the Stamey procedure.

9. **A.** **Rationale:** The Transurethral Resection of the Prostate is the most commonly performed surgical procedure for benign prostatic hypertrophy. Malignancy may be treated with Prostatectomy, radiation, or chemotherapy.

10. **B.** **Rationale:** Impotence is a complication of a Radical Prostatectomy but not for a Nephrectomy.

11. **D.** **Rationale:** The flank or lumbar incision is most commonly used to access a kidney or adrenal gland.

12. **D.** **Rationale:** The adrenal glands are located on the upper pole of the kidneys under the diaphragm, and rib instruments should be available when the surgeon is dissecting in this area.

13. **A.** **Rationale:** Peritoneal dialysis and hemodialysis are methods used to extract waste products of urine when the kidneys have failed.

14. **B.** **Rationale:** The Vasectomy is a sterilization procedure and would require a special permit.

15. **B.** **Rationale:** The Ellik evacuator is used for removing prostatic chips or other debris from the bladder. The double bowl shape provides a means to trap the debris and not return it to the bladder while performing irrigation.

16. **C.** **Rationale:** Ureteral catheters commonly have spiral, olive, or whistle tips. Other tips may include filiform and cone tips.

17. **B.** **Rationale:** A urine specific gravity of 1.020 is within normal limits. This lab value would not indicate glomerulonephritis.

18. **B.** **Rationale:** During Circumcision, the prepuce or foreskin covering the glans penis is removed.

19. **A.** **Rationale:** Extracorporeal Shock Wave Lithotripsy is a nonsurgical method used to break up calculi in the renal pelvis.

20. **C.** **Rationale:** Filiforms and followers are instruments used to bypass severe strictures of the urethra. The filiform is very slender and has a spiral tip to pass through very narrow openings. Once passed, a series of progressively larger followers are screwed onto the filiform to dilate the stricture and drain urine proximal to the stricture.

21. **C.** **Rationale:** A 22fr, 2-way, 30-cc latex Foley catheter is a common urinary drainage catheter found in the OR. It is the only combination presented that is valid.

22. **C.** **Rationale:** Jackknife position is not commonly used for genitourinary procedures.

23. **B.** **Rationale:** Pedicle clamps are commonly used during a nephrectomy to clamp the renal artery and vein before they are sutured and divided.

24. D. **Rationale:** A nephroureterectomy is performed to treat irrepairable hydronephrosis. The kidney and ureter are damaged beyond healing and dilated, which permits pooling of urine and infection.

25. D. **Rationale:** The 30- and 70-degree telescopes are the two most common lenses for cystoscopy. The 30-degree telescope permits visualization of most of the bladder wall, while the 70-degree telescope permits looking at the bladder wall near the bladder neck.

26. D. **Rationale:** A #10 blade does not fit onto a #4 handle; therefore, it cannot be used.

27. B. **Rationale:** An Ileal Conduit involves implanting the ureters into an isolated segment of ileum.

28. A. **Rationale:** The procedure for urinary stress incontinence during which Cystoscopy is performed is the Stamey procedure. Cystoscopy is performed to guide needle placement.

29. D. **Rationale:** 4-0 Dexon is used to close the ureter to prevent postoperative calculus formation.

30. A. **Rationale:** The ileum is the tissue of choice to replace the urinary bladder following Cystectomy.

31. A. **Rationale:** The plastic surgery procedure to change the urethral meatus from the ventral surface of the penis to its normal position at the tip of the penis is the Hypospadius Repair. The ventral side of the penis is the surface that lays against the scrotum when the penis is not erect.

32. C. **Rationale:** An Orchiopexy is the procedure used to treat cryptorchidism, an undescended testicle which fails to travel the inguinal canal during growth and development or fails to remain in the scrotum after birth.

33. D. **Rationale:** No incision is used to perform a TURP. The resectoscope is passed to the prostate through the urethra.

34. D. **Rationale:** Stirrups are not used for positioning aides during Nephrectomy.

35. B. **Rationale:** The procedure performed for the treatment of Wilms' tumor is a Radical Nephrectomy.

36. B. **Rationale:** The term for the surgical crushing of a stone is lithotripsy.

37. C. **Rationale:** The urethra cannot be seen on a KUB. KUB stands for kidney, ureter, and bladder.

38. A. **Rationale:** During kidney transplantation, the renal artery and vein are anastamosed to the iliac artery and iliac vein because the new kidney is positioned in the iliac fossa.

39. C. **Rationale:** During kidney transplantation, the blood vessels are irrigated with heparin solution, an anticoagulant, to prevent blood from clotting in the lumen.

40. A. **Rationale:** van Buren sound
41. (J) renal cortex
42. (B) calyx
43. (K) renal pelvis
44. (N) ureter
45. (O) urethra
46. (H) kidney
47. (A) bladder
48. (M) testis
49. (G) epididymis
50. (E) ductus deferens or vas deferens
51. (L) seminal vesicle
52. (F) ejaculatory duct
53. (I) prostate
54. (C) corpus cavernosum
55. (D) corpus spongiosum
56. (P) urethral meatus

Part II: Deciphering a Surgical Schedule

The following mock surgery schedule will be used to answer several questions pertaining to genitourinary surgery. The same schedule, or a similar one, will be used in subsequent chapters to ask questions about the content of the chapter.

Rm# time	Surgeon	Procedure	Anest.	Rm# time	Surgeon	Procedure	Anest.
Rm00				**Rm07**			
OC	Dr. Z	Rt. Knee Arthroscopy	Gen.	7:00	Dr. M	Laparoscopic appendectomy	Gen.
OC	Dr. C	Craniotomy	Gen.	TF	Dr. M	Lipoma removal	MAC
OC	Dr.Z	Angioplasty	Gen.				
Rm01				**Rm08**			
7:00	Dr. X	Hemorrhoidectomy	Gen.	11:00	Dr. E	Bovine Thrombectomy	MAC
TF	Dr. X	Colostomy	Gen.				
TF	Dr. X	Bowel resection	Gen.				
Rm02				**Rm09**			
7:00	Dr. B	Splenectomy	Gen.	8:30	Dr. T	Cholecystectomy	Gen.
TF	Dr. B	Gastrectomy	Gen.	TF	Dr. T	Palatoplasty	Gen.
Rm03				**Rm10**			
7:00	Dr. A	Cystoscopy	MAC	7:00	Dr. K	Nephrectomy	Gen.
TF	Dr. A	Cystoplasty	Gen.	TF	Dr. K	Choledocholithotripsy	MAC
12:30	Dr. F	Pyelolithotomy	MAC	TF	Dr. K	Hepatic resection	Gen.
3:00	Dr. F	Cystocele repair	Gen.				
Rm04				**Rm11**			
7:00	Dr. Y	Circumcision	Gen.	7:00	Dr. L	Orchidectomy	Gen.
TF	Dr. Y	Radical suprapubic prostatectomy	Gen.	12:00	Dr. L	Hypospadasis repair	Gen.
Rm05				**Rm12**			
7:00	Dr. G	Vasectomy	Gen.	7:00	Dr. W	Trans-metatarsal amputation	Gen.
TF	Dr. G	Trans-urethral resection of the prostate	Gen	TF	Dr. W	Osteotomy	Gen.
TF	Dr. G	Marshall-Marchetti procedure	Gen.	TF	Dr. W	Arthrocentesis	Gen.
Rm06				**Rm13**			Gen.
7:00	Dr. R	Lumbar Laminectomy	Gen.	7:00	Dr. O	Hysterectomy	

The following questions should be answered using the surgery schedule above

1. A patient is scheduled for a Marshall Marchetti procedure in Room 5. What is the purpose for this procedure?

    A. Recurrent kidney infections
    B. Urinary incontinence
    C. Testicular cancer
    D. Torsion of the vas deferens

2. The patient in Room 11 is undergoing a Hypospadasis repair. What age is this patient most likely to be?

    A. 12 months to school age
    B. Early 20s

C. Late teens

D. Geriatric

3. The patient undergoing a circumcision in Room 4 is 45 years old. What instrument is the surgeon likely to use to grasp the prepuce?

A. Curved Kocher

B. Straight mosquito

C. Curved Kelly

D. Penetrating towel clip

4. A TURP is scheduled for Room 5. What will be used to evacuate resected tissue from the bladder?

A. Number 9 Frazier suction

B. Randall stone forceps

C. Toomey Syringe

D. Resecting loop

5. Room 11 has an Orchidectomy scheduled first. During this procedure, which structures will be cross clamped and divided?

A. Vas deferens and Spermatic cord

B. Spermatic artery and vein

C. Testicular duct and spermatic vein

D. Scrotal artery and the vas deferens

6. Which muscle(s) will be cut during the nephrectomy that is scheduled in Room 10?

A. Rectus and Subcapularis

B. Latissimus dorsi and oblique

C. Oblique and transverse

D. Transverse and Subcapularis

7. The nephrectomy will require the rib to be resected. What instrument should the Surgical Technologist have on hand to hand to the surgeon?

A. Sternal saw

B. Lebsche Knife

C. Bailey

D. Bethune

8. During the nephrectomy, the surgeon will need to clamp the pedicle. Which Instrument should the Surgical Technologist have ready?

A. Herrick

B. Vorse

C. Statinsky Clamp

D. DeBakey Sidewinder

9. What is the most likely position for the patient undergoing the radical prostatectomy in Room 4?

A. Trendelenburg

B. Lithotomy

C. Reverse trendelenburg

D. Lateral

10. Room 3 has scheduled a pyelolithotomy at 12:30. The renal pelvis will need to be irrigated after the stone is removed. What fluid should the Surgical Technologist have on hand for the irrigation?

A. Cold Sterile Water

B. Warm Sterile Water

C. Cold Sterile Saline

D. Warm Sterile Saline

Answers & Rationales

1. **B. Rationale:** The Marshall-Marchetti-Krantz procedure is also known as a vesicourethral suspension. It is performed to treat urinary incontinence in the female patient. Answers C and D can immediately be discarded as they are performed on male patients. An alternative procedure, a suburethral sling is also used to treat this condition in female patients.

2. **A. Rationale:** Hypospadasis is a birth defect that is fairly common and associated with chordee, a condition causing the urethra to be shortened. The repair usually is done on younger patients, usually up to school aged.

3. **B. Rationale:** Circumcisions are performed on adult males when the foreskin is unable to be retracted, usually due to irritation. The surgeon will generally clamp the prepuce with straight mosquitoes or hemostats. This is done prior to the dorsal incision and subsequent circumferential incision.

4. **C. Rationale:** Resected pieces of the prostate will be evacuated from the bladder using either an ellick evacuator or a Toomey syringe. These pieces must be kept and sent to pathology.

5. **B. Rationale:** After the testicle is separated from the scrotum, usually through blunt dissection, the spermatic artery and vein are then cross clamped, separated and ligated with a larger absorbable suture.

6. **C. Rationale:** The incision for a nephrectomy will usually end at the rectus muscle, dividing the oblique and transverse muscles. The Subcapularis muscle is located at the anterior shoulder and would not be involved in the dissection. The latissimus dorsi muscle is also located in the shoulder.

7. **D. Rationale:** A Sternal saw would not be used to remove the rib during a nephrectomy. The Lebsche knife likewise is used on the sternum, not a rib. The Bailey is a rib approximator, used to pull the ribs together during closing. Therefore, the Bethune rib shear is the correct choice. There are several instruments that are used for this portion of the procedure, depending on the set pulled and the surgeons preference.

8. **A. Rationale:** Generally the surgeon will require a Herrick pedicle clamp or a similar instrument when clamping the kidney pedicle. The Surgical Technologist should have three clamps ready for use, as triple clamping is commonly done to ensure that the renal artery is completely occluded. The Vorse is a tube occluding clamp, generally used by Perfusionists during bypass, and the Statinsky and DeBakey sidewinder are vascular clamps.

9. **A. Rationale:** While several positions may be used for prostate removal, the schedule shows that this is going to be a suprapubic removal. Generally, this patient will be in the trendelenburg position, and may require shoulder braces. The perineal approach will place the patient into exaggerated lithotomy for access to the perineum and anus.

10. **D. Rationale:** Warm sterile saline will be required for irrigation of the renal pelvis. If the Surgical Technologist has sterile saline on the table, it most likely will have cooled during the procedure. The ST should receive fresh, warmed saline form the circulator, and should ensure that the temperature is neither too hot nor too cold.

Head and Neck Surgery

15 chapter

Otorhinolaryngology is the branch of medicine and surgery that deals with conditions of the ear, nose, and throat. Some neck and dental procedures are included in this section for the sake of clarity, although other specialists perform them.

I. **Surgery of the Ear**

   A. **Special features of otologic surgery**

   1. *Close proximity of the following:*

   a. Cranial nerves VII (Facial) and VIII (Vestibulocochlear) to the middle and inner ear

   b. Meninges of the temporal lobe of the brain to the middle ear

   c. Internal carotid artery, jugular vein, and lateral sinus of the dura mater to the middle ear (*Note:* Injury to these structures produces meningitis and venous thrombosis, which could cause morbid or even lethal complications.)

   2. *Hearing loss may be associated with the following:*

   a. *Otosclerosis:* bony ankylosis (adhesions) of the stapes, characterized by tinnitus (ringing in the ears) and chronic progressive bone conduction hearing loss

   b. *Perforated eardrum:* caused by trauma

   c. *Otitis media:* accumulation of fluid and infection in the middle ear

   d. *Cholesteatoma:* cystlike mass that develops from chronic middle ear infection

   e. *Acoustic neuroma:* benign tumor of the vestibular portion of Cranial Nerve VIII

   f. *Perceptive or sensorineural loss:* associated with the nerve, receptor cells, or brain

   3. *Diagnostic audiogram:* measurement of hearing loss

   4. *Anesthesia:* local anesthesia may be used for minor procedures; general anesthesia commonly is used to prevent patient movement.

   a. Anesthesiologist sits to the side of the patient while the surgeon is positioned at the head of the table (the bed is turned after anesthesia induction).

   b. A bloodless field may be created, especially during microsurgery, with the use of hypotensive anesthesia using vasodilator drugs.

   c. Epinephrine is often used locally to control bleeding (this can present a problem for day-surgery patients who may bleed after they go home and the effects of epinephrine have worn off).

   5. *Positioning:* patient is positioned on the OR bed with head at the foot end to allow the surgeon to sit with legs under the table and the microscope base to fit under the table

   6. *Skin prep:* hair may be shaved 11/2 inches from incision site, if ordered; ear is cleaned with mild soap solution.

   7. *Draping:* three folded towels are draped around the ear and one split sheet is used to cover patient (plastic incise drape may be used before towels). (*Note:* To avoid granuloma, drapes should be lint free and gloves powder free. To facilitate breathing and decrease patient anxiety during local procedures, the drapes may be placed across a Mayo stand placed close to the patient's face.)

   8. *Equipment:* operating microscope is positioned over the patient's head; room is darkened

   9. *Instrumentation*

   a. Delicate microsurgery instruments are handled with care, kept on the sterile field in protective racks, cleansed of blood and tissue after each use with special wipes; delicate suction tips are cleansed frequently with water and a syringe

   b. **Drills:** Ototome with small burrs are frequently used; require continuous irrigation to remove bone dust, prevent clogging of burrs, and keep tissue cool

   c. **Suction:** small Frazier or needle suction tips; suction-irrigation system may be used, especially during use of the drill

d. Special ear instruments include aural speculum, bayonet and angled forceps, mastoid self-retaining retractor, and Kerrison rongeur; alligator-type forceps and various picks are used

e. Cottonoids moistened with normal saline are used instead of sponges and are counted

10. Hemostasis provided by bone wax, LASER, epinephrine, absorbable hemostatic sponge, oxidized cellulose, or electrosurgical unit

11. Autogenous tissue grafts (commonly taken from the temporalis fascia) are used as tympanic membrane grafts; they are placed on a drying block to allow them to "stiffen" before insertion

12. Prosthetic devices are extremely delicate and should be left in their sterilizing case until needed and then handled carefully

13. Nerve stimulator used to identify facial and vestibulocochlear nerves (circulator frequently observes the patient's face and/or nerve monitor)

14. Pressure dressing with head bandage may be used

15. **Postoperative considerations**: patient is advised to
    a. Keep the ear canal dry for 10 days to 2 weeks.
    b. Avoid blowing the nose and coughing; if sneezing occurs, keep the mouth open.
    c. Vertigo (severe dizziness) may occur.
    d. Avoid air travel for 2 weeks.

B. **Surgical procedures and related pathology**
    1. *Myringotomy:* incision into the eardrum; PE (pressure-equalizing) tubes are frequently inserted and left in place
        a. *Indications:* otitis media with effusion (fluid in the middle ear)
        b. *Procedure:* ear speculum is inserted, wax is removed with curette and alligator forceps, eardrum is incised with a myringotomy knife, fluid is suctioned with Frazier suction, cultures are taken (if indicated), tube is inserted with alligator forceps or tube applier, and otic drops (antibiotic and/or steroid) are instilled.
    2. *Mastoidectomy:* removal of mastoid air cells for chronic mastoiditis; the Facial (VII) Nerve travels along the roof of the mastoid process and may be injured during Mastoidectomy
        a. *Simple Mastoidectomy:* mastoid process is approached through a postaural (behind the ear) incision and drilled with small burrs.
        b. *Modified Radical Mastoidectomy:* Simple Mastoidectomy plus removal of the posterior wall of the ear canal to facilitate drainage
        c. *Radical Mastoidectomy:* removal of mastoid cells, malleus, incus, and tympanic membrane; opens the mastoid antrum and middle ear to create one cavity
    3. *Tympanoplasty:* repair of defects in the eardrum and middle ear to restructure the sound-conduction pathway; classified into five types
        a. *Type I:* Myringoplasty; use of an autogenous graft (temporalis fascia or vein) to "patch" the perforated eardrum; graft may be supported by gelfilm during healing
        b. *Type II:* use of an autogenous graft to repair the perforated eardrum for erosion and replacement of the malleus
        c. *Type III:* replacement of the tympanic membrane, malleus, and incus with a homograft or implant—PORP (partial ossicular replacement prosthesis)
        d. *Type IV:* homograft transplantation of the tympanic membrane and ossicles (the footplate of the stapes may be intact); may also implant PORP or TORP (total ossicular replacement prosthesis)
        e. *Type V:* use of a homograft to seal off the middle ear and provide sound protection for the round window when otosclerosis has resulted in fixation of the stapedial footplate. (*Note:* Once a graft or prosthesis has been placed, nitrous oxide should not be given as an anesthetic

gas since it can cause bubbles to form in the middle ear, displacing the graft or prosthetic device.)
4. *Stapes mobilization:* freeing the footplate of the stapes from an adhered position
    a. *Indication:* otosclerosis
    b. *Procedure (microsurgery):* chisels and picks are used to free the footplate of the stapes from its ankylosed site; a prosthetic device may be used.
5. *Stapedectomy:* removal of the stapes
    a. *Indication:* otosclerosis
    b. *Purpose:* to correct hearing loss
    c. *Procedure:* incision is made deep in the ear canal (endaural); eardrum is folded over, and stapes is disconnected with fine microinstruments and removed; window is sealed by a graft of vein, fascia, fat, perichondrium, or an absorbable hemostatic sponge; prosthesis is inserted and connected to the incus and the graft. (*Note:* Various types of prostheses are available.)
6. *Labyrinthectomy:* removal of the vestibular labyrinth to correct incapacitating vertigo
7. *Endolymphatic sac shunt:* through a mastoidectomy approach, the endolymphatic sac behind the semicircular canals is opened, the inner ear is drained into the mastoid or subarachnoid space, and a tube is inserted; performed to treat Ménière's Disease—vertigo, ringing in the ears (tinnitus), and sensorineural hearing loss
8. *Cochlear prosthetic implant:* done for sensorineural deafness
9. *Otoplasty:* cosmetic procedure of the external ear to correct microtia (small ears) or macrotia (large ears)

II. **Surgery of the Nose and Paranasal Sinuses**
    A. **Special features of nasal surgery**
        1. Rhinoscopy and Sinusoscopy as well as computerized tomography are used to diagnose conditions related to the nose and paranasal sinuses.
        2. **Medications**
            a. Local anesthesia is frequently used.
            b. Topical 4% to 10% cocaine may be sprayed or applied with soaked sponges or cottonoids for topical anesthesia and vasoconstriction to lessen bleeding (never injected).
            c. 1% to 2% lidocaine hydrochloride (Xylocaine) with epinephrine may be used as a local anesthetic and hemostatic; phenylephrine (Neo-synephrine) may also be used to decrease bleeding.
            d. All solutions must be clearly labeled.
        3. When general anesthesia is used, aspiration of blood is prevented by placing a pack in the pharynx after the patient is intubated.
        4. Instruments must be sterile, as tissues underlying the mucosa and paranasal sinuses are sterile.
        5. Endoscopes, suction irrigators, and LASERs should be checked prior to use.
        6. To enhance hemostasis, nasal packing is left in place following nasal surgery. (*Note:* Packing may not be needed following endoscopic sinus surgery or LASER procedures because there is minimal postoperative bleeding with LASERs and excellent visualization is possible with endoscopic surgery to assure hemostasis.)
        7. Patients are taught to breathe through the mouth, avoid blowing the nose, and open the mouth to sneeze.
        8. **Procedure**
            a. *Position:* supine with the head supported on a headrest
            b. *Prep:* nose, face, and neck to shoulders and to bed line; eyes are protected with ointment and lids are closed; towel may be used to cover the eyes for additional protection

c. *Draping:* drape sheet with two towels placed under the head, with upper towel wrapped around head and secured with a towel clip; split sheet is applied

d. *Special nasal instruments:* Joseph nasal saw, nasal chisels and rasps, Freer septum elevator, Takahashi forceps, Cottle single-prong and Joseph double-prong skin hooks, nasal knives, Ballinger swivel knife, nasal scissors, nasal speculum, septal forceps, antrum curettes, and nasal snare and wires

B. **Surgical procedures and related pathology**

1. Cauterization and nasal packing for epistaxis (nosebleed) (*Note:* Bleeding generally occurs at the arterial plexus in the anterior nasal septum and may be associated with trauma, hypertension, bleeding disorders, or arteriosclerosis.)

    a. Local vasoconstriction by cooling and pressure may be sufficient.

    b. Bleeder may be cauterized with the electrosurgical unit, chemical hemostatic agent, or LASER.

    c. Nasal packing may be accomplished by rolled gauze with a string secured to the center, gauze lubricated with an antibiotic, a balloon catheter, Rhinorocket (commercially prepared packing), or an absorbable gelatin sponge (Gelfoam)

    d. Ligation of the internal maxillary artery, a branch of the external carotid, may be done when other methods fail to control epistaxis.

2. *Turbinectomy:* endoscopic LASER vaporization or cauterization of the middle or inferior turbinates (concha) to treat chronic engorgement, nasal congestion, and rhinorrhea to improve breathing

3. *Polypectomy:* excision of a polyp

    a. Polyp is a benign tumor that grows on mucous membranes.

    b. Polyps obstruct ventilation, interfere with the sense of smell (anosmia), and frequently become infected.

    c. Polypectomy may be accomplished with a wire-loop snare or LASER.

4. *Nasal fracture reduction:* under anesthesia, the bone is elevated and cartilage is realigned and a splint applied

5. *Rhinoplasty:* correction of nasal deformity; may be done by otorhinolaryngologist or plastic surgeon and involves major restructuring and molding; rigid shield applied for protection; ecchymosis (black eye) results from operative trauma but is temporary

6. *Septoplasty:* repair of nasal septum

    a. May be called Septal Reconstruction or Submucous Resection (SMR)

    b. Performed to correct a deviated septum, which interferes with drainage from paranasal sinuses and breathing

    c. **Procedure:** mucous membrane and perichondrium are reflected with elevators, and some septal cartilage is excised; bone fragments are excised with a punch, rongeur, cutting forceps, or osteotome and mallet; intranasal incision is sutured; Rhinorocket or petrolatum gauze packing is inserted; dressing is placed over the nose; sometimes a metal or plastic splint is used for protection against accidental bumping

7. *Caldwell-Luc operation (antrostomy):* creation of a nasoantral window in the maxillary bone, above the canine teeth; limited to adults, and designed for aeration and permanent drainage of the maxillary sinus by gravity into the nasal fossa; diseased tissue is removed, sinus is packed with antibiotic ointment-covered gauze; one end of packing left accessible for easy removal during office visit; oral incision is closed. (*Note:* Intranasal antrostomy may also be performed by passing an antral rasp through the nasal opening leading to the maxillary sinus.)

8. *Ethmoidectomy:* drainage procedure for diseased tissue of the middle turbinate or another part of the ethmoid bone; may be approached through intranasal incision, sinuscope, or external incision from the eyebrow alongside the nose

9. *Frontal sinus surgery:* incision is made above the eye; frontal sinus trephination is performed to drain pus or fluid accumulation; further surgery may be required to remove the lining of the sinus and reconstruct the nasofrontal duct to improve drainage; sinus cavity may be packed with a fat graft.

10. *Functional endoscopic sinus surgery (FESS)*
    a. Used to visualize paranasal sinuses and lateral nasal walls, for removal of polyps, to establish drainage procedures, and to repair the septum or turbinate
    b. Performed under topical and local anesthesia
    c. Provides optimum light through fiberoptics and small scope
    d. Suction/irrigation device permits unobstructed viewing
    e. Inserted intranasally and advanced to frontal, ethmoid, or sphenoid sinuses or through the canine fossa to the maxillary sinus; may use navigation system to aid in identification of pathology
    f. Hemostasis is controlled with epinephrine, ESU, or a LASER
    g. Packing may not be necessary

III. **Surgery of the Oral Cavity and Throat**

A. **Special features**
    1. Mouth is not a sterile area, but the best possible aseptic technique should be followed.
    2. Anesthesiologist is working in the same general area.
    3. Patient placed in the supine position; arms may be tucked at the side or extended on an armboard; head may be slightly raised or a rolled sheet or towel placed under the shoulders to extend the neck.
    4. **Skin preparation:** generally not required
    5. **Draping:** folded sheet with two towels under the head, with top one drawn up to cover the hair and eyes and clipped in place; one sheet covering the body
    6. Suction and electrosurgical unit must be available; moist pack is often placed in the pharynx if patient has an endotracheal tube in place.
    7. Postoperative bleeding necessitates positioning patient to allow blood to flow out of the mouth before consciousness is regained (on side with patient in slight Trendelenburg position).
    8. If topical anesthesia is used, the patient may be in a sitting position for surgery.
    9. Extreme care is taken to avoid leaving a sponge in the pharynx, as it could occlude the airway.

B. **Surgical procedures**
    1. *Uvulopalatopharyngoplasty (UPPP):* resection of the uvula, palatine tonsils, and mucosa from the posterior margin of the soft palate to correct obstructive sleep apnea (during sleep, the soft tissue falls back to obstruct the patient's airway). Table setup is similar to that for a Tonsillectomy.
    2. *Adenoidectomy:* removal of adenoids (pharyngeal tonsils found in nasopharynx)
        a. Common procedure in children; may be combined with Tonsillectomy (T&A)
        b. **Indications:** recurrent otitis media and chronic adenoiditis/adenoid hypertrophy—enlarged and inflamed tissue blocks the nasopharyngeal meatus of the Eustachian tubes
        c. **Anesthesia:** general with endotracheal intubation
        d. Adenoids are resected with an adenotome, curette, or punch; may be vaporized with a CO_2 LASER.
        e. Bleeding is controlled with ESU and pressure of gauze sponges, which may be soaked in epinephrine.

3. *Tonsillectomy:* surgical removal of the palatine tonsils in the oropharynx
   a. *Indications:* hypertrophied or chronically infected tonsils
   b. *Position:* supine, slight Trendelenburg
   c. *Anesthesia:* general with endotracheal tube
   d. Adult may be positioned in semi-Fowler and given local anesthesia; throat is anesthetized with a topical spray and local infiltration
   e. *Procedure:* mouth is retracted with a mouth gag; tongue is depressed (adenoids are removed first in a combined procedure), tonsils are grasped, dissected free; fossa is packed with a tonsil sponge to tamponade bleeding. (*Note:* dissection may be done with a snare, knife, ESU, or Harmonic Scalpel.)
   f. Special T&A instruments include mouth gags (Jennings, Davis, McIver, Denhart), Hurd tonsil dissector/Pillar retractor, uvula retractor, adenotome, tonsil snare and wire, fisher knife or #7 handle with #12 blade, adenoid curettes, and tonsil hemostats (Schnidt)
4. *Laryngoscopy:* direct visualization of the larynx with a laryngoscope; biopsy may be taken, polyps removed, secretions aspirated, and bleeding controlled
5. *Microlaryngoscopy:* use of a microscope and microsurgical instruments for minor surgery of the vocal cords; accommodates use of the CO_2 LASER (all LASER precautions should be taken)
6. *Bronchoscopy:* direct visualization of the bronchi with a flexible or rigid bronchoscope; performed under local anesthesia; bronchial washings, removal of foreign bodies, or biopsies may be done through the scope; rigid scope is commonly used for retrieval of foreign body; Lukens trap is useful in collecting specimens by connecting to suction tubing
7. *Esophagoscopy:* direct visualization of the esophagus through a flexible or rigid scope inserted through the mouth to the esophagus. Indications are diagnosis, removal of a foreign body or polyp, and dilation of strictures.
8. *Glossectomy/Hemiglossectomy:* surgical removal of the tongue for malignancy; may be done with CO_2 LASER to reduce blood loss
9. *Mandibulectomy:* partial or total removal of the lower jaw for extension of tumor into bone. It may be performed with Glossectomy and Radical Neck Dissection (Commando's operation).

IV. **Surgery Related to the Neck**
   A. **Related anatomy and physiology**
      1. *Larynx (voice box)*
         a. Located in upper part of the neck, between the pharynx and trachea
         b. Functions: passageway for air and voice, and to close off air passage during swallowing (epiglottis)
         c. Composed of nine separate cartilages (thyroid, cricoid, epiglottic, and two each arytenoid, corniculate, and cuneiform)
      2. *Vocal cords:* controlled by intrinsic muscles; innervated by the recurrent laryngeal nerve branch of the Vagus (X) Nerve. (*Note:* Paralysis or division of both recurrent laryngeal nerves causes a total airway obstruction, necessitating a tracheostomy.)
      3. *Glottis:* space between vocal cords

SURGERY HINT

Many surgical procedures on the throat or larynx are done with the surgeon at the head of the table. Generally, anesthesia will be on one side, and the ST will pull up on the opposite side. Make sure that the back table is set up with this configuration in mind.

Any surgical intervention that enters both the mouth and the neck should have separate setups for each stage. The mouth is considered a "dirty" area, while neck dissection must remain sterile.

4. Blood is supplied from branches of the external carotid and subclavian arteries

5. *Laryngeal ligaments:* connect the larynx to the hyoid bone and the different laryngeal cartilages to each other

6. Tongue is connected to the hyoid bone; during swallowing, the larynx is pulled upward and closed off by the epiglottis.

7. *Trachea (windpipe):* extends from larynx to the carina (bifurcation of the trachea into the right and left bronchi)
   a. Contains C-shaped cartilage rings, with incomplete section resting against the esophagus (cartilage keeps the airway patent)
   b. Cricoid cartilage of the larynx serves as the first tracheal ring, is complete, and is used (by pressure) to close off the esophagus to prevent aspiration in an unconscious person—Sellick's maneuver
   c. Thyroid gland isthmus is anterior to the upper trachea
   d. Brachiocephalic and left common carotid arteries lie close to the trachea, posing a surgical hazard

8. *Salivary glands:* located in the walls of the oral cavity; produce saliva, which is carried by ducts into the oral cavity to moisten food; facilitate deglutition (swallowing); and begin digestion of starches
   a. *Sublingual:* paired salivary glands which lie beneath the tongue
   b. *Submandibular:* lies beneath the posterior half of the mandible
   c. *Parotid:* largest; lies alongside the ear. Stensen's duct pierces the buccinator muscle of cheek to enter the mouth; Facial Nerve (VII) passes through it, and blood is supplied by the superficial temporal artery and branches of the external carotid artery

9. *General structures of the neck*
   a. **Platysma:** muscle sheet lies beneath the subcutaneous skin of the neck from the anterior chest to the mandible and corners of the mouth
   b. Deep cervical fascia surrounds the neck and attaches to the trapezius and sternocleidomastoid muscles
   c. Pretracheal fascia lies within the strap muscles (sternothyroid, sternohyoid, and omohyoid) and fuses with the carotid sheath (surrounds the carotid arteries and Vagus (X) Nerve)
   d. Cervical lymph glands: closely associated with salivary glands, jugular veins, larynx, and thyroid
   e. **Thyroid gland:** located in the anterior neck on either side of the trachea; united by the isthmus, which lies over the trachea; has four major blood supplies (superior thyroid arteries branch off the external carotids, and the inferior thyroid arteries ascend from the subclavians); essential for the body's metabolism
      i. **Hyperthyroidism:** Graves' Disease
      ii. **Hypothyroidism:** deficiency of thyroid hormone (myxedema in adults, cretinism in children)
      iii. **Goiter:** enlarged thyroid due to deficiency of iodine, a mineral essential in the production of thyroxin
      iv. Deficiency of hormones is treated by administration of hormones.
      v. Hyperactivity is treated by surgical removal, medication, or administration of radioactive iodine to decrease function.
   f. **Parathyroid glands:** four small glands embedded in the posterior thyroid (two on each side); may be as many as 10 located along the neck
      i. **Function:** regulation of calcium and phosphorus metabolism
      ii. Primary hyperparathyroidism is associated with hypercalcemia (secondary to kidney, skeletal, or GI disease).

B. **Preparation for surgery**
   1. *Position:* supine with shoulder roll, head hyperextended
   2. *Prep:* male patients shave, skin prep begins with neck and extends to hairline, to nipples, and bed line

3. *Anesthesia:* general; for certain radical procedures (Laryngectomy) anesthesia is administered directly into trachea through a Tracheotomy
4. *Instrumentation:* minor set plus specialty instruments
5. *Draping:* crushed towels on either side of the neck, head drape, and split sheet

C. **Surgical procedures and related pathology**
   1. *Supraglottic Laryngectomy*
      a. Surgical removal of the epiglottis, false cords, and hyoid bone
      b. **Indications:** tumor of the epiglottis
      c. **Temporary Tracheotomy:** done before excision of diseased tissue to avoid aspiration and combat effects of postoperative edema
   2. *Hemilaryngectomy:* removal of one true cord, one false cord, arytenoid, and half of thyroid cartilage
   3. *Total Laryngectomy*
      a. Removal the larynx, hyoid bone, cricoid cartilage, two or three tracheal rings, and strap muscles
      b. **Indication:** malignancy of the larynx
      c. Permanent Tracheostomy with closure of pharyngeal opening to trachea
         i. Patient breathes through a stoma at the base of the neck. (Air is no longer humidified by the nose, and olfactory sense is lost.)
         ii. Temporary nasogastric feeding tube is necessary.
      d. Loss of voice; prosthesis for speech can be used
      e. **Surgical hazard:** rupture of the carotid artery
   4. *Tracheotomy:* opening into the trachea with insertion of a cannula to provide a patent airway or bypass a mechanical obstruction
      a. Emergent or elective procedure
      b. **Procedure:** transverse incision (better cosmetic effect) between the cricoid cartilage and suprasternal notch; thyroid isthmus is retracted or divided; trachea is incised and suctioned; tracheotomy tube, with obturator, is inserted; obturator is removed, liner is inserted, and outer cannula is suctioned; wound edges may be closed; split dressing is applied around the tracheotomy tube, and outer cannula secured around the neck with tape (snug, but not tight); procedure may also be performed pericutaneously
      c. **Precautions:** a tracheotomy set and sterile tube; identical to the one inserted; must accompany the patient from the OR; only sterile equipment is used to suction the tracheotomy; suction is applied only during withdrawal of the suction catheter; humidified air is essential. (*Note:* Any patient having extensive surgery on the face or neck must have a tracheotomy set, with all essential equipment, at the bedside for 24 to 48 hours postoperatively.)
   5. *Subtotal Thyroidectomy:* removal of approximately five-sixths of the thyroid gland to treat hyperthyroidism
   6. *Thyroid Lobectomy:* excision of an entire lobe for benign tumor or toxic diffuse goiter
   7. *Thyroidectomy:* removal of the thyroid gland for malignancy or to relieve compression on the trachea or esophagus
      a. *Transverse incision:* "collar" incision made in the crease of the neck 1 inch above the suprasternal notch (silk suture may be pressed against

---

SURGERY HINT

When the tracheotomy is being performed, the endotracheal tube will be removed. Until the tracheotomy is inserted, the patient airway is compromised. If retracting with tracheal hooks, care must be taken that the hooks remain in the position placed. If retraction is lost, the patient airway is also lost. For patients on a vent, the vent will be connected to the tracheotomy.

the neck to mark the line of incision); bleeding is controlled with curved hemostats or the electrosurgical unit

  b. *Procedure:* platysma muscle is incised and retracted; strap muscles are separated with blunt and sharp dissection; thyroid lobe is elevated with a Lahey tenaculum, and the sternocleidomastoid muscle is retracted with Green retractor; inferior and middle thyroid vein and the superior and inferior thyroid arteries are identified, clamped, and ligated; care is taken to identify and preserve the recurrent laryngeal nerve; thyroid gland is freed from the trachea and delivered as a specimen; strap muscles are approximated with an interrupted suture; Penrose drain may be inserted in the thyroid bed and brought to the outside; platysma is approximated; skin is closed with staples, or a nonabsorbable suture and a collar-type dressing is applied

  c. *Special thyroid instruments:* Lahey tenaculum, Green thyroid (loop) retractor, Lahey thyroid retractor, and Beckman self-retaining retractor

  d. *Surgical hazards*
    i. Accidental removal of parathyroid glands with resulting tetany
    ii. Damage to one or both recurrent laryngeal nerves with paralyzed vocal cord(s) and completely obstructed airway
    iii. Thyroid storm from excessive manipulation of a toxic gland
    iv. Hemorrhage from major arteries in the neck
    v. Tracheal edema with resultant obstructed airway

  e. *Postoperative position:* Fowler

8. *Parathyroidectomy:* removal of one or more parathyroid glands for adenoma or hypersecretions of parathormone

9. *Thyroglossal duct cystectomy:* removal of a pretracheal cystic pouch attached to the hyoid bone and, when present, the sinus tract, an embryological remnant from the descent of the thyroid gland into the anterior neck. Surgical setup similar to that for a Thyroidectomy

10. *Scalene node biopsy:* incision is made just above the clavicle, and biopsy is taken to determine the spread of tuberculosis or cancer from the lungs.

11. *Radical neck dissection/modified radical neck dissection:* excision of all lymph tissue from the midline to the trapezius muscle and clavicle, deep cervical fascia, and platysma muscle (except carotid artery system), jugular vein, spinal accessory nerve, sternocleidomastoid muscle, and submandibular gland. Several incisions are used depending on the location of nodes. Macfee, Latyschvsky, freund, babcock, martin, and crile are several of the incisions implemented during radical neck dissection surgery.

  a. **Indication:** malignant tumors of the mouth or pharynx or skin cancer in the head or neck region

  b. Closed vacuum drainage system used postoperatively

  c. Tracheotomy may be performed.

  d. Feeding tube may be inserted.

  e. **Complications of surgery:** injury to a major vessel or thoracic duct and emotional problems related to disfigurement from surgery

12. *Excision of submaxillary gland*

  a. *Incision* is made in the neck beneath the chin

  b. *Indication:* mixed tumors or multiple calculi

  c. *Procedure* similar to Parotidectomy

13. *Parotidectomy*

  a. **Incision:** Y-type on either side of the ear

  b. Fine-toothed forceps and scissors used to elevate the skin, which is retracted with a suture

  c. Blunt dissection is used to identify and protect the superficial temporal artery and vein, external jugular vein, and Facial (VII) Nerve.

  d. Nerve stimulator is used to identify all branches of the facial nerve to avoid inadvertant damage.

  e. Drain may be left in place and pressure dressing applied.

V. **Maxillofacial Surgery**

  A. **Fractures of the face and cranium require multidisciplinary teams led by the plastic surgeon**

  B. **Midface advancement:** neurosurgeon and plastic surgeon work together to separate the facial skeleton from the cranial base, advance it in three dimensions, and stabilize it with a plating system or wire it into position; performed for facial deformities.

  C. **Midfacial fracture**

   1. Suspected when the patient complains of pain, malocclusion of the jaws, or diplopia (double vision)

   2. **Le Fort classification of facial fractures**

    a. *Le Fort I:* transverse fracture of the maxilla with fractures to the palate and alveoli, sometimes referred to as a "moustache" fracture

    b. *Le Fort II:* fracture of the frontal process of the maxillae, nasal bones, and orbital floor

    c. *Le Fort III:* fracture of both zygomas, maxillae, nasal, ethmoid, sphenoid, and other orbital bones

   3. Fractures must be reduced and immobilized

   4. **Priorities:** airway, cervical spine injury, and hemorrhage

  D. **Reduction of nasal fractures:** may accompany other fractures; depressed bone is raised with nasal packs and an external splint

  E. **Reduction of zygomatic fracture:** common; involves orbital bones which are unstable; internal reduction is accomplished with counterpressure below the arch; micro plates and screws **commonly used for** fixation; also called Malar fractures

  F. **Intermaxillary fixation of a fracture:** immobilized with interdental wiring if the patient has upper and lower teeth. (*Note:* Edentulous patients would have open reduction and skeletal fixation by circumferential wiring over an intraoral splint or screws and connecting bars. Maxillary and mandibular fractures are usually immobilized by interdental wiring.)

   1. Nasal intubation is performed for delivery of general anesthesia.

   2. **Erich arch bars** are shaped and placed along the dental arches.

   3. Wires (#25 or #26) are passed between the teeth to anchor the arch bars. Wires should be loaded onto a Rubio needle driver

   4. Elastic bands are placed around lugs (projections) of upper and lower arch bars to hold teeth together.

   5. Pair of heavy scissors must accompany the patient from OR and remain at bedside until wires and bands are removed (used to cut the elastics if the patient vomits or has respiratory difficulty).

  G. **Mandibular fracture:** can be immobilized transorally with compression plates and screws

  H. **Orthognathic surgery:** reshaping or repositioning of the jaws to correct a malocclusion or for cosmetic purposes

   1. *Indications:*

    a. *Prognathism:* jaw projecting forward

    b. *Retrognathism:* receding chin

    c. *Apertognathia:* open bite created by the back teeth coming together first, thus preventing closure of the front teeth

    d. *Micrognathia:* dental arch is too small to accommodate the teeth, causing them to be pushed out of alignment or crowded together.

    e. *Asymmetry:* imbalance between the right and left side of the face due to a discrepancy in the size, shape, or position of the jaws

I. *Temporomandibular joint (TMJ) syndrome*
   1. *Associated with stress:* related to bruxism (grinding of teeth), position of teeth, trauma, arthritis, or malocclusion
   2. *Diagnosis:* CT scan, MRI, and arthroscopy
   3. *Arthroscopy:* 1.7- or 1.9-mm scope with camera attached is inserted into TMJ through an incision in the joint capsule; continuous inflow and out-flow of Ringer's solution used to distend the joint for visibility and for irrigation; synovectomy, partial meniscectomy, and lysis of adhesions may be accomplished through the scope.
   4. *Arthroplasty:* the TMJ may be reshaped or resurfaced through a preauricular or postauricular incision. The TMJ may also be replaced with a prosthesis.

VI. **Dental Surgery**

A. **Terminology**
   1. *Alveoloplasty:* surgical contouring of alveolar processes and repair of the tooth sockets in preparation for dentures
   2. *Apertognathia (apert: to open; gnathia: jaw):* open bite
   3. *Bruxism:* unconscious grinding of the teeth
   4. *Edentulous:* without teeth
   5. *Gingivectomy:* surgical excision of a portion of the gums to remove deep pockets of inflamed tissue or plaque
   6. *Malocclusion:* misfit of upper and lower teeth
   7. *Odontectomy:* surgical excision of a tooth or teeth (*Note:* In surgery, Odontectomy usually refers to the removal of impacted third molars—"wisdom" teeth.)
   8. *Oral surgeon:* one who removes teeth and performs minor surgery in the oral cavity; some perform dentofacial procedures
   9. *Orthodontist:* one who straightens teeth and corrects malocclusions and associated facial problems
   10. *Orthognathia (orth/o: straight; gnathia: jaw):* branch of oral medicine dealing with bones of the jaw
   11. *Periodontist:* one who treats diseases of the gums and alveoli surrounding the teeth
   12. *Prosthodontist:* one who restores intraoral and external facial structures with prostheses

B. **Special considerations**
   1. **Anesthesia:** general
   2. **Position:** supine
   3. **Drape:** head drape and sheet—as for a Tonsillectomy
   4. Pharynx is packed with saline-moistened packing (ensure removal upon completion of the procedure).
   5. Hemostasis is provided by local injection of epinephrine, suctioning, suturing of the gum, and packing.
   6. **Instruments:** minor set and dental instruments (elevators, picks, probes, forceps, and mouth props); drill used to fracture impacted teeth for removal

Show What You Know

Directions
Each of the numbered items or incomplete statements in this section is followed by answers or by completions of the statement. Select the ONE lettered answer or completion that is BEST in each case.

1. The incision used for a Thyroidectomy is:
   A. postaural
   B. eyebrow
   C. Y-type incision on either side of the ear
   D. collar

2. The knife used to make an opening into the eardrum is:
   A. scalpel with #12 blade
   B. Fisher knife
   C. Myringotomy knife
   D. Ballinger swivel knife

3. Careful dissection around the Facial (VII) Nerve and its branches is essential in which of the following procedures?
   A. Parotidectomy
   B. Thyroidectomy
   C. Caldwell Luc Procedure
   D. Turbinectomy

4. With which of the following procedures should a patient be instructed to avoid blowing the nose, coughing, sneezing, swimming, and air travel?
   A. Stapedectomy
   B. Thyroglossal Duct Cystectomy
   C. Radical Neck Dissection
   D. Parathyroidectomy

5. Which of the following statements is true of cocaine hydrochloride?
   A. a 5% solution of cocaine may be injected as a local anesthetic
   B. it is used topically as an anesthetic and to lessen bleeding
   C. it is mixed with epinephrine and given IV
   D. it is applied to the postoperative dressing

6. A disease associated with bone conduction hearing loss whereby the stapes become fixed is:
   A. Epistaxis
   B. Acoustic Neuroma
   C. Ménière's Disease
   D. Otosclerosis

7. Benign tumors that grow on a stalk and can be found on mucous membranes are called:
   A. turbinates
   B. polyps
   C. adenoids
   D. scalene nodes

8. The surgical procedure done to straighten a deviated septum in the nose is a/an:
   A. Antrostomy
   B. Sphenoidectomy
   C. Submucous Resection
   D. Mastoidectomy

9. Immediately following surgery of the mouth or pharynx, before consciousness is regained, the patient is positioned:
   A. in the lateral position with slight Trendelenburg
   B. in the supine position with arms extended
   C. in a high Fowler position
   D. in the prone position

10. The surgical procedure done to correct sleep apnea (absence of breathing for periods during sleep) is:
    A. Laryngectomy
    B. Tracheotomy
    C. Rhinoplasty
    D. Uvulopalatopharyngoplasty

11. The laryngeal cartilage which serves as the first tracheal ring and completely encircles the trachea is the:
    A. thyroid cartilage
    B. cricoid cartilage
    C. epiglottis
    D. arytenoid cartilage

12. The salivary glands located alongside the ear and drained by Stenson's duct into the mouth are:
    A. sublingual
    B. submandibular
    C. tonsils
    D. parotids

13. Patients having neck surgery are more likely to encounter respiratory problems from edema. The equipment to accompany these patients from surgery is:
    A. suction
    B. tracheotomy set
    C. oxygen
    D. packing

14. A Tracheotomy would precede which of the following surgical procedures?
    A. Laryngectomy
    B. Parathyroidectomy

C. Labyrinthectomy

D. Turbinectomy

15. Surgical hazards associated with a Thyroidectomy include all of the following *except:*

A. damage to one or both recurrent laryngeal nerves

B. damage to the facial nerve

C. accidental removal of the parathyroid glands

D. hemorrhage from major arteries in the neck

16. Surgical contouring of the teeth sockets in preparation for dentures is:

A. Alveoloplasty

B. Dermabrasion

C. Cheiloplasty

D. Blepharoplasty

17. For which of the following fractures would Erich arch bars and 25-gauge wire be applied?

A. maxillary fracture

B. nasal fracture

C. pharyngeal fracture

D. zygomatic fracture

18. The drill used for ear surgery is a/an:

A. auraltome

B. ototome

C. auricotome

D. osteotome

19. Basic instrumentation for a Myringotomy would include all of the following *except:*

A. ear speculum

B. curette

C. myringotomy knife

D. Yankauer suction tip

20. The transparent, absorbable sponge used to support a graft in the ear is:

A. gelfoam

B. thrombin

C. surgicel

D. Gelfilm

21. The anesthetic agent NOT used during middle ear surgery after graft placement is:

A. nitrogen

B. nitrous oxide

C. oxygen

D. sevoflurane

22. The type of Tympanoplasty which involves malleus damage and a graft placed between the tympanic membrane and the incus is:

A. Type I

B. Type II

C. Type III

D. Type V

23. Tissue used for a graft over the tympanic membrane is the:

A. transversalis fascia

B. conjunctiva

C. periosteum of the mastoid bone

D. temporalis fascia

24. The nerve which may be injured during Mastoidectomy is the:

A. Facial Nerve

B. Trigeminal Nerve

C. Ocular Nerve

D. Olfactory Nerve

25. The major nerve supply to the nose is the:

A. Olfactory Nerve

B. Facial Nerve

C. Trigeminal Nerve

D. Acoustic Nerve

26. The medication used during nasal surgery which shrinks mucous membranes and relieves pain is called:

A. Neosynephrine

B. cocaine HCl

C. lidocaine HCl

D. vasopressin

27. The surgical procedure to open the maxillary sinus by way of the canine fossa for removal of the sinus contents is referred to as:

A. Sinupolypectomy

B. Rhinoplasty

C. Caldwell Luc

D. Submucous Resection

28. Excision of a concha for improved ventilation is called:

A. Submucous Resection

B. Ethmoidectomy

C. Sinus Trephination

D. Turbinectomy

29. The treatment for persistent epistaxis is:

A. Ethmoidectomy

B. Submucous Resection

C. Internal Maxillary Artery Ligation

D. none of the above

30. A Turbinectomy is performed for which of the following conditions?

A. epistaxis

B. chronic rhinorrhea

C. vertigo

D. otosclerosis

31. The major blood vessel that is in close proximity to the ear is the:

    A. aorta
    B. internal carotid artery
    C. basilic artery
    D. femoral artery

32. An accumulation of fluid in the middle ear is called:

    A. otosclerosis
    B. rhinitis
    C. otitis media with effusion
    D. tinnitus

33. The medication used during ear surgery to reduce bleeding is:

    A. heparin sodium
    B. ephedrine
    C. bupivicaine HCl
    D. epinephrine

34. The prosthesis that replaces the malleus and incus is called a/an:

    A. Partial Ossicular Replacement Prosthesis
    B. Austin Moore Prosthesis
    C. Neer Prosthesis
    D. Tragus Fascia Prosthesis

35. Which of the following procedures is *not* done for the treatment of otosclerosis?

    A. Tympanoplasty Type V
    B. Stapedectomy
    C. Labyrinthectomy
    D. Stapes Mobilization

36. Which of the following instruments is *not* used during nasal surgery?

    A. Freer elevator
    B. Ballinger swivel knife
    C. Antrum curettes
    D. aural speculum

37. Which of the following is true of an autogenous tissue graft taken from the temporalis fascia for use on the tympanic membrane?

    A. placed on a drying block to allow it to stiffen before insertion.
    B. obtained with a Kerrison rongeur and alligator forceps
    C. flattened with a bayonet
    D. polished with an ototome

38. The procedure usually performed for the diagnosis of carcinoma of the tongue would include:

    A. Hemiglossectomy
    B. Axillary Node Dissection

    C. Mandibulotomy
    D. Sialolithectomy

39. Salivary glands include which of the following?

    A. submental
    B. frontal
    C. parotid
    D. lingual

40. A sampling of the lymph nodes in the neck region is referred to as a:

    A. Modified Neck Dissection
    B. Scalene Node Biopsy
    C. Carotid Node Biopsy
    D. Lingual Tonsillectomy

41. The subcutaneous neck muscle that covers the anterior portion of the neck region from the jaw to the clavicle is called the _____ muscle.

    A. platysma
    B. deltoid
    C. sternocleidomastoid
    D. buccinators

42. Tonsillar fossa bleeders encountered during Tonsillectomy are ligated with:

    A. nylon
    B. silk
    C. prolene
    D. surgical gut

43. Preoperative testing which should be reported for the patient undergoing Tonsillectomy would be:

    A. PTT—7 minutes
    B. WBC—8,700
    C. U/A—pH 6
    D. Hematocrit—13

44. The embryologic structure of the tongue/neck region that may remain open, form a cystic pouch, and become infected is the:

    A. parathyroid duct
    B. parotid duct
    C. scalene node duct
    D. thyroglossal duct

45. To create a Tracheostomy, a transverse incision is created in the neck, just below the _____.

    A. suprasternal notch
    B. hyoid bone
    C. cricoid cartilage
    D. corniculate cartilage

46. The parotid glands are located:

    A. under and in front of each ear
    B. on the inner surface of the mandible

C. deep in the floor of the mouth

D. in the sublingual area

47. The procedure resulting in the patient's permanent loss of the ability to speak normally is a:

A. Parotidectomy

B. Tracheostomy

C. Total Laryngectomy

D. Radical Neck Dissection

48. The tissue that may be accidentally resected during a Thyroid Lobectomy is:

A. a scalene node

B. the larynx

C. parathyroid gland(s)

D. a cervical lymph node

49. The facial bone which makes up the bony structure of the outer aspect of cheek is the:

A. zygomatic

B. vomer

C. maxilla

D. mandible

50. The midface fracture which results in a "moustache" fracture is classified as a:

A. Le Fort I fracture

B. Le Fort II fracture

C. Le Fort III fracture

D. Le Fort IV fracture

51. A malar fracture is a fracture primarily involving which bone?

A. maxilla

B. zygoma

C. mandible

D. vomer

52. When performing interdental wiring for fracture fixation, which of the following is true?

A. Remove the throat pack before placement of the elastic bands on the approximating appliance (arch bars).

B. Wires are used to approximate the maxilla and the mandible against one another.

C. Potts scissors should accompany the patient at all times.

D. Oral intubation is used for delivery of general anesthesia.

53. The condition where the dental arch is too small to accommodate the teeth, causing them to be pushed out of alignment or to be crowded together, is called:

A. prognathism

B. retrognathism

C. apertognathia

D. micrognathia

Instrument Identification

54.

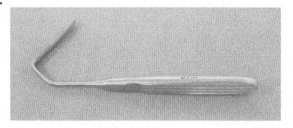

A. van Buren sound

B. Aufricht retractor

C. Hegar dilator

D. Bougie

55.

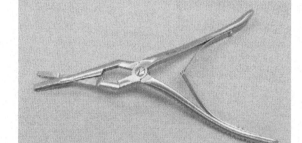

A. Takasahi forceps

B. Aufricht retractor

C. Jansen-Middleton forcep

D. nasal speculum

56.

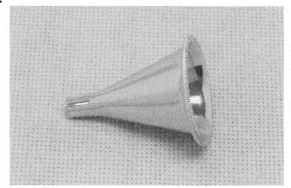

A. aural speculum
B. nasal speculum
C. vaginal speculum
D. Cottle elevator

57.

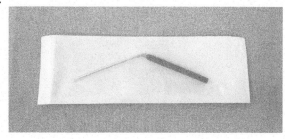

A. van Buren sound
B. Aufricht retractor
C. Hegar dilator
D. Myringtomy knife

58.

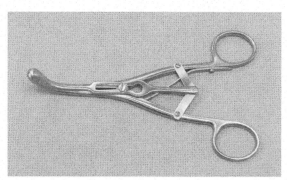

A. nasal speculum
B. Aufricht retractor
C. tracheal spreader
D. mastoid retractor

59.

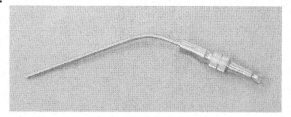

A. Ballenger swivel knife
B. Frazier suction tip
C. Myringotomy knife
D. Bougie

60.

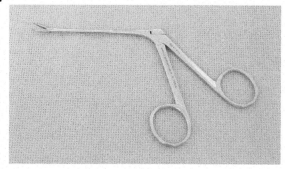

A. Frazier suction tip
B. Myringotomy knife
C. Bayonet forcep
D. Alligator forcep

Anatomy Review

Head and Neck

61–72.

A. frontal bone
B. inferior nasal concha
C. mandible
D. masseter
E. maxilla
F. middle nasal concha
G. nasal bone
H. platysma
I. sternocleidomastoid
J. temporal bone
K. trapezius
L. zygoma

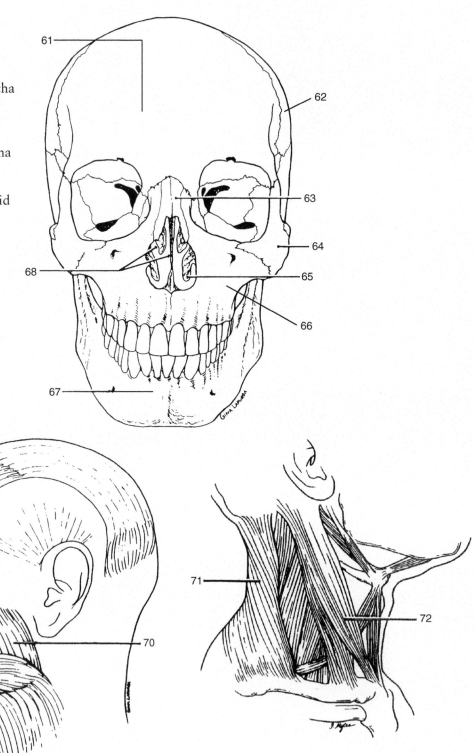

Answers & Rationales

1. **D.** **Rationale:** The collar incision made 1 inch above the suprasternal notch for removal of thyroid or parathyroid tissue provides the best cosmetic results.

2. **C.** **Rationale:** A Myringotomy knife is used to incise the eardrum (myrinx: eardrum; otomy: incision).

3. **A.** **Rationale:** The Facial (VII) Nerve penetrates the parotid gland and sends out six branches. Dissection of this nerve is the most time-consuming part of the procedure and requires the use of a nerve stimulator.

4. **A.** **Rationale:** Following ear surgery, such as a Stapedectomy, the patient must be instructed to avoid air travel, swimming, blowing the nose, coughing, and sneezing, as it would increase pressure and disrupt the anatomical revisions.

5. **B.** **Rationale:** Cocaine hydrochloride (5% solution) is used as a topical anesthetic and hemostatic in ENT surgery. It is *never* injected!

6. **D.** **Rationale:** Otosclerosis is a disease whereby the stapes become fixed (ankylosed) to the oval window. It is corrected by a Stapedectomy with prosthesis, graft replacement, or stapes mobilization.

7. **B.** **Rationale:** Polyps are benign tumors which grow on a stalk on mucous membranes and can be found in the nose.

8. **C.** **Rationale:** A Submucous Resection (SMR) is the correction of a deviated nasal septum. It may also be called a Septoplasty or Septal Reconstruction.

9. **A.** **Rationale:** Unconscious patients, especially those with bleeding in the mouth or pharynx, should be positioned on their side in a slight Trendelenburg (head-down) position to allow blood secretions to flow out. Swallowed blood can result in nausea.

10. **D.** **Rationale:** Sleep apnea occurs when excessive amounts of soft tissue surrounding the soft palate fall back to obstruct respiration during sleep. The procedure done to correct sleep apnea is a Uvulopalatopharyngoplasty.

11. **B.** **Rationale:** The cricoid cartilage is one of nine laryngeal cartilages, connects the larynx with the trachea, and completely encircles it. To block off the esophagus to prevent aspiration from stomach contents, pressure is applied to the cricoid cartilage (Sellick's maneuver), as the esophagus lies directly behind it.

12. **D.** **Rationale:** The parotid glands are located alongside the ear, produce saliva, are the most common location for mumps, and are the largest salivary glands.

13. **B.** **Rationale:** A tracheotomy set should accompany patients leaving the OR following procedures on the neck because of the serious complications of respiratory embarrassment, which may occur in the event of severe cervical edema.

14. **A.** **Rationale:** Prior to a Laryngectomy, a Tracheotomy is performed so that the anesthesiologist can intubate the trachea for administration of anesthesia. It will also remain as a permanent tracheotomy after the larynx has been removed.

15. **B.** **Rationale:** Surgical hazards associated with a Thyroidectomy include thyrotoxicosis (thyroid storm), accidental removal of the parathyroids, accidental injury to major arteries in the neck, and damage to the recurrent laryngeal nerves. The Facial (VII) Nerve does not extend to the neck.

16. **A.** **Rationale:** Alveoli are sockets in the mandible and maxilla into which teeth fit. When teeth are removed and one is fitted for dentures, the alveoli need contouring to make the dentures fit.

17. **A.** **Rationale:** Erich arch bars and 25-gauge wire will usually be used for interdental wiring to permit immobilization of the jaw when fractures occur in the maxilla or mandible. Heavy scissors should accompany the patient from the operating room, should vomiting require cutting the alignment elastics.

18. **B.** **Rationale:** The ototome is a drill used for ear surgery.

19. **D.** **Rationale:** Basic instrumentation for a Myringotomy would include all except a Yankauer suction tip.

20. **D.** **Rationale:** Gelfilm is the transparent, absorbable sponge used to support a graft in the ear.

21. **B.** **Rationale:** Nitrous oxide is not used during middle ear surgery after graft placement because it can form bubbles in the middle ear, displacing the graft.

22. **B.** **Rationale:** Type II Tympanoplasty involves malleus damage and a graft placed between the tympanic membrane and the incus.

23. D. **Rationale:** Temporalis fascia is commonly used for a graft over the tympanic membrane.

24. A. **Rationale:** The Facial (VII) Nerve travels along the roof of the mastoid process and may be injured during Mastoidectomy.

25. A. **Rationale:** The Olfactory (I) Nerve is the major nerve supply to the nose.

26. B. **Rationale:** Cocaine hydrochloride is the medication used during nasal surgery which shrinks mucous membranes and relieves pain. Neo-Synephrine is only a vasoconstrictor and Xylo-caine, without epinephrine, is only an anesthetic.

27. C. **Rationale:** Caldwell Luc is the procedure where the maxillary sinus contents are removed by accessing the sinus through the canine fossa.

28. D. **Rationale:** A Turbinectomy is a procedure where the turbinate or concha is removed to improved breathing.

29. C. **Rationale:** Internal Maxillary Artery Ligation is the procedure of choice to treat persistent epistaxis (nosebleed).

30. B. **Rationlae:** A Turbinectomy is performed for the diagnosis of chronic rhinorrhea; (rhin/o = nose and –rrhea = discharge or flow).

31. B. **Rationale:** The internal carotid artery is one of the major blood vessels located close to the ear.

32. C. **Rationale:** Otitis media with effusion is an accumulation of fluid in the middle ear.

33. D. **Rationale:** Epinephrine is used during ear surgery. It is a vasoconstrictor that is applied topically to reduce bleeding.

34. A. **Rationale:** The Partial Ossicular Replacement Prosthesis or PORP is the prosthesis used to replace the malleus and incus.

35. C. **Rationale:** A Labyrinthectomy is not a procedure done to treat otosclerosis.

36. D. **Rationale:** An aural speculum is used for ear procedures, not for nasal procedures.

37. A. **Rationale:** An autogenous tissue graft taken from the temporalis fascia would be placed on a drying block to allow it to stiffen before insertion.

38. A. **Rationale:** Hemiglossectomy is performed for the diagnosis of cancer of the tongue.

39. C. **Rationale:** The parotid gland is one of the three salivary glands.

40. B. **Rationale:** A Scalene Node Biopsy is sampling of the lymph nodes in the neck region.

41. A. **Rationale:** The subcutaneous neck muscle that covers the anterior portion of the neck region from the jaw to the clavicle is called the platysma muscle.

42. D. **Rationale:** Tonsillar fossa bleeders encountered during Tonsillectomy are ligated with surgical gut, an absorbable suture.

43. A. **Rationale:** A PTT (partial thromboplastin time) of 7 minutes is abnormal and indicates bleeding problems. This should be reported to the surgeon because one of the complications of tonsillectomy is postoperative bleeding. The other laboratory values are within normal limits.

44. D. **Rationale:** The thyroglossal duct is an embryologic structure of the tongue/neck region that may remain open, form a cystic pouch, and become infected.

45. C. **Rationale:** To create a Tracheostomy, a transverse incision is created in the neck, below the cricoid cartilage.

46. A. **Rationale:** The parotid glands are located under and in front of each ear.

47. C. **Rationale:** Total Laryngectomy is the only procedure listed that results in the patient's permanent loss of the ability to speak normally. Patients with tracheostomy tubes may be able to speak if a fenestrated tube is used.

48. C. **Rationale:** The tissue that may be accidentally resected during a Thyroid Lobectomy is one or more parathyroid glands.

49. A. **Rationale:** The zygomatic bone makes up the outer aspect of the cheek. The maxilla and mandible make up the jaw, and the vomer is located in the nasal area.

50. A. **Rationale:** The Le Fort I fracture is a midface fracture often referred to as a "moustache" fracture.

51. B. **Rationale:** A malar fracture is a fracture involving the zygoma.

52. A. **Rationale:** When performing interdental wiring for fracture fixation, remove the throat pack before placement of the elastic bands on the approximating appliance. Elastics are used to approximate the jaw, heavy scissors should accompany the patient, and a nasal intubation is performed for the delivery of general anesthesia.

53. D. **Rationale:** Micrognathia is the condition where the dental arch is too small to accommodate the teeth, causing them to be pushed out of alignment or to be crowded together.

54. **B.** **Rationale:** Aufricht retractor
55. **C.** **Rationale:** Jansen-Middleton forcep
56. **A.** **Rationale:** aural (ear) speculum
57. **D.** **Rationale:** Myringtomy knife
58. **C.** **Rationale:** tracheal spreader
59. **B.** **Rationale:** Frazier suction tip
60. **D.** **Rationale:** alligator forcep
61. **(A)** frontal bone
62. **(J)** temporal bone
63. **(G)** nasal bone

64. **(L)** zygoma
65. **(B)** inferior nasal concha
66. **(E)** maxilla
67. **(C)** mandible
68. **(F)** middle nasal concha
69. **(H)** platysma
70. **(D)** masseter
71. **(K)** trapezius
72. **(I)** sternocleidomastoid

Part II: Deciphering a Surgical Schedule

The following mock surgery schedule will be used to answer several questions pertaining to head and neck surgery. The same schedule, or a similar one, will be used in subsequent chapters to ask questions about the content of the chapter.

Rm# time	Surgeon	Procedure	Anest.	Rm# time	Surgeon	Procedure	Anest.
Rm.00				**Rm07**			
OC	Dr. Z	Rt. Knee Arthroscopy	Gen. Gen.	7:00	Dr. M	Laparoscopic appendectomy	Gen.
OC	Dr. C	Parathyroidectomy	Gen.	TF	Dr. M	Lipoma removal	MAC
OC	Dr.Z	Angioplasty	Gen.				
Rm.01				**Rm08**			
7:00	Dr. X	TMJ	Gen.	11:00	Dr. E	Bovine Thrombectomy	MAC
TF	Dr. X	Le Fort II	Gen.				
TF	Dr. X	Tracheotomy	Gen.				
Rm02				**Rm09**			
7:00	Dr. B	Splenectomy	Gen.	8:30	Dr. T	Parotidectomy	Gen.
TF	Dr. B	Gastrectomy	Gen.	TF	Dr. T	Palatoplasty	Gen.
Rm03				**Rm10**			
7:00	Dr. A	Cystoscopy	MAC	7:00	Dr. K	Nephrectomy	Gen.
TF	Dr. A	Cystoplasty	Gen.	TF	Dr. K	Choledocholithotripsy	MAC
12:30	Dr. F	Pyleogram	MAC	TF	Dr. K	Hepatic resection	Gen.
3:00	Dr. F	Cystocele repair	Gen.				
Rm04				**Rm11**			
7:00	Dr. Y	Carpal tunnel release	Gen.	7:00	Dr. L	Colposcope	Gen.
TF	Dr. Y	Whipple	Gen.	12:00	Dr. L	Mastectomy	Gen.
Rm05				**Rm12**			
7:00	Dr. G	Radical Neck Dissection	Gen.	7:00	Dr. W	Trans-metatarsal amputation	Gen.
TF	Dr. G	Tonsillectomy	Gen	TF	Dr. W	Osteotomy	Gen.
TF	Dr. G	Turbinectomy	Gen.	TF	Dr. W	Arthrocentesis	Gen.
Rm06				**Rm13**			
7:00	Dr. R	Scalene node biopsy	Gen.	7:00	Dr. O	Thyroidectomy	Gen.

The following questions should be answered using the surgery schedule above

1. The patient in Room 6 is having a scalene node biopsy. While this procedure is sometimes classified as a thoracic procedure, it may be performed by the surgeons of this specialty. Where is the incision usually made during this procedure?

    A. Midline neck
    B. Approximately 2 cm above the clavicle
    C. Approximately 2 cm below the clavicle
    D. Midline thoracic

2. There is a Parathyroidectomy in On Call status. The skin and superficial flaps will be retracted with which instrument?

    A. Weitlaner
    B. Double skin hooks
    C. Army navy retractors
    D. Alm

3. The patient in Room 9 undergoing a Parotidectomy has been positioned, and the surgeon is dissecting the neck. What structure must be identified before removing the parotid?

    A. Facial nerve
    B. Sternocleidomastoid muscle
    C. Thyroid gland
    D. Carotid artery

4. Room 5 has a radical neck dissection scheduled. What positioning device may be required for the patient?

    A. Chest rolls
    B. Mayfield
    C. Arm boards
    D. Shoulder braces

5. Before the Turbinectomy in Room 5 begins, the Surgical Technologist should have this medication ready for the surgeon.

    A. Antibiotic irrigation
    B. 0.25% bupivicaine plain
    C. 1% Lidocaine with epinephrine
    D. Heparin

6. Before the tonsillectomy begins, which instrument should the Surgical Technologist have ready for the surgeon?

    A. Mouth gag
    B. Local anesthetic
    C. Tonsil snare
    D. 2-0 vicryl

7. The Le Fort II in Room 1 will require arch bars. The Surgical Technologist should pre load 24- or 26-gauge wires onto which instrument?

    A. McGee wire crimping forceps
    B. Rubio needle driver
    C. Sternal needle holder and wire twister
    D. Hegar needle driver

8. When performing the tracheotomy scheduled in Room 1, what instrument will be placed by the surgeon before incising the trachea?

    A. The obturator
    B. Mastoid retractor
    C. Trousseau tracheal dilator
    D. Tracheal hooks

9. When placing the arch bars on the patient undergoing Le Fort II, which retractor should the Surgical Technologist hand the surgeon for retraction?

   A. Sweetheart retractor
   B. Army navy
   C. Mastoid retractor
   D. Lothrop uvula retractor

10. Which type of incision is not used in a radical neck dissection?

   A. Kocher incision
   B. Freund incision
   C. Crile incision
   D. MacFee incision

Answers & Rationales

1. **B. Rationale:** The incision for a scalene node biopsy is made approximately 2 cm above the collar bone. The nodes that will be biopsied are located near the scalene fat pads. This procedure is generally performed to check for malignancies associated with several types of cancer, including lung cancer.

2. **B. Rationale:** Generally, the surgeon will request double skin hooks to retract the skin during this procedure. The Surgical Technologist should have two ready to hand the surgeon at his request. Extreme caution must be used in handling and passing the hooks, to prevent tearing or puncturing gloves and drapes.

3. **A. Rationale:** The facial nerve must be identified before the surgery progresses. The sternocleidomastoid muscle will be retracted during the procedure, but the nerve must be identified and preserved.

4. **B. Rationale:** The patient may be positioned with a Mayfield head rest or a doughnut. A shoulder roll may be placed to aid in the hyperextension of the neck. The patient's arms will be tucked.

5. **C. Rationale:** Prior to beginning the case, the surgeon will request local anesthetic with epinephrine. Generally, the most widely used

medication for this procedure is 1% Lidocaine with epinephrine.

6. **A. Rationale:** The surgeon will request a mouth gag before the procedure begins. There are various gags available for use, so the Surgical Technologist should understand that surgeon's preferences and the components of the set will help decide which gag will be used.

7. **B. Rationale:** The Rubio needle driver is specially designed for the placement of arch bars. There would be no need for the other instruments listed. The Surgical Technologist should have the wire cutters ready for the surgeon after placement.

8. **D. Rationale:** The surgeon will carefully place the trachea hook(s) to ensure that the airway remains stable during insertion of the tracheotomy tube. The Surgical Technology must remember to test the balloon for leaks, as well as remember that the obturator must be sent to the floor with the patient.

9. **A. Rationale:** Generally, the surgeon will request a sweetheart or similar retractor to allow for visualization while placing arch bars.

10. **A. Rationale:** Macfee, freund, and crile incisions are all radical neck incisions.

PEARSON
myhealthprofessionskit™

Use this address to access the interactive Companion Website created for this book. Simply select "Surgical Technology" from the choice of disciplines. Find this book and click to enter.

16 Plastic and Reconstructive Surgery

Plastic and reconstructive surgery is a specialty concerned with restoring, restructuring, correcting, or improving the shape and appearance of body parts that are defective, damaged, or misshaped by growth and development, injury, or disease. Most people are familiar with cosmetic plastic surgery, but the specialty has a wide range with complex procedures. Many plastic surgeons specialize in reconstructive procedures that result from genetic abnormalities affecting children, to accidental disfigurements. This specialty is wide reaching and calls for the Surgical Technologist to be familiar with multiple procedures and the anatomy accompanying them.

CHAPTER OUTLINE

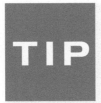

Answering questions about plastic surgery can be challenging because of the wide range of procedures involved in the specialty. When faced with these questions, first you must decipher the procedure that will be performed. This requires using medical terminology to first understand the essence of the procedure. The second step, which is similar to the other specialties, is to remember the anatomy associated with the procedure. Once this is deciphered, it then becomes easier to answer these questions. Distinctions have to be made to be successful. For example, there is a large difference in a palatoplasty and a cheiloplasty. While these surgeries are often combined, one is much more intricate than the other. To repair a cleft lip, without the cleft palate, is much less involved and does not involve the bones. This procedure may be done for cosmetic reasons, rather than for the survival of an infant. These distinctions are instrumental in answering questions related to this unique specialty.

Example:
A procedure to tighten excess skin on the lower face and neck is a

a. Rhinoplasty
b. Blepharoplasty
c. Rhytidectomy
d. Rhizotomy

To answer the question correctly, the Surgical Technologist must first look at the type of procedure being performed. A procedure to remove or tighten the skin of the lower face and neck is a facelift. Once that is established, knowledge of medical terminology is all that is required to answer the question correctly. Rhizo- is the medical term for root, in this instance; it is referring to the resection of the dorsal root of a spinal nerve, a procedure used to relieve chronic pain. Even if the ST is unfamiliar with this procedure or term, the process of elimination can work well for this question. Blepharo- is the combining word for eyelid, so this term would be used for a procedure on the eye, not the lower face. Rhino- is the word meaning nose, again, not a term used for a facelift. That would leave two possible answers: Rhytidectomy and Rhizotomy. If you recall that Rhytid- means wrinkle, you have the answer, even if you are unfamiliar with the surgical procedure.

I. Terminology

   A. *Alloplasty:* plastic surgery with nonhuman tissue

   B. *Autograft:* tissue transplanted from one part of the body to another

   C. *Blepharoplasty (blephar/o: eyelid; plasty: mold, shape):* plastic surgery on the eyelids

   D. *Cheiloplasty (cheil: lip; plasty: shape, mold):* plastic surgery on the lips

   E. *Contracture: (drawn together):* a complication in the healing of thermal burns where scar tissue prevents movement

   F. *Debridement:* excision of nonviable tissue

   G. *Dermabrasion:* "sandpapering" skin by mechanical means

   H. *Eschar:* scab or slough produced by thermal burns

   I. *Heterograft (xenograft):* porcine (pigskin) or synthetic skin graft used to protect burns during the early phase of healing

   J. *Homograft:* graft of tissue between individuals of the same species

   K. *Liposuction (lip/o: fat):* surgical removal of adipose tissue through a suction cannula

   L. *Mammopexy/Mastopexy:* surgical fixation of pendulous breasts

M. *Mentoplasty: (ment/o: chin; plasty: mold, shape):* plastic surgery on the chin

N. *Paresthesia:* prickling or tingling sensation

O. *Polydactyly:* excess number of fingers and toes

P. *Preauricular:* in front of the ear

Q. *Replantation:* reattachment of a structure or organ

R. *Rhytidectomy (rhytid: wrinkle; ectomy: surgical removal):* a face-lift

S. *Stent dressing:* cotton or fluffed gauze placed over a graft site and preplaced sutures drawn across the dressing and tied

II. **Plastic and Reconstructive Surgery**

A. **Special features**
    1. Patient anxiety
    2. Feelings and perception of physical deformity
    3. Social acceptance

B. **Preparation for surgery**
    1. *Preoperative skin preparation*
       a. Special attention should be paid to the fingernails of patients undergoing hand surgery.
       b. Special attention should be paid to the hair of the patient having surgery of the head, face, or neck (many surgeons require that the patient scrub or shower from head to toe with an antimicrobial soap the night before or morning of surgery).
       c. Oral hygiene is essential when the procedure involves the mouth.
       d. Shaving is avoided; eyebrows and eyelashes are left intact.
       e. Nonstaining prep solutions are generally used; prevent prep solutions from getting into patient's eyes.
    2. *Positioning:* access to all operative sites must be considered; adequate padding is essential for long procedures.
    3. *Draping*
       a. Wide area may be required to expose both sides for comparison.
       b. More than one incision site is frequently necessary.
       c. **Head drape:** barrier sheet with two towels is placed beneath the head, with top towel clipped around the head; diagonal towels are placed and secured alongside the neck; full sheet is used to cover the patient from head to foot.
       d. **Hand drape:** two barrier sheets are used to cover the hand table, with one forming a cuff proximally; stockinette is used to cover the involved extremity; folded sheet is placed over the upper part of the body to the stockinette and secured with clips around the upper arm; additional sheets are used to cover the remainder of the body.
    4. *Dressings*
       a. Applied while the patient is still anesthetized
       b. Used to immobilize, apply even pressure, collect drainage, provide comfort, and protect the wound
       c. Closed wound suction drains or catheters may be used, such as Jackson-Pratt, Hemovac, or butterfly cannula to rubber-tipped tube
       d. Dressings include nonadherent gauze (Adaptic, Xeroform), petrolatum gauze, Telfa, Webril, Kling, Kerlix, adhesive bandage, skin closure tape, Coban, and plaster supplies.
       e. **Stent dressings:** sutures tied over dressing to maintain position of a graft
       f. **Biological dressings:** homografts or heterografts used as temporary cover for denuded skin to help control infection, prevent serum loss, decrease pain, and stimulate growth of new tissue

5. *Anesthesia:* local, topical, regional, or intravenous sedation. Local infiltration anesthesia is given with 26- to 30-gauge needles.
6. *Effects of aspirin and smoking:* patients are asked to avoid aspirin (anticoagulant) and smoking (vasoconstrictor) for at least 2 weeks after surgery because of their effects on bleeding and wound healing.
7. *Use of photography:* photographs may be taken and/or displayed during surgery to assure symmetry and effective cosmesis.
8. *Cosmetic wounds:* cosmetic wound is enhanced by the following:
   a. Marking the incision site with sterile marking pen or sterile dye (brilliant green, methylene blue, gentian violet)
   b. Making the incision along natural body lines and contours
   c. Meticulous approximation of tissue
   d. Adequate hemostasis
   e. Small scalpel blade (#11 or #15)
   f. Small suture sizes (2-0 to 7-0); for microsurgery (8-0 to 11-0); generally synthetic nonabsorbable (nylon/polypropylene) or absorbable (Vicryl) is used; swaged needles
9. *Instrumentation, equipment, and supplies*
   a. *Instruments:* delicate, such as Iris or Stevens tenotomy scissors, mosquito hemostats, fine-tipped forceps (Brown-Adson), skin hooks or Senn retractors, and Webster needle holder
   b. *Equipment:* nerve stimulator, microscope or loupes, bipolar electrosurgical unit, and pneumatic tourniquet
   c. *Implant materials:* silicone (gel, adhesive, or performed), Dacron, Marlex, Teflon, or metals (stainless steel, Vitallium, titanium, tantalum), or ceramics
      i. Usually come with packaged sterile
      ii. Handle carefully to avoid contamination; kept lint free, oil free, and powder free; inspected for defects
      iii. Follow manufacturer's guidelines when sterilizing is necessary.
   d. *Dermatomes:* used for split-thickness skin grafts (STSGs)
      i. Knife dermatomes
      ii. **Drum-type manual dermatomes (Reese and Padgett-Hood):** restricted to use on flat or open areas but provide uniform thickness for STSG
      iii. **Motor-driven dermatomes (Brown, Padgett):** have oscillating blades that work like hair cutters with power supplied by electricity or compressed air
      - For use on firm areas such as the thighs
      - Opened up and kept on separate sterile table
      - Foot pedal is placed at surgeon's feet when ready for use and removed immediately after use.
      - Blade is inserted into the carrier, generally by the surgeon, and adjusted for desired thickness.
      - Sterile mineral oil is applied to the donor site, and the assistant holds tissue taut with a sterile tongue blade.
   e. *Skin graft mesher:* enlarges graft two to three times by making multiple uniform slits in the skin graft
      i. Used for expanding skin to cover large denuded areas
      ii. Skin, removed by a dermatome, is stretched out over plastic disposable dermacarrier and passed through rollers of the skin graft mesher.
      iii. Scrub or assistant grasps edges of the skin with Adson forceps as it is advanced.
      iv. Skin is left on the carrier and kept moist with saline until the recipient site is ready.

     f. Immediately after skin is removed, the donor site is covered with moist sponges soaked in a solution of 20 mg of Neosynephrine to 1000 ml of normal saline or sprayed with topical thrombin for hemostasis.

     g. Donor site is dressed with nonadherent gauze, moist dressings, or covered with bio-occlusive dressing.

     h. Skin may be sutured or stapled in place on the recipient site.

III. Burns

A. Types of burns
1. Thermal
2. Chemical
3. Electrical
4. Mechanical

B. Classification of burns
1. *First-degree burn:* involves epidermis; characterized by redness of skin (erythema) swelling, pain; first-aid treatment is to rinse in cold water
2. *Second-degree burn:* involves epidermis and part of dermis; characterized by redness, swelling, pain, and blisters; open for infection and loss of body fluid
3. *Third-degree burn:* involves injury to full thickness of the skin; characterized by anesthetic surface which is dry, pearly white, and/or charred; destroyed skin will slough and form eschar; requires skin grafts
4. *Fourth-degree burn:* extended beyond skin into subcutaneous tissue, muscle, or bone; requires full-thickness grafts

C. Assessment of burn damage
1. *Rule of Nines:* 9% for head and neck, and each upper extremity; 18% for anterior trunk, posterior trunk, and each lower extremity; and 1% for perineum
2. *Lund and Browder chart:* percentage of burn is based on age and anatomical location; useful in estimating burn damage in children, where percentages of body surface vary greatly

D. Initial burn care
1. Open airway is ensured; smoke-induced edema of the respiratory tract may necessitate endotracheal intubation or Tracheotomy; Bronchoscopy is routine on patients with burns around the face.
2. Venous access for IV fluids, plasma, blood, and electrolytes is established.
3. Urinary drainage for hourly output and urine checks is established.
4. Wound is cleansed; aseptic technique is essential, using mild cleansing agent in warm sterile saline or water.
5. Percentage and depth of burn is estimated.
6. Patient history is taken.

E. Operative treatment for burns
1. *Goal:* prevent infection, promote healing, and address psychological needs
2. *Excisional therapy:* debridement with scalpel, skin graft knife, dermatome, electrosurgical knife or LASER
3. Temporary application of homograft or heterograft
4. *Tangential excision:* removal of burned tissue until the normal tissue is reached; frequently used on hands, arms, and legs to minimize contractures, reduce infection and mortality, and shorten hospitalization
5. *Escharectomy:* excision of full-thickness eschar down to the fascia; denuded areas are covered with a biological dressing and later grafted with full-thickness autografts; biological dressings are not used on face, neck, or over joints

6. *Escharotomy:* bilateral incisions through eschar which has produced a tourniquet effect on an extremity or the chest; done to improve circulation
7. *Fasciotomy:* bilateral incision through the fascia to release a tourniquet effect on an extremity or the chest when Escharotomy is not adequate
8. *Grafts*
   a. *Full-Thickness Skin Graft (FTSG):* contains both epidermis and dermis, causes minimal contractures, can be used near joints, adds padding, and is more aesthetic than STSG; donor site must be closed primarily; referred to as composite or free-tissue grafts
   b. *Split-Thickness Skin Graft (STSG)*
      i. Contains epidermis and only a portion of dermis
      ii. Donor site heals more readily and can be used again as a donor site
      iii. Some postgraft contracture occurs
   c. *Flaps:* tissue for grafting removed from one part of the body and transferred to another location with its blood supply left intact
      i. Used for recipient sites with poor blood supply or to cover exposed bone, tendon, or nerve
      ii. Retains more normal skin properties
      iii. Gives bulky appearance
      iv. Classification of flaps
         • *Pedicle flap:* skin and underlying muscle rotated into distant defects
         • *Advancement flaps:* pedicle graft cut and advanced to reconstruct a defect in a nearby area
         • *Rotation flap:* pedicle flap that is widened by curving the edges of the flap
         • *Omental flap:* omentum mobilized from the peritoneal cavity and rotated to cover a defect in the chest wall
         • *Transverse Rectus Abdominis Myocutaneous (TRAM) Flap:* single-stage breast reconstruction with a flap of the rectus abdominis muscle
   d. *Tips for tissue autografts*
      i. Separate sterile setup for donor site.
      ii. Dermatome is kept on a separate small table.
      iii. Grafts must be kept moist with normal saline; avoid loss.
      iv. Free flap should be placed in iced saline slush until the recipient site is ready.
      v. Recipient site is covered with a sterile towel until ready for graft or flap.
      vi. Donor and recipient sites are prepped and draped separately and concurrently.
      vii. Patient should be kept warm.
   e. *Environmental control for the burn patient*
      i. Transported to surgery in own bed, which may be a special frame to facilitate turning with minimal pain
      ii. Reverse isolation is practiced.
      iii. Strict adherence to aseptic technique; anything touching the burned area of the patient must be sterile
      iv. Hypothermia is prevented by
         • Raising the room temperature and lowering the humidity
         • Using hyperthermia or warm blanket
         • Monitoring the patient's temperature
         • Warming the IV, irrigating, and prep solutions. (*Note:* Some prep solutions may be damaged by warming.)
      v. Physical and emotional status of the patient is considered

IV. **Surgical Procedures**

A. **Cosmetic and reconstructive procedures**

1. *Blepharoplasty:* excision of redundant skin or fat from the eyelids
    a. *Indications*
        i. **Blepharochalasis:** loss of elasticity of the skin of the eyelids
        ii. **Dermatochalasis:** hypertrophy of the skin of the upper eyelids
        iii. Protrusion of infraorbital fat into the eyelids
        iv. Hypertrophy of the orbicularis oculi muscle (horizontal bulge at the lower lid margin)
    b. *Anesthesia:* local
    c. Performed by plastic surgeon or ophthalmologist

2. *Otoplasty:* correction of external ear deformities
    a. **Indications**
        i. **Microtia:** small ears; prosthesis is available
        ii. **Macrotia:** large ears are reduced
        iii. **Trauma**
        iv. **Malignancy**

3. *Rhinoplasty:* restructuring or reshaping the nose
    a. **Indications**
        i. **Cosmetic** alteration
        ii. **Defects** following excision of malignancy

4. *Mentoplasty:* restructuring the shape and size of the chin; prosthesis is available

5. *Liposuction:* removal of adipose tissue for cosmesis with a blunt hollow metal cannula connected to suction

6. *Abdominoplasty:* excision of excess skin and adipose tissue with tightening of the abdominal wall

7. *Augmentation mammoplasty:* insertion of prosthetic implants under breast tissue or underlying muscle
    a. **Implants**
        i. Inflatable silicone sac—filled with sterile saline
        ii. Contoured sac of silicone gel
    b. **Incisions:** periareolar, transaxillary, or inframammary
    c. Bilateral augmentary mammoplasty for cosmesis; unilateral for replacement following Mastectomy

8. *Reduction mammoplasty:* excision of excess skin and glandular and adipose tissue of the breast
    a. **Indications**
        i. Hyperplasia, gigantomastia, or macromastia, which causes back pain and deep grooves in the shoulder from the weight of the breast
        ii. Asymmetry following Mastectomy

9. *Gynecomastia:* enlarged male breast tissue

10. *Cleft Lip Repair (Cheiloplasty):* rearrangement of the tissue of the lips of an infant due to a congenital anomaly
    a. *Indications:* cosmesis, sucking difficulties

11. *Cleft Palate Repair (Palatoplasty):* performed on toddlers with a congenital defect in the midline of the palatine bone to prevent the escape of air through the nose during speech, keep food and liquids out of the nose, and facilitate sucking and eating

12. *Repair of Syndactyly:* surgical separation of webbed fingers or toes

13. *Dermabrasion:* "sandpapering" of acne scars; performed with high-speed dermabrader with a rotating tip

14. *Scar revision:* excision of scars with realignment of tissue to improve appearance

15. *Excision of skin lesions:* sometimes associated with flap or grafts
    a. **Verruca:** wart
    b. **Nevus:** mole

    c. **Basal-Cell Carcinoma (BCC):** spreads but does not metastasize

    d. **Squamous-Cell Carcinoma (SCC):** capable of distant metastasis

    e. **Malignant Melanoma:** begins with a nevus which has changed in color and appearance

    f. May be performed by plastic surgeon or dermatologist

    g. Accomplished by

        i. Excision with scalpel; closed with sutures, flaps, or grafts

        ii. Electrosurgical curettage and electrodesiccation

        iii. LASER surgery

        iv. Cryosurgery

        v. Radiation therapy

16. *Rhytidectomy (facelift):* excision of redundant facial and neck skin; hypotensive anesthesia and meticulous hemostasis help decrease incidence of hematoma formation; closed-wound drainage frequently used

17. *Excision of pressure sores (decubitus ulcer):* removal of the ulcer and underlying bony prominence, followed by a skin graft (local flap) to the denuded area

    a. Occurs most frequently over the sacrum, greater trochanter, and ischial tuberosities

    b. Occurs in paraplegics or patients who lack normal sensation and lie or sit in one position for prolonged periods of time

B. Hand surgery

1. *Purpose:* restore function

    a. Replace lost tissue

    b. Restore bony structure

    c. Restore motor unit (tendon repair, graft, or transfer)

    d. Replant severed digits

    e. Repair severed nerves

2. *Surgical anatomy*

    a. *Metacarpals:* bones of the hand

    b. *Phalanges:* bones of the fingers and thumbs

        i. *MP joint:* metacarpophalangeal joint

        ii. *DIP joint:* distal interphalangeal joint

        iii. *PIP joint:* proximal interphalangeal joint

    c. *Carpals:* wrist bones (scaphoid, lunate, triquetrum, pisiform, trapezium, trapezoid, capitate, and hamate)

        i. *Radial side:* lateral aspect

        ii. *Ulnar side:* medial side

        iii. *Dorsal:* back

        iv. *Volar or palmar:* anterior

    d. *Muscle and tendons:* provide for flexion, extension, abduction, and adduction

    e. *Nerves:* motor and sensory; radial, median, and ulna

    f. *Blood supply:* radial and ulnar arteries form the palmar arch

3. *Special equipment*

    a. Pneumatic tourniquet

    b. Hand table; surgeon and assistant sit during surgery

    c. Disposable sterile system for lavage and debridement of tissue

4. *Anesthesia:* intravenous regional—Bier block

    a. Pneumatic tourniquet with double cuff (along with control valves and tubing) is needed.

    b. Esmarch bandage is used to exsanguinate the extremity; proximal cuff of the tourniquet inflated; Esmarch is removed and 0.5% lidocaine is injected IV; prepping and draping is done.

    c. Second cuff is inflated and proximal cuff is deflated to reduce patient discomfort.

5. *Dressing and immobilization*
   a. Wound healing is enhanced by elevation and immobilization
   b. Support and splinting is provided by proper immobilization of the entire hand (fingers, wrist, and distal two-thirds of the forearm) for 3 to 4 weeks postoperatively
   c. Dressing and immobilization secured while the patient is still anesthetized
   d. Steps in applying the hand dressing
      i. Assistant supports affected hand.
      ii. Nonadherent gauze is applied over the incision.
      iii. Gauze sponges (thin and of uniform thickness) are placed between the fingers, and a thicker sponge is placed between the thumb and the index finger.
      iv. Soft bulky material is placed in the hand to support PIP and DIP joints and placed across the volar and dorsal surface.
      v. Rolled gauze is wrapped around the hand and forearm with MP joints in 90° flexion, and PIP and DIP joints are extended.
      vi. Fingertips are left exposed.
      vii. Adhesive tape is applied vertically to prevent a tourniquet effect.
6. *Surgical procedures*
   a. *Open Reduction and Internal Fixation (ORIF):* for treatment of fractures
      i. Need plastic hand instrument set, Kirschner wire, mini or maxi driver, marking pen, and Esmarch bandage
      ii. **Procedure:** incision site is marked; tourniquet is inflated; incision is made to expose the fracture; fracture is reduced; Kirschner wire is driven into the bone; x-ray is taken; Kirschner wire is trimmed and twisted with needle-nosed pliers, and skin is closed; hand dressing is applied.
   b. *Tendon repair:* 3-0 or 4-0 double-armed nonabsorbable suture on Keith needles commonly used.
   c. *Flexor tendon graft:* palmaris longus tendon in the wrist and forearm is used as free graft to repair flexor tendon.
   d. *Peripheral nerve repair and grafting:* need jeweler's forceps, Castro-viejo scissors and needle holder, von Graefe muscle hook, microsurgical blade, nerve stimulator, Esmarch bandage, marking pen, loupes or operating microscope, and very fine nonabsorbable nylon sutures (7-0 to 10-0)
   e. *Implant arthroplasty:* for traumatic or rheumatoid arthritis; diseased area of joint is reamed out using Swanson burrs; prosthetic joint is placed, joint capsule is repaired, skin is closed, and dressing is applied
   f. *Palmar fasciectomy:* Z-plasty incision is made to lengthen the involved skin of the finger and palm; part of the palmar fascia is excised; tourniquet is released, and incision is closed; full-thickness skin graft may be required. Indications: Dupuytren's Contracture (progressive disease of the palmar fascia which causes severe flexion contractures—"trigger finger").
   g. *Microsurgery:* operating microscope and special instruments are used for tissue replantation; this is a long procedure, requiring microvascular sutures.

SURGERY HINT

Always test the mini or maxi driver before handing to the surgeon. Face the driver away from the field and any personnel in the room when testing. Be familiar with the Jacobs chuck and key before loading wires.

Show What You Know

Directions
Each of the numbered items or incomplete statements in this section is followed by answers or by completions of the statement. Select the ONE lettered answer or completion that is BEST in each case.

1. When tissue is taken from one part of the body and grafted to another, it is called a/an:

   A. xenograft
   B. autograft
   C. allograft
   D. heterograft

2. The scab or slough produced by a thermal burn is called:

   A. contracture
   B. plume
   C. paresthesia
   D. eschar

3. The medical term for a facelift is:

   A. Rhytidectomy
   B. Lipectomy
   C. Mentoplasty
   D. Rhizotomy

4. All of the following are hand procedures *except*:

   A. Release of Dupuytren's Contracture
   B. Carpal Tunnel Release
   C. Palmar Fasciotomy
   D. Le Fort III

5. Homografts or heterografts used as temporary coverings for denuded skin are called:

   A. biological dressings
   B. stent dressings
   C. hand dressings
   D. flaps

6. The removal of devitalized tissue is:

   A. dermabrasion
   B. escharotomy
   C. fasciotomy
   D. debridement

7. A burn patient is brought to the OR with an arm greatly charred and distended with cyanotic fingers. Which of the following procedures would you anticipate?

   A. full-thickness skin graft
   B. escharotomy
   C. dermabrasion
   D. conization

8. Tissue transfer from one part of the body to another with the graft tissue's blood supply left intact is called a/an:

   A. split-thickness skin graft
   B. pedicle graft
   C. full-thickness skin graft
   D. xenograft

9. Blepharoplasty would be indicated for a patient with:

   A. microtia
   B. macromastia
   C. hypertrophy of the orbicularis oculi
   D. strabismus

10. Special fine-tipped forceps used in plastic surgery include:

    A. Senn
    B. Brown-Adson
    C. Webster
    D. Stevens

11. Which of the following skin closure materials would be most appropriate for use in hand surgery?

    A. staples
    B. 0 chromic gut on a cutting needle
    C. 5-0 nylon on a cutting needle
    D. 2-0 Vicryl on a taper needle

12. What supplies would be needed for a STSG?

    A. heparin, 5-0 chromic suture
    B. Marlex mesh, Lugol's solution
    C. methylene blue, cryoprobe
    D. mineral oil, wooden tongue blade

13. The device used to expand a skin graft by making multiple uniform slits is a:

    A. Reece dermatome
    B. Marlex mesh
    C. skin graft mesher
    D. dermabrader

14. A TRAM flap would be used for which type of surgery?

    A. Breast Reconstruction
    B. Repair of Syndactyly
    C. Palatoplasty
    D. Cheiloplasty

15. Release of a "trigger finger" due to contraction of the palmar fascia is technically referred to as a/an:

    A. Metacarpal Arthroplasty
    B. Dupuytren's Contracture Release
    C. Carpal Tunnel Release
    D. Bankart Procedure

16. During Peripheral Nerve Repair, which of the following sutures would commonly be used?

    A. chromic gut
    B. silk
    C. nylon
    D. stainless steel

17. Another name for an intravenous regional anesthetic block is:

    A. Bier Block
    B. Le Fort Block
    C. TMJ Block
    D. Esmarch Block

18. Another name for a "mole" is a:

    A. verruca
    B. nevus
    C. microtia
    D. dermatochalasis

19. A burn that involves the epidermis and part of dermis layers of the skin and is characterized by redness, swelling, pain, and blisters is called a:

    A. first-degree burn
    B. second-degree burn
    C. third-degree burn
    D. fourth-degree burn

20. Surgery to change the shape of the chin is called:

    A. Rhytidectomy
    B. Cheiloplasty
    C. Mastopexy
    D. Mentoplasty

21. Burns are assessed using which of the following assessment techniques?

    A. Rule of Nines
    B. Brown and Sharp
    C. STSG
    D. ORIF

22. Brown and Padgett are examples of which type of equipment used for skin grafting?

    A. knife dermatome
    B. drum dermatome
    C. motor dermatome
    D. mesher

23. Otoplasty is performed for which of the following diagnoses?

    A. otosclerosis
    B. microtia
    C. blepharochalasis
    D. syndactylism

24. Which of the following bones is NOT one of the carpal bones?

    A. pisiform
    B. hamate
    C. scapula
    D. scaphoid

25. A xenograft for human skin replacement most commonly comes from which animal?

    A. horse
    B. cow
    C. goat
    D. pig

Answers & Rationales

1. **B.** **Rationale:** When tissue is grafted from one part of the body to another, it is called an autograft.

2. **D.** **Rationale:** Eschar is the scab which is produced from devitalized tissue which is sloughed from thermal burns.

3. **A.** **Rationale:** Rhytidectomy is derived from two words, rhytid/o = wrinkles, and –ectomy = to remove surgically. The general term used for rhytidectomy is *facelift*.

4. **D.** **Rationale:** Le Fort III is a procedure classification given to facial fractures in which both zygomas, maxillae, nasal, ethmoid, sphenoid, and other orbital bones are fractured. Release of Dupuytren's Contractures, Carpal Tunnel Release, and Palmar Fasciotomy are all approached from the volar surface of the hand or wrist.

5. **A.** **Rationale:** Biological dressings are composed of homografts or heterografts used as temporary dressing on denuded areas of skin to control infection, prevent loss of serum, decrease pain, and stimulate growth of new tissue.

6. **D.** **Rationale:** Removal of devitalized or nonviable tissue, or debridement, may be accomplished by a scalpel, skin graft knife, dermatome, electrosurgical knife, or LASER.

7. **B.** **Rationale:** An escharotomy is a bilateral incision through eschar, which completely encircles an area such as an extremity or chest, causing a constricting or tourniquet effect and cutting off circulation. An escharotomy relieves the constricting effect, and the wounds are left open.

8. **B.** **Rationale:** A pedicle graft is a transfer graft of tissue from one part of the body to another with the graft tissue's blood supply remaining intact.

9. **C.** **Rationale:** Blepharoplasty, revision of the eyelids, is indicated when the orbicularis oculi muscle is overdeveloped (hypertrophied), the skin of the eyelids has lost its elasticity (blepharochalasis), the skin of the eyelids hypertrophies (dermatochalasis), and infraorbital fat protrudes into the eyelid.

10. **B.** **Rationale:** Brown-Adsons are fine-tipped forceps used in plastic surgery. Senns are rake retractors, Websters are needle holders, and Stevens are tenotomy scissors.

11. **C.** **Rationale:** A small-gauge nylon suture with a cutting needle is preferred by plastic surgeons because it is monofilament (less wicking action), has elasticity (stitches stretch as tissue swells during the inflammatory phase), and provides better cosmetic results. A cutting needle is essential in suturing the skin of the hand.

12. **D.** **Rationale:** During a split thickness skin graft, mineral oil is applied to the donor site, and the skin is held taut with a sterile wooden tongue blade when taking the graft.

13. **C.** **Rationale:** The skin graft mesher expands a skin graft by making multiple uniform slits.

14. **A.** **Rationale:** A Transverse Rectus Abdominis Myocutaneous (TRAM) Flap is used during breast reconstruction following Mastectomy.

15. **B.** **Rationale:** A Dupuytren's Contracture Release is the technical name for the release of a "trigger finger" due to contraction of the palmar fascia.

16. **C.** **Rationale:** Nylon suture is the material commonly used to repair peripheral nerves. Stainless steel is too difficult to work with and might damage the nerve; silk is braided and would drag on the delicate tissues, and chromic gut causes adhesions to form due to the reaction of the tissue to its presence.

17. **A.** **Rationale:** A Bier Block is a method for the delivery of intravenous regional anesthetic.

18. **B.** **Rationale:** Nevus is another name for a mole. A verruca is a wart.

19. **B.** **Rationale:** A burn that involves the epidermis and part of dermis layers of the skin and is characterized by redness, swelling, pain, and blisters is called a second-degree burn.

20. **D.** **Rationale:** A Mentoplasty is a surgical procedure that involves changing the shape of the chin (ment/o = chin).

21. **A.** **Rationale:** The rule of nines is used to assess burns; there are 11 sections, each of which comprises 9% of the total adult body surface. The perineum comprises the last 1%.

22. **C.** **Rationale:** Brown and Padgett are motor dermatomes used for skin grafting.

23. **B.** **Rationale:** Otoplasty is performed for the diagnosis of microtia (micro– = small, ot/o = ear, –ia = condition of).

24. **C.** **Rationale:** The pisiform, hamate, and scaphoid are all carpal bones. The scapula is a bone of the shoulder girdle.

25. **D.** **Rationale:** Porcine (pig) grafts are xenografts commonly used for human skin replacement.

Part II: Deciphering a Surgical Schedule

The following mock surgery schedule will be used to answer several questions pertaining to plastic and reconstructive surgery. The same schedule, or a similar one, will be used in subsequent chapters to ask questions about the content of the chapter.

Rm. # time	Surgeon	Procedure	Anest.	Rm. # time	Surgeon	Procedure	Anest.
Rm.00				**Rm07**			
OC	Dr. Z	STSG	Gen.	7:00	Dr. M	Laparoscopic	Gen.
OC	Dr. C	Craniotomy	Gen.	TF	Dr. M	appendectomy	MAC
OC	Dr.Z	Angioplasty	Gen.			Lipoma removal	
Rm.01				**Rm08**			
7:00	Dr. X	Hemorrhoidectomy	Gen.	11:00	Dr. E	Abdominoplasty	MAC
TF	Dr. X	Colostomy	Gen.				
TF	Dr. X	Bowel resection	Gen.				
Rm02				**Rm09**			
7:00	Dr. B	Reduction mammoplasty	Gen.	8:30	Dr. T	FTSG	Gen.
TF	Dr. B	Breast augmentation	Gen.	TF	Dr. T	Palatoplasty	Gen.
Rm03				**Rm10**			
7:00	Dr. A	Cystoscopy	MAC	7:00	Dr. K	Nephrectomy	Gen.
TF	Dr. A	Cystoplasty	Gen.	TF	Dr. K	Choledocholithotripsy	MAC
12:30	Dr. F	Pyleogram	MAC	TF	Dr. K	Hepatic resection	Gen.
3:00	Dr. F	Cystocele repair	Gen.				
Rm04				**Rm11**			
7:00	Dr. Y	Carpal tunnel release	Gen.	7:00	Dr. L	Rhytidectomy	Gen.
TF	Dr. Y	Whipple	Gen.	12:00	Dr. L	Blepharoplasty	Gen.
Rm05				**Rm12**			
7:00	Dr. G	z-plasty for Dupuytrens	Gen.	7:00	Dr. W	Trans-metatarsal	Gen.
TF	Dr. G	contracture		TF	Dr. W	amputation	
TF	Dr. G	TRAM	Gen	TF	Dr. W	Osteotomy	Gen.
		Bletharoplasty	Gen.			Arthrocentesis	Gen.
Rm06				**Rm13**			
7:00	Dr. R	Lumbar Laminectomy	Gen.	7:00	Dr. O	Hysterectomy	Gen.

The following questions should be answered using the surgery schedule above

1. The TRAM scheduled in Room 5 will utilize which muscle to reconstruct the patient's breast?
   A. Internal oblique
   B. Pectoralis
   C. Transverse Rectus
   D. External oblique

2. Dr. T has scheduled a FTSG. Why would he opt for this instead of STSG?
   A. It will be grafted near a joint
   B. It will heal more quickly
   C. It will cause more contracture
   D. It contains less padding tissue than STSG

3. There is a STSG on call. What instrument should the Surgical Technologist have available for the surgeon to enlarge the graft?
   A. Adson forceps
   B. Mesher
   C. Dermatome
   D. Iris scissors

4. Dr. G will be performing a z-plasty. What is the reason for this procedure?

   A. To lengthen the skin
   B. To repair a tendon
   C. To repair the flexor tendon
   D. To shorten the skin

5. Dr. B has scheduled a reduction mammoplasty. What will the Surgical Technologist do with excess breast tissue?

   A. Send it to pathology
   B. Dispose of it in the kick bucket
   C. Pass it off to the circulator
   D. Place tissue from each breast into a separate container to be weighed

6. All of the following incisions may be used for the breast augmentation EXCEPT

   A. Periareolar
   B. Transaxillary
   C. Inframammary
   D. Midline

7. The most likely suture to be used in the augmentation skin closure will be

   A. Silk
   B. PDS
   C. Chromic Gut
   D. Monocryl

8. There is an Abdominoplasty scheduled for Room 8. What are the prep parameters for this procedure?

   A. Nipple to groin
   B. Neck to groin
   C. From the umbilicus to pelvis
   D. From umbilicus to knees

9. What is going to be used to prepare the skin during the skin graft?

   A. Betadine
   B. Alcohol
   C. Mineral oil
   D. Chlorohexidine

10. Room 11 has a Rhytidectomy. What position will the patient most likely be in for this procedure?

    A. Lounge chair
    B. Lateral
    C. Prone
    D. Supine

Answers & Rationales

1. **C.** **Rationale:** A TRAM flap is a common reconstructive procedure following a mastectomy. It uses the transverse rectus abdominal muscle to reconstruct the breast. This may be followed by tattooing of the aereola for cosmetic reasons.

2. **A.** **Rationale:** Using a full-thickness skin graft allows for more padding and is commonly used near a joint. The other statements are true of the split thickness grafts.

3. **B.** **Rationale:** While all of these instruments may be used during a STSG, the Mesher is the instrument that will be used to enlarge the graft before placement.

4. **A.** **Rationale:** Z-plastys are performed to lengthen skin area. They are commonly used in scar revision and to reduce the appearance of scars.

5. **D.** **Rationale:** The surgeon may request that excess breast tissue be weighed to ensure that the same amount of tissue is being removed from each breast. The Surgical Technologist must ensure that he or she does not contaminate the glove or arm of the gown when placing the tissue into the container.

6. **D.** **Rationale:** Most surgeons use a specific incision based on individual patient needs. Generally, they will be an Inframammary, Transaxillary, or Periareolar incision.

7. **D.** **Rationale:** Plastic surgery skin closures tend to be made with the goal of minimal scarring. Chromic gut would be an unlikely choice, as would PDS and silk.

8. **A.** **Rationale:** The parameters of the skin prep for an Abdominoplasty should incorporate the incision site, as well as a large area surrounding the site.

9. **C.** **Rationale:** Regardless of the skin prep solution used, the surgeon will most likely prep the donor skin with mineral oil before it is harvested.

10. **A.** **Rationale:** This procedure requires the surgeon to have several views of the operative site. Generally, the preferred position is a lounge chair or modified beach chair position with the head in a Mayfield or doughnut.

PEARSON
myhealthprofessionskit™

Use this address to access the interactive Companion Website created for this book. Simply select "Surgical Technology" from the choice of disciplines. Find this book and click to enter.

Orthopedic Surgery

Orthopedics is a branch of medicine that deals with disorders of the musculoskeletal systems, including fractures, congenital anomalies, joint diseases and injuries, neoplasms, and muscular or postural disabilities. The Surgical Technologist should have a great understanding of the skeletal system as well as tendons and ligaments. A working knowledge of saws, drills, reamers, and plating systems is also a necessity when working in this specialty. It is important to note that many times patients with fractures and joint issues have special needs. Many geriatric patients are seen with hip fractures, and the field is seeing an increase in obese patients with joint problems so severe that they require a replacement. When dealing with special populations, the Surgical Technologist must keep the particular issues in mind when positioning and padding these patients.

CHAPTER OUTLINE

Orthopedic surgery has many instruments that are specific to the specialty. The knowledge and understanding of these instruments can make or break an individual on the certification examination. While the Surgical Technologist must understand the procedures, many students and professionals stumble on the instrumentation. Knowing the accessory items in an orthopedic case is of vital importance. The vast number of instruments can be intimidating to the student and ST alike. Tip one is "DON'T PANIC!" When confronted with numerous trays for total joint replacements, many people feel overwhelmed. Remember, each tray contains numerous trial prosthetics that will not necessarily be used in the case. Understanding the order of use is the key to managing these cases.

Example:
During an ORIF, the order of instrumentation is

a. Tap, drill, plate, screw
b. Drill, tap, plate, screw
c. Plate, drill, tap, screw
d. Drill, tap, screw, plate

To answer this question, think logically. You cannot place the screw before the plate, as there would be no way of holding the plate to the bone. Knowing this, you can discard answer D. You also cannot tap a hole that has not been drilled, so question A can also be discarded from possible answers. This leaves two possibilities: answers B and C. Knowing that a plate is the end result of the surgical intervention, allows the ST to visualize the procedure. Generally, the surgeon will drill the hole; prepare it with the tap, place the plate, then screw the plate into place. Therefore, the correct answer would be B. Once the ST understands that orthopedics is a very precise specialty, the panic that some experience begins to subside.

I. Special Features of Orthopedic Surgery
   A. Diagnostic procedures
      1. **X-rays:** views include A/P (anterior/posterior), lateral (side-to-side), and oblique (at an angle)
      2. Computerized tomography (CT)
      3. Magnetic resonance imaging (MRI)
      4. Biopsy
      5. Arthroscopy
   B. Surgical pathology
      1. *Injuries*
         a. **Fractured bones:** break in continuity
         b. **Avulsion:** tearing away of ligament or tendon at the insertion site
         c. **Torn cartilage, ligament, or tendon**
         d. **Ruptured or herniated intervertebral disc**
         e. **Joint dislocation or subluxation (partially out of joint)**
            i. One or more bones at a joint are out of place.
            ii. Results from traumatic injury
            iii. Results from stretched or torn ligaments, tendons, or muscles
            iv. Causes damage to nerves, blood supply, and joint capsule
            v. Generally treated by closed reduction
            vi. Open reduction may be necessary for recurrent dislocation as may occur in the shoulder.
      2. *Congenital deformities*
         a. *Talipes equinovarus:* clubfoot
         b. *Coxa vara:* dislocated hip
         c. *Kyphosis:* forward curvature of the spine (hunchback)

      d. *Lordosis:* backward curvature of the spine (swayback)

      e. *Scoliosis:* abnormal lateral curvature of the spine

  3. *Neoplasms*

      a. *Osteoma:* tumor of bone

      b. *Osteochondroma:* tumor of bone and cartilage

      c. *Osteosarcoma:* malignant tumor of bone

      d. *Exostosis:* excess growth of bone

  4. *Degenerative joint disease (DJD)*

      a. *Chondromalacia:* softening of the articulating cartilage (autoimmune)

      b. *Arthritis:* degenerative/osteoarthritis and rheumatoid (autoimmune)

      c. *Osteoporosis:* bone becomes porous due to loss of calcium; commonly seen in postmenopausal women

  5. *Contracture:* shortening (drawing up) of distal extremities following injury or improper use of a tourniquet

  6. *Atrophy (a = without; trophy = development):* a wasting away

  7. *Ankylosis:* immobility and consolidation of a joint

  8. *Spondylosis:* ankylosis of the vertebral joint

  9. *Strain:* overstretched muscles

 10. *Sprain:* tendon or ligament pulled from its insertion site

C. **Complications of orthopedic surgery**

  1. *Osteomyelitis:* inflammation of the bone marrow that may last a lifetime

      a. Antibiotics

         i. Are administered IV if procedure is expected to last over 2 hours (e.g., broad-spectrum cephazolin preoperatively and every 6 hours for several doses)

        ii. Added to wound irrigation when an orthopedic implant is used (bacitracin/aerosporin most common; broad-spectrum against *Staphlococcus aureus*)

      b. Meticulous asepsis is essential.

      c. Strict policy regarding skin prep

      d. Antiseptic-impregnated incise drapes

      e. Double or heavy-weight gloving

      f. Laminar airflow, ultraviolet lights, or special exhaust system

      g. Traffic controlled in operating room

  2. *Pain*

      a. Involved extremities are elevated and ice is applied

      b. Injured parts are supported—cast/splint

      c. Care in transferring patient to minimize pain and prevent further injury

      d. Transcutaneous electric nerve stimulator (TENS) may be used for post-operative analgesia.

      e. Epidural catheter or patient-controlled analgesia (PCA) pump for pain medication administration

  3. *Immobilization Issues:* short- and long term

      a. Skin breakdown

      b. **Urinary tract problems:** infection and stones

      c. **Lung complications:** pneumonia

      d. Thrombophlebitis (DVT—Deep vein thrombosis or blood clots)

      e. **Emotional depression:** patient may require occupational therapy, counseling, or psychotherapy

      f. Loss of muscle mass and strength (atrophy) with nonuse

      g. **Nonunion/delayed union of fracture:** bone does not heal or takes longer to heal than expected

      h. **Malunion:** healing with fragments in a faulty position to cause malfunction or cosmetic defect

      i. **Avascular necrosis:** death of tissue, such as the femoral or humeral head, due to lack of a blood supply

D. Protection for the surgical team
1. **Radiation:** x-ray and fluoroscopy—time, distance, shielding, and monitoring (x-ray badges)
2. Irrigating fluids
   a. Knee-high, fluid-proof boots or shoe covers
   b. Fluid-proof gowns
   c. **Face shield:** also protects from blood and spray from saws and drills
3. Sharps
   a. Types
      i. Instruments
      ii. Bone edges
   b. Protection
      i. Double gloving or heavy-weight gloves for extra protection
      ii. Sharp instrument technique to avoid injury to self or others

E. Instrumentation
1. Concepts
   a. Large, bulky, heavy, numerous, wide variety, and constantly changing
2. Types
   a. *Cutting instruments for bone:* osteotomes, gouges, chisels, curettes, rongeurs, rasps, reamers, files, drills, saws, and bone-cutting forceps
   b. *Grasping instruments:* bone hooks, bone-holding forceps (Lane, Lowman, Kern), and meniscus clamp
   c. *Exposing instruments:* periosteal elevators (Langenbeck, Freer, Chandler, Key) and retractors (Bennett, Hibbs, Cobra, Hohmann)
   d. *Implants and related instruments:* drivers, extractors, and impactors; special for each type of implant
   e. *Power-driven instruments*
      i. Drilling—rotary drill
      ii. Cutting
         • Oscillating/sagittal—"side-to-side" cut
         • Reciprocating—"in-and-out" cut
      iii. Shaping/contouring bone
         • Drill reamer
         • High-speed drills: Midas Rex or Anspache; burr protected by collar due to high speed of rotation of burr
   f. *Suction irrigators (pulse lavage):* used for debridement of bone in joint revisions and replacements, traumatic wounds, and open fractures and for cleaning and irrigating contaminated wounds and soft tissue; often used with antibiotic irrigation
   g. *Bone wax:* used for hemostasis of bone.

F. Bone and tissue grafts
1. Bone
   a. Autogenous bone
      i. Donor sites
         • *Iliac crest:* cancellous bone (spongy bone) or cortical bone (compact bone)
         • *Tibia:* cortical bone
      ii. Concepts
         • Bone may be harvested before the recipient site is entered.
         • Change of gown and gloves by the team is required if bone is harvested after the recipient site is opened.
   b. **Cadaveric bone:** bone from bone bank; homogeneous (freeze-dried); obtained, slightly thawed, cultured, washed in antibiotic solution, and placed in fractured site. (*Note:* Never shake a bottle of freeze-dried bone; it will shatter.)

2. Tendon/ligament/cartilage
   a. Soft-tissue allografts
      i. Source:
         • *Patient:* similar tissue from another area in body
         • *Cadaver:* same or similar tissue taken from cadaver

G. **Fixation devices**
   1. Screws
      a. Types
         i. *Cortical:* dense bone
         ii. *Cancellous:* spongy bone
         iii. *Compression:* impacts two bone fragments together
         iv. *Cannulated:* hole in the shaft to pass screw over guide pins
      b. Parts
         i. Shaft
            • Gliding/nonpurchasing
            • Purchasing
         ii. Thread
         iii. Head
            • Hex
            • Slot
            • Other
      c. Screw placement
         i. *Drill:* drill bit and drill
         ii. *Measure:* depth gauge
         iii. *Tap (if indicated):* correct size to perform thread pathway
         iv. *Insert screw:* screwdriver
   2. Plates
      a. Shape
         i. Tubular
         ii. Flat
         iii. T-plate
         iv. Other
      b. Holes—used to "size" the plate
   3. Pins
      a. Types
         i. Plain/smooth
         ii. Threaded
      b. Sizes
         i. Kirschner wires (K-wires)—0.035–1/8 diameter
         ii. Steinmann pins—larger than 1/8
   4. Rods/Nails
      a. *Intramedullary placement in long bones:* humerus, femur, tibia, fibula
      b. *Types*
         i. Locking
         ii. Nonlocking
      c. *Examples:* Enders, Kuntschner, Rush
      d. *Procedure:* medullary canal is entered by drill and awl, nail length is determined, nail is driven into the shaft under fluoroscopy, and the wound is irrigated and closed
   5. **Staples:** secure soft tissue to bone

H. **Prosthetic Implants**
   1. Used to replace joints, bones, or tendons
   2. Made of metal, silicone, or polyethylene
   3. Infection around prosthesis carries high morbidity and permanent disability; should be sterilized according to manufacturer's guidelines

I. **Tourniquet**
   1. Used to exsanguinate limb during surgery; creates a "bloodless" field for better visualization and decreased blood loss
   2. Generator, sterile/unsterile cuffs of various sizes, padding
   3. **Use: unsterile**
      a. Place padded cuff around limb and attach to generator.
      b. Use Esmarch bandage and gravity to remove blood from limb.
      c. Inflate tourniquet to pressure determined by diastolic blood pressure and diameter of limb.
      d. **Set alarms for one hour**—after 1 hour, alert the surgeon as to elapsed time, reset alarms for every 15 minutes; maximum cuff inflation time **11/2 to 2** hours; may need to deflate and allow blood flow to limb for 5–10 minutes, then reinflate.
      e. Deflate cuff at the time of wound closure or after application of pressure dressing.
      f. Document cuff placement, pressure setting, inflation/deflation/duration times, generator serial number.
   4. **Use: sterile**
      a. Skin prep is performed.
      b. Sterile sheets placed under limb to maintain sterility
      c. Sterile padding and cuff placed
      d. Sterile tubing passed to circulator for connection to generator
      e. Remainder of sterile draping is performed.

J. **Sutures**
   1. Nonabsorbable sutures and cutting needles needed for tough fibrous tissue (muscles, tendons, and ligaments)
   2. Absorbable suture is generally used on periosteum and soft tissues (muscle, adipose); they heal readily due to good blood supply.

K. **Limb prep**
   1. Limb is elevated during prep.
   2. Unsterile tourniquet cuff applied and protected from solutions/fluids
   3. Scrub
      a. When the surgical incision involves a joint, the skin prep includes areas to the joint above and below.
      b. When the incision is located between two joints, the skin prep should be extended beyond the joint above and below.
   4. Antimicrobial incise drape may be used to cover skin—source of microbes that can cause osteomyelitis

L. **Surgical draping**
   1. Standardized packs with sterile drapes, towels, and stockinettes for extremities are generally used.
   2. Steri-drape or iodophor-impregnated adhesive drapes; applied after other drapes, the incision is made through the drape; removed before placement of skin stitches or staples

M. **Dressings**
   1. Bulky dressing commonly used to absorb drainage and give compression
   2. Soft dressing material placed between skin surfaces to prevent skin-to-skin contact
      a. Digits (fingers/toes)—kerlix or 4×4 gauze
      b. Axilla for shoulder procedures—abdominal pads (ABDs)
   3. Common types
      a. Nonadherent material (Adaptic, Xeroform, povidone-iodine gauze)
      b. Kerlix fluff, 4×4 gauze
      c. Rolled gauze—kerlix, kling
      d. Ace/elastic bandage for compression

e. Immobilization
   i. *Casts:* complete immobility
   ii. *Sling and swathe:* bones of the shoulder joint immobilized against the torso
   iii. *Splints/braces:* partial or complete immobilization, depending on type and application

N. Casts
  1. External molds used to immobilize a joint or fractured bone(s)
  2. Types of casts
     a. *Short limb*
        i. *Leg:* from knee to toes; for fractures of the ankle or foot
        ii. *Arm:* from below the elbow to fingers; used to treat wrist fractures
     b. *Long limb*
        i. *Leg:* from the groin to toes, for fractures of the fibula, or tibia
        ii. *Arm:* from above the elbow to fingers, used for fractures of elbow or forearm (radius, ulna)
     c. *Cylinder cast:* from the groin to ankle; used to immobilize the knee to treat a fractured patella
     d. *Spica*
        i. *Hip cast:* from the waist to toes on the affected side and to the knee on the unaffected side; for femoral shaft fractures
        ii. *Shoulder cast:* body cast from the waist to involved shoulder and arm to fingers; for humeral fractures
     e. *Body cast:* encircles the torso; used to treat spinal conditions
     f. *Walking:* heel incorporated into casting material
     g. *Splints:* provide support without encircling the limb
  3. Padding under casts
     a. Sterile padding applied to wounds prior to casting
     b. **Purpose:** protect bony prominences and the skin
     c. **Materials**
        i. *Stockinette:* knitted cotton tubing, fits contour snugly
        ii. *Sheet wadding:* glazed cotton bandage, used over or in place of a stockinette
        iii. *Soft roll:* thin soft roll of cotton with some stretch
        iv. *Felt sheets of wool blend, rayon, or cotton in variable thicknesses:* applied over sheet wadding and used for adherence of plaster to avoid slippage
        v. *Webril:* lint-free soft cotton bandage with smooth surface so that each spiral adheres to the next
  4. Cast materials
     a. Types
        i. Plaster
           • Materials
             1. Plaster of paris (gypsum)
             2. Anhydrous calcium sulfate-impregnated crinoline
           • Available in bandages or strips—1–6" wide
           • **Three types:** slow setting (up to 18 minutes), medium setting (up to 8 minutes), and fast setting (4 to 5 minutes)
           • Principles of handling plaster casts
             1. Protect the floor and furniture with disposable drapes.
             2. Protect the patient's hair with cap.
             3. Use a plastic liner in the plaster bucket.
             4. Wear disposable gloves to protect skin.
             5. Plaster bucket is filled with water at room temperature.
             6. Prepare rolls as needed, not in advance.

7. With both hands, submerge bandage under water in vertical position (to provide for escape of air bubbles) and with edge of roll held in fingers.
8. Remove from water when bubbles cease and squeeze gently to remove excess water.
9. Strips should be fanfolded when being submerged in water.
10. When plaster is placed in water, heat is generated by a chemical reaction (exothermic reaction); the plaster hardens as it dries.
11. Imprints in the "wet" cast must be avoided by using palms of hands instead of fingers and supporting the cast with pillows.
12. Plaster fragments are cleaned off the patient and equipment as soon as possible (before they dry).
13. Plaster water is not poured down regular drains as it may lead to clogging.

ii. **Fiberglass:** lighter, thinner, stronger, more porous; not destroyed by wetting; provides better ventilation than gypsum, and is penetrable by x-rays; preferred by some orthopedists
- Made of woven fiberglass tape impregnated with a water-activated polyurethane resin
- Generally preferable to plaster as it is lighter, stronger, more porous for better ventilation, and penetrable by x-rays
- Polypropylene stockinette is applied over skin and a webril wrap is used as extra padding over bony prominences and pressure points.
- Water may be cold or warm (physician preference); cast sets quicker with warm water; soap/cream may be coated onto cast to enhance smoother application.
- Gloves are worn during cast application to protect skin from resin.
- Applied in the same manner as plaster

b. Changing, trimming, or removing casts
i. Casts may be bi-valved (cut on either side for easy removal) in the cast room or in the patient's room and removed in surgery. (*Note:* Care must be taken to avoid airborne contamination when removing casts in the operating room). Casts may also be bi-valved after surgery to allow for swelling and prevent Compartment Syndrome—compression of the nerve and blood vessels resulting in ischemia to the distal extremity.

c. Accessory equipment
i. Casts may be cut with plaster knives, plaster scissors, or an electric cast cutter; a special carbide steel blade is needed for fiberglass casts.
ii. **Cast spreader:** long instrument with serrated jaws used to pry a cast open once it has been bivalved
iii. **Cast cart:** wheeled cart supplied with various types of cast materials and padding which is brought into the room when cast application or removal is anticipated

II. **Fracture Management**

A. **Fracture management is a challenge not only to the surgeon but to the entire surgical team, as no two fractures are exactly alike, and fixation devices and equipment are continually being added to the operating room inventory.**

B. **Types of fractures**
1. Closed versus open
   a. *Closed (simple):* skin is unbroken
   b. *Open (compound):* bone protrudes through the skin; carries high morbidity

2. Traumatic versus pathologic
   a. *Traumatic (accidental injury):* may be open or closed
   b. *Pathologic (spontaneous):* caused by bone disease, such as osteoporosis or bone neoplasms; bone cement may be used to increase strength or fill a defect

C. **Fracture by design and/or location**
   1. *Greenstick:* one side of the bone broken with another side bent; common in children
   2. *Comminuted:* splintered or crushed
   3. *Depressed:* broken bone portion is pressed inward, common in skull fractures
   4. *Compression/impacted:* bone fragments are driven into each other causing a "collapse" of the bone structure
   5. *Longitudinal:* lengthwise
   6. *Spiral:* fracture "twists" up the bone forming a climbing pattern
   7. *Transverse:* at right angle to the bone axis
   8. *Epiphyseal:* a fracture across the growth plate
   9. *Colles':* a transverse fracture of the distal radius
   10. *Pott's:* a fracture of the distal fibula

D. **Principles of facture treatment**
   1. Distal fragments are brought in line with the proximal fragment by the surgeon.
   2. Fractures in lower extremities are realigned to provide stability for weight bearing.
   3. Problems associated with open fractures are infection, damage to blood vessels and nerves, severe damage to soft tissue, and contracture.
   4. Fractured extremities are handled gently with support above and below the site of injury.
   5. General medical treatment precedes surgical management.
   6. Ready availability of trained personnel and proper equipment to treat shock and control hemorrhage are necessary.
   7. Meticulous surgical asepsis is necessary to prevent infection.
   8. Pneumatic counterpressure device (MAST trousers), traction, and splints are removed by or under the direction of the orthopedic surgeon.
   9. Patient's comfort must be considered.

E. **Steps in fracture healing**
   1. Stages in osteogenesis
      a. *Hematoma formation:* blood clot formation; the clot serves as a fibrin meshwork for fibroblasts/osteogenic cells
      b. *Callus stage:* fibroblasts/osteogenic cells invade the fibrin meshwork to form fibrous connective tissue and cartilage
      c. *Osteoid:* osteoblasts and deposits of calcium form a collagen matrix that unites the bone fragments
      d. *Remodeling stage:* excess callus is reabsorbed
   2. Alterations in healing
      a. *Malunion:* bone heals with deformity, causing impaired function or cosmetic defect
      b. *Nonunion:* bone does not heal
      c. *Delayed union:* healing does not take place in the usual amount of time

F. **Treatment of fractures**
   1. *Goals:* reduction, immobilization, and rehabilitation
   2. *Types*
      a. *Closed reduction:* fracture is manipulated into alignment without an incision
         i. Generally done under anesthesia in the cast room or emergency room
         ii. Immobilized by a molded plastic fracture brace, cast brace, or cast (plaster or fiberglass)

b. *Skeletal traction*
   i. Steinmann pins, Kirschner wires, or tongs are inserted in the bone distal to the fracture site using a small sterile setup (scalpel, hand drill with chuck key, wires or pins, bolt cutter, ruler, dressing, and traction bow).
   ii. Pulleys and weights are attached to apply traction (constant force) until the bone heals.
   iii. Sharp ends of wires or pins are protected by corks or plastic tips.
   iv. Example: balanced suspension with a Thomas or Pearson attachment
c. *Skin traction (Buck's extension or Russell-Zells traction):* pulleys and weights are attached to bandages around an extremity.
d. *External fixation*
   i. **Uses:** pelvic or extremity fracture with marked instability with/without tissue loss
   ii. **Components:** pins or wires for anchoring to bone, rods for external support, and clamps or rings as connectors
   iii. Applied with the patient under anesthesia
   iv. X-ray/image intensification used to visualize bone alignment
   v. **Equipment needed:** soft tissue instrument set, suction irrigator, power drill, external fixation device, and pin cutter
e. *Internal fixation:* used when closed reduction and stabilization does not maintain bone fragment alignment
   i. *Closed reduction with internal fixation (CRIF):* fracture is reduced without exposure of the fracture site; bone fragments are aligned and stabilized using an implant placed under image intensification (C-arm) guidance.
      • *Devices*
         1. Intramedullary rods/nails, such as Ender nails, placed through small distal incisions into the canal of a long bone
         2. Closed interlocking nail fixation such as the Grosse-Kempf or Russell-Taylor systems
      • *Advantages:* bone stability, decreased incidence of infection—fracture site is not exposed, and minimal damage to blood vessels and other soft tissue
   ii. *Open reduction and internal fixation (ORIF):* bone fragments are manually aligned through an incision, and fragments are secured with plates and screws, pins, wires, or nails.
      • Used when fracture management by closed reduction has been ruled out
      • Patients are not confined to bed.
      • May carry a higher incidence of infection and nonunion due to exposure of the fracture site and placement of an implant
      • May be accompanied by bone grafting or bone growth stimulators
      • May be performed percutaneously (e.g., K-wires placed during Boxer's Fracture management—metacarpal fracture)
      • Uses: treat bone defects, some congenital anomalies, in cases of nonunion, or when there is a risk of nonunion

SURGERY HINT

When positioning a patient on the fracture table, the surgeon will need to be in charge of positioning the fractured limb.

When using the fracture table, make sure that all accessories are brought into the room. Pad the post with Kerlix or under cast padding

III. **Joint Reconstruction**

A large number of people are afflicted with joint disease—the older population with degenerative disease, the very young with congenital deformities, and young adults with traumatic injury.

A. **Principles of joint function**

1. Joint function depends on the quality of its structures.
2. Bones are held securely in place by ligaments and the joint capsule.
3. The synovial membrane lining the joint capsule secretes synovial fluid to lubricate the joint.
4. Articular cartilage covers the ends of the bones where they meet to form a joint.

B. **Types of joint reconstruction**

1. *Arthrodesis:* joint fusion
   a. *Purpose:* following excision of neoplasms, to relieve pain from osteoarthritis, to stabilize a joint, or to correct a deformity
   b. *Procedure:* articular surfaces are removed and a bone graft or fixation implant secured in place; joint is immobilized until bone fusion is complete
2. *Arthroplasty*
   a. Cup arthroplasty of the hip
      i. Hip joint is disarticulated.
      ii. Femoral head is smoothed into spherical shape.
      iii. Acetabulum is reamed to hemisphere configuration.
      iv. Metallic cup is implanted in the acetabulum, and the femoral head is made to fit.
   b. Femoral or Humeral Head Replacement
      i. *Purposes of prosthesis*
         • Replace head in the case of neck/proximal shaft fracture.
         • Replace head in cases of nonunion or avascular necrosis.
         • Mobilize arthritic joint.
      ii. *Procedure:* prosthesis has a shaft which is driven into the medullary canal and a head which is fitted into the joint.
         • *Femoral head surface replacement:* metal shell is cemented over the femoral head.
   c. Total joint arthroplasty/replacement
      i. **Purposes:** alleviate pain and create functional stability and patient mobility
      ii. Designed for weight bearing, stress, and kinetics
      iii. Bones on both sides of the joint are replaced or resurfaced
      iv. Prosthesis fixation methods
         • *Press-fit fixation:* threads, pegs, or screws on the prosthesis fix it to the bone
         • *Biofixation:* implant with irregular, beaded surface which allows in-growth of tissue; prosthetic coated with hydroxyapatite to promote bone in-growth
         • *Polymethylmethacrylate fixation:* bone cement
            1. Bone cement is mixed immediately before use by a sterile person following manufacturer's instructions.
            2. Fume evacuator should be used.
            3. Solvent should be kept off gloves.
            4. Injected into the medullary canal from a syringe when the proper consistency is reached
            5. Excess cement is commonly removed with a small curette while still soft.
            6. Room and component temperature will affect the setting time—cold = prolonged setting time, warm = shorter setting time.

> ## SURGERY HINT
>
> When doing joint replacements, there may be multiple trays involved. Pick instruments from the trays before stacking to reduce the number of moves necessary. Selecting correct instruments will come with practice and familiarity with the various systems
>
> Always mix cement close to the time it will be used. Keep watch on the time that you begin mixing
>
> Have a freer elevator or small cup curette to hand to the surgeon after a cemented prosthesis has been placed. Have a moist sponge ready to accept excess cement.
>
> Never use cell saver after bone cement has been used as the Methyl Methylcrylate will contaminate blood already collected.

d. **Bone graft:** used to replace bone loss

e. Care of prosthesis
   i. Avoid dents and scratches, glove powder, and lint.
   ii. Use instruments specifically designed for the prosthesis.
   iii. Open the sterile prosthesis after the orthopedist has determined the size and style; check boxes carefully before opening to be sure correct size/side, etc.
   iv. Prosthesis is usually sterile when it arrives from the manufacturer.

f. Considerations of joint arthroplasty
   i. Nitrogen/compressed air—used with air-powered reamers, saws, or drills; if in tanks, check the pressure before the operation begins and ensure that 500 psi or more is available
   ii. Suction tubing is kept patent and containers changed as necessary to accommodate irrigation.
   iii. Blood loss is closely monitored and may be salvaged through a cell saver for autotransfusion.
   iv. Closed-wound vacuum drainage should be available.
   v. Ultraclean (laminar flow) air system may be used.
   vi. Operating room traffic should be minimized.
   vii. Implant label is affixed to the patient's chart.

3. *Arthroscopy:* visualization of a joint—common joints include knee, shoulder, ankle, elbow
   a. *Uses:* diagnosis or treatment of defects in ligaments, cartilage, and meniscus
   b. *Procedure:* sterile irrigating solution (Ringer's solution or normal saline) is used to distend the joint; small stab wounds are made for irrigation inflow, arthroscope, and outflow; irrigation pressure may be regulated by a pressure pump; telescope attached to fiberoptic light cord and source, video camera and closed-circuit monitors used to visualize joint; exploration and interventions performed using probes, hooks, scissors, knives, punches, and grasping forceps; LASER, power-driven shavers, radio frequency (RF) ablation probes remove damaged tissues
   c. *Checks on equipment by scrub during setup:* optics unbroken and lens clean; irrigation ports and stopcocks working; cutting instruments working; correct parts and sizes available for power equipment
   d. *Checks by circulator:* projection lamp, video equipment, LASER, camera and cable, two to four 3000-ml containers of irrigating fluid at room temperature available, and fluid outflow setup functioning

4. *Repair/Reconstruction of tendons and ligaments*
   a. **Purpose:** ligaments are replaced, repositioned, or sutured to permit support of joint during range of motion.
   b. **Example:** anterior cruciate ligament (ACL) reconstruction of knee
   c. Tendons may be lengthened, shortened, transferred, or repaired
   d. Artificial tendons are available.

IV. **Surgical Procedures**

    A. **Shoulder and upper extremities:** rehabilitation of the shoulder joint is the most difficult because of its great range of motion with numerous muscle attachments

        1. *Shoulder arthroscopy*

           a. Diagnostic arthroscopy

           b. **Operative arthroscopy:** subacromial decompression, arthroscopic rotator cuff repair—see knee arthroscopy (p. 392)

        2. *Acromioclavicular (AC) joint separation*

           a. Frequently seen in athletes from acute injury

           b. **Purpose of surgery:** re-establish relationship of the clavicle with the coracoid process of the scapula

           c. **Incision:** anterior curvilinear over the distal clavicle

           d. **Procedure:** replace the coracoclavicular ligament with a heavy suture or screw through the clavicle into the coracoid; Steinmann pin across acromium process into the clavicle may be used to further stabilize the joint

        3. *Correction of rotator cuff tear*

           a. Occurs in the humerus at the insertion site of four muscles (infraspinous, supraspinous, teres minor, and subscapularis)

           b. May follow trauma or degenerative joint disease

           c. Problems with abduction of the arm at the shoulder

           d. Treated with splints and braces or surgery

           e. **Procedure:** torn edges are sutured with a heavy nonabsorbable suture if tear is simple; massive tears require insertion of torn edges into the bone by a wedge osteotomy or by drilling holes

        4. *Recurrent anterior dislocation of the shoulder*

           a. **Objective:** strengthen the joint capsule weakened by frequent dislocations

           b. **Position:** supine or semi-Fowler (beachchair) with affected shoulder raised

           c. **Incision:** over the shoulder joint in the anterior axillary fold

           d. *Operative procedures*

               i. *Bankhart:* heavy sutures are used to reattach the weakened anterior capsule to the rim of the glenoid fossa.

              ii. *Putti-Platt:* subscapularis tendon is overlapped and shortened.

             iii. *Bristow:* a screw is used to secure the coracoid process onto the neck of the glenoid cavity.

        5. *Clavicular fracture*

           a. Very common; generally treated by immobilization in a figure-eight splint

           b. Because of the close proximity of the brachial plexus and major vessels, displaced clavicular fractures require ORIF.

        6. *Humeral head fracture/neer/total shoulder arthroplasty*

           a. ORIF required for comminuted fracture

           b. Prosthetic replacement is required for a severely comminuted, neck, or proximal shaft fracture or degenerative arthritis of the shoulder.

        7. *Humeral fracture:* generally treated by closed reduction and immobilization; more difficult fractures require nails, compression plates, or lag screws, or bone grafts

        8. *Distal humeral fractures:* are managed with Kirschner wire and screw, dynamic compression plate (DCP), or semitubular plate and immobilized with a cast

        9. *Correction of olecranon fracture:* larger fragments are managed by ORIF (screws, Kirschner wires, Steinmann pins) or figure-eight wires

       10. *Transposition of the ulna nerve*

           a. Ulna nerve damage occurs from trauma and results in hand atrophy and sensory loss, or claw-hand deformity.

           b. **Procedure:** incision is made in the lateral elbow, and the ulna nerve is freed (neurolysis) and placed in the brachialis flexor muscle origin; a long-arm cast is applied with elbow flexed 90 degrees.

11. *Excision of the radial head:* in adults, a damaged radial head resulting from a severe comminuted or unstable fracture is treated by excision and immobilization.

12. *Total elbow replacement:* done for severe pain and instability resulting from traumatic injury or degenerative arthritis

13. *Fractures of the radius and ulna*
    a. Occur frequently in children and are generally corrected by closed reduction and immobilization
    b. Adults with displaced fragments require ORIF (plate and screws)

14. *Colles' fracture:* fracture of the distal radius; managed by closed reduction and immobilization, external fixation, or internal fixation with Kirschner wires for a comminuted fracture

15. *Excision of Ganglion*
    a. **Ganglion:** fluid-filled synovial sacs protruding between the carpal bones
    b. May resolve or be excised for cosmesis or discomfort

16. *Carpal tunnel release (CTR)*
    a. **Indications:** carpal tunnel syndrome (CTS), compression of the median nerve which causes pain and paresthesia in the thumb, index finger, long finger, and the radial half of the ring finger due to thickening of the transverse carpal ligament
    b. Carpal tunnel is located on the volar surface of the wrist through which the median nerve, superficial and deep finger flexor, and long thumb tendon pass.
    c. **Procedure:** tourniquet is inflated; incision is made across volar wrist surface; carpal ligament is incised; Tenosynovectomy (excision of synovial tissue surrounding the tendons that pass through the carpal tunnel) may be performed; incision is closed and hand dressing is applied; may be performed endoscopically —telescope and cutting device placed into tunnel via small wrist incision after dilation of the tunnel, blade cuts upward to divide ligament, skin incision is closed

17. *Metacarpal arthroplasty:* use of a prosthesis, such as a Swanson, to replace an arthritic joint in the metacarpophalangeal (MP) joint to relieve pain and stabilize joints; postoperative weakness of grasp and pinch action, along with disease progression, is a major concern

B. **Hip and lower extremities**
    1. *Fracture of the acetabulum:* internal fixation is required for severe displacement or presence of loose bodies but is delayed until the patient is clinically stable
    2. *Correction of hip fractures*
        a. Intertrochanteric (between the greater and lesser trochanters of the proximal femur)
            i. Generally occurs in geriatric patients
            ii. Internal fixation is necessary to prevent malunion when external rotation occurs at the fracture site.
            iii. Referred to as Compression Hip Plating or Hip Nailing
            iv. **Procedure:** patient is secured on the fracture table in the supine position, and a lateral incision is made, beginning at greater trochanter; guide pin is placed in the neck and head of the femur and checked under fluoroscopy; lag screw channel is reamed over guide pin; lag screw and angled compression plate are inserted into the channel with side of plate secured to the femoral shaft with cortical bone screws; further impaction is accomplished by placing a compressing screw through the lag screw; wound is closed and pressure dressing is applied.
        b. Femoral neck fracture
            i. To avoid aseptic necrosis and nonunion, internal fixation is necessary.

      ii. Universal cannulated screws or pins are designed for fixation of the femoral neck.

      iii. Slipped capital femoral epiphysis in growing children is stabilized as with femoral neck fractures

      iv. **Procedure:** resembles fixation of the intertrochanteric fracture

  c. Femoral head prosthesis replacement

      i. *Indications:* aseptic necrosis, nonunion, degenerative arthritis, and a displaced femoral neck that cannot be manipulated into position

      ii. *Prostheses available:* Austin-Moore, Thompson, and bipolar endoprosthesis

      iii. *Procedure:* femoral head and neck excised, medullary canal is opened and reamed to accommodate the stem of the prosthesis, prosthesis is secured with or without bone cement, vacuum drain is positioned, and wound is closed

3. *Total hip arthroplasty*
   a. Common orthopedic procedure
   b. Indicated for degenerative joint disease (DJD)
   c. **Prostheses:** acetabulum, femoral head and neck, femoral stem; may be modular—each component consisting of several pieces to allow for "custom fit" at the surgical field
   d. **Procedure:** femoral neck is exposed through a lateral incision and the capsule is opened; hip is dislocated, femoral head and neck excised and acetabulum exposed, reamed, and tested for proper fit, with holes drilled in the ilium, ischium, and pubis for implant anchoring; acetabulum is lavaged, dried, and prepared for prosthesis; a canal is made in the femoral neck for the implant; femoral component is inserted (bone plug may also be used if prosthesis is cemented); femoral head is positioned onto the stem and the joint is reduced; wound is closed over vacuum drains, and abduction pillow is secured between patient's legs; may be performed using minimally invasive incisions and fluoroscopy

4. *Correction of congenital hip dislocation*
   a. Femoral head is displaced upward and laterally.
   b. Can lead to contractures of the hip muscles, deformed joint, scoliosis, or knee problems
   c. **Treatment methods:** closed reduction, application of a spica cast, or surgery
   d. Surgical corrective procedures
      i. *Open reduction:* joint is opened, soft tissue is excised from the acetabulum, and the femoral head is reduced to correct position and held by sutures placed in the capsule.
      ii. *Derotational osteotomy:* femur is divided and the distal fragment is rotated externally, to place the foot straight ahead, and immobilized.
      iii. *Innominate osteotomy:* ilium is divided and wedged down with a bone graft or heavy wires to increase the depth of the acetabulum.

5. *Correction of femoral shaft fractures*
   a. **Etiology:** high-impact injuries or bone disease such as cancer or osteoporosis

---

SURGERY HINT

Use caution when handling the prosthesis. It must be handled as little as possible before insertion. Once the size has been determined, the prosthesis will be opened and presented to the ST. Keep the prosthesis in the packaging until the surgeon is ready for it.

Have the impactor and a clean laparotomy sponge ready to hand to the surgeon.

Hand the impactor with a mallet.

---

b. Treatment methods
   i. Skeletal traction for 4 to 6 weeks followed by immobilization
   ii. **Surgical:** insertion of an intramedullary nail
      • Methods of nail insertion
         1. **Closed:** nail is driven over a guidewire inserted from the proximal end of the bone; preferred method
         2. **Open nailing:** requires two incisions—one for nail insertion and one over the fracture site
      • Nail is inserted into the medullary canal and interlocked with screws placed in the proximal and/or distal end of the nail

6. *Knee arthroscopy*
   a. Diagnostic arthroscopy
   b. **Operative arthroscopy:** synovial biopsy, resection of the plicae, removal of loose bodies or synovium, repairs of the meniscus or the anterior or posterior cruciate ligament, partial or complete meniscectomy, and patella shaving

7. *Correction of Tibial Plateau or Femoral Condyle Fractures:* open reduction is required for displaced fractures, and fixation is accomplished with angled plates and/or cancellous screws.

8. *Patellectomy:* surgical removal of the knee cap may be required for degenerative arthritis or comminuted fracture.
   a. Chondromalacia (cartilage softening) may be shaved or excised to improve the range of motion; chronic dislocation of the patella may predispose the patient to this condition
   b. Knee fractures may be reduced with a screw or tension band wiring.
   c. Recurrent dislocation of the knee: more common in teenagers; the lateral quadriceps tendon is incised, and the insertion of the patella tendon is shifted medially or distally on the tibia

9. *Repair of Cruciate or Collateral Ligament Tears*
   a. Common injuries to the knee include tears of the medial meniscus, anterior cruciate ligament, and medial collateral ligament, resulting in instability of the joint.
   b. May be repaired with arthroscopy or arthroscopy-assisted repair
   c. Arthrotomy may be indicated when there is a combination of tears.

10. *Baker's (popliteal) Cyst Excision*
   a. Ganglion-like cyst in popliteal fossa (behind the knee)
   b. May be associated with a torn medial meniscus or rheumatoid arthritis
   c. Patient is placed in the prone position; oblique incision is made in the popliteal region; cyst is removed, and knee is immobilized in extension.

11. *Total knee arthroplasty*
   a. *Prostheses:* femoral cap, tibial platform, posterior patellar surface; may be modular—each component consisting of several pieces to allow for "custom fit" at the surgical field
   b. *Procedure:* with a pneumatic tourniquet in place, anterior longitudinal incision is made over the knee, bone surfaces are cut with "jigs" to accommodate prosthetics; tibial, femoral, and patellar components are implanted; wound is irrigated and closed over a drain, and knee is immobilized; may be performed through a small minimally invasive lateral incision

12. *Correction of Tibial Shaft Fractures*
   a. Open fractures are more common; delayed union, nonunion, and infection are possible complications.
   b. ORIF is indicated when soft tissue is caught between fragments, when fracture is severely rotated or unstable, or with delayed treatment.

  c. Compression plates and screws or interlocking intramedullary nails (ORIF or CRIF)
     i. *Nail procedure:* patient is supine on a fracture table with hip and knee flexed, and a calcaneal pin is inserted and traction applied for rotational alignment; incision is made in the front of the knee; medullary canal is opened and reamed, and a rod is placed over a guidewire under fluoroscopy.
13. *Correction of an ankle (malleolar) fracture:* achieved with pins, screws, and plates with screws (especially Rush rods, long cancellous bone screws, and Steinmann pins), and a short leg cast is applied
14. *Triple arthrodesis:* fusion of the talocalcaneal, talonavicular, and calcaneocuboid joints
    a. **Indications:** inversion or eversion deformities, as in poliomyelitis, rheumatoid arthritis, or clubfoot
    b. **Procedure:** articular bone surfaces are removed; bones are secured with bone grafts, bone staples, or compression plates
    c. Cast or external fixation device is applied
15. *Bunionectomy*
    a. **Hallux valgus (bunion):** a bony mass on the medial side of the first metatarsal or a mass of soft tissue
    b. **Etiology:** structural defect of the foot frequently associated with wearing high heels/narrow-toed shoes (females), heredity, muscle imbalance, or a longer first toe
    c. **Surgical procedure for Bunionectomy:** Keller or McBride—most common
    d. **Objective:** cosmesis, resect abnormal tissue, realign bones of foot and improve function
16. *Hammer toe correction:* flexion deformity of the toes that leads to callus formation on the dorsal surface, caused by contraction of flexor tendons causing digits to rub against the tops of the shoes; the long extensor tendons are incised, and the middle joints are fused and stabilized with Kirschner wires
17. *Amputation of extremities*
    a. May be done by orthopedic or general surgeon
    b. **Indications:** malignancy, massive trauma, extensive infection, vascular insufficiency as may occur in the atherosclerotic gangrene due to diabetes
    c. Types
       i. Above-the-knee amputation (**AKA**)
       ii. Below-the-knee amputation (**BKA**)
    d. **Instrumentation:** Gigli, amputation saw (Satterlee) or oscillating power saw, absorbable suture, bulky pressure dressing (fluffs with ace bandage), with stump elevated on a pillow
    e. **Postoperative considerations:** phantom limb sensations, contractures, stump care, ambulation, and rehabilitation
C. **Surgery of the vertebral column**
   1. *Discectomy:* surgical excision of an intervertebral disk
      a. *Indications:* herniated nucleus pulposa (HNP)—"ruptured" or "slipped" disk
      b. *Methods of diagnosis:* MRI, CT, or myelography (x-ray of the spinal cord)

SURGERY HINT

Be prepared to amputate further than planned depending on the severity of the infected bone. The bone may be more infected than previously thought, and more bone may need to be removed to uncover healthy tissue.

Depending on the physiology of the patient, this procedure may be done with a spinal instead of general anesthesia.

SURGERY HINT

For a prone patient on a Wilson frame have standing stools available in sufficient numbers for the surgical team.

   c. *Procedures*
       i. *Lumbar laminectomy:* with the patient in the prone position, a vertical midline incision is made over the involved lumbar vertebrae; soft tissue is retracted; ligamentum flavum is incised; spinous processes and laminae are removed with a rongeur to expose intervertebral spaces; disk and fragments are removed.
       ii. *Microdiscectomy:* under an operating microscope, one-level unilateral discectomy is performed.
       iii. *Percutaneous lumbar discectomy:* under local anesthesia, IV sedation, and fluoroscopy, a nucleotome is inserted through a cannula, and the HNP is excised and aspirated.
       iv. *Anterior cervical discectomy:* with the patient in the supine or Trendelenburg position, an incision is made along the lateral aspect of the neck; the carotid artery/jugular vein/esophagus/trachea are retracted; the disk is removed, and a bone dowel with plates and screws is inserted to fuse the vertebra.
2. *Spinal stabilization*
   a. *Indications:* chronic degenerative disease of the spine, scoliosis, or spinal injury
   b. *Methods*
       i. *Spinal fusion:* bone grafts, with or without internal fixation devices (cages), are used to bridge the intervertebral spaces or spinous processes to stabilize the spine; autografts or homogeneous grafts may be used.
       ii. *Internal fixation of the spine:* several systems are available
       • Harrington rods
       • Luque segmental spinal rods
       • Wisconsin compression system
       • Cotrel-Dubousset system
       • Texas Scottish Rite Hospital (TSRH) crosslink system
       • Dwyer instrumentation with anterior spinal fusion
       • Zielke instrumentation with anterior spinal fusion
3. *Kyphoplasty:* injection of polymethylmethacrylate "cement" into the vertebral body to treat compression fractures

Show What You Know

Directions
Each of the numbered items or incomplete statements in this section is followed by answers or by completions of the statement. Select the ONE lettered answer or completion that is BEST in each case.

1. An abnormal lateral curvature of the spine for which a stabilization procedure may be done is:
   A. scoliosis
   B. osteoporosis
   C. exostosis
   D. herniated nucleus pulposa

2. Death of bone tissue due to the lack of circulation is:
   A. arthritis
   B. avascular necrosis
   C. malunion
   D. osteomyelitis

3. Equipment used to debride and clean infected wounds and joints is:
   A. periosteal elevator
   B. drill/reamer
   C. suction irrigator
   D. impactor

4. The most likely donor site for an autogenous bone graft is the:
   A. femur
   B. ischium
   C. scapula
   D. ilium

5. In orthopedic surgery, absorbable suture would most likely be used on:
   A. tendons
   B. periosteum
   C. ligaments
   D. bone

6. The patient would be placed in the prone position for which of these procedures?
   A. Excision of a Baker's Cyst
   B. AK Amputation
   C. Knee arthroscopy
   D. Triple Arthrodesis of the Ankle

7. When assisting with the application of a plaster cast, you would do all of the following *except:*
   A. secure a bucket of hot water
   B. prepare only one plaster bandage or strip at the time
   C. gently squeeze excess water from the plaster bandage after bubbles have ceased to rise
   D. clean plaster from the patient and equipment as soon as possible

8. The type of fracture that includes splintered or crushed bone is:
   A. Colles'
   B. greenstick
   C. compound
   D. comminuted

9. The general term for joint reconstruction is:
   A. osteotomy
   B. arthrodesis
   C. osteoarthritis
   D. arthroplasty

10. All of the following are guides to be followed when using polymethylmethacrylate (bone cement) *except:*
    A. mix immediately before use
    B. use a fume evacuator
    C. mix with a gloved hand
    D. supply to the surgeon in a syringe for injection into the medullary canal

11. Heavy suture is used to reattach a weakened anterior capsule to the glenoid fossa to correct recurrent dislocation of the shoulder in which procedure?
    A. Excision of Ganglion
    B. Keller Procedure
    C. Bankhart Procedure
    D. Kyphoplasty

12. Removal of a fluid-filled sac protruding between wrist joints for cosmesis or discomfort describes which procedure?
    A. Excision of Ganglion
    B. Patellectomy
    C. McBride Procedure
    D. Metacarpal Arthroplasty

13. Use of a prosthesis to replace arthritic joints in the hand is referred to as a/an:
    A. Triple Arthrodesis
    B. Carpal Tunnel Release
    C. Bankhart Procedure
    D. Metacarpal Arthroplasty

14. The excision of the kneecap for degenerative arthritis is called a/an:
    A. Bristow Procedure
    B. Patellectomy
    C. Putti-Platt Procedure
    D. Rotator cuff correction

15. Bone retrieved from the patient for bone grafting is called _____ bone.

    A. cadaveric
    B. autogenic
    C. xenogenic
    D. allogenic

16. The placement of fixation pins through the skin into the bone proximal and distal to the fracture site, which are then connected to stabilizing bars, is called:

    A. external fixation
    B. skeletal fixation
    C. internal fixation
    D. compression fixation

17. The fixation device(s) most commonly used for intratrochanteric fractures of the femur include(s):

    A. compression plates and screws
    B. hinged replacement prosthesis
    C. rods/nails
    D. Kirschner wires

18. When a tourniquet is inflated during surgery, the surgeon is notified at which recommended time intervals?

    A. at the half hour, and every 15 minutes thereafter
    B. at the half hour, and every half hour thereafter
    C. at the hour, and every 15 minutes thereafter
    D. at the hour, and every half hour thereafter

19. Screws come in which type(s)?

    A. cortical only
    B. cortical and Kirschner
    C. cancellous and cortical
    D. trochanteric and Kirschner

20. Polymethylmethacrylate is commonly known as:

    A. a material implants are made from
    B. material used to coat implants when placing a noncemented prosthesis
    C. a material soft tissue allografts are made of
    D. material used to hold the prosthesis when placing a cemented prosthesis

21. The implant used on small bone fragments or as part of skeletal traction is called:

    A. cancellous screw
    B. steinmann pin
    C. cortical screw
    D. nail

22. When performing a skin prep for surgery on the tibia, the skin prep would extend:

    A. from above the hip joint to the toes
    B. from above the knee joint to the toes
    C. from the incision site down to the toes
    D. from the hip joint to the knee joint

23. The dressing applied at the end of an orthopedic procedure which gives compression to the wound is a/an:

    A. kerlix fluff
    B. xeroform
    C. ace or elastic bandage
    D. fiberglass or plaster cast

24. The sterile tourniquet cuff is applied:

    A. before the skin prep begins
    B. during draping but before other drapes are placed over the upper extremity
    C. at the end of the draping procedure
    D. never; tourniquet cuffs do not come sterile

25. The x-ray views usually obtained during orthopedic surgery include all of the following except:

    A. sagittal
    B. oblique
    C. anterior/posterior
    D. lateral

26. After shoulder surgery:

    A. the unaffected arm is immobilized against the torso of the patient
    B. the affected arm is not immobilized, as the patient will not move it due to postoperative discomfort
    C. the affected arm is not immobilized, as the patient needs to begin range of motion in the joint immediately
    D. the affected arm is immobilized against the torso of the patient, and padding is placed between skin surfaces which will contact one another

27. Casting material can be made from all of the following materials except:

    A. hydroxyapatite
    B. gypsum
    C. anhydrous calcium sulfateimpregnated crinoline
    D. fiberglass

28. An open fracture, where bone protrudes through the skin, is also referred to as a _____ fracture.

    A. greenstick fracture
    B. closed traumatic fracture
    C. comminuted fracture
    D. compound fracture

29. A fracture where the tendonous attachments of the bone are torn away is called a/an:

    A. tendon fracture
    B. epiphyseal separation
    C. avulsion
    D. compound fracture

30. The stage of osteogenesis where there is a prolif-
    eration of cells from the fracture site into the
    fibrin to form fibrous connective tissue and carti-
    lage is called:

    A. osteoid stage
    B. blood clot formation stage
    C. remodeling stage
    D. callus stage

31. The method of fracture treatment where a pull-
    ing force is exerted directly on the bone itself via
    a pin in the bone using a system of weights and
    pulleys is called:

    A. Buck's traction
    B. external fixation
    C. open reduction internal fixation (ORIF)
    D. skeletal traction with balanced suspension

32. Principles of joint reconstruction include all of
    the following *except:*

    A. joint function depends on the quality of its
       structures
    B. bones are held loosely in place by ligaments
       and the joint capsule
    C. the synovial membrane lining the joint capsule
       secretes synovial fluid to lubricate the joint
    D. articular cartilage covers the ends of the
       bones where they meet to form a joint

33. A loosening of a joint with some displacement of
    the articular surface from the joint capsule is
    called a/an:

    A. dislocation
    B. avulsion
    C. fracture
    D. subluxation

34. Reconstruction of a joint to restore or improve
    range of motion and stability or to relieve pain is
    referred to as an:

    A. arthrotomy
    B. arthroplasty
    C. arthrogenesis
    D. arthroscopy

35. Methods of prosthetic fixation and stabilization
    include all of the following *except:*

    A. biofixation using hydroxyapatite
    B. biofixation using polymethylmethacrylate
    C. polymethylmethacrylate cement fixation
    D. direct bone contact with a press-fit prosthesis

36. Concepts concerning polymethylmethacrylate
    use on the surgical field include all of the follow-
    ing *except:*

    A. room and component temperature will affect
       the setting time
    B. contact of the polymer and your skin may
       cause a dermatitis reaction

    C. avoid excessive exposure to the vapors pro-
       duced during mixing of the polymer and the
       powder
    D. polymethylmethacrylate should be prepared
       at the beginning of the case, so it is ready at
       the desired time of use

37. Visualization of a joint for diagnosis and con-
    servative treatment of joint disease is called:

    A. arthroplasty
    B. arthrotomy
    C. arthroscopy
    D. arthrorrhaphy

38. An overgrowth of bone is referred to as an:

    A. exostosis
    B. osteoblast
    C. osteocyte
    D. osteoclast

39. The "freeing up" of an entrapped nerve is
    referred to as a/an:

    A. neuropexy
    B. kyphosis
    C. neurolysis
    D. kyphoplasty

40. Excision of a tendon sheath and its associated
    synovium is referred to as a:

    A. tenorrhaphy
    B. tenotomy
    C. tendopexy
    D. tenosynovectomy

41. The yellow, elastic tissue connecting the lamina
    is called the:

    A. nucleus pulposa
    B. anterior cruciate ligament
    C. ligamentum flavum
    D. coraco-acromion ligament

42. A rotator cuff tear occurs in which region of the
    body?

    A. knee
    B. shoulder
    C. vertebrae
    D. ankle

43. A fracture where healing has not taken place in
    the usual amount of time is referred to as a/an:

    A. nonunion
    B. malunion
    C. delayed union
    D. subluxation

44. The patient position for a Bristow Procedure is:

    A. semi-Fowler
    B. prone
    C. Sims
    D. lithotomy

45. An Austin Moore prosthesis is used at which joint?

    A. knee
    B. hip
    C. shoulder
    D. ankle

46. A Colles' fracture occurs in which bone(s)?

    A. radius
    B. humerus
    C. tibia/fibula
    D. clavicle/acromion

47. Positioning for procedures include all of the following combinations *except:*

    A. supine in traction for a Compression Hip Nailing
    B. lateral for a Total Hip Arthroplasty
    C. semi-Fowler for a Bristow Procedure
    D. prone for a Total Knee Arthroplasty

48. The bony process which can be involved in an ankle fracture is the:

    A. medial malleolus
    B. medial meniscus
    C. lateral trochanter
    D. calcaneous

49. The procedure which consists of excision and fusion of the middle phalangeal joint of the foot with incision of the flexor tendon is:

    A. Bunionectomy
    B. Triple Arthrodesis
    C. Correction of Hammer Toe Deformity
    D. Metacarpal Arthroplasty

50. The fracture commonly treated with angled blade plates or a long cancellous screw would be:

    A. patella fracture
    B. tibial plateau fracture
    C. humeral shaft fracture
    D. femoral shaft fracture

51. A Triple Arthrodesis does not include fusion of which bones?

    A. calcaneocuboid joint
    B. metacarpophalangeal joint
    C. talocalcaneal joint
    D. talonavicular joint

52. Which position is the patient placed in for an Anterior Cervical Discectomy and Fusion?

    A. supine
    B. prone
    C. Sims
    D. Kraske

53. Long cancellous screws placed with a gliding hole for the shaft provide:

    A. compression of bone fragments
    B. approximation of bone fragments

C. distraction of bone fragments
D. subluxation of bone fragments

54. A potential complication of ischemia of the femoral head is:

    A. intermittant claudication
    B. intussusception
    C. avascular necrosis
    D. chondromalacia

55. A fracture commonly found in children is a:

    A. comminuted
    B. greenstick
    C. Colles'
    D. longitudinal

56. A fracture requiring debridement and closure prior to casting would be a:

    A. comminuted
    B. greenstick
    C. compound
    D. spiral

57. A surgical procedure designed to stiffen or fuse a joint is called:

    A. Arthropexy
    B. Arthroplasty
    C. Arthrotomy
    D. Arthrodesis

58. A tear in the lateral or medial knee cartilage is repaired by performing a/an:

    A. Synovectomy
    B. Menisectomy
    C. Patellectomy
    D. Arthrodesis

59. Chronic dislocation of the patella may predispose the patient to a condition called:

    A. osteomyelitis
    B. chondromalacia
    C. rheumatoid arthritis
    D. osteoporosis

60. Baker's cysts are found in the:

    A. popliteal fossa
    B. interdigital fossa
    C. intercarpal fossa
    D. olecranon fossa

61. Which of the following would *not* be used for cast padding?

    A. webril
    B. felt
    C. Esmarch bandage
    D. stockinette

62. A hemostatic agent used to control bleeding from an open bone is:

    A. heparin sodium
    B. protamine sulfate

C. methylene blue

D. bone wax

63. The power drill or saw used to divide bone with a "side-to-side" cutting action is a/an:

A. reciprocating saw

B. rotary drill

C. oscillating saw

D. drill/reamer

Questions 64 and 65 refer to the following scenario.

Mr. Smith, a 27-year-old patient, is admitted directly to the OR with a fractured femur. The surgeon plans to perform an ORIF with plates and screws.

Instrument Identification

66.

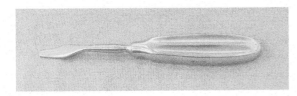

A. Key elevator

B. Ferris Smith forcep

C. Chandler elevator

D. Ballenger swivel knife

67.

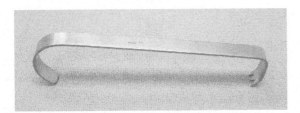

A. Bennett retractor

B. Richardson retractor

C. Cobra retractor

D. Hibbs retractor

68.

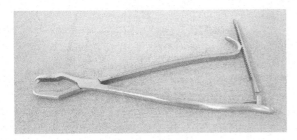

A. Lane bone holding forcep

B. Lowman bone holding forcep

C. Castroviejo forcep

D. Russian tissue forcep

64. Which one of the following is the correct order for screw placement?

A. drill, measure, tap, place

B. drill, tap, measure, place

C. tap, drill, measure, place

D. tap, measure, drill, place

65. When implanting plates and screws, what medication is used on the surgical field?

A. heparin sodium for anticoagulation

B. polymixin for decreasing edema

C. Hypaque for hemostasis

D. Bacitracin for antimicrobial prophylaxis against osteomyelitis

69.

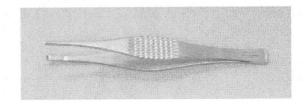

A. DeBakey forcep

B. Ferris Smith forcep

C. Russian forcep

D. Kerrison rongeur

70.

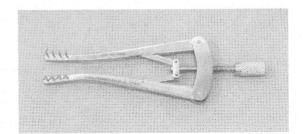

A. Alm retractor

B. Senn retractor

C. Cushing retractor

D. Pituitary rongeur

Anatomy Review

Musculoskeletal System

71–100.

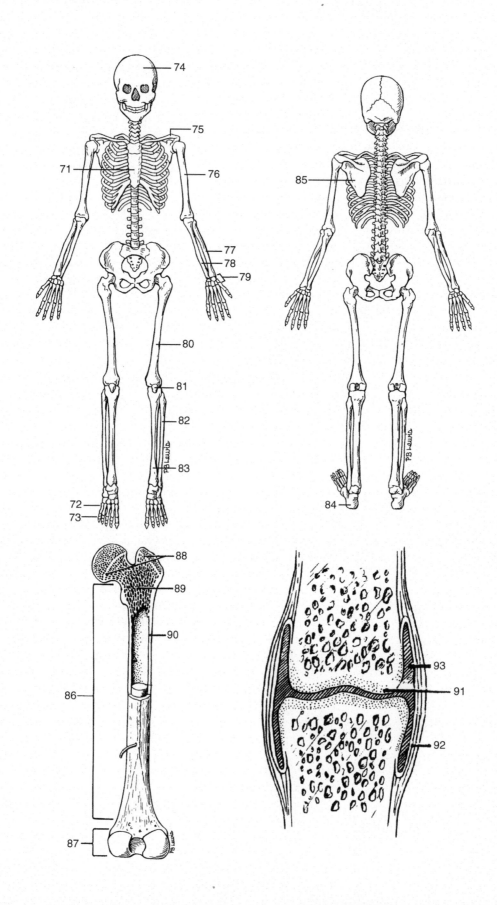

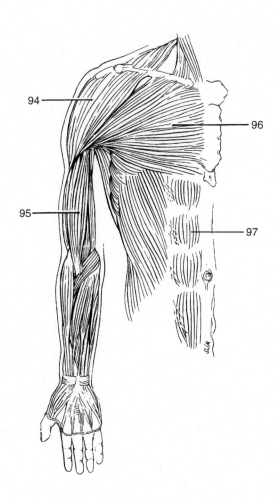

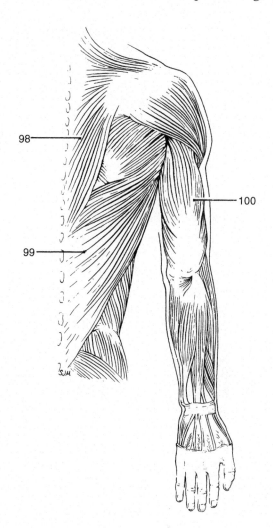

A. articular cartilage
B. biceps brachii
C. calcaneus
D. cancellous bone
E. carpals
F. clavicle
G. cortical bone
H. deltoid
I. diaphysis
J. epiphyseal plates
K. epiphysis
L. femur
M. fibula
N. humerus
O. joint cavity

P. latissimus dorsi
Q. metatarsals
R. patella
S. pectoralis major
T. phalanges
U. radius
V. rectus abdominis
W. scapula
X. skull or cranium
Y. sternum
Z. synovial membrane
AA. tibia
BB. trapezius
CC. triceps brachii
DD. ulna

Answers & Rationales

1. **A.** **Rationale:** Scoliosis is an abnormal lateral curvature of the spine. Osteoporosis is a loss of bone substance (calcium). Exostosis is excess growth on a bone. Herniated nucleus pulposa pertains to the intervertebral disks.

2. **B.** **Rationale:** Avascular necrosis is the death of bone or other tissue which occurs when the blood supply had been cut off.

3. **C.** **Rationale:** A suction irrigator, such as a pulse lavage, is used for cleaning, irrigating, and debridement of wounds.

4. **D.** **Rationale:** Both cancellous and cortical bone can be obtained from the iliac crest, an area of the ilium. Cortical bone may also be obtained from the tibia.

5. **B.** **Rationale:** Absorbable suture is generally used on the periosteum because of its rapid healing. Tendons, ligaments, and bones are tougher tissues and generally require use of a nonabsorbable suture.

6. **A.** **Rationale:** A Baker's cyst is associated with a torn meniscus or rheumatoid arthritis and occurs behind the knee; the patient would be placed in the prone position for excision. Above-the-Knee Amputation, Triple Arthrodesis of the Ankle, and Knee arthroscopy are performed with the patient in the supine position.

7. **A.** **Rationale:** Because of the exothermic reaction of gypsum in water, the chemical reaction would be increased even more if it were placed in hot water. It is generally recommended that water be at room temperature when submerging plaster bandages or strips.

8. **D.** **Rationale:** A comminuted fracture is one that is splintered or crushed, is more difficult to treat, and frequently requires ORIF. A Colles' fracture occurs in the distal radius, a greenstick facture is a partial fracture in young bones, and a compound fracture is one that is open with bone protruding through the skin.

9. **D.** **Rationale:** *Arthroplasty* is a general term denoting revision or repair of the articulating surfaces of a joint. Osteotomy is an incision into bone; arthrodesis is joint fusion, and osteoarthritis is a degenerative disease of the articulating surfaces of a joint.

10. **C.** **Rationale:** When using bone cement, the scrub person mixes it immediately before use; a fume evacuator or some type of scavenging system is used to minimize staff exposure to the potentially harmful fumes; the cement is poured into a syringe to be injected into the medullary canal but is shaped manually for hinged joints. The solvent should not be allowed to contact surgical gloves, as it can diffuse through latex to cause an allergic dermatitis.

11. **C.** **Rationale:** The Bankhart Procedure (use of heavy suture to reattach the anterior capsule to the glenoid cavity) is done to strengthen the shoulder joint capsule to prevent recurrent dislocation.

12. **A.** **Rationale:** Excision of Ganglion is the removal of a fluid-filled sac of synovium protruding between wrist joints.

13. **D.** **Rationale:** Metacarpal Arthroplasty is the replacement of arthritic metacarpophalangeal (MP) joints in the hand.

14. **B.** **Rationale:** Patellectomy is the surgical removal of the kneecap; it may be done for degenerative arthritis.

15. **B.** **Rationale:** Bone retrieved from the patient for bone grafting is called autogenic bone. Cadarveric bone comes from cadavers; xenografts come from animals, usually pigs or cows; and allografts are like structures taken from other parts of the body or from a donor.

16. **A.** **Rationale:** The placement of fixation pins through the skin into the bone proximal and distal to the fracture site, which are then connected to stabilizing bars, is called external fixation. Skeletal traction involves attachment to balanced suspension; internal fixation and compression fixation require exposure of the fracture site.

17. **A.** **Rationale:** The fixation device most commonly used for intratrochanteric fractures of the femur is a compression plate and screws. Kirschner wires are too fine to stabilize this type of fracture; rods and nails are intramedullary devices; and a hinged prosthesis can be used in Knee Arthroplasty.

18. **C.** **Rationale:** The recommended time intervals for tourniquet use include notifying the surgeon after an hour has passed and every 15 minutes thereafter.

19. **C.** **Rationale:** Cancellous screws are used on spongy bone, and cortical screws are used on hard, dense bone.

20. **D.** Rationale: Polymethylmethacrylate is commonly known as a material used to hold the prosthesis when placing a cemented prosthesis. Implants are made of polyethylene, stainless steel, or other metals. Hydroxyapetite is used to coat biofixation implants to promote bone ingrowth. Soft tissue allografts are not made of artificial materials.

21. **B.** Rationale: The implant used on small bone fragments or as part of skeletal traction is called a Steinmann pin. While screws can be used on small bone fragments, they are not used as part of skeletal traction. Nails are intramedullary devices used on long bones.

22. **B.** Rationale: When performing a skin prep for surgery on the tibia, the skin prep would extend from above the knee joint to the toes.

23. **C.** Rationale: The dressing applied at the end of an orthopedic procedure which gives compression to the wound is an ace or elastic bandage. Kerlix fluff provides absorption and padding, xeroform covers the incision with a nonadherent dressing, and a cast provides immobility.

24. **B.** Rationale: The sterile tourniquet cuff is applied during draping but before other drapes are placed over the upper extremity. This permits the cuff to be applied in a sterile manner while allowing the cuff to be placed directly onto the limb. An unsterile cuff is applied prior to beginning the skin prep.

25. **A.** Rationale: Anterior/posterior (A/P), lateral, and oblique x-ray views permit visualization of the bones in a three-dimensional relationship.

26. **D.** Rationale: After shoulder surgery, the affected arm is immobilized against the torso of the patient, with padding placed between skin surfaces which will contact one another.

27. **A.** Rationale: Casting material can be made from gypsum, anhydrous calcium sulfate–impregnated crinoline, or fiberglass. Hydroxyapatite is used to promote bone ingrowth on implanted prostheses.

28. **D.** Rationale: A compound fracture is an open fracture, where bone protrudes through the skin. A closed fracture does not involve bone fragments protruding through the skin. A greenstick fracture is a partial fracture in young bones, and a comminuted fracture is one where the bone is broken into three or more pieces.

29. **C.** Rationale: An avulsion is a type of fracture where the tendonous attachments of the bone are torn away. Tendons are soft tissues that do not "fracture"; rather they tear. An epiphyseal separation is a fracture at the growth plate of a long bone. A compound fracture is one where the bone protrudes through the skin.

30. **D.** Rationale: The callus stage is the stage of osteogenesis where there is a proliferation of cells from the fracture site into the fibrin to form fibrous connective tissue and cartilage.

31. **D.** Rationale: Skeletal traction with balanced suspension is the method of fracture treatment where a pulling force is exerted directly on the bone itself via a pin in the bone using a system of weights and pulleys. Buck's traction is skin traction.

32. **B.** Rationale: The principles of joint reconstruction include the concepts that joint function depends on the quality of its structures, that bones are held tightly in place by ligaments and the joint capsule, that the synovial membrane lining the joint capsule secretes synovial fluid to lubricate the joint, and that articular cartilage covers the ends of the bones where they meet to form a joint.

33. **D.** Rationale: A loosening of a joint with some displacement of the articular surface from the joint capsule is called a subluxation. A dislocation is where the articular surfaces are completely displaced. A fracture is a discontinuity of a bone, and avulsion is the "tearing away" of a tendon or ligament insertion.

34. **B.** Rationale: Reconstruction of a joint to restore or improve range of motion and stability or to relieve pain is referred to as an arthroplasty.

35. **B.** Rationale: Bofixation involves the ingrowth of bone to stabilize a prosthesis. Polymethylmethacrylate, or bone cement, does not permit bone ingrowth.

36. **D.** Rationale: Polymethylmethacrylate is prepared immediately before use, as it hardens quickly, usually within 5 to 10 minutes, depending on the temperature of the components.

37. **C.** Rationale: Arthroscopy is the procedure where the joint is visualized and conservative treatment of disease is carried out.

38. **A.** Rationale: An exostosis is an overgrowth of bone. Osteoblasts, osteocytes, and osteoclasts are types of bone cells.

39. **C.** Rationale: The term *neurolysis* refers to the "freeing up" of an entrapped nerve.

40. **D.** Rationale: The excision of a tendon sheath and its associated synovium is referred to as a tenosynovectomy.

41. **C.** **Rationale:** The ligamentum flavum is the yellow, elastic tissue connecting the lamina that is divided during Posterior Laminectomy.

42. **B.** **Rationale:** A rotator cuff tear occurs in the shoulder region, involving a tearing of tendons that make up the rotator cuff, including the infraspinous, supraspinous, teres minor, and subscapularis muscles.

43. **C.** **Rationale:** A fracture where healing has not taken place in the usual amount of time is referred to as a delayed union. A nonunion occurs when the bone does not heal and a malunion occurs when the bone heals in such a manner that it is not functional or cosmetically appealing.

44. **A.** **Rationale:** A Bristow Procedure, a procedure involving the shoulder, is performed in the semi-Fowler or beach chair position.

45. **B.** **Rationale:** An Austin Moore prosthesis is a type of hip prosthesis used to replace the femoral head and neck for certain types of intertrochanteric fractures.

46. **A.** **Rationale:** A Colles' fracture is a fracture of the distal radius.

47. **D.** **Rationale:** A Total Knee Arthroplasty is performed with the patient in the supine position. All of the remaining procedures/positions are correct.

48. **A.** **Rationale:** The medial malleolus, a projection of the tibia, is involved in an ankle fracture.

49. **C.** **Rationale:** A Correction of Hammer Toe Deformity is the procedure which consists of excision and fusion of the middle phalangeal joint of the foot with incision of the flexor tendon. Bunionectomy is the correction of a hallux valgus of the first metatarsal. Triple Arthrodesis involves the ankle joint. A Metacarpal Arthroplasty involves the hand.

50. **B.** **Rationale:** A tibial plateau fracture is commonly treated with an angled blade plate and cancellous screws. Femoral and humeral shaft fractures are commonly treated with plate and screws or intramedullary rods/nails. Patellar fractures are not treated with an angled blade plate.

51. **B.** **Rationale:** A Triple Arthrodesis does not include fusion of the metacarpophalangeal joint, located in the hand.

52. **A.** **Rationale:** During Anterior Cervical Discectomy and Fusion, the patient is placed in the supine position.

53. **A.** **Rationale:** Long cancellous screws placed with a gliding hole for the shaft provide compression of bone fragments.

54. **C.** **Rationale:** Avascular necrosis is a potential complication of ischemia of the femoral head. Intermittant claudication is pain in the lower extremities during walking due to ischemia from peripheral vascular disease. An intussusception is an "in-folding" of the bowel causing an obstruction of the lumen. Chondromalacia is an abnormal softening of the articular cartilage of a bone.

55. **B.** **Rationale:** A greenstick fracture is a fracture commonly found in children due to the softness of their immature bones.

56. **C.** **Rationale:** A compound fracture is one that results in a bone fragment protruding through the skin. This requires that the wound be debrided and closed before a cast is applied. A comminuted (multifragmented), a greenstick (incomplete fracture), and a spiral fracture usually do not require debridement before casting.

57. **D.** **Rationale:** An arthrodesis involves the removal of articulating surfaces of cortical bone, with the placement of a bone graft, resulting in a fusion or stiffening of a joint.

58. **B.** **Rationale:** Menisectomy involves the removal of the lateral or medial knee cartilage, called the lateral or medical meniscus.

59. **B.** **Rationale:** Chronic dislocation of the patella may result in an abnormal wearing and softening of the articulating cartilage, a condition called chondromalacia. Osteomyelitis is an infection of the bone marrow. Rheumatoid arthritis is an autoimmune disease resulting in the body's destruction of its own articular cartilage. Osteoporosis is the loss of bone density, which can result in fractures.

60. **A.** **Rationale:** Baker's cysts are found in the popliteal fossa, behind the knee joint.

61. **C.** **Rationale:** An Esmarch bandage is used to exsanguinate a limb prior to tourniquet cuff inflation. Webril, felt, and stockinette are all materials that can be used for cast padding.

62. **D.** **Rationale:** Bone wax is a hemostatic agent used to control bleeding from an open bone. When applied, the bone wax fills the bone matrix, forming a "plug" that stops blood flow. Bone wax, when applied to the end of a bone, will prevent osteogenesis.

63. **C.** **Rationale:** The oscillating saw is used to divide bone using a "side-to-side" cutting action. A reciprocating saw uses an "in and out" action, and the drill and drill/reamer use a rotary action.

64. **A.** **Rationale:** The correct order for screw placement is drill, measure, tap, and place.

65. **D.** **Rationale:** Bacitracin is an antibiotic added to wound irrigation on the sterile field when implants are used to reduce the risk of osteomyelitis.

66. **C.** **Rationale:** Chandler elevator

67. **D.** **Rationale:** Hibbs retractor

68. **A.** **Rationale:** Lane bone holding forcep

69. **B.** **Rationale:** Ferris Smith forcep

70. **A.** **Rationale:** Alm retractor

71. (Y) sternum

72. (Q) metatarsals

73. (T) phalanges

74. (X) skull or cranium

75. (F) clavicle

76. (N) humerus

77. (U) radius

78. (DD) ulna

79. (E) carpals

80. (L) femur

81. (R) patella

82. (M) fibula

83. (AA) tibia

84. (C) calcaneus

85. (W) scapula

86. (I) diaphysis

87. (K) epiphysis

88. (J) epiphyseal plates

89. (D) cancellous bone

90. (G) cortical bone

91. (A) articular cartilage

92. (Z) synovial membrane

93. (O) joint cavity

94. (H) deltoid

95. (B) biceps brachii

96. (S) pectoralis major

97. (V) rectus abdominis

98. (BB) trapezius

99. (P) latissimus dorsi

100. (CC) triceps brachii

Part II: Deciphering a Surgical Schedule

The following mock surgery schedule will be used to answer several questions pertaining to orthopedic surgery. The same schedule, or a similar one, will be used in subsequent chapters to ask questions about the content of the chapter.

Rm# time	Surgeon	Procedure	Anest.	Rm# time	Surgeon	Procedure	Anest.
Rm.00				**Rm07**			
OC	Dr. Z	Rt. Knee Arthroscopy	Gen.	7:00	Dr. M	Laparoscopic appendectomy	Gen.
OC	Dr. C	Craniotomy	Gen.	TF	Dr. M	Lipoma removal	MAC
OC	Dr.Z	ORIF left fibula	Gen.				
Rm.01				**Rm08**			
7:00	Dr. X	Hemorrhoidectomy	Gen.	11:00	Dr. E	Bankart Rt Shoulder	MAC
TF	Dr. X	Colostomy	Gen.				
TF	Dr. X	Bowel resection	Gen.				
Rm02				**Rm09**			
7:00	Dr. B	Splenectomy	Gen.	8:30	Dr. T	Cholecystectomy	Gen.
TF	Dr. B	Gastrectomy	Gen.	TF	Dr. T	Palatoplasty	Gen.
Rm03				**Rm10**			
7:00	Dr. A	Cystoscopy	MAC	7:00	Dr. K	Nephrectomy	Gen.
TF	Dr. A	Cystoplasty	Gen.	TF	Dr. K	Choledocholithotripsy	MAC
12:30	Dr. F	Pyelogram	MAC	TF	Dr. K	Hepatic resection	Gen.
3:00	Dr. F	Cystocele repair	Gen.				
Rm04				**Rm11**			
7:00	Dr. Y	Keller	Gen.	7:00	Dr. L	Total Knee Arthroplasty	Gen.
TF	Dr. Y	Arthroscopy Lt knee	Gen.	12:00	Dr. L	Total Hip Arthroplasty	Gen.
Rm05				**Rm12**			
7:00	Dr. G	Trans-sphenoidal Adenectomy	Gen.	7:00	Dr. W	Trans-metatarsal amputation	Gen.
TF	Dr. G	Trans-urethral resection of the prostate	Gen	TF	Dr. W	Osteotomy	Gen.
				TF	Dr. W	Arthrocentesis	Gen.
TF	Dr. G	Bletharoplasty	Gen.				
Rm06				**Rm13**			
7:00	Dr. R	Posterior Lumbar Laminectomy with fusion	Gen.	7:00	Dr. O	Right ACL	Gen.

The following questions should be answered using the surgery schedule above

1. There is an on call ORIF. The surgeon will require which instruments to perform this procedure?

   A. Drill, saw, plate, screws, depth gauge
   B. Drill, plate, depth gauge, tap
   C. Saw, plate, depth gauge, screws
   D. Drill, plate, screws, reamer

2. The patient in Room 11 is undergoing a total Knee Arthroscopy. The surgeon will need a tourniquet for this procedure. How long can it be inflated before permanent damage may occur?

   A. 1 hour
   B. 1.5 hours
   C. 2 hours
   D. 2.5 hours

3. Before the tourniquet is inflated, the surgeon wants to exsanguinate the limb. What is the most likely way that this will be done?

   A. Eschmark bandage will be wrapped from the proximal leg to the distal point
   B. Eschmark will be wrapped from the distal point to the proximal parameter
   C. Surgeon will elevate the limb for 5 minutes before inflating the tourniquet
   D. Stockinette will be applied

4. The surgeon performing the total knee replacement will be using a cemented prosthesis. What instrument should the Surgical Technologist hand to the surgeon to remove excess polymethylmethacrylate?

   A. Lambotte osteotome
   B. Key elevator
   C. Curette
   D. Chisel and mallet

5. What position will the patient in Room 8 be placed in?

   A. Lateral
   B. Prone
   C. Supine
   D. Beach chair

6. The Surgical Technologist has been assigned to Room 11 for the day. Which piece of equipment or supply will be used for the first procedure but NOT for the second?

   A. Saw
   B. Bone wax
   C. Osteotome
   D. Tourniquet

7. The Surgical Technologist assigned to Room 4 has an arthroscopy scheduled. How will he adjust the stopcocks on the instruments that he hands to the surgeon?

   A. He will open them
   B. He will close them
   C. He will hand them either open or closed depending on the instrument
   D. He will attach the cords and open the stopcocks before handing them to the surgeon

8. Room 6 has a lumbar laminectomy scheduled. The surgeon has requested a crosslink system. Which fixation system should the Surgical Technologist have available?

   A. Dwyer
   B. Zielke
   C. TSRH
   D. Small fragment set

9. The Surgical Technologist in Room 4 has a Keller scheduled. What is this procedure for?

   A. Dupuytrens contracture
   B. Colles fracture treatment
   C. Hammer Toe
   D. Bunion

10. The Surgical Technologist who has been assigned to Room 13 has an ACL repair. What are the most likely prep parameters for this case?

   A. Elbow to neck, circumferentially
   B. Knee to ankle, circumferentially
   C. Upper thigh to ankle, circumferentially
   D. Wrist to neck, circumferentially

Answers & Rationales

1. **B.** **Rationale:** An ORIF is a procedure to reduce a fraction and fixate it with plates and screws. The use of a drill is necessary, as are the depth gauge, plate, and screw. The use of a saw is generally not necessary for most ORIF procedure.

2. **C.** **Rationale:** The surgeon will want to be advised of tourniquet time after 1 hour. However, it may remain inflated on a lower extremity for 2 hours. If more time is necessary, the tourniquet will be deflated for 5 to 10 minutes before being re-inflated. The Surgical Technologist must be aware that blood flow will be restored to the surgical site for that time, and should be ready with lap sponges and suction to manage the field.

3. **B.** **Rationale:** An Eschmark bandage or ACE bandages are commonly used to exsanguinate a limb prior to inflation of the tourniquet. The surgeon will begin wrapping at the distal portion of the limb and continue wrapping to the proximal point. After the Eschmark has been applied, the tourniquet is inflated and surgery may begin.

4. **C.** **Rationale:** Generally, a small curette or a freer-elevator is handed to the surgeon to remove excess bone cement after the prosthetic is placed. The Surgical Technologist should have a lap or towel ready to clean the instrument tip after each pass.

5. **D.** **Rationale:** For proper visualization of the shoulder, the patient is commonly placed in the beach chair or modified beach chair position with the affected arm free so that manipulation of the arm can be done throughout the procedure.

6. **D.** **Rationale:** The first procedure in this room is a knee Arthroplasty, which will require a tourniquet. The second procedure will focus on the hip, making the tourniquet useless. It may remain in the room or be removed to an equipment room before the second case begins.

7. **B.** **Rationale:** Stopcocks should be closed by the Surgical Technologist before passing them to the surgeon.

8. **C.** **Rationale:** Dwyer and Zielke are anterior spinal fusion sets that would not be used during a posterior fusion. The small fragment set would be used in an ORIF, not a spinal fusion. The TSRH, or Texas Scottish Rite system is a crosslink system commonly used in lumbar spinal fusions.

9. **D.** **Rationale:** Keller procedures are commonly used to repair Hallux valgus, or bunion.

10. **C.** **Rationale:** The ACL is the anterior cruciate ligament, located in the knee. Therefore, both preps that include the arm would not be utilized in this case. Likewise, a prep that starts at the knee would be inappropriate for this surgical procedure.

PEARSON
myhealthprofessionskit

Use this address to access the interactive Companion Website created for this book. Simply select "Surgical Technology" from the choice of disciplines. Find this book and click to enter.

Neurosurgery 18 chapter

Neurosurgery became a specialty less than a century ago under the leadership of Dr. Harvey Cushing and deals with conditions of the brain, spinal cord, and nerves. Its diversity and challenges are based on the fact that both the brain and spinal cord, encased in bony cavities, send their branches (nerves) to all parts of the body to control our very awareness of and response to the world around us. Many surgeons are specialized in a specific area of neurosurgery, such as the brain or the spinal cord. Specialists in the brain generally do procedures such as aneurysm clippings and tumor removals, while those specializing in the spine may do fusions and Laminectomies.

CHAPTER OUTLINE

Questions dealing with neurosurgical specialties are complex and wide ranging. Not only does the Surgical Technologist need to be familiar with certain orthopedic instrumentation, they must also work with neurosurgical instrumentation and microscopes. The delicate structures where procedures are performed are covered with bone, which must be removed prior to starting the procedure. Generally, this is achieved with drills, Rongeurs, Kerrisons, and other bone instruments. The brain and spinal cord are also covered with meninges, the three-layered membrane protecting these delicate tissues. Knowing how to expose the site is as important as knowing the steps of the procedure.

Example:
Which instruments are used to incise and open the Dura Mater?

A. #7 Handle, #15 Blade, curved mayo scissors
B. #7 Handle, #11 Blade, Metzenbaum scissors
C. #3 Handle, #15 Blade, Metzenbaum scissors
D. #7 Handle, #15 Blade, Metzenbaum scissors

We know that although the dura mater is a tough fibrous tissue layer, the area is still extremely delicate. Knowing this, the Surgical Technologist will be able to narrow down the questions to the most likely. We can throw out the answer that has the blade loaded onto the #3 handle. Next, we know that curved mayo scissors are used on thicker tissue, such as muscle, so we can discard A. This leaves answer B and D. While an 11 blade is used for many things, it would not be a smart choice for this incision as it may puncture underlying brain tissue. This leaves one option. The correct answer would be D.

I. **Special Features of Neurosurgery**
   A. **Diagnostic procedures**
      1. *CT scanning:* with the use of contrast media, computers, and x-ray technology, a series of images of the brain and spinal cord differentiate between normal and abnormal tissues.
      2. *MRI:* with the use of radiofrequency and magnetic waves to capture images of the brain and spinal cord with less risk to patients, a variety of pathological conditions can be identified. Although expensive, MRI is replacing a number of other diagnostic procedures because of safety factors.
      3. *Isotope brain scan:* visual display of ultrasonographic images following IV injection of a radioactive isotope which concentrates in brain tissue to demonstrate lesions
      4. *Echoencephalography:* use of ultrasonic waves and a transcranial doppler device to measure blood flow to the brain
      5. *CT-guided stereotactic biopsy:* obtaining a specimen of brain tissue for analysis with the use of the stereotactic frame (a system which is attached to the skull to allow orientation of anatomical relationships in three intersecting planes using geometric coordinates for an exacting approach to deep structures within the brain)
      6. *Evoked potential:* noninvasive placement of electrodes over nerves or sensory organs to assess the status of the central nervous system
      7. *Diagnostic procedures once favored but now rarely used are:*
         a. *Cerebral angiography:* injection of a contrast medium into blood vessels to detect vascular lesions
         b. *Venography:* studies of venous sinuses in the brain with injection of contrast medium followed by x-rays

    c. *Ventriculography:* injection of air into lateral ventricles of the brain through burr holes in the skull for x-ray studies to determine blockage in the flow of cerebrospinal fluid

    d. *Pneumoencephalography:* injection of air into the subdural space of the spinal cord to determine if the pathway of cerebrospinal fluid is patent

    e. *Myelography:* x-ray study of the spinal cord following injection of a contrast medium

    f. *Lumbar puncture (spinal tap):* placement of a needle between the lumbar vertebrae to the subdural space to obtain a specimen of cerebrospinal fluid for analysis, to measure pressure, or to inject medications

B. Surgical pathology

1. Congenital anomalies

    a. *Hydrocephalus:* accumulation of cerebrospinal fluid (CSF) in the ventricles of the brain, due to obstructed flow through the ventricular system or overproduction of CSF by the choroid bodies/plexus

    b. *Craniosynostosis:* premature closure of sutures in the skull

    c. *Arteriovenous malformation (AVM):* fistula-type connections between arteries and veins in the brain which gradually enlarge under pressure, divert blood from other tissue, and lead to scarring and multiple small hemorrhages

    d. *Meningocele:* protrusion (hernia) of meninges through a defect in the skull or vertebral column

    e. *Meningoencephalocele:* herniation of the meninges and brain through a skull defect

    f. *Myelomeningocele:* herniation of the meninges and spinal cord through a defect in the vertebral column

    g. *Spina bifida:* congenital defect in the vertebrae/bone surrounding the spinal canal preventing closure and protection of the vertebral column and meninges

2. Neoplasms

    a. *Encephaloma:* brain tumor (glioma, glioblastoma multiforme [GBM], astrocytoma, acoustic neuroma, neuroma, angioma, pituitary tumor, metastatic tumor)

    b. *Meningioma:* tumor of the meninges (covering of the brain and spinal cord)

    c. *Myeloma:* spinal cord tumor

3. Vascular pathology

    a. *Aneurysm:* weakened arterial wall that allows for an area of distention; frequently occurs in the circle of Willis (communicating arterial system at the base of the brain), internal carotid, or middle cerebral artery

    b. *Hemorrhage*

    c. *Occluded arteries:* result from embolism or thrombosis and may occur at various locations

4. Injuries

    a. **Scalp lacerations:** bleed heavily due to excellent blood supply

    b. **Skull fractures:** surgery is required for depressed or compound fracture.

    c. **Intracranial hematomas**

        i. *Epidural:* tear in the middle meningeal artery or one of its branches, resulting in bleeding between the skull and dura mater; generally requires emergency burr holes to relieve pressure

        ii. *Subdural:* bleeding between the dura mater and arachnoid; may be acute, subacute, or chronic; blood mixes with cerebrospinal fluid

        iii. *Intracerebral hematoma* generally occurs in the anterior temporal or frontal lobes of the cerebrum

    d. **Severed nerves:** can occur anywhere in the body

e. **Cervical/vertebral fractures:** with damaged spinal cord; may require skeletal traction with application of halo traction

f. Head trauma (sharp or blunt) resulting in skull fracture and leakage of spinal fluid from the ear (otorrhea) and the nose (rhinorrhea)

g. Intractable pain

h. Trigeminal neuralgia (tic douloureux)

i. **Sciatica:** pain in the sciatic nerve

j. **Dopamine-deficient diseases:** Parkinson's, Huntington's, or Alzheimer's

k. Ruptured or herniated intervertebral disk—protruding herniated nucleus pulposa (HNP) compresses spinal nerves

5. **Complications of neurosurgery and preventive measures**

　a. **Hemorrhage:** meticulous hemostasis is essential.

　b. Increased intracranial pressure (ICP)

　　i. Close monitoring of ICP

　　ii. Decrease cerebral edema

　　iii. Gentle tissue handling

　　iv. IV osmotic diuretic (mannitol)

　　v. Position with head elevated if possible

　　vi. Administration of anti-inflammatory agents (steroids)

　　vii. Meticulous hemostasis

　　viii. Induced hypothermia

　　ix. Induced hypotension

　c. **Neurological defects:** paralysis, muscle weakness, paresthesia (partial paralysis), gait disturbances, aphasia (inability to express thoughts verbally), and ataxia (lack of coordination)

　d. Gentle handling of the extremely delicate neural tissue is essential.

　　i. Spoons or spatula retractors

　　ii. Ligature clips instead of sutures

　　iii. Cottonoid pledgets/patties instead of gauze for sponging

　　iv. Fine suction tip protected by cottonoid pledgets/patties is used with neural tissue.

　　v. Bipolar coagulation/suction coagulator

　e. Prevent sudden movements of the patient or around the surgeon.

　f. **Occluded cerebral circulation with thrombosis or embolism:** closely monitor somatosensory evoked potential.

　g. **Seizures:** use extreme care in tissue handling.

　h. **Venous air embolism with associated ventricular dysrhythmias and fibrillation:** use central venous pressure line with precordial monitoring when head or neck surgery is being done while the patient is in the sitting position.

　i. **Infection**

　　i. Meticulous asepsis

　　ii. Prophylactic antibiotic use

　　iii. Irrigation with antibiotic solution during surgery

C. **Equipment**

1. **Operating microscope**—floor or ceiling mounted; may include camera, closed-circuit television with monitor

2. Ceiling or wall source of nitrogen or compressed air to operate air-powered equipment

3. Monitors for EKG and EEG

4. Operating room bed with attachments and headrests and/or skull clamps (**AMSCO multipurpose, Mayfield, or Gardner**)

5. **Mayfield table:** neurosurgical overbed instrument table or two large Mayo stands, with standing stools or platforms

6. Cooling/heating unit with two blankets, temperature-monitoring devices, and thermostatic probes

7. Monopolar and bipolar electrosurgical unit

SURGERY HINT

Make sure that the Mayfield is inspected before each case. A malfunctioning Mayfield can have serious and even life-threatening complications for patient safety. If skull pins are used, the surgeon may need suture to close skin.

8. Fiber-optic headlight, lighted retractors, and telescopes
9. IV control units (IVACs), nerve stimulator, and solution warmer
10. **Drills:** Hall air drill, air drill 100, craniotome C-100, or Midas Rex/Anspache with attachments
11. **LASERs:** used for hemostasis, vaporization, or shrinkage of tissue by precise dissection; especially useful in microvascular surgery to occlude vessels, as for AVM or aneurysms; types used are carbon dioxide, argon, Nd:YAG, and tunable dye lasers
12. **Ultrasonic aspirator (CUSA):** used to emulsify and remove benign tumors
13. **Cryosurgical unit:** used to freeze and destroy tissue for the treatment of brain tumors, pituitary gland tumors, or for psychosurgery
14. **Stereotactic unit:** attached to the skull for stabilization of the head, collecting computerized data, localizing lesions, and providing an avenue through a burr hole into the skull for surgery to remove lesions in an otherwise inaccessible area of the brain; framed and frameless units

D. **Neurosurgical specialty instruments**
   1. **Drills** with burrs, perforators, guide, key, and bits
   2. **Craniotome (Hudson Brace-manual drill)**
   3. **Rongeurs:** double action and single action, Kerrison, alligator, and pituitary
   4. **Punches:** Cloward and Raney
   5. **Penfield (1–4),** Janson, and Freer dissectors and dura separator
   6. **Retractors:** mastoid, Weitlaner, brain spoons, or spatulas, Leyla-Yasargil self-retaining retractor
   7. **Scalp clips** (Adson, Raney), appliers, and removers
   8. **Forceps:** bayonet, Cushing, and Adson
   9. **Elevators:** Freer, Cushing, and Adson (joker)
   10. **Needles:** aspirating, aneurysm, and ventricular
   11. **Suction tubing and tips** (Frazier, Adson)
   12. **Ligating clips and appliers**
   13. **Irrigating syringes:** bulb, Asepto, syringe/angiocath

E. **Patient preparation and monitoring**
   1. *Foley catheter:* essential for long procedures, when mannitol (osmotic diuretic) is given, when excessive bleeding is anticipated, when hypothermia or hypotension is induced, and for assessment of kidney function
   2. *Central Venous Pressure (CVP) line:* useful for management of air embolism for the patient in the upright position during head or neck surgery
   3. *Induced hypotension:* lowering blood pressure with IV medications to lessen bleeding during intracranial vascular surgery
   4. *Antibiotics:* given IV preoperatively and used intraoperatively (added to irrigation)
   5. *Electroencephalogram:* either scalp or sterile subdermal needle electrodes used; connected to monitor to assess brain activity
   6. *Doppler ultrasound:* transducers placed over the heart for the patient in a sitting position to detect air embolism in the right atrium
   7. *Intracranial pressure (ICP) monitoring*
      a. *Causes of ICP:* increased volume in the brain (edema, increased CSF, or increased cerebral blood flow)
      b. *Normal ICP:* 10 to 20 mm Hg
      c. *Problems associated with ICP:* inadequate perfusion of cerebral cortex when sustained ICP is allowed

  d. *Methods of ICP monitoring*
   i. *Subarachnoid screw:* placed in the subdural space and connected to a monitor
   ii. *Ventricular catheter:* most accurate, inserted into the ventricle through a burr hole
   iii. *Epidural sensor:* implanted in the epidural space through a burr hole

F. Special psychological and emotional needs must be addressed, especially when brain surgery is anticipated

G. Skin preparation
 1. Hair
  a. Head hair removed in surgery holding area; clipped with electric clippers, placed in a special container labeled with the patient's name, and kept with the patient
  b. **For patients with surgery on the cervical spine:** long hair is secured on top of the head, and neck hair is removed with clippers to the top of the ear.
  c. Depilatory or clipping of hair just before surgery may be ordered for the patient undergoing surgery of the thoracic or lumbar spine
 2. Skin lesions are observed and reported to the surgeon.
 3. Surgical scrub is carried out after the patient is anesthetized and positioned.
 4. Incision line may be marked with marking pencil or dyes, such as indigo carmine, gentian violet, or brilliant green (**never with methylene blue—irritates neural tissues**).
 5. Local anesthetic or saline may be injected at incision sites used to decrease bleeding during incision by creating additional pressure within the tissue; or Raney clips may be used

H. **Positioning**
 1. *General considerations:* protect the eyes, maintain joint alignment, avoid pressure on superficial nerves and vessels, and ensure patency of tubes and catheters.
 2. *Fowler (sitting)*
  a. Modified "beach chair" with back of table elevated to full sitting position
  b. **Uses:** infratentorial surgery (posterior cranial fossa) or Posterior Cervical Laminectomy
  c. **Advantages:** optimum visibility and decreased blood loss
  d. **Disadvantages:** drop in arterial pressure, negative venous pressure in the head and neck, which may lead to air embolism, compromise of the airway from neck flexion, and venostasis in the lower extremities
  e. Preparation for the sitting position
   i. Application of sequential compression device, from toes to groin to help prevent venostasis
   ii. Extra padding for the feet
   iii. Stabilizing of the shoulders and torso, with the head in the headrest, to prevent flexion of the neck

SURGERY HINT

Raney clips must be applied to the scalp quickly. Have them ready and be prepared to load with as much speed as possible.

  Most facilities count Raney clips during opening and closing counts, so be prepared to retrieve them as they are removed post operatively.

SURGERY HINT

The patient in the prone position will be induced and intubated on the stretcher and then "log rolled" into the prone position for the surgical procedure.

Once the procedure has concluded, the patient will be rolled back to the stretcher before extubation.

3. *Supine or dorsal recumbent with modifications:* used for Supratentorial Craniotomy, Anterior Cervical Fusion, Subtemporal Decompression, and Lumbar Sympathectomy
4. *Prone position with modifications:* may be used for procedures of the back or posterior fossa of the cranium (infratentorial)
   a. Preparation for the modified prone position
      i. Sequential compression device used on the legs
      ii. Patient anesthetized on stretcher before being positioned for surgery
      iii. Special supports (**chest and axillary rolls**) to permit lung expansion; **Wilson or Andrews** laminectomy frame
      iv. **Horseshoe or Mayfield headrest** may be used.
      v. Concerns with the prone position
         - Increased bleeding caused by increased venous pressure
         - Peripheral venostasis
         - Decreased vital (lung) capacity
         - Pressure on male genitals/female breasts
         - Pressure on brachial plexus caused by hyperextension of the shoulders
         - Abduction of the arms with occlusion of the subclavian and axillary arteries
         - Pressure, scratches, and chemical burns to the eyes

I. Draping
   1. *Towels:* may be secured with silk suture on a heavy cutting needle, disposable staples, or small towel clips. (*Note:* If towels are sutured; needles, needle holder, scissors, forceps, and/or stapler are discarded from sterile field.)
   2. *Plastic adhesive:* placed either before or after towels (skin must be dry); used to prevent "strike-through" due to continuous drainage of CSF intraoperatively
   3. *Large drape sheet:* used to cover the patient and Mayfield table

J. Visibility and hemostasis
   1. **Irrigation/suctioning**
      a. Irrigation with normal saline or Ringer's solution at body temperature is provided by the scrub using a bulb syringe; used to enhance visibility of the operative site
      b. Suction with Frazier tip is used to remove CSF, blood, and irrigation fluid.
      c. Suction is never applied directly to normal neural tissue; tissue is protected with cottonoid pledgets/patties.
   2. **Retractors**
      a. *Scalp:* self-retaining (Greenburg, Leyla)
      b. *Dura mater:* traction sutures (4-0 silk, braided nylon, or Vicryl)
      c. *Brain tissue:* blunt spatulas or spoons
      d. Lighted retractors helpful for intracranial procedures
   3. **Hemostatic agents and methods**
      a. Lidocaine with epinephrine or normal saline may be injected at the intended skin incision site to reduce bleeding from the skin edges.
      b. Bone wax is applied to the cranial bone edges.

c. Cottonoid pledgets/patties (not gauze) soaked in normal saline or Ringer's solution are used on neural tissue; must be counted and displayed on a fluid-proof surface.

d. Scalp wound edges are lined with gauze sponges and secured with scalp clips.

e. Microfibrillar collagen (Avitene) is applied dry.

f. Absorbable gelatin sponge, moistened with normal saline or thrombin solution

g. Ligating clips for larger vessels

h. **Electrosurgery:** bipolar forceps with suction; fulguration tip may be used to stop bleeding in the brain, spinal cord, dura mater, periosteum, or galea

i. **LASER:** argon, carbon dioxide, or Nd:YAG may be used to control bleeding.

j. **Cryosurgery:** stops bleeding by freezing tissue

II. **Cranial Procedures**

A. *Craniotomy:* incision into the skull

1. *Types:* frontal, parietal, occipital, temporal, or a combination

2. *Procedure for craniotomy*

a. With digital pressure over radiopaque sponges, an incision is made through the skin and galea (aponeurosis of the scalp).

b. Scalp clips are applied to flap edges, grouped in segments, and secured with rubber bands, and bleeding is controlled.

c. Soft tissue is removed from the periosteum; scalp flap is turned and covered with moist sponges.

d. Periosteum is stripped, and bone wax is applied to bleeders.

e. Burr holes are drilled through the cranial bone(s)—irrigation and suctioning performed to remove bone dust and counteract heat.

f. Dura mater freed with a Penfield dissector

g. Sawing between drill holes frees the bone flap, while irrigation and suction is continued; bone flap is protected with moist sponges

h. **Dura mater is opened:** dura elevated with a dura hook; scalpel is used to nick the dura, and the edges are grasped and elevated; brain is protected with moist cottonoid pledgets/patties, and traction sutures are applied and held with bulldogs or mosquito clamps; dural veins are ligated, clipped, or coagulated

i. Brain is retracted with spoons, kept moist with Ringer's solution or saline, and bleeding is controlled with bipolar coagulation.

j. Upon completion of anatomical revisions, the brain is irrigated with an antibiotic solution.

k. Dura may be left open or closed with a 4-0 silk, black braided nylon, or polyglycolic acid/polyglactin suture; a drain may be left in place.

l. Holes are drilled in the bone flap (if it is to be replaced) and skull for placement of wire suture or plates/screws (dura protector or spoon is used on the skull side).

m. Muscle, galea, and periosteum are closed with a 2-0 or 3-0 synthetic absorbable suture; skin is closed with staples or nonabsorbable suture.

3. Intracranial procedures

a. *Intracranial Aneurysm Repair*

i. May be approached from frontal, frontotemporal, or bifrontal craniotomy if the aneurysm is in the circle of Willis

ii. Managed by placement of an aneurysm clip to occlude it or by chemical coating with polymethylmethacrylate to prevent rupture. (*Note:* Aneurysm clips should never be compressed between the fingers, only when in their appliers. Clips that have been compressed should be discarded because they may slip or be sprung.)

 b. *Arteriovenous Malformation (AVM) Repair*
  i. Incision may be supratentorial or infratentorial
  ii. Feeding arteries are located and occluded by clipping, ligating, or coagulating
 c. *Intracranial Revascularization*
  i. Occluded portion of the internal carotid or middle cerebral artery is revascularized by anastomosis of the superficial temporal artery to the middle cerebral artery
  ii. Procedure may also be used to bypass a large aneurysm
 d. *Transphenoidal Hypophysectomy/Adenectomy*
  i. **Indications:** pituitary tumor, Cushing's syndrome (overactive pituitary), acromegaly (enlarged extremities), malignant exophthalmus (protruding eyes), hypopituitarism, metastatic cancer of the breast or prostate, or severe diabetes insipidus
  ii. Pituitary gland is removed by a rhinoseptal approach
  iii. **Position:** semi-Fowler with head against headrest
  iv. **Prep:** face, mouth, and nasal cavity
  v. **Anesthesia:** general plus infiltration of local anesthetic with epinephrine into the gingiva and nasal mucosa
  vi. **Drape:** sterile adhesive plastic drape over the face plus additional drapes for the field
  vii. **Incision:** upper gum margin through the maxilla and sphenoid sinus to the sella turcica (depression in the sphenoid bone containing the hypophysis/pituitary gland) and dura mater
  viii. Operating microscope and portable image intensifier used to identify anatomy
  ix. Following excision of the gland, the floor (sella turcica) is reconstructed with cartilage from the nasal septum; nasal packing with antibiotic applied, and gingiva is closed.
  x. *Note:* Pituitary tumors may also be approached by frontal, bifrontal, or frontotemporal incision.
 e. *Craniectomy:* removal of bone from the skull (burr holes)
  i. **Indications:** decompression of the brain (following trauma), tumors of the skull, scars, hematomas, infection, or craniosynostosis
  ii. Position and surgical approach dependent upon pathology and choice of the neurosurgeon
 f. *Subtemporal Craniectomy for Trigeminal Rhizotomy*
  i. **Indications:** severe pain of the face because of pathology of the fifth Cranial (Trigeminal) nerve; known as tic douloureux
  ii. Supine position with a vertical temporal incision and burr hole (enlarged with rongeurs)
  iii. Microscope provides light and magnification.
  iv. Mandibular and maxillary sections of the nerve root are divided.
  v. Absolute (100%) alcohol may be injected into the divided nerve.
 g. *Subtemporal Craniectomy for Ménière's disease*
  i. **Ménière's disease:** severe attacks of vertigo, nausea, vomiting, and tinnitus with progressive hearing loss
  ii. Cerebellum is approached through an incision behind the ear, eighth Cranial Nerve is exposed, and vestibular fibers in the anterior half of the nerve are divided.
 h. *Cranioplasty:* repair of a skull defect with an autogenous bone graft or synthetic or titanium prosthesis
 i. *Trephination:* making an opening (burr holes) into the skull with a trephine or drill
 j. *Micro-Neurosurgical procedures*
  i. Excision of an Acoustic Neuroma, a tumor of eighth Cranial (Vestibulocochlear) Nerve

      ii. Decompression of Cranial Nerves
     iii. Cerebral Revascularization
     iv. Excision of an Arteriovenous Malformation
      v. Occlusion of Aneurysms
     vi. Stereotactic Procedures
    vii. Aspiration of cysts, abscesses, or hematomas
   viii. Biopsy
     ix. **Electrostimulation:** electrodes implanted to control intractable pain or epilepsy

k. *Radiofrequency Trigeminal Rhizotomy:* for the treatment of tic douloureux

l. *Thalamotomy:* destruction of a selected portion of the thalamus for relief of pain, epileptic seizures, involuntary tremor, rigidity of muscles (Parkinson's disease), or emotional disturbances

m. *Cingulotomy:* disruption of the pathways of connecting fibers in the cerebral hemisphere between the frontal and temporal lobes to control severe chronic pain, addiction, or some intractable psychoses

n. *Intracranial Vascular Lesion Management:* thrombosis or AVM can be vaporized or cauterized with LASER, occluded with a silicone bead, or clipped through stereotactic instrumentation

o. **Intracranial Neoplasm Excision with LASER vaporization**

p. *Cryohypophysectomy:* use of a cryoprobe to treat pituitary tumors

q. *Interstitial Radiation:* implantation of radioactive substances into malignant brain tumors

r. *Interstitial Hyperthermia:* destruction of tumors with heat conducted through sensors

s. *Gamma Knife Radiation:* noninvasive stereotaxis to identify the location of tumors and direct a high dose of gamma radiation to stop growth

t. *Shunt operations:* diversion of CSF from ventricles in the brain to other body cavities for absorption; used to treat hydrocephalus
      i. **Types**
        • *Communicating:* overproduction of CSF by the choroid bodies of the ventricles or abnormal absorption from the subarachnoid space
        • *Noncommunicating:* obstruction of flow within the ventricular system
     ii. **Procedures**
        • *Ventriculoatrial (VA) shunt:* ventricular catheter is placed, through a burr hole, in the right lateral ventricle and connected to a reservoir; a tunnel is made from the burr hole and reservoir to a neck incision and the atrial catheter (passed through the jugular vein to the right atrium) is pulled through and connected to the reservoir; a valve, such as a Holter, may be used.
        • *Ventriculoperitoneal (VP) shunt:* CSF is shunted from the right ventricle through the ventricular puncture site beneath the scalp and tissues of the neck, chest, and abdomen to the peritoneal cavity.

u. *Control of epilepsy (seizures)*
      i. *Cortical Resection:* removal of epileptogenic tissue from the anterior temporal lobe
     ii. *Corpus Callostomy:* severing the corpus callosum (white matter connecting the right and left hemispheres of the brain)
    iii. *Vagal Nerve Stimulator Implantation:* used to stimulate the Vagus Nerve, reducing seizures in patient who cannot undergo brain surgery
    iv. *Autologous Adrenal Medulla Transplant:* transfer of tissue from the adrenal medulla to the brain (near the right lateral ventricle) to enhance production of dopamine (neurotransmitter) and treat Parkinson's disease

III. **Spinal Procedures**

A. *Laminectomy: excision of one or more laminae to expose the spinal cord*

1. *Indications:* treat compression fractures, herniated nucleus pulposus (HNP), dislocations, spinal cord tumors, insertion of infusion pump for pain control, or insertion of subarachnoid shunts for pseudotumor cerebri or hydrocephalus

2. *Positioning:* based on physician's preference and specific area of disease. Modified prone position is generally used for Thoracic or Lumbar Laminectomy, whereas a Cervical Laminectomy may be done with the patient in the sitting, prone, or lateral position.

3. *Laminectomy instruments:* include pituitary and Kerrison rongeurs; retractors (Beckman-Adson, Taylor, Scoville, Love nerve root, Adson self-retaining cerebellar), Key periosteal elevators, Penfield and Freer dissectors, ring and angled bone curettes

4. *Surgical procedure for ruptured disk (HNP)—Laminectomy/Discectomy*
   a. Midline vertical incision is made over involved pathology and hemostasis is secured.
   b. Weitlaner or Gelpi retractor is inserted to enhance visibility.
   c. Fascia is incised to expose spinous processes.
   d. Periosteum and paraspinous muscles are stripped, and gauze sponges with periosteal elevator are used for blunt dissection and hemostasis.
   e. Taylor, Scoville, or Beckman-Adson retractor is positioned, and hemostasis is provided by cottonoid pledgets/patties.
   f. Lamina edge is defined with a curette, and ligamentum flavum is grasped and incised as the dura is protected.
   g. Dura and nerve root are retracted with Love nerve root retractor to expose the disk space.
   h. Pituitary ronguers are used to remove nucleus pulposus, and Scoville curettes are used to clean the interspaces.
   i. Interspaces are irrigated; hemostasis is obtained with cottonoid pledgets/patties; and the wound is closed.

5. *Laminectomy for spinal cord tumor*
   a. Dura is incised, incision is lengthened, and a 4-0 nylon suture is placed on the dura edge for traction.
   b. Tumor is dissected free and removed, and hemostasis is secured with bipolar coagulation or an absorbable gelatin sponge with topical hemostatic agent.
   c. Wound is irrigated with Ringer's solution or saline, and dura is closed with 4-0 to 5-0 silk, black braided nylon, or polyglactin suture.
   d. Incision is closed with 0 polyglactin or 2-0 silk suture.

6. *Laminectomy for Meningocele*
   a. Congenital anomaly which may be associated with spina bifida (incomplete closure of the vertebral canal)
   b. Nerve stimulator and pediatric instruments are needed.
   c. Effort is made to protect neural elements.

7. *Laminotomy with Microdiskectomy:* a minimally invasive approach to a herniated disk; use of the operating microscope allows a smaller incision and less tissue dissection.

SURGERY HINT

During a laminectomy and fusion, take care to keep any bone the surgeon may remove. Secure the bone fragments on the back table, remove any soft tissue, and morselize the bone with a rongeur that is not in use. This bone may be used to fuse the patient and must be free of any debris. Keep moist with a damp sponge until the surgeon requests it.

Hand bone to the surgeon in a medicine cup or other container with a Russian forcep.

B. *Cervical Cordotomy:* division of spinothalamic tract (the section of the spinal cord which carries messages to the brain) for treatment of intractable pain
   1. *Rhizotomy:* interruption of the spinal nerve roots
      a. Anterior (motor) root for relief of spasms
      b. **Posterior Cervical Rhizotomy:** division of posterior cervical roots (sensory) for relief of intractable pain

C. *Anterior Cervical Discectomy with Fusion (Cloward Procedure)*
   1. *Indications:* relief of pain in the neck, shoulder, and arm caused by herniated disk or spondylosis (degenerative disease of the vertebrae) with ankylosis (stiffness)
   2. *Procedure*
      a. Patient is in supine position with right hip elevated to expose the iliac crest (if autogenous graft is harvested)
      b. Instruments: minor dissecting set plus Cloward self-retaining retractors, bone graft holder, bone graft impactor, hand retractor, vertebral spreaders, and ronguers; drill guards; spinal fusion curettes; and mallet
      c. Transverse incision is made on the side of the neck, the involved disk is exposed, and an x-ray is taken to verify the level
      d. Bone (autogenous or cadaveric) is grafted between the cervical vertebrae (may be secured in place with plates/screws) and the incision is closed.

D. *Carotid Artery Ligation:* occlusion of internal carotid artery to control hemorrhage during intracranial surgery for vascular anomalies; tied off with heavy silk or gradually occluded with a carotid clamp

E. *Kyphoplasty:* injection of polymethylmethacrylate "cement" onto the vertebral body for treatment of compression fractures

IV.   Peripheral Nerve Procedures

A. *Sympathectomy:* division of a portion of the spinal root ganglion and nerve fibers of the sympathetic division
   1. Variations include:
      a. *Upper Cervical Sympathectomy:* to increase blood supply through the internal carotid arteries
      b. *Cervicothoracic Sympathectomy:* to relieve chronic vasoconstrictive processes as those caused by Raynard's disease (vascular deficiency of the upper extremities)
      c. *Thoracic Sympathectomy:* for relief of chronic or intractable pain from biliary and pancreatic diseases
      d. *Thoracolumbar Sympathectomy:* for treatment of essential hypertension
      e. *Lumbar Sympathectomy:* for relief of intermittent claudication— vasospastic disease in the lower extremities
      f. *Truncal Vagotomy:* excision of a portion of the Vagus (tenth cranial) Nerve below the diaphragm to treat Peptic Ulcer Disease (PUD)
      g. *Presacral Neurectomy:* excision of a portion of the presacral nerve for intractable pain such as in dysmenorrhea

B. *Neurorrhaphy:* surgical repair of divided nerves; use of microscope and fine instruments is essential; multiple fine sutures are placed through the nerve sheath and epineurium

C. *Neurolysis:* release of adhesions from around a nerve to relieve pain and restore function

Show What You Know

Directions: Each of the numbered items or incomplete statements in this section is followed by answers or by completions of the statement. Select the ONE lettered answer or completion that is BEST in each case.

1. Which of the following diagnostic procedures utilizes a contrast medium, a computer, and x-ray technology to show differences between normal and abnormal tissues?

    A. echoencephalography
    B. evoked potential
    C. pneumoencephalography
    D. CT scan

2. A herniation of the brain and its coverings through a defect in the skull is:

    A. Meningoencephalocele
    B. Myelomeningocele
    C. Encephaloma
    D. Aneurysm

3. Bleeding that has occurred between the skull and the outer covering of the brain is a/an:

    A. epidural hematoma
    B. subdural hematoma
    C. intracerebral hemorrhage
    D. arteriovenous malformation

4. Venous air embolism would be a surgical complication more likely to occur in patients having a/an:

    A. Lumbar Laminectomy for a ruptured disk
    B. Repair of a Meningocele with the patient in the prone position
    C. Anterior Cervical Dissectomy in the supine position
    D. Posterior Fossa Craniotomy in the sitting position

5. Of the following equipment, which would least likely be used for neurosurgery?

    A. Mayfield table attachment
    B. insufflation tubing
    C. hypothermia unit
    D. bipolar electrosurgical unit

6. Which of the following positions would be most likely used for performing a Lumbar Laminectomy?

    A. Fowler
    B. modified prone
    C. modified supine
    D. left lateral

7. Which of the following instruments would be considered contaminated during a Craniotomy?

    A. craniotome used for burr holes in skull
    B. Penfield dissector used to separate dura from the skull

C. Cushing forceps used in placement of traction sutures in the dura
    D. needle holder used when securing drape towels

8. During a Craniotomy, the brain is protected with:

    A. cottonoid pledgets/patties
    B. 4×4 sponges
    C. laparotomy tapes
    D. Telfa

9. All of the following procedures would usually require a craniotomy incision *except:*

    A. Intracranial Clipping of an Aneurysm
    B. Transphenoidal Hypophysectomy
    C. Anteriovenous Malformation Repair
    D. Excision of an Acoustic Neuroma

10. Equipment used to emulsify and remove a benign tumor is a/an:

    A. cryosurgical unit
    B. ultrasonic aspirator
    C. Midas Rex/Anspache with attachments
    D. craniotome

11. Hydrocephalus is treated by which surgical procedure?

    A. Craniectomy
    B. Laminectomy
    C. Ventriculoperitoneal Shunt Placement
    D. Cranioplasty

12. A herniated nucleus pulposus is treated with which surgical procedure?

    A. Craniectomy
    B. Laminectomy
    C. Ventriculoperitoneal Shunt Placement
    D. Cordotomy

13. Craniosynostosis is treated with which surgical procedure?

    A. Craniectomy
    B. Cordotomy
    C. Ventriculoperitoneal Shunt Placement
    D. Cranioplasty

14. The diagnostic test used to measure electrical activity of the brain is called:

    A. echoencephalography
    B. electroencephalography
    C. isotope brain scanning
    D. cerebral angiography

15. Stereotaxis provides:
    A. the location of a fixed point in space using geometric coordinates
    B. images of the vascular structures of the brain
    C. images of the outlines of the ventricles to assess for obstruction
    D. a sample of cerebrospinal fluid for analysis

16. The meningeal layer located proximal to the brain tissue is the:
    A. pia mater
    B. subarachnoid
    C. dura mater
    D. arachnoid mater

17. Dopamine-deficient diseases include all of the following except:
    A. Parkinson's Disease
    B. Huntington's Disease
    C. Alzheimer's Disease
    D. Cushing's Syndrome

18. Cranial Nerve X is the:
    A. Trochlear
    B. Olfactory
    C. Vagus
    D. Trigeminal

19. What is the position of choice for supratentoral craniotomy?
    A. "beach chair"
    B. prone
    C. lateral
    D. dorsal recumbent

20. The hemostatic clips applied on the scalp following the skin incision are called _____ clips.
    A. Rolando
    B. Raney
    C. Penfield
    D. Mayfield

21. The instrument used to remove a herniated nucleus pulposus during Laminectomy/Discectomy is the:
    A. pituitary rongeur
    B. Penfield dissector
    C. Kerrison rongeur
    D. Midas Rex or Anspache

22. Hemostatic agents used in neurosurgery include all of the following except:
    A. saline
    B. bone wax
    C. absorbable gelatin sponge
    D. protamine sulfate

23. One of the solutions used to moisten cottonoid pledgets/patties during surgery includes:
    A. sterile water
    B. Lactated Ringer's solution
    C. mannitol/glycine solution
    D. 5% dextrose in water solution

24. The CUSA probe is used for:
    A. freezing destruction of tissue
    B. emulsification and aspiration of tissue
    C. cauterization of tissue
    D. drainage of excessive cerebrospinal fluid

25. The tissue encountered under the skin of the scalp is the:
    A. dura mater
    B. arachnoid space
    C. galea/aponeurosis
    D. periosteum

26. Closure of the dura mater would be accomplished using any of the following suture materials except:
    A. silk
    B. polyglycolic acid/polyglactin
    C. chromic gut
    D. braided nylon

27. The treatment of arteriovenous malformation includes all of the following techniques except:
    A. coagulation using LASER
    B. coating with methylmethacrylate resin
    C. ligation with clips
    D. implantation of silicone beads

28. A congenital defect in the vertebral canal without herniation of the meningeal tissues is referred to as a/an:
    A. meningocele
    B. spina bifida
    C. hydrocephalus
    D. arteriovenous malformation

29. Shunts placed for the treatment of hydrocephalus commonly drain into the:
    A. peritoneum and left atrium
    B. peritoneum and right atrium
    C. right or left atrium
    D. peritoneum or portal vein

30. The procedure for the treatment of chronic pain which involves surgery on the nerve root is referred to as:
    A. Rhizotomy
    B. Cingulotomy
    C. Kyphoplasty
    D. Neurolysis

31. Which of the following is a dye that should not be used to mark the skin prior to neurosurgical procedures?
    A. gentian violet
    B. indigo carmine
    C. methylene blue
    D. brilliant green

32. The headrest used for neurosurgical cases is called the _____ headrest.
    A. Mayfield
    B. Penfield

C. Penrose

D. Raney

33. The area of cerebral circulation where the basilar arteries feed into is referred to as the:

A. Circle of Magendie

B. Circle of Sylvius

C. Circle of Willis

D. Circle of Raney

34. Dural traction sutures are secured with:

A. bulldogs

B. Allises

C. Oschners

D. Kellys/peans

35. The medication used during Transsphenoidal Hypophysectomy to aid incisional hemostasis would be:

A. lidocaine hydrochloride with ephedrine

B. dexamethasone

C. lidocaine hydrochloride without epinephrine

D. cocaine hydrochloride

36. The tissue responsible for the secretion of cerebrospinal fluid is the:

A. cerebellum

B. pia mater

C. choroid bodies/plexus

D. subarachnoid space

37. Lumbar Sympathectomy is performed for the diagnosis of:

A. intermittent claudication

B. myocardial ischemia

C. Peptic Ulcer Disease

D. empyema

38. The tissue/structure found in the sella turcica is the:

A. corpus callosum

B. fourth ventricle

C. pituitary gland

D. pineal gland

39. Tumors of the brain include all of the following *except:*

A. pheochromocytomas

B. meningiomas

C. astrocytomas

D. gliomas

40. The meningeal layer space where bleeding most commonly occurs following trauma is the:

A. epipial space

B. subpial space

C. subarachnoid space

D. subdural space

Anatomy Review

Nervous System

41–54.

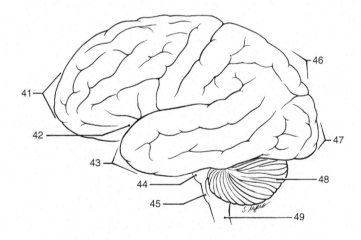

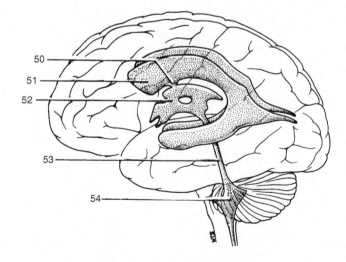

A. aqueduct of Sylvius

B. cerebellum

C. fourth ventricle

D. frontal lobe

E. intraventricular foramen of Monro

F. lateral fissure

G. lateral ventricle

H. medulla oblongata

I. occipital lobe

J. parietal lobe

K. pons

L. spinal cord

M. temporal lobe

N. third ventricle

Cranial Nerves

List the cranial nerves in order.

55. CN I: _____

56. CN II : _____

57. CN III : _____

58. CN IV: _____

59. CN V: _____

60. CN VI: _____

61. CN VII: _____

62. CN VIII: _____

63. CN IX: _____

64. CN X : _____

65. CN XI: _____

66. CN XII : _____

Answers & Rationales

1. **D.** **Rationale:** CT scan (computerized tomography) utilizes a contrast medium, a computer, and x-ray technology to demonstrate a difference between normal and abnormal tissue.

2. **A.** **Rationale:** Meningoencephalocele is a herniation of the brain and its coverings through a defect in the skull. Myelomeningocele is a herniation of the spinal cord and its coverings through a defect in the vertebral column. An aneurysm is a weakness in the wall of an artery, and an encephaloma is a tumor of the brain.

3. **A.** **Rationale:** An epidural hematoma is the presence of blood between the dura and skull resulting from trauma.

4. **D.** **Rationale:** Venous air embolism is a complication more commonly occurring with head or neck surgery when performed with the patient in the sitting position. Preventive measures include doppler and central venous pressure monitoring.

5. **B.** **Rationale:** Insufflation tubing is not used by neurosurgeons, since they are used to create pneumoperitoneum during minimally invasive surgery (laparoscopic procedures). The Mayfield instrument table, hypothermic unit, and bipolar electrosurgical unit are commonly used equipment in neurosurgery.

6. **B.** **Rationale:** The modified prone position with a Wilson or Andrews frame is most frequently used for a Lumbar Laminectomy. A Posterior Cervical Laminectomy may be done with the patient in the sitting or prone position.

7. **D.** **Rationale:** When drape towels are sutured in place, the needles, needle holder, forceps, and scissors used are considered contaminated.

8. **A.** **Rationale:** Cottonoid pledgets/patties are used to protect delicate nerve and brain tissue.

9. **B.** **Rationale:** Transphenoidal Hypophysectomy is the removal of the pituitary gland and is accomplished with the use of a microscope by a rhinoseptal approach with the incision above the front teeth.

10. **B.** **Rationale:** The ultrasonic aspirator is used to emulsify and remove benign tumors. The Midas Rex or Anspache is used for sawing and drilling, the craniotome for incising the skull, and cryosurgery for freezing tissue for removal.

11. **C.** **Rationale:** A Ventriculoperitoneal Shunt Placement is performed for the treatment of hydrocephalus.

12. **B.** **Rationale:** A Laminectomy is performed for the treatment of a herniated nucleus pulposus.

13. **D.** **Rationale:** A Cranioplasty is performed for the treatment of craniosynostosis.

14. **B.** **Rationale:** The diagnostic test used to measure electrical activity of the brain is called electroencephalography.

15. **A.** **Rationale:** Stereotaxis provides the location of a fixed point in space using geometric coordinates.

16. **A.** **Rationale:** The meningeal layer located proximal or closest to the brain tissue is the pia mater.

17. **D.** **Rationale:** Parkinson's Disease, Huntington's Disease, and Alzheimer's Disease are all dopamine-deficient diseases. Cushing's Syndrome is a disease of the adrenal cortex that overproduces cortisol.

18. **C.** **Rationale:** The Vagus Nerve (CN X) is the tenth cranial nerve. The Olfactory Nerve is

CN I, the Trochlear is CN IV, and the Trigeminal is CN V.

19. D. **Rationale:** The dorsal recumbent position is the position of choice for supratentoral craniotomy.

20. B. **Rationale:** Raney clips are applied on the scalp following the skin incision to reduce bleeding from the scalp edges.

21. A. **Rationale:** A pituitary rongeur is used to grasp and extract the nucleus pulposus from the intervertebral disk space during Laminectomy/Discectomy.

22. D. **Rationale:** Hemostatic agents used in neurosurgery include the use of saline injected into the scalp prior to incision for hemostasis, bone wax applied to the edges of the bone, and absorbable gelatin sponge for topical application on delicate tissues. Protamine sulfate is an anticoagulant and heparin antagonist.

23. B. **Rationale:** Lactated Ringer's solution is one of the solutions of choice to moisten cottonoid pledgets during surgery. Sterile water is not used as it is a hypotonic solution. Mannitol/glycine and 5% dextrose solution are sugar-based and are not used for this purpose.

24. B. **Rationale:** The CUSA probe is used to emulsify and aspirate delicate tissues in neurosurgery.

25. C. **Rationale:** The galea/aponeurosis is the tissue layer found under the skin of the scalp.

26. C. **Rationale:** The dura mater would be closed with silk, Vicryl/Dexon, or braided nylon. Dura would not be closed using chromic gut due to the potential for irritation of the meninges from the presence of the foreign protein.

27. B. **Rationale:** The treatment of arteriovenous malformation includes coagulation using LASER, ligation with clips, and occlusion with silicone beads. Coating an AV malformation with methylmethacrylate resin would not prevent shunting of arterial blood into the venous system.

28. B. **Rationale:** Spina bifida is a congenital defect in the vertebral canal without herniation of the meningeal tissues. A meningocele involves herniation of the coverings (meninges) of the brain and/or spinal cord.

29. B. **Rationale:** Shunts placed for the treatment of hydrocephalus commonly drain into the peritoneal cavity or the right atrium.

30. A. **Rationale:** Rhizotomy is the procedure of choice for the treatment of chronic pain where the nerve root is divided, preventing the transmission of pain impulses to the brain.

31. C. **Rationale:** Methylene blue should never be used on neurosurgical procedures as it may cause irritation if it contacts delicate neural tissues.

32. A. **Rationale:** The Mayfield headrest is the headrest most commonly used for neurosurgical cases.

33. C. **Rationale:** The circle of Willis is the area of cerebral circulation at the base of the brain supplied by the basilar and internal carotid arteries. This is a common site for cerebral aneurysms to occur.

34. A. **Rationale:** Dural traction sutures are used to retract the dura without injuring this delicate tissue layer. Once placed, the sutures are secured with bulldogs, which provide slight traction on the sutures, holding the dura away from the surgical site. The other instruments listed would provide too great a pull on the dura, risking tearing this delicate tissue layer.

35. D. **Rationale:** Of the medications listed, only cocaine hydrochloride would provide incisional hemostasis. Dexamethasone is an anti-inflammatory agent used to control postoperative swelling. Lidocaine without epinephrine would provide pain relief, but not hemostasis. Epinephrine, not ephedrine, can be combined with lidocaine for incisional hemostasis.

36. C. **Rationale:** The choroid bodies, located within the four ventricles of the brain, are responsible for the secretion of cerebrospinal fluid.

37. A. **Rationale:** Lumbar Sympathectomy, a division of the sympathetic chain of the autonomic nervous system, is performed for the diagnosis of intermittent claudication, a condition of cramping and pain in the lower extremities during exercise due to ischemia from peripheral vascular disease and vasospasm. Peptic ulcer disease may be surgically treated with Vagotomy. Empyema is the formation of pus in the pleural space.

38. C. **Rationale:** The sella turcica, a depression in the sphenoid bone, contains the hypophysis or pituitary gland.

39. A. **Rationale:** Meningiomas, astrocytomas, and gliomas are all types of brain tumors. Pheochromocytomas are tumors of the adrenal glands.

40. D. **Rationale:** The subdural space contains the arachnoid, a meningeal layer that contains many spider-web–like blood vessels. Injury to this layer can result in bleeding.

41. (D) frontal lobe

42. (F) lateral fissure

43. (M) temporal lobe

44. (K) pons
45. (H) medulla oblongata
46. (J) parietal lobe
47. (I) occipital lobe
48. (B) cerebellum
49. (L) spinal cord
50. (E) intraventricular foramen of Monro
51. (G) lateral ventricle
52. (N) third ventricle
53. (A) aqueduct of Sylvius
54. (C) fourth ventricle
55.   Olfactory Nerve

56. Optic Nerve
57. Oculomotor Nerve
58. Trochlear Nerve
59. Trigeminal Nerve
60. Abducens Nerve
61. Facial Nerve
62. Vestibulocochlear Nerve
63. Glossopharyngeal Nerve
64. Vagus Nerve
65. Spinal Accessory or Accessory Nerve
66. Hypoglossal Nerve

Part II: Deciphering a Surgical Schedule

The following mock surgery schedule will be used to answer several questions pertaining to neuro surgery. The same schedule, or a similar one, will be used in subsequent chapters to ask questions about the content of the chapter.

Rm.#time	Surgeon	Procedure	Anest.	Rm#time	Surgeon	Procedure	Anest.
Rm.00				**Rm07**			
OC	Dr. Z	Rt. Knee Arthroscopy	Gen.	7:00	Dr. M	Subdural hematoma evacuation	Gen.
OC	Dr. C	Craniotomy	Gen.	TF	Dr. M	AVM repair	Gen
OC	Dr.Z	Angioplasty	Gen.				
Rm.01				**Rm08**			
7:00	Dr. X	Hemorrhoidectomy	Gen.	11:00	Dr. E	Bovine Thrombectomy	MAC
TF	Dr. X	Colostomy	Gen.				
TF	Dr. X	Bowel resection	Gen.				
Rm02				**Rm09**			
7:00	Dr. B	Splenectomy	Gen.	8:30	Dr. T	Cholecystectomy	Gen.
TF	Dr. B	Gastrectomy	Gen.	TF	Dr. T	Palatoplasty	Gen.
Rm03				**Rm10**			
7:00	Dr. A	Cystoscopy	MAC	7:00	Dr. K	Nephrectomy	Gen.
TF	Dr. A	Cystoplasty	Gen.	TF	Dr. K	Choledocholithotripsy	MAC
12:30	Dr. F	Pyleogram	MAC	TF	Dr. K	Hepatic resection	Gen.
3:00	Dr. F	Cystocele repair	Gen.				
Rm04				**Rm11**			
7:00	Dr. Y	Carpal tunnel release	Gen.	7:00	Dr. L	Rhizotomy	Gen.
TF	Dr. Y	Whipple	Gen.	12:00	Dr. L	microdiskectomy	Gen.
Rm05				**Rm12**			
7:00	Dr. G	Trans-sphenoidal Adenectomy	Gen.	7:00	Dr. W	ACDF	Gen.
TF	Dr. G	Aneurysm clipping	Gen	TF	Dr. W	Sympathectomy	Gen.
TF	Dr. G	Laminectomy/ diskectomy	Gen.	TF	Dr. W	VP shunt	Gen.
Rm06				**Rm13**			
7:00	Dr. R	Lumbar Laminectomy and fusion	Gen.	7:00	Dr. O	Hysterectomy	Gen.

The following questions should be answered using the surgery schedule above

1. The Surgical Technologist scheduled in Room 7 knows that Dr. M prefers a manual drill for hematoma evacuations. Which instrument should he have available for the first case?

    A. Acorn burr loaded onto the Midas Rex
    B. Hudson Brace
    C. CUSA
    D. Hall

2. The aneurysm clipping in Room 5 will require a self retaining retractor. What should the Surgical Technologist have ready?

    A. Hudson –Brace
    B. Scoville retractor
    C. Williams Retractor
    D. Leyla yasargil

3. The aneurysm exposure will need to make an incision through the scalp. What should the Surgical Technologist have prepared?

    A. 2-0 silk suture
    B. Raney clips
    C. Cloward punch
    D. Hemoclips

4. There is a Rhizotomy scheduled for Room 11. Why is this procedure being performed?

    A. Chronic pain
    B. Tumor treatment
    C. Graves disease complications
    D. HNP

5. The patient scheduled for an ACDF has arrived in Room 12. In what position will the patient be placed?

    A. Prone
    B. Beach chair
    C. Lateral
    D. Supine

6. Dr. G, who is performing a lumbar laminectomy in Room 5, needs to retract the nerve root to expose the disk. What will the Surgical Technologist hand her?

    A. Cloward retractor
    B. Penfield 2
    C. Love retractor
    D. Leyla-yasargil

7. After the HNP is exposed, what should the Surgical Technologist hand to Dr. G?

    A. Kerrison
    B. 4-0 nylon suture
    C. Curette
    D. Pituitary Rongeur

8. Dr. W is performing a VP shunt in Room 12 following his Sympathectomy. Where will the CSF be shunted?

    A. The right atrium
    B. The right jugular
    C. The peritoneum
    D. The pulmonary vein

9. The surgeon is preparing to close the Dura after evacuating the hematoma from the patient in Room 7. What suture should the Surgical Technologist have ready?

A. 3-0 silk
B. 4-0 nylon
C. 4-0 prolene
D. 4-0 cotton

10. Dr. G will need to enlarge the flap at the site of the removed bone. What instruments should the Surgical Technologist have prepared for the surgeon?

A. Periosteal elevator and pituitary rongeur
B. Pituitary rongeur and Kerrisons
C. Kerrisons and double action rongeur
D. Double action rongeur and Penfield 1

Answers & Rationales

1. **B. Rationale:** The Hudson Brace drill is a manual hand held drill. The Midas Rex and the Hall are powered drills, and the CUSA is used to remove benign tumors.

2. **B. Rationale:** Scoville and Williams retractors are used in spinal procedures, not cranial procedures. The Hudson Brace is a drill. The Leyla Yasargil is a neuro self-retaining retractor that is commonly used in cranial procedures.

3. **B. Rationale:** Raney clips placed on the appliers are commonly used to attain hemostasis. The Surgical Technologist should pre-load the clips onto the applier and be prepared to re-load as quickly as possible. There is a reusable gun available with an available disposable clip cartridge that allows the surgeon to clip quickly before a reload is necessary.

4. **A. Rationale:** Rhizotoyomies may be performed for chronic pain if other treatment methods have failed. It may be performed on cranial or spinal nerves.

5. **D. Rationale:** The procedure calls for visualization of the anterior neck. The patient will be placed in a supine position with the head padded with a doughnut or Mayfield head rest. Prone position is used for posterior spinal surgeries.

6. **C. Rationale:** The love nerve root retractor is commonly used to retract the nerve root,

exposing the disk to be removed. Cloward retractors are generally used in ACDF cases, Leyla-yasargil retractors are used for cranial retraction, and the Penfield is used for cutting or dissecting smaller structures such as vessels or nerves, not for retraction.

7. **D. Rationale:** Generally the surgeon will use a pituitary rongeur to grasp and remove the herniated disk. They are available in several angles, including up biting and down biting as well as straight. The surgeon may need to use several different pituitaries to remove the disk in question.

8. **C. Rationale:** When performing a VP shunt, the shunt is tunneled through the neck and chest and allowed to drain into the peritoneal cavity. A VA shunt will drain into the right atrium.

9. **B. Rationale:** The Dura is generally closed with either a 4-0 or 5-0 suture, most commonly a braided nylon.

10. **C. Rationale:** Most bone enlargements are done with a double action or single action rongeur, such as the Leksell or Cushing for larger bites, followed by the Kerrisons for smaller bits of bone. The Periosteal elevator is used to strip periosteum from bone, the pituitary is used to extract disk material, and the Penfield is a dissector.

Ophthalmic Surgery

Ophthalmology is the branch of medicine concerned with the diagnosis and treatment of diseases and defects of the eye and its related structures. Most ophthalmic procedures are done in an outpatient facility. Eye instruments are extremely delicate and must be handled very carefully. Often, the procedure is done with the surgeon looking through the microscope during the procedure.

CHAPTER OUTLINE

Many ophthalmic procedures use multiple medications on the back table, and they must be carefully monitored by the Surgical Technologist. Understanding these medications and their use is a major concern for students. Questions related to eye surgery may also deal with specific procedures, anatomy, and specialty instrumentation and equipment, so the student must be familiar with these aspects of the surgeries.

Example:
An example of an ophthalmic sponge that may be utilized during a Scleral buckle procedure is

a. Weck sponge
b. Micro-cottonoid sponge
c. Eye pad
d. Cellulose sponge

To answer this question, the student has to have an understanding of the supplies used during eye surgeries. Cottonoids are generally used in microsurgical procedures of the nervous system, and are not commonly used during eye procedures. An eye pad is used as dressing after the procedure has completed, and cellulose, while used in ophthalmic procedures, is not common on Scleral buckle cases. They are commonly used during corneal transplants.

I. Terminology

   A. *Accommodation:* adaptation for near and far vision and focus

   B. *Amblyopia:* dim vision

   C. *Anterior chamber:* space between the cornea and the iris filled with aqueous humor

   D. *Aphakia:* absence of the lens, due to congenital abnormality, trauma, or surgical removal

   E. *Blepharoptosis:* drooping of the upper eyelid because of a weakness or absence of the levator palpebra muscle

   F. *Canthus:* angle at the fissure on either side of the eyelids; corner of the eye

   G. *Conjunctiva:* the thin transparent vascular membrane overlying the sclera and continuing on the undersurface of the upper and lower lids

   H. *Cycloplegic:* drug capable of paralyzing the ciliary body which results in a dilated pupil and loss of accommodation (inability to focus)

   I. *Extracapsular cataract extraction (ECCE):* surgical removal of the lens nucleus and cortex via an incision in the anterior surface of the capsule, leaving the posterior capsule surface intact

   J. *Extrinsic eye muscles:* six pairs of muscles connecting the globe to the eye orbit to allow movement

   K. *Intracapsular cataract extraction (ICCE):* removal of the entire lens, including the capsule and the nucleus

   L. *Intrinsic eye muscles:* smooth muscles inside the eye connected to the ciliary body which control the size of the pupil (amount of light entering the back of the globe) and the shape of the lens (accommodation)

   M. *Intraoccular lens (IOL):* an implantable device placed in the anterior or posterior chamber of the eye to aid in light refraction; made of acrylic or silicone

N. *Limbus:* junction of the cornea and sclera

O. *Miotic:* drug capable of constricting the pupil

P. *Mydriatic:* drug capable of dilating the pupil

Q. *Myopia:* nearsighted

R. *OD:* oculus dexter; right eye

S. *OS:* oculus sinister; left eye

T. *OU:* oculus uterque; both eyes

U. *Pars plana:* anterior attachment of the retina

V. *Phacoemulsification:* a method of breaking up and aspirating the nucleus of the cataract lens using a low-frequency ultrasonic handpiece

W. *Posterior chamber:* space between the iris and lens into which aqueous humor flows

X. *Retinopathy:* disease of the retina

Y. *Tarsal plate:* cartilage plate forming the eyelids

Z. *Trephine:* instrument for removing a buttonhole section, generally from the cornea

II. **Pathology of the Eye and Associated Structures**

A. *Cataract:* opacification of the crystalline lens of the eye

B. *Chalazion:* inflammation of the meibomian glands or hair follicles of the tarsal plate of the lid; a sty

C. *Ectropian:* turning outward of the margin of the eyelid, resulting in a constant drainage and irritation of the lid

D. *Entropian:* turning inward of the margin of the eyelid, causing the eyelashes to rub against the cornea

E. *Glaucoma:* a group of diseases resulting in increased intraocular pressure (IOP), which over time can damage the retina resulting in blindness; can be due to overproduction of aqueous humor, obstruction of the drainage system, or a congenital membrane covering the pupil; types include:
   1. *Narrow- or closed-angle glaucoma:* iris mechanically obstructs the flow of aqueous humor, causing an increase in IOP; is very painful and requires early surgical intervention
   2. *Wide- or open-angle glaucoma:* chronic type caused by the hypersecretion of or decreased ability to absorb aqueous humor; generally treated by medication

F. *Macular degeneration (MD):* destruction of the cells of the retina at the area of central vision (macula); types include
   1. *Atrophic or dry MD:* comprises 90% of MD; develops slowly and usually causes mild vision loss with a dimming of vision when reading
   2. *Exudative or wet MD:* the result of the abnormal growth of new blood vessels under the macula that are extremely fragile and are easily broken; bleeding results in separation of the macula from the choroid

G. *Ptygerium:* a benign, fleshy encroachment of opacified conjunctiva that grows over the cornea and can block the visual pathway

H. *Retinal detachment:* a separation of the retina from the choroid, resulting in death of the retina in that area

I. *Strabismus:* a failure to coordinate bilateral eye movements so that both eyes focus in the same direction; convergent/esotropia—eyes turn inward; divergent/exotropia—eyes turn outward

J. *Pathology of the visual pathway*
   1. *Emmetropia:* normal vision
   2. *Myopia:* nearsightedness

3. *Hyperopia/presbyopia:* farsightedness associated with aging
4. *Astigmatism:* an irregular surface on the cornea or lens, resulting in a distorted or blurred image being transmitted to the macula

III.   Medications, Equipment, Instrumentation, and Supplies

A. *Medications*
1. Mydriatics and Cycloplegics
    a. *Action:* constriction of the iris resulting in dilation of the pupil
    b. *Uses:* permits examination of the retina, testing for refraction, and facilitates easy removal of the lens
    c. *Agents*
        i. *Mydriatics:* most commonly used is phenylephrine (NeoSyn-ephrine) 2%, 5%, or 10%; patient can still focus
        ii. *Cycloplegics:* most commonly used are tropicamide (Mydriacyl) 1%, atropine 1%, cyclopentolate (Cyclogyl) 1%, and scopolamine hydrobromide (Isopto-Hyoscine) 0.25%; patient will be unable to focus when cycloplegics are used
2. Miotics
    a. *Action:* constricts the pupil by relaxing the iris
    b. *Uses:* treatment of glaucoma, decreasing IOP by enhancing escape of aqueous humor from the eye, and preventing vitreous rupture following cataract extraction
    c. *Agents*
        i. *Pilocarpine 1% to 4%*
        ii. *Acetylcholine (Miochol):* used during surgery for rapid constriction of the pupil following a lens implant. (*Note:* Miochol is prepared immediately before use as it deteriorates quickly.)
        iii. *Eserine ointment:* is applied topically after surgery, prior to dressing application
        iv. *Carbochol (Miostat):* 0.01% used intraoperatively
3. Corticosteroids
    a. *Action:* anti-inflammatory agents
    b. *Uses:* decrease inflammation; not used in presence of infection, as they mask symptoms
    c. *Agents*
        i. Methylprednisolone (Depo-Medrol, Depo-Kenalog)
        ii. Dexamethasone (Decadron)
        iii. Betamethasone (Celestone)
4. Hyperomostics/Diuretics
    a. *Action:* increase concentration of serum, shrink vitreous body, reduce IOP, and induce diuresis
    b. *Uses:* preoperative medication before ophthalmic surgery or to treat uncontrolled glaucoma
    c. *Agents*
        i. Osmitrol (mannitol)
        ii. Diamox (acetazolamide)
5. Dyes
    a. *Action:* stain tissues
    b. *Uses:* detect abrasions of the cornea, assess the patency of the nasolacrimal ductal system, check for leaks around the sutures of a corneal transplant
    c. *Agents*
        i. Fluorescein sodium: a stain used for detecting foreign bodies or corneal abrasions; also used IV for retinal angiography
        ii. Rose bengal
        iii. Indocyanine green

6. Zonulysis agents
   a. *Action:* an enzyme
   b. *Uses:* to dissolve the zonules holding the lens in place prior to an intracapsular cataract extraction (ICCE)
   c. *Agent:* alpha-chymotrypsin (Alpha-Chymar)
7. Anesthetic agents
   a. *Action:* prevents transmission of nerve impulses; regional anesthesia immobilizes the globe and lowers IOP
   b. *Uses:* local or regional anesthesia
   c. *Agents*
      i. Proparacaine hydrochloride (Ophthaine) 0.5%
      ii. Tetracaine hydrochloride (Pontocaine) 0.5%
      iii. Lidocaine hydrochloride (Xylocaine) 2%
      iv. Bupivicaine hydrochloride (Marcaine/Sensorcaine) 0.25%–0.75%
   d. Methods of administration
      i. *Topical:* Ophthaine and Pontocaine
      ii. *Injection:* Xylocaine and Marcaine; used together in combination with sodium hyaluronidase (Wydase) for retrobulbar (behind the globe) injection
      iii. *Instillation:* placement in the anterior chamber
8. Irrigating fluids
   a. *Action:* irrigation
   b. *Uses:* keep cornea moist and irrigate anterior chamber
   c. *Agents*
      i. Balanced Salt Solution (BSS) (*Note:* 2 ml of Epinephrine 1:10,000 added to 50 ml of BSS; used for hemostasis and to keep pupil dilated.)
9. Lubricants/Viscoelastic agents
   a. *Action:* jelly-like lubricant
   b. *Uses:* prevent the formation of adhesions, avoid damage to cornea when the anterior capsule is opened
   c. *Agents:*
      i. sodium hyaluronate—Healon, Amvisc, Viscoat
10. Antibiotic agents
    a. *Action:* reduces microbe count and risk for infection
    b. *Uses:* to prevent infection
    c. *Agents:*
       i. ointment (topical) and injection
       ii. gentamycin sulfate
       iii. erythromycin ointment
11. Other medications related to eye surgery
    a. *Hyaluronidase (Wydase):* enzyme which softens fibers of tissue to enhance spread of local anesthesia
12. Considerations of ophthalmic medications
    a. Medications play a critical role in surgical procedures of the eye.
    b. Most ophthalmic procedures require the use of different medications than those used for other types of surgical procedures.
    c. Medications used in eye surgery are required to be extremely pure.
    d. All medications injected into the globe should be labeled "for ophthalmic use" to assure proper purity and concentrations.
    e. Eye medications are extremely potent and generally come in low concentrations.
    f. Medications used during the eye procedure are usually colorless but have a specific function.
    g. All syringes and containers must be labeled with the name and strength of the medication to prevent medication errors.

       h. All medications on the sterile field should be double checked before they are passed for administration.

       i. If improperly administered, some medications may cause irreversible damage to the eye or its structures.

  13. Considerations when instilling eye drops

      a. Wash hands before administering.

      b. Use sterile ophthalmic drops.

      c. Verify correct medication, correct strength, correct patient, correct eye(s), exact number of drops, and precise intervals (read label carefully).

      d. If patient is awake, explain the procedure.

      e. With patient's head back and looking upward, the lower lid is pulled down and drops are released into the middle of the lower lid (conjunctival sac); the excess is gently blotted to avoid drainage into the tear duct; application of pressure over the medial canthus (corner of the eye nearest the nose) also diverts fluid from the nose.

      f. Do not allow dropper to touch the globe or lid.

      g. A single-use disposable vial is used for each patient.

      h. For patients under local anesthesia, a drop of topical anesthetic in each eye helps prevent burning from prep solution.

B. *Equipment*

  1. *Operative microscope*

      a. Floor or ceiling mounted

      b. Usually uses a 175–200 mm focal distance lens

      c. Foot controls allow for microscope adjustment/focusing by the surgeon while working

      d. Care of optics (after each procedure)

         i. Remove loose particles with a clean soft brush or ear syringe.

        ii. Using a circular motion, remove blood solutions with a cotton-tipped applicator moistened with distilled water.

        iii. Special cleaning solution is needed for removing oil or fingerprints.

  2. *Phacoemulsification unit*

      a. Designed to fragment, irrigate, and aspirate (vacuum) lens material from within the lens capsule, as well as perform anterior vitrectomy and hydrodissection

      b. Phacoemulsification hand piece consists of a hollow ultrasonic fragmenting tip and irrigation sleeve

      c. Irrigation/aspiration hand piece—irrigation and vacuum only

      d. Optional ocutome/vitrector for removal of vitreous humor, if indicated

      e. Can be programmed to the specific parameters of ultrasonic force, irrigation flow rate, and aspiration pressure desired

      f. Balanced Salt Solution, with or without epinephrine, is instilled into the globe by the phacoemulsification unit to maintain IOP during the procedure and to serve as a liquid medium for fragmented lens aspiration.

  3. *Cryoprobe*

      a. Used to freeze cells of tissues, causing adhesion or cell death

      b. Liquid or gaseous nitrogen is used to create an "iceball" at the end of a sterile hand piece/metal tip

      c. Used to treat retinal detachment and glaucoma or to aid in cataract removal

  4. *LASERs*

      a. **Advantages**

         i. Decreased chance of infection

        ii. Conducive to ambulatory surgery

        iii. Useful for the poor-risk operative patient

        iv. Minimal pain and requires only topical anesthesia

        v. Precisely cauterizes tissue and blood vessels

b. **Types and uses**
  i. **Blue-green argon:** for retinal detachment, lesion, or tear; trabeculoplasty; iridotomy
  ii. **Red-yellow krypton:** for retinal vascular disease or vessel aberrations of the choroid
  iii. **Invisible pulsed neodymium yttrium-aluminum garnet (Nd:YAG):** for preoperative anterior capsulotomy, posterior capsulotomy, lysis of adhesions, and retinal disorders
5. *Honan balloon:* used to massage the eye following administration of retrobulbar anesthetic block; decreases IOP

C. *Instrumentation*
1. *Concepts*
  a. Instruments are small, with fine, delicate tips
    i. Tips and cutting surfaces need to be protected—usually stored in special instrument container to prevent damage
    ii. Points are inspected under magnification
    iii. Instruments are not allowed to touch each other or metal surface
  b. Instrument cleaning
    i. Instruments wiped with distilled water on the sterile field
    ii. Ultrasonic cleaning with distilled water used to dislodge any particles not wiped
    iii. Instruments may be **"milked"**—lubricant used to keep functioning smoothly
2. *Basic eye instruments:* include eye speculum and/or lid retractors, muscle hooks, knife handles (#3 and micro-beaver), scissors (Stevens tenotomy scissors, Wescott scissors), forceps (fine and heavy Bishop-Harmon), calipers, needle holders (micro and heavy), and irrigating cannula (bulb tipped—for BSS; 27g angled blunt—for instilling intraocular medications/air)
3. *Specialty eye instruments*
  a. *Schiotz tonometer:* measures intraocular pressure
  b. *Castroviejo corneal scissors:* right and left
  c. *Vannas scissors:* delicate intraocular structures
  d. *De Wicker iris scissors:* "butterfly"-shaped scissors usually used to perform iridectomy/iridotomy
  e. *Castroviejo suturing and tying forceps:* 0.3- and 0.12-mm tying platforms
  f. *Lid clamps:* hemostasis during lid procedures
  g. *Muscle hooks and clamps:* used during extrinsic muscle procedures

D. *Prep*
1. Tenotomy or iris scissors with a thin film of water-soluble lubricant is used to clip eyelashes, if ordered by the physician, before skin preparation is begun.
2. Care is taken to avoid getting the prep solution in the ears or eyes.
3. Lid margins, lashes, eyelids, eyebrows, and surrounding skin of both eyes are cleansed with an antimicrobial solution using cotton swabs for the lid margins and sponges for the larger skin surfaces.
4. Globe is irrigated with normal saline, using a bulb syringe, from inner to outer canthus; one drop of half-strength povidone-iodine solution may be instilled into the eye before irrigation.

E. *Draping*
1. Drapes should be free of lint or other particles.
2. The head drape is the first to be applied, with an adhesive strip placed just above the brow line and secured anterior to the ears.
3. Adhesive towel is applied and secured over the nose if general anesthesia is used.

4. Patient and OR bed are covered with a split sheet with operative eye isolated.

5. Clear plastic adhesive drape is placed over the operative eye, secured, and arranged to collect irrigating fluid. (*Note:* If the patient is apprehensive about having drapes over the face, a Mayo stand is used to elevate the drape; oxygen, set at 6 to 8 L/min, is delivered through nasal prongs placed beneath the drape.)

F. *Hemostasis*
   1. Bipolar ESU
   2. Microforceps
   3. Wet-field eraser tip
   4. Disposable hot-tip wire cautery unit

G. *Sponges*
   1. *Lint-free sponges*
      a. *Squares:* used in place of 4×4s
      b. *Spears:* tiny, spear-shaped absorbable sponges for use on the globe
   2. *Applicator sticks/Q-tips:* remove blood from non-globe structures

H. *Corneal/Scleral shield:* plastic, cup-shaped device that fits over the cornea of the globe protecting it from injury during procedures of the lid and conjunctiva

I. *Suture materials—ophthalmic sutures*
   1. Range from 4-0 to 10-0; on swaged, side-cutting needles
   2. Gut sutures are rinsed before use.
   3. Absorbable suture is generally used to close the conjunctiva but may be sealed with ESU.
   4. Selection of suture varies with surgeon and procedure.

J. *Intraocular lens (IOL)*
   1. Made of polymethylmethacrylate with polypropylene haptex (curved, wirelike suture material to stabilize the lens until it adheres to the surrounding tissues)
   2. **Diopters:** measurement of focusing strength of lens; selected individually based on measurements taken of the globe (A scan) and anticipated lens position
   3. **Types**
      a. *Anterior chamber:* lens positioned in front of the pupil; haptex are fixed to the iris
      b. *Posterior chamber:* lens positioned into the empty capsular "bag" of the lens
      c. *LASER ridge:* able to dissolve the posterior capsule after lens excision; performed with Nd:YAG LASER to treat opacification of the posterior capsule
   4. **Insertion**
      a. Intraocular lens (IOL) should be soaked and rinsed in BSS to remove any impurities.
      b. Usually lubricated with viscoelastic agent to prevent damaging tissues during lens insertion
      c. Never touched by gloved hands—glove powder may be damaging to the eye tissues and should be removed before beginning setup (scrub) or draping (surgeon) by wiping gloves with a wet sponge that is then discarded

K. *Dressing material*
   1. *Uses:* prevent movement of the eyelid, absorb blood and tears, and protect the eye
   2. *Types:* eye pad, eye shield (Fox) (secured with plastic or paper tape)
   3. *Procedure*
      a. Saline sponges are used to clean around the eye.

b. Antibiotic ointment is placed in the subconjunctival sac to prevent adhesion to bandages.

c. When a pressure dressing is desired, a gauze roller bandage is applied over the initial dressing, encircling the head.

d. The eye shield is used to prevent external pressure on the eye following intraocular procedures.

IV. Special Features of Eye Surgery

A. Environment

1. A calm, quiet environment is maintained during surgery.
2. Verification of proper patient and proper eye is essential.
3. Scrupulous aseptic technique is enforced.
4. Proper padding for the patient is essential for long procedures, especially under regional anesthesia.
5. Do not pass instruments or supplies directly over an exposed globe.
6. The scrub may be responsible for irrigating the cornea with BSS every 10–15 seconds to prevent drying of the tissues.
7. Instruments need to be placed in a working position in the surgeon's hand as they may not look away from the microscope.
8. Patients are instructed to avoid anything that increases IOP, such as bending over, straining, or coughing; and to report any pain, swelling, or redness.

B. Complications of eye surgery

1. *Loss of vitreous:* escape of vitreous into the anterior chamber can cause wound prolapse, severe inflammation, or up-drawn pupil and generally requires immediate removal with a vitreotome/ocutome
2. *Hemorrhage:* Beaver or Wheeler knife is required for fast cut down into pars plain area and an 18-gauge needle or cannula on a syringe to aspirate blood and reduce pressure to avoid loss of vision
3. *Instrument failure:* hand aspiration devices should be immediately available
4. Systemic reaction to medication or local anesthesia leading to cardiac arrest

V. Extraocular Surgery

A. *I&D of a Chalazion*

1. *Chalazion:* small lump on the eyelid resulting from chronic inflammation of a meibomian (sebaceous) gland; sometimes referred to as a meibomian or tarsal (edge of eyelid) cyst
2. *Procedure:* the affected lid is everted, cruciate (shaped like a cross) incision is made on the inner surface and contents of cyst removed, and a pressure dressing is applied.

B. *Ectropian/Entropian repair*

1. Definitions

a. *Ectropion:* eyelid turns outward (sagging); causes tearing, conjunctivitis, and irritation; may result from facial paralysis

b. *Entropion:* eyelid margin turns inward; results in lashes rubbing against the cornea causing inflammation

2. Procedure

a. V-shaped wedge of tissue excised from lid (ectropian) or skin lateral to the lateral canthus; sutured to reposition lid

---

SURGERY HINT

Make sure that gloves are completely free of all powder.
Keep towels to a minimum on the field as they may contain lint which can cause complications.

C. *Blepharochalasis:* eyelid hangs down over the eye to obstruct vision; excess tissue is excised by making an elliptical incision in the fold of the upper eyelid, redundant tissue is removed, skin edges are sutured, and dressing is applied.

D. *Blepharoplasty:* plastic surgery to correct faulty position of the eyelids, ptosis, drooping, or sagging; similar to blepharochalasis

E. *Pterygium Excision*
   1. *Pterygium:* winglike benign growth which begins at the medial canthus and extends over the conjunctiva to the cornea
   2. *Procedure:* pterygium with the underlying conjunctiva is freed from the cornea, dissected from the sclera, and the conjunctiva defect is closed; chemotherapeutic agent may be applied to prevent regrowth.

F. *Dacryocystorhinostomy (DCR)*
   1. *Lacrimal apparatus:* consists of a lacrimal gland (tear gland with ducts) located on the superior lateral aspect of each eye, lacrimal canals located at the medial canthus (opening to lacrimal canals called puncta), a lacrimal sac located on the medial orbit, and a nasolacrimal duct which carries tears into the nasal cavity.
   2. *Specialty items:* fluorescein dye; lacrimal duct probes and dilators, trephine, silastic tubing
   3. *Procedures*
      a. *Lacrimal duct probing/dilation:* probes in graduated sizes are introduced into the duct system to enhance drainage of tears; patency verified by irrigating the canals/duct with fluorescein-stained BSS irrigation—dye should appear in the nasal cavity if patent.
      b. *Dacryocystectomy (dacry/o: tear; cyst: sac):* surgical excision of the tear sac for chronic dacryocystitis
      c. *Dacryocystorhinostomy:* creation of an opening from the lacrimal sac into the nasal cavity due to obstruction related to trauma or congenital malformation; silastic stent tubing placed from puncta to nare and soft tissue closed over it; may need to create a new opening in nasal bone with trephine (circular drill for hollow bones); epithelialization of the pathway occurs to create a new drainage system

G. *Resection and recession*
   1. *Strabismus:* extraocular muscles are not coordinated to permit eyes to position correctly for stereoscopic sight due to inequality of muscle strength; types include:
      a. *Esotropia:* convergent strabismus; eyes turn medially—"cross-eyes"
      b. *Exotropia:* divergent strabismus; eyes turn laterally
   2. *Procedures:* involve weakening strong muscles and tightening weak muscles; both eyes are draped out so that the surgeon can compare their appearance intraoperatively
   3. *Specialty items:* calipers for measuring distances; muscle clamps and hooks; absorbable suture for muscle reattachment
   4. *Procedures*
      a. *Resection:* strengthening a muscle by removal of a section; lid speculum is inserted, and conjunctiva is incised; affected muscle is grasped with muscle hook, a double-armed suture is preplaced, the muscle anterior to the suture is excised; stump of muscle is sutured to the old insertion site; conjunctiva is closed and dressing applied
      b. *Recession:* weakening a muscle by moving the insertion site farther back on the globe

H. *Orbital fractures/blowout fracture:* fracture of the floor of the orbit; silastic sling is inserted over the fracture site to prevent the globe and periorbital tissues from being trapped/damaged

I. *Evisceration/Enucleation/Exenteration*
  1. *Specialty items:* heavy scissors—optic nerve; conformers and spheres—prosthetics
  2. *Procedures*
     a. *Enucleation:* removal of the globe (eyeball) with preservation of muscle stumps to form a pocket into which a prosthesis is secured
     b. *Evisceration:* removal of the contents of the globe, leaving sclera and muscles intact to accommodate a prosthesis
     c. *Exenteration:* removal of all orbital contents, including periorbital fat, for treatment of malignant tumors

VI. **Intraocular Surgery**

  A. Keratoplasty/Corneal transplant
    1. Classification
       a. *Lamella:* partial-thickness graft
       b. *Penetrating:* full-thickness graft
    2. *Procedures:* Keratectomy
       a. *"Peeling the cornea"*
       b. *Indications:* corneal opacity from degenerative changes, perforated ulcers, or complications of ocular surgery
       c. *Donor tissue criteria:* healthy eye from young donor (legal consent required), enucleated within 4 to 6 hours of death, and properly preserved by eye bank
    3. Separate sterile table set for preparation of donor tissue where the cornea is trephined, washed in neosporin solution, and kept moist in saline; grafts and sutures are preplaced
    4. *Procedure:* trephine is used to remove buttonhole section from the recipient eye, peripheral iridotomy (incision into the iris) may be performed, prepared button graft from donor eye is anchored in place with 10-0 nylon suture, and antibiotic ointment and dressing with shield are applied

  B. **Corneal reshaping (Refractive Keratoplasty)**
    1. *Indications:* correct or minimize visual problems
       a. *Myopia:* nearsightedness
       b. *Hyperopia:* farsightedness
       c. *Astigmatism (a: without; stigma: point):* light does not focus on the retina
       d. *Aphakia (a: without; phakia: lens):* absence of the lens
       e. *Keratoconus (kerat: cornea; conus: cone):* conical cornea
    2. *Procedures*
       a. *Radial Keratotomy:* multiple radial incisions are made in the cornea to allow flattening in treatment of myopia.
       b. *Keratophakia:* a slice of donor cornea is shaped, curved, and inserted between layers of the recipient's cornea to modify refractivity of light.
       c. *Epikeratophakia:* donor button of corneal tissue is sutured onto the recipient's cornea following the removal of the corneal epithelium; performed for severe refractive problems.
       d. *Corneal sculpturing:* reshaping the corneal surface with a LASER for an irregular or scarred surface

  C. **Cataract extraction**
    1. *Lens:* biconvex, 1-cm, oval-shaped transparent structure suspended behind the iris by zonules which connect it to the ciliary muscles; it expands and retracts to provide accommodation for near and far vision; the aging process causes the lens to harden and loose elasticity, which results in opacity (cataract) and presbyopia (old vision or farsightedness) caused by the inability of the lens to accommodate and focus light on the macula lutea

2. *Cataracts*
   a. *Pathophysiology:* made of layers—like a "peanut M & M"—peanut is hard and fractured into small pieces and removed with suction, chocolate is soft and vacuumed away, candy shell remains
   b. *Types*
      i. *Primary*
         • Congenital (at birth)
         • Senile (acquired in old age)
      ii. *Secondary:* results from injury or disease
3. *Specialty items*
   a. *Phacoemulsification*
      i. Fragmentation of the lens by ultrasonic vibration and irrigation-aspiration, which permits removal of a cataract through a small incision in the limbus; all functions of the phacoemulsifier can be controlled by a foot pedal; constant flow of BSS prevents heat buildup
      ii. *Advantages:* shorter convalescence, smaller incision, which may be closed with one or no stitches; and retains posterior capsule, which supports IOL
      iii. *Disadvantages:* contraindicated in some conditions, requires special techniques which must be thoroughly mastered, and requires meticulous technical monitoring
   b. *Linear extraction:* a small incision is made at the limbus and anterior capsule, and a cystotome is used to excise a portion of the lens which is irrigated from the anterior chamber.
4. *Procedures for cataracts*
   a. *Extracapsular Cataract Extraction (ECCE):* excision of nucleus and cortex only
      i. *Procedure*
         • Incision is made at the limbus.
         • Anterior capsule is incised with a cystotome.
         • Nucleus is removed by manual expression or phacoemulsification.
         • Remaining cortex is extracted by irrigation and aspiration, preserving the posterior lens capsule.
         • Incision may/may not be sutured.
      ii. *Advantage of ECCE:* posterior lens capsule serves as an anatomical barrier between the anterior and posterior eye segments and protects the vitreous and the retina.
   b. *Intracapsular Cataract Extraction (ICCE):* excision of the lens and the entire capsule
      i. Requires a larger incision at the limbus
      ii. Sector iridectomy or iridotomy is needed to prevent iris prolapse and preserve communication between the anterior and posterior chambers.
      iii. Zonulysis agent instilled into posterior chamber to dissolve zonules
      iv. Lens is grasped with a suction device, mechanical forceps, or cryoextractor (cryoprobe freezes on cataract surface to enhance removal).
      v. Multiple sutures of 10-0 nylon may be required to make a watertight closure.
      vi. Procedure is less common—used for very dense, hard lenses, or presence of other pathology
   c. *Implantation of the Intraocular Lens (IOL)*
      i. Rinsed with BSS to remove any impurities; then coated with viscoelastic agent for ease in insertion
      ii. *Insertion:* inserted through primary incision; during cataract extraction or during future procedures

      iii. *Advantages of IOL:* superior binocular vision, permanent, does not interfere with pupillary dilation

      iv. *Complications of IOL:* prolonged inflammation, infection (foreign body), corneal damage, edema, corneal opacity, and dislocation

D. *Anterior Vitrectomy:* removal of vitreous lost due to trauma or tearing of the posterior capsule during phacoemulsification; fibrous-jelly in nature; uses vitrector or ocutome—guillotine-like hand piece that vacuums in a segment of vitreous, cuts it off, and vacuums it out of the globe

E. *Iridectomy/Iridotomy:* removal of a small peripheral segment or a wedge of iris to permit the flow of aqueous humor from the posterior chamber to the anterior chamber of the anterior segment of the globe; may be performed using argon LASER

F. *Posterior Capsulotomy:* removal of the center portion of the posterior capsule after the lens has adhered to the capsular bag following cataract extraction using ECCE; capsule may become opaque with time; removed using Nd:YAG LASER

G. *Trabeculoplasty/Trabeculectomy:* enlargement of the drainage intertrabecular spaces of the Canal of Schlemm at the limbus to promote drainage of aqueous humor from the anterior chamber to the subconjunctival space; used to treat glaucoma

H. *Scleral Buckle*

  1. *Anatomy:* the retina is a thin transparent membrane lining the posterior part of the eye that receives visual images and converts them into electrical impulses that are sent via the optic nerve to the brain for interpretation; the retina receives oxygen and nutrients through the choroid (vascular middle layer); a separation of the retina from the choroid results in a sudden onset of "floating spots" due to blood pigment in the vitreous and progresses to eventual blindness.

  2. *Surgery for retinal detachment*

    a. *Diathermy coagulation:* application of heat to the sclera over the area of detachment to cause inflammation, which acts to seal the defect

    b. *Cryosurgery:* application of cold to produce adhesions

    c. *Scleral Buckling:* elevating the sclera to contact the retina by implanting a wedge of silicone outside the sclera (extraocular procedure)

    d. Injection of air or gas into the vitreous cavity: to force the retina back into place

    e. *LASER therapy:* use of radiant heat from a LASER for rapid burn to produce adhesions

    f. *Photocoagulation:* sealing off a hole in the retina with a xenon or LASER photocoagulator

    g. *Posterior Vitrectomy*

      i. Removal of the vitreous from its normal location; indicated for severe intraocular trauma, advanced diabetic eye disease, vitreous opacity, and retinal detachment from large retinal tears

      ii. **Procedure:** incision is made in the pars plana; lens, if present, is removed; vitrector (suction-irrigator) is inserted, and vitreous is removed by a combination of diathermy, cryosurgery, irrigation, and suction; vitreous is replaced with BSS or viscoelastic agent; incision is closed; antibiotics and steroids are instilled and an eye patch applied

Show What You Know

Directions
Each of the numbered items or incomplete statements in this section is followed by answers or by completions of the statement. Select the ONE lettered answer or completion that is BEST in each case.

1. The corner of the eye is called the:

   A. canthus
   B. limbus
   C. tarsal plate
   D. pars plana

2. A Radial Keratotomy is done to correct:

   A. glaucoma
   B. retinal detachment
   C. strabismus
   D. myopia

3. Which of the following surgical procedures is an intraocular procedure?

   A. Blepharoplasty
   B. Enucleation
   C. Dacryocystorhinostomy
   D. Iridectomy

4. A cyst or tumor of the meibomian (sebaceous) gland of the eyelid is a:

   A. pterygium
   B. cataract
   C. chalazion
   D. dacryocyst

5. Which of the following procedures would require draping out both eyes?

   A. Recession/Resection of an extraocular muscle for strabismus
   B. Iridectomy for glaucoma
   C. Cataract Extraction
   D. Scleral Buckling for retinal detachment

6. The procedure involving the removal of all orbital contents is called:

   A. Enucleation
   B. Evisceration
   C. Vitrectomy
   D. Exenteration

7. The surgical schedule shows the first operation to be "ECCE with IOL, OD." You will be prepared for:

   A. removal of the right eye with prosthesis replacement
   B. removal of a cataract with lens implant in the right eye
   C. correction of strabismus of both eyes
   D. corneal replacement of the left eye

8. Drapes included in the eye pack are (1) split sheet, (2) plastic eye sheet, (3) head drape. The order in which they will be used is:

   A. 1, 2, 3
   B. 2, 3, 1
   C. 3, 1, 2
   D. 3, 2, 1

9. Preoperative drops administered were recorded as "Cyclogyl gtts ii O.S. q 5 min times 3." This means:

   A. 11 drops of medicine were put in the patient's left eye five times, 3 minutes apart
   B. 2 cc were put in the right eye five times at 3-minute intervals
   C. 2 drops were placed in both eyes three times at 5-minute intervals
   D. 2 drops were placed in the left eye three times at 5-minute intervals

10. The medication which may be added to a local anesthetic to increase absorption and dispersion/spreading is:

    A. sodium hyaluronate (Healon)
    B. hyaluronidase (Wydase)
    C. alpha-chymotrypsin (Chymar)
    D. epinephrine (Adrenalin)

11. All of the following are potential complications during intraocular surgery except:

    A. systemic reaction to drugs
    B. glaucoma
    C. loss of vitreous
    D. hemorrhage

12. Of the following ophthalmic drugs/solutions, which would be used to constrict the pupil immediately following removal of a cataract?

    A. acetylcholine (Miochol)
    B. methylprednisolone (Depo-Medrol)
    C. tropicamide (Mydriacyl)
    D. tetracaine hydrochloride (Pontocaine) 0.5%

13. Astigmatism is:

    A. a defect in the curvature of the cornea or lens
    B. nearsightedness
    C. the absence of the lens in the eye
    D. failure of the eyes to focus in the same direction

14. The procedure of choice for retinal detachment is:

   A. Scleral Buckling
   B. Vitrectomy
   C. Keratotomy
   D. Keratoplasty

15. The purpose for performing a Dacrocystorhinostomy is to:

   A. create an opening into the maxillary sinus
   B. correct an entropion
   C. create an opening for tear flow from the eye
   D. correct a defect in the tarsal plate of the eyelid

16. The term used to describe the eye's ability to adapt for near and far vision is:

   A. accommodation
   B. aphakia
   C. hyperopia
   D. astigmatism

17. The space between the lens and the iris/pupil is called the:

   A. anterior cavity
   B. posterior cavity
   C. anterior chamber
   D. posterior chamber

18. Dilating drops are called:

   A. mydriatics
   B. myotics
   C. corticosteroids
   D. oxytocics

19. Intraocular pressure is measured with a/an:

   A. caliper
   B. tonometer
   C. phacoemulsifier
   D. ocutome

20. Sagging and eversion of the lower lid is termed a/an:

   A. entropion
   B. blepharoptosis
   C. ectropion
   D. pterygium

21. Removal of the entire globe is termed a/an:

   A. Keratoplasty
   B. Exenteration
   C. Enucleation
   D. Evisceration

22. The removal of a portion of an ocular muscle with reattachment is called a/an:

   A. Strabismus
   B. Myomectomy
   C. Recession
   D. Resection

23. Removal of a fleshy encroachment on the cornea is called:

   A. Corneal Transplant
   B. Pterygium Excision
   C. Epikeratophakia
   D. Blepharchalasis

24. Esotropia is:

   A. a defect in the curvature of the cornea or lens
   B. divergent strabismus
   C. hypertrophy and loss of elasticity of the skin of the upper eyelid
   D. convergent strabismus

25. Which of the following cataract extraction methods is false?

   A. extracapsular lens extraction using alpha chymotrypsin
   B. extracapsular lens extraction using phacoemulsification
   C. intracapsular lens extraction using a cryoprobe
   D. intracapsular lens extraction using alpha chymotrypsin

26. The plastic cover used to protect the cornea during certain eye operations is called a/an:

   A. Fox shield
   B. scleral shield
   C. eye pad moistened with BSS
   D. Honan balloon

27. Medications used in ophthalmic surgery require all of the following considerations *except*:

   A. they are required to be extremely pure
   B. should be labeled "for ophthalmic use" to assure proper purity and concentrations
   C. eye medications are extremely potent and generally come in low concentrations
   D. medications used during the eye procedure are usually colored to prevent medication errors

28. The operative microscope in ophthalmic surgery often uses which objective lens distance?

   A. 100
   B. 175
   C. 250
   D. 400

29. Which of the following ophthalmic LASER/use combinations is incorrect?

   A. blue-green argon for Iridectomy/Iridotomy
   B. red-yellow krypton for retinal vascular disease
   C. Nd:YAG for Posterior Capsulotomy
   D. CO2 for Vitrectomy

30. Scissors found in the basic eye instrument tray that are used to cut the conjunctiva are called:

   A. Wescott
   B. Vannas
   C. de Wicker
   D. Bishop Harmon

31. Presbyopia is:

   A. absence of a lens in the eye
   B. nearsightedness
   C. a defect in the curvature of the cornea or lens
   D. farsightedness

32. Eye lubricants which give viscoelastic support to the eye during surgery include:

   A. phenylephrine
   B. carbochol
   C. sodium hyaluronate
   D. betamethasone

33. The classification of medications used to dilate the pupil while inhibiting the ability to focus are:

   A. mydriatics
   B. cycloplegics
   C. hyperosmotic agents
   D. miotics

34. Injectable agents for ophthamologic anesthesia include all of the following *except:*

   A. Xylocaine
   B. Wydase
   C. tetracaine hydrochloride
   D. sodium hyaluronidase

35. The procedure where an eye muscle insertion is removed and reattached more posteriorly on the sclera is called a/an:

   A. Recession
   B. Exenteration
   C. Trabeculoplasty
   D. Resection

36. When suturing the cornea following an intraocular procedure, which material would most commonly be used?

   A. 10-0 chromic gut
   B. 7-0 polyglycolic acid
   C. 10-0 nylon
   D. 7-0 nylon

37. The instrument used to excise vitreous humor is called a/an:

   A. cryoprobe
   B. ocutome
   C. phacoemulsifier
   D. wet-field "eraser"

38. During surgery, the eye is irrigated with _____ to compensate for lack of lid motion and function.

   A. saline
   B. proparacaine hydrochloride
   C. Balanced Salt Solution
   D. Miochol

39. Macular degeneration is:

   A. a defect in the curvature of the cornea
   B. an overproduction or ineffective absorption of aqueous humor
   C. a breakdown of cells in the macula lutea
   D. a complete or partial separation of the retina

40. A "blowout" fracture would be repaired with which device(s)?

   A. plates and cortical screws
   B. plates and cancellous screws
   C. cortical screws only
   D. silastic sling

41. Miotic agents include all of the following *except:*

   A. phenylephrine
   B. acetylcholine
   C. Miostat
   D. pilocarpine

42. Dyes used in ophthalmic surgery include which of the following?

   A. Mannitol
   B. flourescein sodium
   C. alpha chymotrypsin
   D. Carbochol

Anatomy Review

The Eye

43–55.

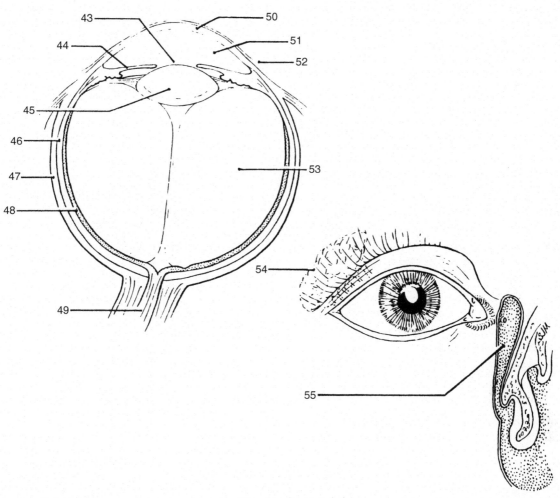

A. aqueous humor
B. choroid
C. conjunctiva
D. cornea
E. iris
F. lacrimal gland
G. lens

H. nasolacrimal duct
I. optic nerve
J. pupil
K. retina
L. sclera
M. vitreous humor

Answers & Rationales

1. **A.** Rationale: The corner of the eye is the canthus, the limbus is the area where the cornea joins the sclera, the tarsal plate is the lid cartilage, and the pars plana is the anterior attachment for the retina.

2. **D.** Rationale: Myopia is a light refraction deformity which can be managed surgically by altering the shape of the cornea.

3. **D.** Rationale: Iridectomy, excision of a section of the iris, is an intraocular procedure. Blepharoplasty is a revision of the eyelid, Enucleation is removal of the globe, and Dacryocystorhinostomy is the creation of an opening between the tear sac and the nose.

4. **C.** Rationale: A chalazion is a cyst or tumor of a meibomian (sebaceous) gland of the eyelid. A pterygium is a benign growth which begins at the medial canthus and extends over the conjunctiva to the cornea, a cataract is an opaque lens, and a dacryocyst is the tear sac.

5. **A.** Rationale: Both eyes would be draped out for strabismus surgery so that the surgeon can compare the appearance of both eyes.

6. **D.** Rationale: Exenteration is the removal of all orbital contents and is generally performed for malignancy.

7. **B.** Rationale: "ECCE with IOL, OD" is interpreted as extracapsular cataract extraction with intraocular lens implant in the right eye.

8. **C.** Rationale: The order in which eye drapes are applied is: head drape is applied with adhesive strip above the brow line, adhesive towel is secured over the nose if general anesthesia is used, split sheet is used to cover the OR bed, and a clear plastic adhesive drape is placed over the operative eye and secured.

9. **D.** Rationale: "Cyclogyl gtts ii O.S. q 5 min times 3" is interpreted as 2 drops of Cyclogyl in the left eye every 5 minutes three times.

10. **B.** Rationale: Hyaluronidase (Wydase) is an enzyme that may be added to a local anesthetic to enhance its spread and absorption.

11. **B.** Rationale: Potential complications during intraocular surgery include systemic reaction to drugs, loss of vitreous, hemorrhage, and instrument failure. Glaucoma is a condition with increased intraocular pressure resulting from obstruction in the flow of aqueous humor.

12. **A.** Rationale: Immediately following the removal of a cataract, the pupil may be constricted with a miotic drug such as acetylcholine (Miochol). Methylprednisolone (Depo-Medrol) is a steroid, tropicamide (Mydriacyl) is a mydriatic used to dilate the pupil, and tetracaine is a local anesthetic.

13. **A.** Rationale: Astigmatism is a defect in the curvature of the cornea or lens. Nearsightedness is myopia, aphakia is the absence of the lens, and strabismus is the failure of the eye to focus together.

14. **A.** Rationale: Scleral Buckling is the procedure of choice for retinal detachment. Keratotomy and Keratoplasty address issues of the cornea, and Vitrectomy involves the vitreous humor.

15. **C.** Rationale: The purpose for performing a Dacrocystorhinostomy is to create an opening for tear flow from the eye.

16. **A.** Rationale: The term used to describe the eye's ability to adapt for near and far vision is *accommodation*. Aphakia is the absence of the lens, hyperopia is farsightedness, and astigmatism is a defect in the curvature of the cornea or lens.

17. **D.** Rationale: The space between the lens and the iris/pupil is called the posterior chamber. The anterior chamber is the space between the cornea and the iris/pupil. Both the anterior chamber and the posterior chamber are contained in the anterior cavity of the eye. The posterior cavity contains vitreous humor.

18. **A.** Rationale: Dilating drops are called mydriatics or cycloplegics. Myotics constrict the pupil. Corticosteroids decrease inflammation, and oxytocics are medications used to stimulate uterine contractions.

19. **B.** Rationale: Intraocular pressure is measured with a Schiotz tonometer. A caliper is used to measure distances, the phacoemulsifier breaks the lens into small pieces for evacuation from inside the lens capsule, and the ocutome is used to remove vitreous.

20. **C.** Rationale: Sagging and eversion of the lower lid is termed an ectropion. Blepharoptosis involves sagging of the upper lid. An entropion is the inversion of a lid and a pterygium is a fleshy growth over the cornea.

21. **C.** Rationale: Removal of the entire globe is termed enucleation. Evisceration is removal of

the globe contents, exenteration is removal of all of the orbital contents, and keratoplasty involves just the cornea.

22. **D.** **Rationale:** A Resection is the removal of a portion of an ocular muscle with reattachment. It is performed as part of the procedure to correct strabismus. Recession is the reinsertion of a muscle further back on the globe, strabismus is the pathology that leads to Recession and Resection, and Myomectomy is a procedure to remove fibroids from the uterus.

23. **B.** **Rationale:** A Pterygium Excision is the removal of a fleshy encroachment on the cornea. Corneal Transplant and Epikeratophakia involve replacement or reshaping of the cornea, and Blepharochalasis is a condition of "droopy" eyelids.

24. **D.** **Rationale:** Esotropia is also referred to as convergent strabismus. Exotropia is divergent strabismus.

25. **A.** **Rationale:** The cataract extraction method that is incorrect is the extracapsular lens extraction using alpha chymotrypsin. Extracapsular extraction is performed with the lens capsule intact. The use of alpha chymostrypsin would dissolve the zonules holding the lens in place.

26. **B.** **Rationale:** A scleral shield is used to protect the cornea during certain eye operations. A Fox shield is used to cover the orbit after a procedure is complete. Eye pads are not placed on the cornea or sclera. A Honan balloon is used to reduce intraocular pressure.

27. **D.** **Rationale:** Medications used during the eye procedure are usually clear. They are required to be extremely pure, should be labeled "for ophthalmic use" to assure proper purity and concentrations, are extremely potent, and generally come in low concentrations.

28. **B.** **Rationale:** The operative microscope in ophthalmic surgery often uses a 175-mm objective lens. A 100-mm objective lens would require the microscope to be too close to the patient. A 250-mm objective lens is used for ear procedures, and a 400-mm lens is used for Microlaryngoscopy.

29. **D.** **Rationale:** The CO_2 LASER is not used for eye surgery since the CO_2 LASER is a "water-loving" LASER and would coagulate the vitreous. The argon LASER is a pigmented tissue LASER that passes through clear structures, such as the cornea, without damage. The krypton LASER is designed to work directly on the fine retinal tissues. The Nd:YAG LASER is a focal LASER that affects tissue at a precise distance.

30. **A.** **Rationale:** Wescott scissors are basic eye scissors used to cut tissue such as conjunctiva, lid adipose, and extrinsic eye muscles. Vannas and de Wicker scissors are very delicate and are used for intraocular application. Bishop Harmon is a type of forceps found in basic eye instrumentation.

31. **D.** **Rationale:** Presbyopia is another term for farsightedness. Myopia is nearsightedness, aphakia is the absence of the lens, and astigmatism is a defect in the curvature of the cornea or lens.

32. **C.** **Rationale:** Sodium hyaluronate is an eye lubricant which gives viscoelastic support to the eye during surgery. Carbochol is a diuretic, phenylephrine is a mydriatic, and betamethasone is a corticosteroid.

33. **B.** **Rationale:** The classification of medications used to dilate the pupil while inhibiting the ability to focus is called cycloplegics. Mydriatics dilate the pupil but permit focusing while miotics cause the pupil to constrict. Hyperosmotic agents are diuretics.

34. **C.** **Rationale:** Pontocaine (tetracaine hydrochloride) is a topical anesthetic agent used for eye anesthesia. Xylocaine and Wydase are both injectable, and sodium hyaluronidase is an agent that aids in the spread of anesthetic agents injected around the Optic Nerve.

35. **A.** **Rationale:** A Recession is a procedure where an eye muscle insertion is removed and reattached more posteriorly on the sclera. Exenteration is removal of the orbital contents, including the globe; Trabeculoplasty is the modification of the Canal of Schlemm to permit more aqueous humor to pass into the subconjunctival space; and Resection is the excision of a segment of muscle, with reattachment to the original insertion site on the globe.

36. **C.** **Rationale:** 10-0 nylon is commonly used to suture the cornea following intraocular procedures, when indicated. 7-0 sutures are too large to use on this delicate structure, and chromic gut can cause an inflammatory reaction and scarring.

37. **B.** **Rationale:** The ocutome is used to excise vitreous. The cryoprobe creates an "iceball" that can freeze and destroy the ciliary body for treatment of glaucoma. The phacoemulsifier breaks up the nucleus of the lens during

ECCE, and the wet-field eraser is a cautery used for conjunctival bleeders.

38. **C.** **Rationale:** During surgery, the eye is irrigated with Balanced Salt Solution to compensate for the lack of lid motion and function, which normally keeps the cornea moist. Normal saline has a slightly different concentration of salt than does BSS. Proparacaine hydrochloride is Opthaine, a topical anesthetic. Miochol is a miotic agent.

39. **C.** **Rationale:** Macular degeneration is a breakdown of cells in the macula lutea. Astigmatism is a defect in the curvature of the cornea or lens, glaucoma is an overproduction or ineffective absorption of aqueous humor, and retinal detachment is a complete or partial separation of the retina from the choroid.

40. **D. Rationale:** A silastic sling would be used to repair a "blowout" fracture of the floor of the orbit. Plates and screws would cause irritation and possible entrapment of perioribtal tissues during eye movements.

41. **A.** **Rationale:** Miostat (acetylcholine) and pilocarpine are miotic agents, used to constrict the pupil. Neosynephrine (phenylephrine) is a mydriatic, used to dilate the pupil.

42. **B.** **Rationale:** Flourescein sodium is a dye used in ophthalmic surgery to assess patency of the lacrimal duct system. Mannitol is a diuretic, alpha chymotrypsin is a zonulysis agent, and Carbochol is a miotic.

Anatomy

43. (J) pupil
44. (E) iris
45. (G) lens
46. (B) choroid
47. (L) sclera
48. (K) retina
49. (I) optic nerve
50. (D) cornea
51. (A) aqueous humor
52. (C) conjunctiva
53. (M) vitreous humor
54. (F) lacrimal gland
55. (H) nasolacrimal duct

Part II: Deciphering a Surgical Schedule

The following mock surgery schedule will be used to answer several questions pertaining to ophthalmic surgery. The same schedule, or a similar one, will be used in subsequent chapters to ask questions about the content of the chapter.

Rm.# time	Surgeon	Procedure	Anest.	Rm. # time	Surgeon	Procedure	Anest.
Rm.00				**Rm07**			
OC	Dr. Z	Rt. Knee Arthroscopy	Gen.	7:00	Dr. M	IOL	Gen.
OC	Dr. C	Craniotomy	Gen.	TF	Dr. M	Enucleation	MAC
OC	Dr.Z	Angioplasty	Gen.				
Rm.01				**Rm08**			
7:00	Dr. X	Hemorrhoidectomy	Gen.	11:00	Dr. E	Scleral buckle	MAC
TF	Dr. X	Colostomy	Gen.				
TF	Dr. X	Bowel resection	Gen.				
Rm02				**Rm09**			
7:00	Dr. B	Excision of Chalazion	Gen.	8:30	Dr. T	Iridectomy	Gen.
TF	Dr. B	Orbital decompression	Gen.	TF	Dr. T	Palatoplasty	Gen.
Rm03				**Rm10**			
7:00	Dr. A	Cystoscopy	MAC	7:00	Dr. K	Nephrectomy	Gen.
TF	Dr. A	Cystoplasty	Gen.	TF	Dr. K	Choledocholithotripsy	MAC
12:30	Dr. F	Pyleogram	MAC	TF	Dr. K	Hepatic resection	Gen.
3:00	Dr. F	Cystocele repair	Gen.				
Rm04				**Rm11**			
7:00	Dr. Y	Resection of lateral	Gen.	7:00	Dr. L	Colposcope	Gen.
TF	Dr. Y	muscle OS		12:00	Dr. L	Mastectomy	Gen.
		phacoemulsification	Gen.				
Rm05				**Rm12**			
7:00	Dr. G	Trans-sphenoidal Adenectomy	Gen.	7:00	Dr. W	Trans-metatarsal amputation	Gen.
TF	Dr. G	Trans-urethral resection of the prostate	Gen	TF	Dr. W	Osteotomy	Gen.
TF	Dr. G	Bletharoplasty	Gen.	TF	Dr. W	Arthrocentesis	Gen.
Rm06				**Rm13**			
7:00	Dr. R	ICCE	Gen.	7:00	Dr. O	Posterior Vitrectomy	Gen.

The following questions should be answered using the surgery schedule above

1. Room 2 has a Chalazion excision scheduled. What type of incision will be used in this procedure?
   A. Cruciate (cross-shaped)
   B. Single median
   C. Transverse
   D. H shape

2. What type of dressing should the Surgical Technologist have prepared following the IOL procedure in Room 7?
   A. Telfa and tape
   B. Steristrips
   C. Kling rolls
   D. Fox eye shield

3. An ICCE is planned for Room 6. What instrument is used to grasp the lens?

    A. Castroviejo clamp
    B. Suction device
    C. DeBakey forceps
    D. Serrafines

4. For the resection procedure scheduled in Room 4, what will the Surgical Technologist hand to the surgeon to grasp the muscle?

    A. Muscle hook
    B. Hunt clamp
    C. Jewelers forcep
    D. McPherson tying forceps

5. Dr. E. in Room 8 will be using a LASER to seal the retinal tear. He would like a LASER that performs photocoagulation. Which LASER should the Surgical Technologist have ready?

    A. Argon
    B. ND:Yag
    C. xenon
    D. KPT

6. After the Posterior vitrectomy has been completed in Room 13, the surgeon will need an agent to replace the vitreous fluid. Which agent is the most likely to be used?

    A. Normal Saline
    B. Healon
    C. Ophthaine
    D. Wydase

7. The patient in Room 7 is undergoing an Enucleation. Which structure(s) will the surgeon leave in place?

    A. The cornea
    B. The muscle stumps
    C. The sclera
    D. The contents of the globe

8. Dr. Y will need to place a stitch after the phacoemulsification procedure. What stitch should the Surgical Technologist have ready?

    A. 6-0 side cutting
    B. 3-0 side cutting
    C. 6-0 taper
    D. 6-0 blunt

9. Dr. T will use a LASER for the iridectomy in Room 9. Which LASER should the Surgical Technologist have available?

    A. Argon
    B. Xenon
    C. KTP
    D. Nd:YAG

10. The patient undergoing the resection is beginning to hemorrhage. What should the Surgical Technologist have ready to hand to the surgeon?

    A. 21G needle and syringe
    B. 12 G needle and syringe
    C. 18 G needle and syringe
    D. Frazier tip

Answers & Rationales

1. **A** **Rationale:** The most common incision when excising Chalazion is a cross-shaped (cruciate) incision.

2. **D** **Rationale:** A Fox eye shield or its equivalent will be used to reduce pressure following intraocular procedures. It will be secured with paper or plastic tape.

3. **B** **Rationale:** Of these choices, the suction device is the one most likely to be selected.

4. **A** **Rationale:** Generally, the muscles will be grasped by the muscle hook before being divided and then reconnected to strengthen the muscle.

5. **C** **Rationale:** LASERS are commonly used in eye surgeries. The argon LASER, while used to seal retinal tears, is a possible choice; the surgeon has specifically requested a LASER that performs photocoagulation. Nd:YAG is used for breaking up adhesions, and Xenon is used for photocoagulations.

6. **B** **Rationale:** Generally, lost vitreous will be replaced with either balance saline solution (BSS) or a viscoelastic agent. In this case, BSS was not a listed option. Therefore, Healon will be the best option available to the Surgical Technologist.

7. **B** **Rationale:** The muscle stumps will be preserved to help form a pocket that will be used to secure a prosthetic eye.

8. **A** **Rationale:** Generally, suture used in eye surgeries will be 4-0 to 10-0 suture swaged onto a side-cutting needle.

9. **A** **Rationale:** The argon LASER would be the most likely LASER chosen for this procedure.

10. **C** **Rationale:** Hemorrhaging is a possible complication in eye procedures. Generally, the surgeon will need to aspirate blood in a timely manner. Therefore, the Surgical Technologist should have an 18 G needle and syringe available for this situation.

PEARSON
myhealthprofessionskit™

Use this address to access the interactive Companion Website created for this book. Simply select "Surgical Technology" from the choice of disciplines. Find this book and click to enter.

20

Thoracic, Cardiac, and Vascular Surgery

Thoracic, cardiac, and vascular surgery are combined in this chapter due to the overlapping of concepts and techniques of chest and cardiac surgery, on the one hand, and of cardiac and peripheral vascular surgery on the other. Thoracic surgery is performed for disorders of the lungs, mediastinum, chest wall, diaphragm, and thoracic esophagus. Cardiac and peripheral vascular surgery deals with congenital and acquired conditions of the circulatory system. Cardiac surgery experienced a renaissance in the 1960s with the first open heart and transplant procedures. Several surgeons have emerged as leaders in the field, and have lent their names to the instruments that they helped develop. Dr. DeBakey, who recently passed away at age 99, was one of these pioneers. With the invention of the heart-lung machine, the surgeries have become more common, with millions of Americans undergoing heart surgery each year.

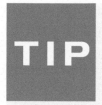

The number of cardiac surgeries has exploded in modern times, with multiple procedures being performed daily in the United States. This specialty, perhaps more than any other, is considered the most elite in the Operating Room. The procedures performed tend to be highly specialized and open to only a few Surgical Technologists. Many hospitals do not perform these surgeries, and they may only be found in larger facilities. However, with the number of cases increasing, more and more STs are being trained to scrub these cases. One of the more common procedures is the CABG (coronary artery bypass graft). Knowledge of the specialty instrumentation and procedures is necessary for answering questions about cardiothoracic and vascular surgery successfully. Peripheral vascular deals mainly with the veins and arteries, and is generally separate from cardiac procedures. Vascular grafts and vascular bypasses are commonly performed in peripheral vascular specialties, but generally do not include the heart. Thoracic procedures generally include the lungs, the mediastinum, and the diaphragm. Questions can range from procedure to accessory equipment used in any of the surgical interventions.

Example:
During a Thoracotomy, the ribs are retracted by using a

A. Allison
B. Finochetto
C. Bethune
D. Bailey

While all of these instruments may be used in thoracic surgical procedures, only one is used to retract, or spread, the ribs. An Allison is used to retract lung tissue, not the ribs. A Bethune is a rib shear, used to cut and remove a rib during exposure. A bailey is a rib contractor, used to approximate the ribs during closure. Therefore, the correct answer would be B, the Finochetto. This is a self-retaining rib retractor commonly used in thoracic procedures.

I. Terminology

A. *Aneurysm:* sac-like dilation and thinning of an artery wall that can lead to rupture of the vessel

B. *Angina pectoris:* pain in the chest due to decreased blood flow to the myocardium

C. *Ascites:* accumulation of fluid in the abdomen

D. *Bifurcation:* branching or forking into two

E. *Claudication:* symptoms of arterial obstruction—pallor, pain on exercise, and coolness

F. *Collateral circulation:* physiological formation of alternative pathways around occluded vessels

G. *Cyanosis:* bluish discoloration due to oxygen deficiency

H. *Defibrillation:* use of electrical, chemical, or physical means to stop the irregular, quiver-like beating of a heart; consists of generator with external (unsterile) or internal (sterile) paddles

I. *Dyspnea:* difficulty in breathing

J. *Embolism:* mass of undissolved matter carried in the bloodstream

K. *Extracorporeal:* outside the body

L. *Fibrillation:* rapid, ineffective heartbeat

M. *Ischemia:* reduced blood supply to tissue resulting in insufficient oxygenation of that tissue

N. *Plaque:* buildup of cellular debris on the lining of the artery (tunica intima)

O. *Pneumothorax:* air in the chest; may occur from a bleb (blister) that ruptures

P. *Premature ventricular contraction (PVC):* abnormal heart rhythm

Q. *Stenosis:* abnormal narrowing

R. *Tension pneumothorax:* closed pneumothorax in which the positive pressure in the pleural space displaces the mediastinum to the opposite side

S. *Thrombosis:* formation of a clot

II. Thoracic Surgery

A. Diagnostic procedures
1. *Blood gases*
2. *Chest x-ray films:* should be in surgery with the patient
3. *Bronchoscopy*
   a. Indications
      i. Direct visualization of the bronchial tree
      ii. Tissue biopsy and bronchial secretions for analysis
      iii. Removal of foreign bodies or obstructive lesions
   b. Bronchoscope may be rigid or flexible fiberoptic and used with patient under IV sedation and topical anesthesia
      i. adaptable to LASER surgery in treatment of pulmonary lesions, granulomas, neoplasms, or vascular lesions
4. *Mediastinoscopy*
   a. Sterile procedure is performed under general anesthesia with the patient in the supine position with head hyperextended and turned slightly to the right
   b. Scope is introduced through a transverse incision 2 cm above the suprasternal notch
   c. Electrosurgical suction tip is used to control bleeding
   d. Sampling of the lymph nodes surrounding the Great Vessels in the chest area
5. *Thoracoscopy:* visualization inside the chest, middle and lower mediastinum, visceral and parietal pleura, and pericardium
   a. General anesthesia; a double lumen endotracheal tube allows the anesthesiologist to inflate the lung, which would otherwise deflate when an incision is made into the chest
   b. One or more small incisions are made in appropriate intercostal spaces for introduction of the scope with camera and accessories
   c. Thorascope can be adapted for use with LASER, a video camera, and instruments for obtaining biopsies and providing definitive treatment for spontaneous pneumothorax
   d. Chest tubes are inserted and connected to water-seal drainage at the conclusion of the procedure
6. *Scalene (supraclavicular) node biopsy:* excision of lymph tissue to determine the spread of disease from the lungs
7. *Thoracocentesis:* aspiration of fluid from the chest cavity with needle and syringe

B. Surgical pathology
1. *Neoplasms:* most common is bronchogenic carcinoma
2. Pulmonary tuberculosis or fungal diseases
3. Traumatic injuries
4. *Flail chest:* unstable chest wall as a result of broken ribs, which causes a paradoxical effect (involved lung tissue deflates on inspiration and inflates on expiration)
5. *Sucking (open) wound of the chest:* defect in the chest wall through which air is drawn into the pleural space on inspiration, collapsing the lung and causing a mediastinal shift to impair function of the other lung

6. *Bronchiectasis:* chronic dilatation of the bronchi with a secondary infection resulting in halitosis, coughing spells, and thick sputum production
7. *Thoracic outlet syndrome:* compression of the brachial plexus nerve trunks, causing pain in the arm, paresthesia of the fingers, vasomotor symptoms, weakness, and muscle wasting; caused by a drooping shoulder girdle, fibrous band along the first rib, and continued hyperabduction of the arm or compression on the scalenus muscle following injury
8. *Bullous emphysema:* accumulation of air in tissue due to cystic alveolar dilatation (bulla or blebs) of the lungs
9. *Pectus excavatum (funnel chest):* congenital deformity in which the anterior chest wall is pushed back toward the spine
10. *Pulmonary fibrosis:* chronic inflammation and progressive fibrosis of alveolar walls with dyspnea, which may progress to death
11. *Pectus carinatum (pigeon breasted):* congenital deformity in which the sternum is projecting forward
12. *Empyema:* accumulation of pus in the pleural space, compressing the lung
13. *Pleural effusion:* "pouring out" of fluid into the pleural space
14. *Adult Respiratory Distress Syndrome (ARDS):* also known as shock lung or progressive pulmonary insufficiency; complications of chest trauma or diffuse pneumonia characterized by dyspnea, grunting respiration, tachycardia, and cyanosis

C. Special tools
   1. Endoscopes
      a. *Bronchoscope*
         i. *Rigid:* used for removal of foreign objects, a large central mass, or a vascular mass when hemorrhage may pose a problem; side channel is incorporated in a scope which permits aeration of lungs with oxygen or anesthetic gas
         ii. *Fiber optic:* permits visualization of lobar bronchi; can be used in patients with jaw deformities or rigid cervical spines; adaptable to videoendoscopy
      b. *Mediastinoscope:* hollow tube with fiber-optic light carrier
      c. *Accessories for endoscopes:* include light carrier, cord, and illuminator; sponge carrier and sponges, specimen collector (Lukens tube/trap) and aspirating tube; and forceps of different types
   2. LASERs: Nd:YAG, adaptable to bronchoscope, is useful in treating bronchial stenosis or photoradiation of bronchogenic carcinoma
   3. Positioning aids such as beanbag, pillows, shoulder roll, and wide tape
   4. Sterile magnetic pad to go over sterile field to prevent instruments from sliding from the field when the patient is in the lateral position
   5. Instruments
      a. *Scissors:* Nelson, Potts tenotomy and dissecting, and wire cutters
      b. *Retractors:* Volkman rake, Finochietto, large Kelly Richardson, Semb retractor, Davidson scapula, and Bailey rib contractor
      c. *Bone/rib:* elevators (Overhault, Doyen), rongeurs (Sauerbruch, Stille-Luer), Liston-Stille bone-cutting forceps, Bethune rib shears, and Alexander or Matson periosteotome
      d. *Median sternotomy:* sternal saw, Lebsche sternal knife, mallet, sternal spreader and approximator, bone hook, and punch
      e. *Clamping:* Mixter (right angles) and Sarot bronchus clamp
      f. *Holding:* Potts-Smith vascular forceps, Rummel thoracic clamp, and Duval lung-grasping forceps
      g. *Vascular clamps:* Crawford coarctation, patent ductus, and Satinsky and Cooley
      h. *Suturing:* Sarot needle holder, clip appliers with clips, and staples
   6. **Accessories:** electrosurgical unit, bone wax, Asepto irrigating syringe, thoracic catheters, water-seal drainage system, suction tubing, and umbilical tape

D. **Special considerations for chest surgery**
  1. *Chest drainage:* sterile closed water-seal drainage system used to restore airtight pleural cavity and maintain negative pressure
      a. May consist of one-, two-, or three-bottle setup
      b. Disposable chest drainage units—one piece but contains three chambers and operates on the same principle as three-bottle setup
          i. First bottle is the water seal; most critical; tube from the patient's intrapleural space is connected to this bottle to provide escape of air into the water without backflow of air into the chest (essential in achieving and maintaining a negative intrapleural pressure, allows reexpansion of the lung). The level of water in the tube will fluctuate when the patient breathes or coughs and will stop fluctuating when the negative pressure in the intrapleural space has been reestablished.
          ii. Second bottle is for the collection of pleural drainage; collected separately for measurement and so that the level of fluid in the water-seal chamber is unaffected
          iii. Third bottle is the safety valve; necessary when suction is applied to protect the delicate lung tissue from being drawn into the tube. The depth of the tube under the water in this bottle determines the amount of pull and is generally about 10 cc or as ordered by the physician. Increasing suction only increases bubbling sounds without extra pull on the pleura
      c. Chest tubes (26 to 36 French for adults, angled and straight) inserted in pleural space; if more than one is used, they are connected with a Y connector to one drainage system; one is placed near the lung base for fluid evacuation and one at the lung apex for air evacuation; postoperative patient is generally in Fowler position to enhance respiration and allow air to rise to the apex and fluid to drain to the base
      d. **Critical points**
          i. Tubes and closed system must be sterile.
          ii. Tubes are inserted by the physician prior to wound closure and brought through stab wound(s) and sutured for security.
          iii. Tubes are clamped until ready for connection to the water-seal drainage unit and during transport, unless instructions indicate otherwise.
          iv. Sterile saline is used for the underwater seal, and the directions/physicians are consulted regarding the amount of saline for suction control.
          v. Tube connections are secured with tape to avoid leakage of air.
          vi. Drainage system should remain below the patient chest level as much as possible.
          vii. As a precaution, a clamp accompanies the patient from the OR to occlude the chest tube in the event of a break in the continuity of the water-seal drainage system.
          viii. Portable chest x-ray is often done to confirm re-expansion of the lung.
          ix. Instrument, needle, and sponge counts are essential when the chest is opened; extra counts are taken before a cavity is closed (e.g., pericardium); sponges used inside the thorax are passed to the surgeon on long-handled forceps.
          x. Hemostasis is achieved by electrocoagulation and bone wax (ribs and sternum).
          xi. Items coming in contact with the bronchial lining are considered contaminated.
  2. *Surgical incisions*
      a. *Posterolateral:* most commonly used; provides maximum exposure to lungs, esophagus, diaphragm, and thoracic aorta; patient is placed in

the lateral chest position with lower leg flexed and upper leg extended on pillows; anesthesia screen is used to isolate the anesthesiologist; incision extends from the scapula spine to the submammary fold and generally follows the fifth to sixth rib interspace

b. *Anterolateral:* patient is in the semilateral position with pillows beneath shoulder and hip on affected side; incision extends from the sternum to the midaxillary line; used for resection of pulmonary cyst, lung biopsy, or local lesions

c. *Median Sternotomy:* sternum is split vertically with a power saw from the suprasternal notch to xiphoid process (which is removed); patient is placed in the supine position; uses include bilateral pulmonary operations, cardiac or aortic procedures, mediastinal neoplasms, and trauma or access to lower cervical or upper thoracic vertebrae

d. *Thoracoabdominal:* with the patient in the modified supine position, an incision is made through seventh to eighth intercostal space from the posterior axillary line to the abdominal midline; used for Hiatal Hernia Repair, Esophagectomy, high abdominal retroperitoneal tumors, and cardioesophageal lesions

e. *Transaxillary:* with the patient in the modified supine position, a vertical incision is made from the axillary to the submammary fold; used for lung biopsy, Wedge Resection of the Lung, Thoracic Sympathectomy, and Thoracic Outlet Syndrome procedures

f. *Supraclavicular:* with the patient in the supine position and the head turned to the unaffected side, an incision is made parallel to the clavicle; used for Phrenic Nerve Resection, Cervicothoracic Sympathectomy, and Axillary Vein Thrombosis

E. Thoracic procedures
  1. *Correction of pectus excavatum*
    a. **Purpose:** correct mediastinal compression to relieve pressure on heart, great vessels, and lungs or for cosmetic effect
    b. **Procedure:** with the patient in the supine position, a bilateral inframammary or anterior midline incision is made; affected costal cartilages are freed from the sternum, realigned, and fixed; silicone prosthesis may be used to fill the defect if procedure is done only for cosmesis.
    c. May be done endoscopically
  2. *Closed thoracotomy/chest tube insertion:* insertion of a tube into the pleural space through an intercostal incision with the use of a trocar and cannula attached to a water-seal drainage unit done to establish continuous drainage or aid in restoring negative pressure for spontaneous pneumothorax or to treat empyema
  3. *Open thoracotomy*
    a. *Indications:* confirm a diagnosis, determine the extent of a disease, evaluate chest trauma, or control bleeding
    b. *Procedure:* posterolateral thoracotomy, incision is deepened using the electrosurgical pencil, periosteum is lifted from the rib with elevator or raspatory and cut with rib shears (rib is not always removed), bone edges are trimmed with rongeurs or Sauerbruch rib shears, and bone wax is applied to bleeders; wound edges are protected with lap sponges and a Finochietto retractor is positioned; pleura is incised, adhesions are freed, and chest is explored and suctioned as necessary; procedure of choice is performed; irrigation fluid is used to test for air leaks from the lung, and chest tubes are inserted and brought out through stab wounds; ribs are approximated with a Bailey rib contractor and heavy pericostal suture; periosteum is closed with running absorbable suture; muscles, subcutaneous tissue, and skin are closed; tubes are anchored to chest and connected to water-seal drainage system, and dressing is applied, with petrolatum-impregnated gauze around chest tubes to prevent air leaks

4. *Lobe resection of the lung*
   a. *Indications:* bronchiectasis, cysts (blebs), tuberculosis, tumors, or abscesses
   b. *Procedure:* posterolateral thoracotomy, diseased segment identified, blood supply and bronchus clamped, transsected, sutured, and/or stapled; tested for air leaks, pleural space irrigated, and hemostasis secured
5. *Wedge resection of the lung:* excision of wedge-shaped piece of tissue from the lung periphery with use of a stapler to treat peripheral lung tumors and/or blebs/bulla
6. *Lobectomy:* excision of one or more lobes of the lung when disease is confined to lobe(s); bronchus is isolated, stapled, or sutured, and tested for leaks
7. *Pneumonectomy:* removal of an entire lung for extensive disease or malignant neoplasm through a posterolateral incision; mediastinal pleura is entered, and major vessels (pulmonary artery, superior and inferior pulmonary veins) and main stem bronchus are isolated; vagus, phrenic, and recurrent laryngeal nerves are identified; lymph nodes are dissected; vessels are ligated, and lung is delivered; vessels are closed, and bronchus is stapled or sutured, covered with surrounding pleura, and tested for leaks; chest suction is generally not needed; empty space will gradually fill with fluid/fibrotic tissue; potential complications are bronchial stump blowout, bronchopleural fistula, respiratory insufficiency, infection, and cardiac dysrhythmias
8. *Thoracoplasty:* extrapleural resection of one or more ribs to reduce thoracic space for post-pneumonectomy mediastinal shift or chronic empyema
9. *Pulmonary Decortication:* removal of restricting fibrous membrane (secondary to chronic empyema or clotted hemothorax) over the lung to permit reexpansion of an entrapped lung; rib resection may be necessary; fibrous membrane is peeled away from the visceral pleura, resulting in potential for blood loss
10. *Scalenectomy:* resection of the scalenus muscle for the treatment of thoracic outlet syndrome through a supraclavicular incision; first rib may be removed
11. *Fractured ribs, sternum, or clavicle:* stabilized with pins or wires
12. *Lung assist device (intravascular oxygenator)*
    a. *Purpose:* provide temporary assistance for the patient in acute respiratory distress
    b. *Procedure:* device is inserted into the femoral vein and advanced to the vena cava; gas conduit exits the skin for oxygen administration and elimination of carbon dioxide
13. *Lung-Volume Reduction Surgery:* resection of large areas of bulla/bleb formation using reinforced (polytetrafluoroethylene [PTFE] or bovine pericardium strips) staplers; performed through thoracoscopy or open thoracotomy; used for the treatment of end-stage emphysema/chronic obstructive pulmonary disease (COPD)
14. Other thoracic procedures covered earlier include Thymectomy, Esophagectomy, and Diaphragmatic Hernia Repair—Thoracic Approach

F. Complications of thoracic surgery
   1. *Pulmonary insufficiency because of:*
      a. Shallow breathing due to pain on chest expansion
      b. Inadequate coughing to raise secretions
      c. Obstruction from secretions
   2. *Pneumonia:* inflammation of the lungs
   3. *Atelectasis:* inadequate lung expansion because of collapse of a section
   4. *Pneumothorax:* air in the chest secondary to air leaks, hemorrhage, or pleural effusion
   5. *Empyema:* pus or pockets of air or fluid

6. *Bronchopleural fistula:* abnormal connection between the bronchus and pleural cavity

7. **Adult respiratory distress syndrome (ARDS)**

III. **Cardiac Surgery**

A. **Diagnostic procedures**

1. *Noninvasive:* chest x-ray, stress testing, EKG, cardiac output, venous pressure, blood chemistries, pulmonary function studies, echocardiography, radionuclide imaging, and cineradiogram (x-ray of organ in motion)

2. *Invasive*

a. *Arteriogram:* x-ray or fluoroscopy of arteries following injection of contrast media

b. *Angiogram:* study of vessels with use of contrast media

c. *Cardiac catheterization*

i. *Uses:* diagnose coronary artery disease, valvular disease, or congenital anomalies

ii. *Procedure for study of coronary arteries:* performed using surgical asepsis, a single catheter is inserted through a percutaneous puncture into a brachial or femoral artery and advanced to the coronary artery, where contrast media is injected and traced and findings recorded by cineradiograms; incision is closed and pressure dressing is applied.

iii. *Procedure for right heart catheterization:* catheter is inserted into the brachial, femoral, or jugular vein, and advanced to the right atrium, ventricle, and pulmonary artery; tests include oxygen saturation, measurement of cardiac output and chamber pressures, and injection of contrast media to assess anatomical structures and congenital anomalies.

iv. *Potential complications:* air embolus, thrombosis, dysrhythmias, and vascular or cardiac perforation

B. **Surgical pathology**

1. **Congenital anomalies**

a. *Atrial Septal Defect (ASD):* opening in the septum between the right and left atria

b. *Ventricular Septal Defect (VSD):* opening in the septum between the right and left ventricles

c. *Patent Ductus Arteriosus (PDA):* communicating artery between the pulmonary artery and the aorta, essential in the fetus, remains open, shunting blood away from the lungs

d. *Coarctation of the Aorta:* constriction of the aortic arch by the ligamentum arteriosum, a fetal remnant of the bypass from the pulmonary artery to the aorta (ductus arteriosus)

e. *Tetralogy of Fallot (blue baby):* four structural defects of the heart—pulmonary stenosis, VSD, overriding aorta, and right ventricular hypertrophy; most common cyanotic congenital cardiac anomaly

f. *Transposition of the Great Vessels:* pulmonary artery arises from the left ventricle, and the aorta arises from the right ventricle, resulting in cyanosis

2. **Acquired diseases and defects**

a. *Coronary Artery Disease (CAD):* progressive obstruction of coronary arteries by plaque, causing ischemia of the heart muscle resulting in chest pain; plaque can break off and proceed to block the coronary artery (coronary thrombosis) to cause a myocardial infarction (MI, heart attack)

b. *Valvular stenosis:* narrowing of a cardiac valve (aortic, pulmonary, tricuspid, or bicuspid [mitral])

c. *Valvular insufficiency or incompetence:* inability of a valve to close properly, which results in a backflow of blood

      d. *Angina pectoris:* decreased blood flow in coronary arteries because of plaque, stress, or nicotine, which results in chest pain and shortness of breath; treated first with a coronary vasodilator—nitroglycerine

      e. *Heart block:* interruption in the electrical conduction system in the heart

      f. *Ventricular aneurysm:* segmental dilation of the ventricular wall, generally a postinfarction complication

C. **Special tools**

  1. *Cardiopulmonary bypass (extracorporeal circulation):* equipment which serves as the patient's heart and lungs during open heart surgery

    a. *Operator:* perfusionist, sometimes referred to as the "pump technician," a person with specialized training in heart–lung bypass

    b. *Components of the heart–lung machine*

      i. *Oxygenator:* adds oxygen to the blood and removes carbon dioxide from the blood, serves as the "lungs"

      ii. *Heat exchanger:* regulates blood temperature

      iii. *Pump:* rollers which squeeze blood through tubes by a "milking action"; serves as the "heart muscle" responsible for blood movement

    c. *Perfusion*

      i. Pump oxygenator is primed with BSS or lactated Ringer's solution, a cardiopreservative solution with sodium bicarbonate, and a heparinized plasma volume expander

      ii. Venous blood is diverted to the machine through cannulas inserted into the venae cavae.

      iii. Arterial blood is pumped back into the body through an aortic cannula.

    d. Monitoring during perfusion includes arterial and venous pressure, blood gases, electrolytes, temperature, and urinary output

    e. Upon completion of the cardiac repair, air is removed from the heart, the heartbeat is restored, ventilation is re-established, the patient is rewarmed, and perfusion is gradually decreased.

    f. *Myocardial preservation:* motionless heart is needed for surgical repair and is arrested by:

      i. *Aortic cross-clamping:* results from ischemia (deoxygenated blood)

      ii. *Cardioplegia:* hyperkalemic (potassium) solution produces an electromechanical arrest

      iii. *Hypothermia:* cardiac arrest can be induced by lowering the body temperature, which may be achieved by surface cooling (ice slush of saline or Ringer's solution), a cooling blanket, or by adding a cooling perfusate to the heart–lung machine.

    g. *Complications associated with extracorporeal circulation*

      i. Alterations in blood clotting

      ii. Renal tubular necrosis

      iii. Metabolic acidosis

      iv. Hypervolemia

      v. Elevated stress hormones (antidiuretic hormone [ADH], aldosterone) with resulting cerebral edema

      vi. Postpump psychosis, postperfusion lung syndrome, and cardiac tamponade (compression of the heart from fluid collecting in the pericardium)

  2. *Other equipment:* electrical defibrillator, external paddles, external and internal pulse pacemaker generator, epicardial pacemaker leads, fiberoptic headlight and light source, hyper/hypothermia unit, intraaortic balloon pump, cardiotomy suction tips and sump tubes, noncrushing vascular and anastomosis clamps, vessel loops, and umbilical tape, in addition to basic surgical instruments, thoracic instruments, and additional cardiovascular instruments

3. *Suture material:* variety of cardiovascular sutures—synthetic, nonabsorbable, and atraumatic (polypropylene, polyester, polytetrafluoroethylene [PTFE], and Dacron); wire for sternal closure and skin staples

4. *Supplies:* various sizes of tubing, adapters, connectors, and stopcocks; rubber-shod clamps, sponges, tourniquet, catheters, disposable drapes, electrosurgical unit, syringes and needles (for injections, infusions, and blood samples), irrigation cannulas, marking pen, disposable bulldog clamps, autotransfusion supplies, chest tubes, and a chest drainage system

5. *Prosthetic materials:* intracardiac patches, synthetic grafts, and heart valves; manufacturer's guide must be followed for preparation and insertion

D. **Medications for cardiac surgery (in addition to tranquilizers, analgesics, anesthetics, antibiotics, and antiarrhythmics)**

1. *Heparin sodium as an anticoagulant:* given IV before vascular system is opened; used in a solution for flushing vessels—generally 5000 U of heparin in 500 ml of normal saline

2. *Protamine sulfate* as a heparin antagonist

3. *Calcium channel-blocking agent* to decrease the risk of myocardial spasm

4. *Calcium chloride* to increase the force of heart contraction

5. *Sodium bicarbonate* as a buffer for metabolic acidosis

6. *Potassium chloride* as a cardioplegic

7. *Furosemide (Lasix)* and mannitol for diuresis

8. *Epinephrine or phenylephrine (NeoSynephrine)* to strengthen the heartbeat

9. *Nitroglycerine* to dilate coronary arteries

10. *Sodium nitroprusside (Nipride)* to lower blood pressure by relaxing smooth muscles

11. *Lidocaine hydrochloride (Xylocaine)* to treat ventricular arrhythmias and prevent ventricular fibrillation

12. *Papaverine* to prevent vasospasms

E. **Special patient concerns**

1. *Preinduction:* insertion of peripheral arterial and venous lines (may require a cut-down), and insertion of indwelling urinary catheter; children are encouraged to bring a favorite article/toy

2. *Admission to the OR:* proper identification, an attempt to allay apprehension and make the patient comfortable with warm blankets, proper padding, etc.

3. *Monitoring devices:* observed by anesthesiologist include, but are not limited to, blood pressure, pulse oximeter, urinary drainage, temperature probes, left atrial line, arterial line, CVP, and pulmonary artery pressure.

4. *Positioning:* generally supine with arms on padded armboards and legs slightly everted to provide access to the femoral artery and saphenous vein; may use artery/vein of forearm

5. *Skin prep:* when a saphenous vein graft is needed, the cardiac patient is prepped from the jaw to the feet with the torso from the bed line and legs circumferentially; prep stops at the knees when vein graft is not required.

6. *Draping:* sheets are placed under the legs, and perineum is covered with a folded towel; towel is placed across the umbilicus for drape connections, feet are covered with gloves or towels, and sheets are draped around the patient to expose the anterior chest, abdomen, groin, and legs; incision drape may be used to minimize skin exposure.

F. **Other features of cardiac surgery**

1. Principles of thoracic, general, and vascular surgery are applicable.

2. Handling complications requires a dedicated and trained team, time management, and adequate and properly working equipment.

3. Thorough physical and psychological preparation of the patient for surgery, close monitoring during surgery, and comprehensive care following surgery are essential for successful cardiac surgery.

SURGERY HINT

For valve replacement, the ST should not have sterile water on the field. Accidental irrigation with water will cause blood cells to rupture.

Always have a French eye or mayo needle available in case suture needs to be reused.

Careful tracking of intracardiac needles is necessary to prevent incorrect counts and possible patient injury.

4. Methods for volume replacement include intraoperative autotransfusion, blood and blood substitutes (hetastarch), albumin substitute, or platelets.
5. Water-seal drainage is needed for surgery of the mediastinum or chest.
6. Well-supplied crash cart must be readily available.
7. Careful monitoring of medication types and dosages on the surgical field is a must; all medications must be carefully labeled.
8. The scrub must ensure absence of air in tubes, catheters, or cannulas placed in the vascular system. A 10-cc syringe with a 19-gauge needle must be readily available for aspiration of air.

G. Cardiac procedures
   1. *Closed Mitral Commissurotomy:* use of a finger, dilator, or valvulotome to open a stenosed mitral valve; anterolateral incision, and preplaced purse-string suture in the left atrium; incision is made within the purse-string, instrument or finger is introduced to open valve, purse-string is tightened to prevent leakage, and atrium is sutured; heart–lung bypass not required
   2. *Open Mitral Commissurotomy:* mitral valve opened under direct vision with the patient on heart–lung bypass
   3. *Valve Replacement:* various types of valves are available for replacement of bicuspid (mitral), aortic, and tricuspid valves with the patient on bypass; the affected valve is removed and a prosthetic valve inserted; the wound is irrigated with an antibiotic solution; and a temporary pace-maker electrode is sutured to the heart.
   4. *Pericardectomy:* removal of a segment of pericardium, permitting peri-cardial fluid to drain into the pleural space for the treatment of cardiac tamponade
   5. *Coronary Artery Bypass Graft (CABG):* revascularization of coronary arteries to improve blood supply to the myocardium
      a. Single or multiple grafts may be required.
      b. Median sternotomy incision is used.
      c. Bypass (detour) of obstructions in coronary arteries generally requires two teams—while one team is retrieving the autogenous vessel, the other team is opening the sternum and cannulating the venae cavae.
      d. The autograft, once retrieved and its tributaries clipped, is tested for leaks, placed in heparinized saline until ready for use, reversed, and sutured to the coronary artery by end-to-side anastomosis above and below the areas of obstruction; an argon LASER may be used to weld the vascular anastamosis.
      e. Newer techniques include "off pump" CABG and minimally invasive CABG (MID-CABG)
   6. *Internal Mammary Artery Conduit:* one internal mammary artery may be dissected from its origin at the subclavian vein, passed through a notch in the pericardium, and sutured into the coronary artery distal to the obstruction increasing the overall volume of blood supply to the cardiac muscle; microscope magnification or a surgical loupe enhances visibility for the anastamosis.

7. *Coronary Artery Angioplasty:* process of restoring perfusion to a stenosed coronary artery by direct enlargement; the stenosed area is incised and patched with pericardium or saphenous vein
   a. *Endarterectomy:* removal of atherosclerotic plaque and intima from inside the artery with the use of small spatulas, a wire drill, a miniature abrasive drill, or an ultrasonic device
   b. *LASER Angioplasty:* removal of plaque or thrombosis from coronary arteries distal to the anastomosis site with a LASER
   c. *Percutaneous Transluminal Coronary Angioplasty (PTCA):* balloon dilatation of atherosclerotic coronary arteries; introduced through a femoral or brachial artery cut-down; performed under fluoroscopy in a cardiac catheterization lab
   d. Ultrasonic device with tiny drill heads is used in conjunction with PTCA to pulverize plaque with insertion of a stent to maintain arterial patency.
   e. *Transmyocardial Revascularization:* a LASER is used to bore holes in the heart wall to increase blood supply to the muscle for patients who are not candidates for CABG.
8. *Surgical management of cardiac dysrhythmias which do not respond to medical treatment*
   a. *Endocardial resection:* ablation or excision of the focus or site of ventricular arrhythmia or incision to channel electrical impulses from SA node to AV node for atrial focal tachycardia
   b. *Cryoablation:* use of cryosurgery to fuse ends of fibers or ablate the site of ventricular tachycardia
   c. *Balloon electric shock dilation:* a balloon containing electrodes is introduced through an incision in the left atrium, advanced to the left ventricle, and inflated to contact the endocardium for mapping. Shock is delivered to specific sites for ablation.
9. *Ventricular aneurysmectomy:* with the patient on bypass, the aneurysm sac is opened, fibrotic tissue is excised, air is suctioned from ventricle, ventricle is closed, and heartbeat is restored; Batista Procedure—removal of a ventricular flap to decrease the size of the ventricle for the treatment of ventricular hypertrophy
10. *Cardiac transplantation:* transfer of cadaver heart to patient in endstage cardiac disease
11. Mechanical device implanted to provide assistance for life-sustaining cardiac function or in conjunction with another cardiac operation
12. *Cardiac pacemaker insertion:* use of an electronic device to enhance the heart's electrical system; consists of a pulse generator and leads to carry impulses to the heart; performed under local anesthesia using fluoroscopy
    a. **Types**
       i. **Endocardial pacemaker:** pacing generator implanted in a subcutaneus pocket beneath the clavicle with leads inserted through the subclavian or other vein and advanced to the apex of the right ventricle; the leads are directed into the atrium and ventricle and connected to the pulse generator
       ii. **Placement of epicardial electrodes:** by a transthoracic incision and resection of the fifth costal cartilage, two screw-in electrodes are implanted in the myocardium; electrode leads are tunneled under the costal margin to the pulse generator implanted in a subcutaneous pocket in the left upper quadrant (LUQ) of the abdominal wall; if pleura was opened, chest tubes are inserted and connected to a water-seal drainage system
    b. **Precautions with pacemakers:** include avoiding use of the electrosurgical unit during placement of the pacemaker or when the patient with pacemaker is in surgery; keeping the electrosurgical generator at a safe

distance from the pulse generator; placing a grounding pad on the patient's buttock or thigh; placing a magnet over the pacemaker generator when using the monopolar electrosurgical unit; record on the patient's chart the serial number model, manufacturer's name, date of insertion, and rate; warn the patient to avoid close proximity to electromagnetic devices

13. *Cardioverter-defibrillator implantation:* similar to the pacemaker, but capable of detecting life-threatening arrhythmias and delivering a synchronized shock to stop them

14. *Intra-Aortic Balloon Pump (IABP)*
   a. Supportive device for the patient in cardiogenic shock, reversible left ventricular failure, or prolonged myocardial ischemia
   b. May be inserted in the OR in conjunction with open heart surgery for circulation support while the patient is being weaned from pulmonary bypass
      i. Balloon is inserted through the femoral artery into the descending thoracic aorta and connected to a pump console.
      ii. Balloon inflates during diastole to increase coronary perfusion and coronary arterial pressure.
      iii. Balloon deflates during systole, decreasing resistance of the ventricles.
   c. Balloon sizes range from 20 to 40 ml.
   d. **Complications** include ischemia of distal extremities, thrombus, gas embolism, perforation of the artery or aorta, bleeding, and infection.

15. *Ventricular Assist Devices (VAD):* implantation of a mechanical pump to assist or replace the function of the left ventricle while the patient is recuperating from open heart surgery

16. *Patent Ductus Arteriosus (PDA):* using a thoracotomy incision, the mediastinal pleura is incised, the ductus isolated and closed, chest tubes are inserted, and the wound is closed.

17. *Atrial Septal Defect (ASD):* with the patient on heart–lung bypass, the atrial defect is closed with a suture or a patch.

18. *Ventricular Septal Defect (VSD):* with the patient on heart–lung bypass, the defect is closed with a suture or a patch.

19. *Tetralogy of Fallot:* basic repairs
   a. *Blalock-Taussig procedure:* anastomosis of the right subclavian artery to the right pulmonary artery
   b. *Potts-Smith-Gibson procedure:* aorta is connected to the left pulmonary artery by a side-to-side anastamosis.
   c. *Waterston procedure:* posterior aorta is anastomosed to the right pulmonary artery.
   d. *open corrective procedure:* repair of pulmonary valve stenosis and closure of VSD

20. *Transposition of the great vessels:* palliative procedures until the infant can tolerate a corrective procedure are
   a. *Raskind operation:* creation of an atrial septal defect with the aid of a balloon-tipped catheter; may be done in the cardiac catheterization laboratory
   b. *Blalock-Hanlon operation:* creation of an ASD by excision of a septal segment
   c. *Corrective Mustard operation:* remnant of atrial septum is excised and patch is placed in atrial cavities to reverse venous inflow.

21. *Coarctation of the aorta:* resection of coarctation (area of stenosis) with end-to-end anastomosis or aortic graft

H. Complications of cardiac surgery
   1. *Cardiogenic shock:* precipitated by air embolism, pulmonary embolism, myocardial contusion, hypothermia, or mechanical venous obstruction

2. *Hemorrhage*
3. *Cardiac tamponade:* compression of the heart as a result of the pericardial sac filling with blood
4. *Arrhythmia*
5. *Infection:* sternum, mediastinum, cardiac suture line, prosthetic valve, implanted device, or saphenous vein donor site

IV. **Vascular Surgery**

A. **Diagnostic procedures:** include computerized tomography, MRI, carotid phonoangiography, oculoplethysmography (blood flow measurement), sonography, angiography, phlebography (for deep vein thrombosis), angioscopy, and intravenous ultrasonic scanning (ultrasonic probe introduced into a vessel to determine distribution of plaque and thickness of vessel wall)

B. **Surgical pathology**
   1. *Atherosclerosis:* accumulation of plaque or thrombus in arteries with disruption of the tunica intima, results in narrowing, stenosis, and occlusion; generally occurs near bifurcations; most common arterial disease
   2. *Arteriosclerosis:* hardening of the arteries resulting in decreased elasticity with increasing blood pressure
   3. *Aneurysm:* localized dilation due to a weak vessel wall with resulting mechanical pressure; secondary to atherosclerosis or trauma
      a. *Dissecting aneurysm:* separation of the intima from the medial layer caused by necrosis of the media; occurs in abdominal, thoracic, or arch of the aorta
      b. *Ruptured abdominal aortic aneurysm:* requires emergency surgery
   4. *Arterial embolism:* blockage of an artery caused by air, clot particles, fat, a foreign body, or a tumor; results in absence of pulse, pallor, pain, numbness, and ischemic pain in the involved tissue
   5. *Pulmonary Embolism (PE):* obstruction in the pulmonary artery from a mass which originated in the veins of the lower extremities; diagnosed by lung scan, pulmonary angiography, or phlebogram; results in hypoxemia and hypotension
   6. *Varicose veins:* torturous dilated veins with valvular insufficiency due to back pressure; can result in swelling of involved tissue, purplish discoloration, warmth, pain on inactivity, thrombophlebitis, and venous stasis ulcers

C. **Special tools**
   1. *Vascular monitoring equipment*
      a. **Doppler ultrasound:** for blood flow assessment
      b. **Pulse volume recorder:** used to assess blood flow
      c. **Intravascular imaging:** used to measure hemodynamic changes and assess blood flow
      d. **Pulmonary artery pressure (Swan-Ganz catheter):** measures pressure in the pulmonary artery
   2. *Operating microscope or surgical loupes (magnifying glasses)* for small vessel anastomosis
   3. *Vascular instruments*
      a. *Cutting:* #7 scalpel with #11 and 15 blades, straight and angled Potts-Smith vascular scissors
      b. *Clamps:* angled peripheral vascular clamps, aortic occlusion clamps, and Satinsky, DeBakey bulldog, and Fogarty occlusion clamps
      c. *Forceps:* Potts-Smith and DeBakey
      d. *Accessory items:* heparin flushing needles, occlusion clips and appliers, nerve hook, submucous elevators, Fogarty arterial embolectomy catheters, valvulotome, vascular dilators, tunneling instruments, neurosurgical elevators (Freer and Penfield)

SURGERY HINT

If a heparin flush needle is not available, the ST can use an angiocath sheath for this. Make sure that the needle is included in all counts.

4. *Sutures:* synthetic, nonabsorbable, atraumatic double- and single-armed sizes 0 to 8-0; polypropylene, polyester, Dacron, and PTFE (Teflon)
5. *Vascular prostheses*
   a. **Human grafts**
      i. *Saphenous vein graft:* most commonly used autogenous arterial bypass or vein graft
      ii. *In-situ conduit/bypass:* for revascularization in lower extremities; saphenous vein is exposed and left in place; valves are cut to reverse blood flow and anastomosed to the femoral artery proximally and popliteal artery distally
      iii. *Reversed vein graft:* saphenous vein harvested, tested for leaks, reversed, and used as bypass for arterial obstruction
      iv. *Human umbilical cord vein graft:* commercially supplied; must be thoroughly irrigated with heparinized saline or Ringer's solution to remove glutaraldehyde and kept in solution until implanted; only noncrushing forceps should be used
   b. **Synthetic vascular prostheses**
      i. *Knitted polyester (Dacron):* must be preclotted (with 30 cc of the patient's blood in a basin, drawn by the surgeon before administration of heparin)
      ii. *Filamentous velour (polyester):* used across moveable joints; steam sterilized and soaked in a patient's plasma before use
      iii. *Woven polyester:* does not require preclotting; used for aortic replacement
      iv. *Polytetrafluorethylene (PTFE) Gore-Tex, or Impra:* does not require preclotting; available straight, tapered, bifurcated, or with supporting rings to resist compression
      v. *Composite graft:* prosthetic graft (PTFE) is anastomosed to a segment of the saphenous vein as a substitute for insufficient length.

D. **Special considerations and techniques**
   1. Steps must be taken to prevent the most common complications: hemorrhage and thrombus formation.
   2. Procedures may be performed under local or monitored anesthesia care (MAC)/local with sedation
   3. Anticoagulants must be available; IV heparin is administered 3 to 5 minutes prior to incision in a vessel; lumen may be flushed with heparinized saline solution.
   4. Papaverine or lidocaine hydrochloride may be used to prevent vascular spasm.
   5. Topical hemostatic agents should be readily available: absorbable gelatin sponge, microfibrillar collagen, oxidized cellulose, and topical thrombin; vasodilating and vasoconstricting drugs should be readily available.
   6. Vessels are retracted with moistened umbilical tape or vessel loops (long, thin, elastic-like tapes) with clamp attached.
   7. Vessels may be occluded with vascular clamps, rubber-shod clamps, bulldog clamps, or with umbilical tape (ends held together with a clamp and snared over rubber tubing/bolster, which is pressed against the vessel and secured to produce a tourniquet effect).
   8. All air must be removed from tubing prior to intravascular insertion.
   9. **Internal shunts:** temporary bypass to provide continuous circulation during surgical intervention; used in the case of Carotid Endarterectomy

E. Conservative therapy for vascular disease
   1. *Percutaneous Transluminal Coronary Angioplasty (PTCA)*
   2. *LASER Angioplasty*
   3. *Atherectomy:* transluminal pulverization and retrieval of atherosclerotic plaque with high-frequency burrs or cutters
   4. *Thrombectomy:* removal of a clot with a balloon-tipped catheter (Fogarty) under local anesthesia
   5. *Fibrinolytic therapy:* infusion of drugs into an occluded vessel, such as streptokinase or urokinase, which causes clot dissolution; may be infused intraoperatively or used in conjunction with angioplasty

F. Peripheral vascular procedures
   1. *Arterial Bypass:* providing a shunt or detour of blood around an obstruction
      a. *Femoro-Popliteal Bypass:* obstruction is bypassed with in-situ saphenous or artificial graft
      b. *Aorto-Iliac Bypass:* use of a bifurcated synthetic graft to bypass atheromatous obstructions in the distal aorta or proximal iliac arteries
      c. *Aorto-Femoral Bypass:* use of a synthetic bifurcated graft to bypass obstruction in the iliac arteries
      d. *Femoro-Femoral Bypass:* use of a synthetic graft to connect the proximal femoral artery of an ischemic leg with that of the unaffected leg
      e. *Axillo-Femoral Bypass:* use of a graft between the axillary artery and femoral artery of the ischemic leg
   2. *Profundoplasty:* suturing of a patch into an artery wall to widen an area of bifurcation and increase blood flow
   3. *Arterial Embolectomy:* use of a Fogarty catheter to remove blood clots from an artery to restore circulation
   4. *Carotid Endarterectomy:* performed at the bifurcation of the common carotid artery (bifurcates into the internal and external carotid arteries); can be performed under general or regional anesthesia; incision is over the lateral neck area, just behind the angle of the jaw; an intraluminal (inside the artery) shunt may be placed to provide adequate blood flow to the brain during cross-clamping of the artery/removal of the plaque; local anesthesia may be injected into the carotid body (located behind the bifurcation) to prevent inducing hypotension; the arteriotomy is performed with an #11, #15, or #12 scalpel blade and extended with Potts-Smith scissors; the plaque is separated from the tunica intima using a dissector; the vessels are back flushed (clamp released momentarily to flush blood, clot, and debris out of the lumen); arteriotomy is closed with vascular suture; soft tissues are closed and the wound dressing applied
   5. *Pulmonary Embolectomy:* patients not responding to anticoagulant therapy, vasodilators, or sympathetic block may be placed on heart–lung bypass and embolus removed from pulmonary artery by manually squeezing lungs to force clot out or by the use of a balloon catheter.
   6. *Vena Cava Umbrella Filter Placement (Moddin-Udden or Greenfield):* insertion of an umbrella filter under fluoroscopy through the right internal jugular venotomy and advancing it through the right atrium into the inferior vena cava, where it is ejected and fixed below the level of the renal veins; may also be inserted through the femoral vein.

SURGERY HINT

Many surgeons perform carotid endarterectomy under regional anesthesia. Always be aware that the patient can hear conversations among team members.

   Careful tracking of the amounts of local and heparin need to be kept.

---

7. *Ligation and Stripping of Varicose Veins:* a vein stripper is passed through the saphenous vein from ankle level to groin level (branches ligated with vascular clips) and pulled backward to strip out the vein; following wound closure, the entire leg is bandaged from distal to proximal with elastic bandages to provide pressure.

8. *Portosystemic Shunts (included in the general surgery section of the review):* for cirrhosis of the liver; may be done by the vascular surgeon; include Splenorenal, Mesocaval, and Portocaval Shunts.

9. *Arteriovenous Shunt:* insertion of a shunting device (prosthetic loop) between an artery and vein, generally in the arm between the radial artery and the cephalic vein of the nondominant hand to provide for insertion of a large-bore needle to facilitate hemodialysis for patients with end-stage renal disease

10. *Arteriovenous Fistula:* creation of a fistula (communication or opening) between an artery and a vein (direct connection or by implanting the saphenous vein or a prosthesis) for hemodialysis access

11. *Peritoneojugular Shunt:* for palliative treatment of intractable ascites, a shunt is placed from the peritoneal cavity to the jugular vein for the return of ascitic fluid to general circulation.

12. *Venous Access Procedures:* for frequent access to the vascular system such as for the administration of chemotherapy for cancer patients or for hyperalimentation; indwelling catheter is placed, under local anesthesia, into the subclavian, external jugular, or cephalic vein and advanced to the right atrium; catheter can be externalized through a subcutaneous tunnel from the venotomy site—examples include Broviac, Hickman, Ash Split, and Groshong; or internalized to prevent infection—examples include Medi-Port and Port-a-Cath

13. *Abdominal Aortic Aneurysm with Graft (AAA)*
    a. Patient in supine position, prepped from nipple line to knees and draped
    b. Midline incision from xiphoid to symphysis pubis is made and deepened using the electrosurgical pencil, peritoneum is entered, intestines are placed in a moistened plastic bag, and the retroperitoneum is opened
    c. Aneurysm sac is identified and freed with blunt and sharp dissection
    d. Umbilical tape is placed around the aorta above the aneurysm and around both iliac arteries and retracted.
    e. Bifurcated graft size is determined (30 cc of blood is withdrawn from the patient and placed in a basin with graft for preclotting if needed).
    f. Heparin sodium is given IV, followed 3–5 minutes later with clamping of iliac arteries with angled peripheral vascular clamps and of aorta above the aneurysm with Crawford, Satinsky, or Cooley clamp.
    g. Aneurysm is opened with a #11 blade and heavy scissors; plaque is removed
    h. Anterior wall of the aneurysm is trimmed with scissors and vascular forceps.
    i. Bleeding is controlled from lumbar arteries with suture ligatures.
    j. Graft is sutured in place using double-armed nonabsorbable vascular suture and flushed by briefly releasing the aortic clamp to flush out clots and check the security of the suture line.
    k. Distal vessels are inspected for backflow, and the graft is anastomosed to the iliac or femoral arteries.
    l. Protamine sulfate IV may be administered, suture line is inspected, first count is taken, and wounds are closed.

Show What You Know

Directions
Each of the numbered items or incomplete statements in this section is followed by answers or by completions of the statement. Select the ONE lettered answer or completion that is BEST in each case.

1. A mass of undissolved matter carried in the blood is:

   A. thrombus
   B. embolus
   C. ascites
   D. platelets

2. For visualization of the pleurae, lower and middle mediastinum, and pericardium, the surgeon would need a:

   A. thorascope
   B. mediastinoscope
   C. bronchoscope
   D. laryngoscope

3. As the scrub, with which of the following procedures would you anticipate the use of chest tubes and a water-seal drainage system?

   A. Lobectomy
   B. Scalene Node Biopsy
   C. Percutaneous Transluminal Coronary Angioplasty
   D. Cardiac Pacemaker Insertion

4. The surgical incision most likely for open heart surgery is:

   A. anterolateral thoracotomy
   B. posterolateral thoracotomy
   C. median sternotomy
   D. supraclavicular

5. Which of the following retractors would be most useful in a posterolateral Thoracotomy?

   A. Balfour
   B. O'Sullivan-O'Connor
   C. Davidson scapula
   D. Weitlaner

6. Which medication is commonly given intravenously about 3–5 minutes prior to cross-clamping the artery during Arteriotomy?

   A. epinephrine
   B. protamine sulfate
   C. papaverine
   D. heparin

7. With which of the following procedures would you expect the greatest amount of bleeding?

   A. Wedge Resection of the Lung
   B. Decortication of the Lung

   C. Open Thoracotomy for Closure of a Ruptured Bulla
   D. Closure of a Patent Ductus Arteriosus

8. All of the following are sutures used in cardiovascular surgery to suture vessels or vascular grafts *except*:

   A. polytetrafluoroethylene (PTFE or Gore-Tex)
   B. polypropylene (Prolene)
   C. polyester (Dacron)
   D. surgical gut (chromic)

9. Which of the following procedures would commonly require the use of extracorporeal circulation (heart–lung bypass)?

   A. Abdominal Aortic Aneurysmectomy with Graft
   B. Pneumonectomy
   C. Coronary Artery Bypass Graft
   D. Vena Cava Umbrella Insertion

10. Which of the following bypass grafts would require preclotting?

    A. knitted polyester (Dacron)
    B. saphenous vein
    C. human umbilical cord graft
    D. polytetrafluoroethylene (PTFE)

11. The removal of plaque and lining from an artery is called a/an:

    A. Profundoplasty
    B. Endarterectomy
    C. Phlebography
    D. Arteriovenous Fistula Formation

12. The creation of a communication between an artery and a vein for hemodialysis access is called a/an:

    A. Bypass Graft
    B. Aneurysmectomy
    C. Vena Cava Umbrella Filter Placement
    D. Arteriovenous Fistula Formation

13. The removal of a lung is referred to as a/an:

    A. Pneumonectomy
    B. Endarterectomy
    C. Blalock-Hanlon operation
    D. Cryoablation

14. The closing of a defect between the lower heart chambers is a procedure referred to as a:

    A. Closure of a Patent Ductus Arteriosus
    B. Commissurotomy

C. Repair of a Ventricular Septal Defect

D. Transmyocardial revascularization

15. Portosystemic shunts include all of the following *except:*

A. Splenorenal
B. Portorenal
C. Mesocaval
D. Portacaval

16. Facts concerning arteriovenous fistulas and shunts include all of the following *except* that they:

A. are usually performed in the upper arm or leg
B. establish blood flow between the arterial and venous circulation
C. bypass the capillary network
D. are used for vascular access during hemodialysis

17. Vena cava filter devices are inserted to prevent pulmonary emboli by trapping clots from the venous system of the legs and include which of the following?

A. Greenfield filter
B. Debakey filter
C. Statinsky filter
D. LeVeen filter

18. A sac-like dilation and thinning of an artery wall that can lead to rupture of the vessel is a/an:

A. bifurcation
B. claudication
C. aneurysm
D. stenosis

19. The procedure in which a Fogarty catheter is used to remove blockage of a vessel is referred to as:

A. arteriovenous shunt
B. endarterectomy
C. embolectomy
D. ligation and stripping

20. The autogenous graft which is left in place after destruction of the internal valves and then sutured into the arterial system is:

A. in-situ saphenous vein graft
B. human umbilical cord graft
C. PTFE graft
D. ligation and stripping of the saphenous vein

21. Cardiac pacing is indicated for which of the following conditions?

A. atelectasis
B. atherosclerosis
C. congestive heart failure
D. heart block

22. During pacemaker insertion, the pacing generator is placed:

A. in the inferior vena cava via the jugular vein
B. in the ventricle via the femoral vein
C. in the ventricle via the subclavian vein
D. in a subcutaneous pocket on the upper anterior chest wall

23. Specific equipment used during surgery on a patient with a pacemaker in place should include:

A. a magnet
B. mono-polar ESU with its patient return electrode applied to the patient
C. mono-polar ESU without its patient return electrode applied to the patient
D. bi-polar ESU with its patient return electrode applied to the patient

24. The scissors used for intravascular access during endarterectomy are called:

A. Metzenbaum
B. Jameson
C. Potts
D. Tenotomy

25. The medication used to reverse the initial anticoagulant therapy during vascular surgery is:

A. Vitamin K
B. heparin sodium
C. protamine sulfate
D. sodium bicarbonate

26. The artery that carries deoxygenated blood in the adult is the:

A. aorta
B. carotid artery
C. pulmonary artery
D. coronary artery

27. The vessel used to increase the overall blood supply to the heart following CABG is the:

A. saphenous artery
B. brachial artery
C. carotid artery
D. internal mammary artery

28. Which of the following procedures is/are performed under fluoroscopic (C-ARM) control?

A. endarterectomy
B. cardiac pacemaker insertion
C. vena cava filtering device placement
D. both B and C

29. Common artery bypass procedures include all of the following *except:*

A. axillo-popliteal
B. femoro-femoral
C. axillo-femoral
D. femoro-popliteal

30. The procedure which may require the temporary use of an intraoperative bypass shunt is a/an:

    A. Femoro-Popliteal Bypass Graft
    B. Abdominal Aortic Aneurysmectomy
    C. Carotid Endarterectomy
    D. Aortic-Artery Bypass Graft

31. The procedure performed to remove a fibrous covering from the lung following empyema formation is:

    A. Pulmonary Decortication
    B. Thoracostomy
    C. Thymectomy
    D. Aneurysmectomy

32. An outpouching of an alveolar sac which leads to subsequent rupture resulting in a pneumothorax is called a/an:

    A. aneurysm
    B. bleb
    C. atelectasis
    D. arteriovenous fistula

33. The instrument used to approximate the ribs following Thoracotomy is the:

    A. Duval clamp
    B. Bailey rib contractor
    C. Harken-Finochetto retractor
    D. Alexander periosteotome

34. Cervical Rib Resection is performed to relieve:

    A. Thoracic Outlet Syndrome
    B. Thoracic Inlet Syndrome
    C. Adult Respiratory Distress Syndrome
    D. pneumothorax

35. When two chest tubes are placed into the pleural space, the uppermost tube is used to:

    A. evacuate air/re-establish negative pressure
    B. evacuate blood/re-establish positive pressure
    C. evacuate serous fluid/re-establish positive pressure
    D. evacuate pus/re-establish negative pressure

36. When a rib is removed, the remaining bone edges are trimmed with a:

    A. Doyen raspatory
    B. Bethune shear
    C. Lebsche knife
    D. Stille-Luer rongeur

37. When transporting a patient with closed water-seal drainage:

    A. the bottle should be kept at or above the height of the patient's chest
    B. the chest tube should always be clamped

C. chest tube clamps should accompany the patient at all times
    D. the patient should be placed in the Trendelenburg position

38. Mediastinoscopy is usually performed with the patient in what position?

    A. lateral
    B. Sims
    C. dorsal recumbent
    D. prone

39. The diagnostic procedure which permits visualization of the Great Vessels is called:

    A. Bronchoscopy
    B. Mediastinoscopy
    C. Thoracoscopy
    D. Pleuroscopy

40. A decrease in blood supply to tissues is called:

    A. atherosclerosis
    B. ischemia
    C. varicosities
    D. embolus formation

41. Suture material used to place vascular grafts would include:

    A. PDS
    B. Vicryl/Dexon
    C. Prolene
    D. stainless steel

42. A Femoro-Popliteal Bypass is scheduled. Which self-retaining retractor would be used to facilitate exploration of the femoral artery?

    A. Harken
    B. DeBakey
    C. Weitlaner
    D. Gelpi

43. The retraction of fine structures during vascular surgery is accomplished by use of:

    A. Senn retractors
    B. vessel loops
    C. malleable ribbon retractors
    D. penrose drain

44. Which of the following would be placed on an embolectomy setup for the purpose of removing clots through an arteriotomy?

    A. Foley catheter
    B. Fogarty catheter
    C. Swanz-Ganz catheter
    D. Randall forcep

45. A small, spring-like vascular clamp used for occluding peripheral vessels is a:

    A. vessel loop
    B. Harken

C. bulldog
D. Duval

46. The treatment of choice for patent ductus arteriosus is:

A. patch graft
B. suture ligation of the duct
C. Atrial Septostomy
D. Posterior Sagittal Anorectoplasty

47. Removal of air or fluid from the pleural cavity via needle aspiration is:

A. Thoracoscopy
B. Thoracotomy
C. Hemocentesis
D. Thoracentesis

Instrument Identification

48.

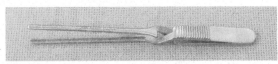

A. DeBakey bulldog clamp
B. Payr clamp
C. Bakes dilator
D. Potts-Smith scissor

49.

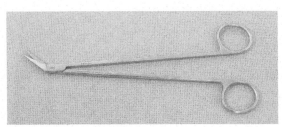

A. Crawford coarctation clamp
B. Payr clamp
C. Tenotomy scissor
D. Potts scissor

50.

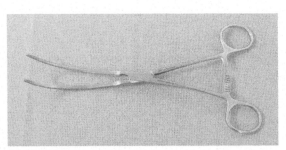

A. Rummel thoracic clamp
B. DeBakey tissue forcep
C. DeBakey peripheral vessel clamp
D. Sarot needle holder

51.

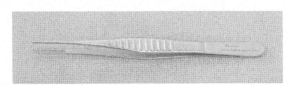

A. DeBakey bulldog clamp
B. DeBakey tissue forcep

C. DeBakey peripheral vessel clamp
D. Duval lung-grasping forceps

52.

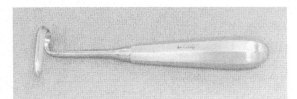

A. Alexander raspatory
B. Doyen rib raspatory
C. Bailey rib contractor
D. Key elevator

53.

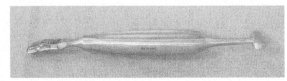

A. Alexander raspatory
B. Doyen rib raspatory
C. Harken rib spreader
D. Lowman clamp

54.

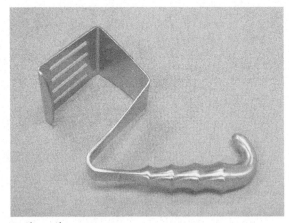

A. Bailey rib contractor
B. Bennett retractor
C. Harken rib spreader
D. Davidson scapula retractor

Anatomy Review

Respiratory and Cardiovascular Systems

55–80.

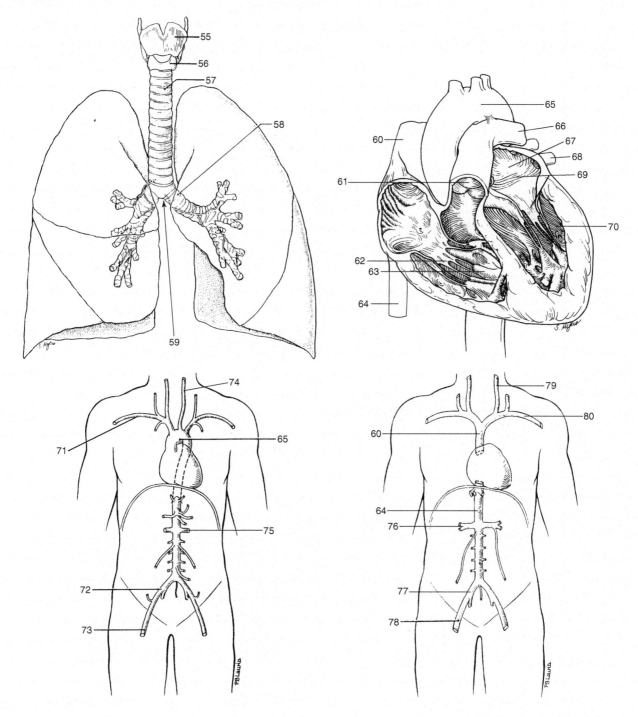

A. aorta
B. bronchus
C. carina
D. carotid artery
E. chordae tendonae
F. cricoid cartilage
G. femoral artery
H. femoral vein
I. iliac artery

J. iliac vein
K. inferior vena cava
L. jugular vein
M. left atrium
N. left ventricle
O. mitral valve
P. papillary muscles
Q. pulmonary artery
R. pulmonary valve

S. pulmonary vein
T. renal artery
U. renal vein
V. subclavian artery
W. subclavian vein
X. superior vena cava
Y. thyroid cartilage
Z. trachea

Answers & Rationales

1. **B.** **Rationale:** An embolus is a mass of undissolved matter circulating in the blood and may consist of fat, air, foreign body, or parts of a clot.

2. **A.** **Rationale:** A thorascope is inserted between the ribs into the chest cavity to view the lungs, pleurae, pericardium, and lower and middle mediastinum. Visualization is limited to the upper mediastinum with a mediastinoscopy. The laryngoscope facilitates visualization inside the larynx, and the bronchoscope is used to visualize inside the bronchi or the trachea.

3. **A.** **Rationale:** Chest tubes are inserted and connected to a water-seal drainage system whenever the pleural space is entered. Lobectomy, removal of a lobe of the lung, requires entry into the pleural cavity. A Scalene Node Biopsy is the removal of tissue from above the clavicle. PTCA is a procedure performed in the cardiac catheterization laboratory where a balloon catheter is inserted into the femoral or brachial artery, advanced to the coronary arteries, and used to dilate an atherosclerotic vessel. A pacemaker generator is implanted in subcutaneous tissue with leads passed through a vein to the heart.

4. **C.** **Rationale:** A median sternotomy is the incision most frequently used for open heart surgery because it provides a more accessible route and patient positioning is much simpler.

5. **C.** **Rationale:** The Davidson scapula retractor is needed to raise the scapula when a posterolateral Thoracotomy is performed. The Balfour is designed for a vertical incision in the abdomen, the O'Sullivan-O'Connor for a transverse incision in the abdomen, and the Weitlaner for superficial surgery.

6. **D.** **Rationale:** Heparin is given intravenously about 3–5 minutes prior to cross-clamping the artery during Arteriotomy, an opening into the vascular system, to prevent blood clot formation which could later obstruct distal vessels.

7. **B.** **Rationale:** Bleeding is to be expected during a decortication of the lung as the fibrosed tissue is peeled off. Little bleeding occurs when staples are used to remove lung tissue. With closure of a patent ductus arteriosus on an infant, bleeding should be minimal.

8. **D.** **Rationale:** Surgical gut is an absorbable suture material and is not recommended for the suturing of vessels and vascular grafts. A non-absorbable, swaged suture is used.

9. **C.** **Rationale:** Extracorporeal circulation is commonly required for the placement of a bypass graft around an obstructed coronary artery. Abdominal Aneurysmectomy is performed through a midline abdominal incision; Pneumonectomy is the removal of a lung, generally by a posterolateral thoracotomy, and a vena cava umbrella is advanced from a percutaneous approach through the jugular or femoral vein.

10. **A.** **Rationale:** A knitted polyester (Dacron) graft requires preclotting. It is porous and enhances in-growth of tissue but could allow leakage of blood through its pores if the graft is not preclotted or pretreated.

11. **B.** **Rationale:** An Endarterectomy is the removal of plaque along with the tunica intima of the affected portion of the artery.

12. **D.** **Rationale:** The creation of a fistula between an artery and vein to create an area for the frequent passage of a large-bore needle for the patient on hemodialysis is an Arteriovenous Fistula Formation.

13. **A.** **Rationale:** Surgical removal of a lung, Pneumonectomy, is performed for extensive lung disease or cancer.

14. **C.** **Rationale:** A ventricular septal defect is managed surgically by closing the defect with suture or, if the defect is large, with a patch.

15. **B.** **Rationale:** Portosystemic shunts include Spleno-renal (between the splenic vein and the renal vein), Meso-caval (between the mesenteric vein and the vena cava), and Porta-caval (between the portal vein and the vena cava) shunts. Shunts are not created between the portal vein and the renal vein due to location and blood volume.

16. **A.** **Rationale:** Arteriovenous fistulas and shunts establish blood flow between the arterial and venous circulation, bypass the capillary network, and are used for vascular access during hemodialysis. They are commonly performed in the lower forearm area.

17. **A.** **Rationale:** Greenfield vena cava filter devices are inserted to prevent pulmonary emboli by trapping clots from the venous system of the legs.

18. **C.** **Rationale:** An aneurysm is a sac-like dilation and thinning of the wall of an artery. A bifurcation is a branching or forking into two. Claudication is a symptom of arterial obstruction. Stenosis is an abnormal narrowing.

19. **C.** **Rationale:** Embolectomy is the procedure in which a Fogarty catheter is used to remove blockage of a vessel. An endarterectomy involves the removal of plaque from the inside of an artery, usually close to an area of bifurcation.

20. **A.** **Rationale:** The autogenous graft which is left in place after destruction of the internal valves and then sutured into the arterial system is an in-situ saphenous vein graft.

21. **D.** **Rationale:** Cardiac pacing is indicated for heart block, a condition of alteration in electrical conductivity of the Bundle of His. Congestive heart failure is treated with diuretics. Atherosclerosis is plaque accumulation in the vessels. Atelectasis is a collapse of the lung due to blockage of the alveoli or bronchioles.

22. **D.** **Rationale:** During pacemaker insertion, the pacing generator is placed in a subcutaneous pocket on the upper anterior chest wall. The leads are placed into the right atrium or ventricle via the subclavian vein and superior vena cava.

23. **A.** **Rationale:** A magnet is used during surgery on a patient with a pacemaker in place. It is placed over the pacemaker generator. The magnet will assist in blocking stray electricity from reaching the pacing generator, since electricity is able either to reprogram or to significantly interfere with the generator's function. The use of mono-polar ESU should be limited and should always be used with a patient return electrode (grounding pad). The use of bipolar ESU does not require use of a patient return electrode.

24. **C.** **Rationale:** Potts scissors are fine, angled scissors used to extend an arteriotomy during vascular surgery. Jameson and Tenotomy have sharp, pointed tips that could damage the inside lining of the vessel, and Metzenbaum's are used for general tissue dissection.

25. **C.** **Rationale:** Heparin sodium is the medication commonly used for anticoagulation during vascular surgery. Protamine sulfate, also an anticoagulant, will bind to the heparin sodium that is present, neutralizing heparin's ability to prevent clotting. Vitamin K is a medication that promotes clot formation, and sodium bicarbonate is a neutralizing or buffering agent used to treat metabolic acidosis.

26. **C.** **Rationale:** The pulmonary artery carries deoxygenated blood in the adult.

27. **D.** **Rationale:** During coronary artery bypass surgery (CABG), the internal mammary artery (IMA) can be dissected from the chest wall and attached to the coronary circulatory system, increasing the overall volume of blood delivered to supply the heart muscle.

28. **D.** **Rationale:** Both cardiac pacemaker insertion and vena cava filter device insertion are percutaneous procedures. The placement of each device is aided by visualization of the anatomical structures where the devices are placed using fluoroscopy. Endarterectomy is performed through an open incision.

29. **A.** **Rationale:** An axillo-popliteal bypass is not commonly performed due to the significant distance the graft must travel through the subcutaneous tunnel which could lead to clot formation in the graft and obstruction of blood flow.

30. **C.** **Rationale:** A Carotid Endarterectomy may require the use of a temporary intraoperative bypass shunt to assist in maintaining an adequate oxygen supply to the brain, decreasing the chance of intraoperative cerebrovascular accident (CVA). One example is the Javid shunt.

31. **A.** **Rationale:** Pulmonary Decortication is the surgical procedure where the fibrous covering over the lung resulting from empyema (pus formation in the pleural space) is removed to permit re-expansion of an entrapped lung.

32. **B.** **Rationale:** A bleb is an area of alveoli that have lost their elasticity and are therefore thin and distended, leading to rupture and leakage of air into the pleural space (pneumothorax), causing the lung to collapse.

33. **B.** **Rationale:** The Bailey rib contractor is the instrument used to approximate the ribs during closure of a Thoracotomy. Duval lung clamps are used to manipulate lung tissue.

34. **A.** **Rationale:** Cervical Rib Resection is performed to relieve compression of the brachial plexus neurovascular bundle, a condition called thoracic outlet syndrome.

35. **A.** **Rationale:** When two chest tubes are placed into the pleural space, the uppermost tube is used to evacuate air. The lower chest tube is used to evacuate fluids, such as blood. The removal of air and fluid collection from the pleural space and re-establishment of negative pressure is necessary to inflate the lungs for proper respiration.

36. **D.** **Rationale:** A Stille-Luer rongeur is used to trim the edges of a rib following rib resection.

37. **C.** **Rationale:** When transporting a patient with closed water-seal drainage, chest tube clamps should always accompany the patient for use in the event that the tube separates from the

drainage device. This separation will permit air to enter the pleural space causing pneumothorax and can be life-threatening. The drainage device should be kept at or below the level of the patient's chest to promote proper drainage. Chest tubes are only clamped when ordered by the physician or in case of separation of the drainage device from the chest tube. Patients with chest tubes should be placed in the semi-Fowler (sitting) position to promote and ease respiratory effort.

38. **C.** **Rationale:** Mediastinoscopy is usually performed with the patient in the dorsal recumbent or semi-Fowler position with the neck hyperextended for access to the area just above the suprasternal notch.

39. **B.** **Rationale:** Mediastinoscopy is a diagnostic procedure that permits access to the cavity between the two lungs, an area that contains the great vessels—the aorta, the vena cavea, and the pulmonary arteries and veins.

40. **B.** **Rationale:** Ischemia is the condition of decreased blood flow to tissue. Ischemia can be caused by atherosclerosis or embolus formation. Varicosities, dilation of veins resulting from prolonged backpressure that destroys the veins' valves, results in venous stasis or pooling of blood in lower extremities.

41. **C.** **Rationale:** When vascular grafts are placed, they are sutured to the vessel with nonabsorbable suture material, preferably monofilament suture. Prolene or polypropylene is a synthetic monofilament, nonabsorbable suture material. Stainless steel, while also monofilament and nonabsorbable, is difficult to work with and could easily tear the delicate vessel wall. PDS and Vicryl/Dexon are all absorbable suture materials.

42. **C.** **Rationale:** The Weitlaner retractor is used to expose the femoral artery by retracting the soft tissues of the groin. The Gelpi retractor is sharp and may damage blood vessels if not carefully placed and monitored.

43. **B.** **Rationale:** Vessel loops are long, thin, elastic-like tapes that can easily be passed around a vessel and are commonly used to manipulate the vessel rather than grasping it with a clamp or forcep.

44. **B.** **Rationale:** The Fogarty catheter is used during Embolectomy to remove clots and debris from an artery. Following exposure and control of the affected artery, a small arteriotomy is performed with a sharp scalpel blade and extended with Potts scissors. The Fogarty catheter is inserted and passed beyond the area of obstruction. The Fogarty catheter balloon is inflated with IV saline, and the catheter is slowly removed, dragging the debris back to the arteriotomy site.

45. **C.** **Rationale:** The bulldog is a small, spring-like vascular clamp used for occluding peripheral vessels. Harken and DeBakey vascular clamps are not spring-like and are used to occlude major vessels. The Duval is a lung clamp used to manipulate lung tissue.

46. **B.** **Rationale:** Patent Ductus Arteriosus (PDA) is a congenital anomaly where the ductus arteriosus, a communication between the pulmonary artery and the aorta during fetal development, fails to close. This communication, in the neonate, permits deoxygenated blood to enter the arterial system. Suture ligation of this duct is performed to eliminate this alternate blood flow pattern.

47. **D.** **Rationale:** Thoracentesis is the procedure performed to remove air or fluid from the pleural space. It is performed by inserting a large gauge (13g or 15g) 3" needle into the pleural space by passing the needle through an intercostal space. A 60-cc syringe is used to withdraw the air or fluid. Once the needle is removed from the chest wall, an air-occlusive dressing is applied.

Instrument Identification

48. **A.** DeBakey bulldog clamp
49. **D.** Potts scissor
50. **C.** DeBakey peripheral vessel clamp
51. **B.** DeBakey tissue forcep
52. **A.** Alexander raspatory
53. **B.** Doyen rib raspatory
54. **D.** Davidson scapula retractor

Anatomy

55. **(Y)** thyroid cartilage
56. **(F)** cricoid cartilage
57. **(Z)** trachea
58. **(B)** bronchus
59. **(C)** carina
60. **(X)** superior vena cava
61. **(R)** pulmonary valve
62. **(E)** chordae tendonae
63. **(P)** papillary muscles

64. **(K)** inferior vena cava

65. **(A)** aorta

66. **(Q)** pulmonary artery

67. **(M)** left atrium

68. **(S)** pulmonary vein

69. **(O)** mitral valve

70. **(N)** left ventricle

71. **(V)** subclavian artery

72. **(I)** iliac artery

73. **(G)** femoral artery

74. **(D)** carotid artery

75. **(T)** renal artery

76. **(U)** renal vein

77. **(J)** iliac vein

78. **(H)** femoral vein

79. **(L)** jugular vein

80. **(W)** subclavian vein

Part II: Deciphering a Surgical Schedule

The following mock surgery schedule will be used to answer several questions pertaining to cardio-thoracic and peripheral vascular surgery. The same schedule, or a similar one, will be used in subsequent chapters to ask questions about the content of the chapter.

Rm#time	Surgeon	Procedure	Anest.	Rm#time	Surgeon	Procedure	Anest.
Rm00				**Rm07**			
OC	Dr. Z	Rt. Knee Arthroscopy	Gen.	7:00	Dr. M	CABG	Gen.
OC	Dr. C	Craniotomy	Gen.	TF	Dr. M	CABGX2	Gen.
OC	Dr.Z	Angioplasty	Gen.				
Rm01				**Rm08**			
7:00	Dr. X	Lobectomy	Gen.	11:00	Dr. E	Bovine Thrombectomy	MAC
TF	Dr. X	Pneumonectomy	Gen.				
TF	Dr. X	Scalene node biopsy	Gen.				
Rm02				**Rm09**			
7:00	Dr. B	Wedge Resection R Lung	Gen.	8:30	Dr. T	AV fistula	local
TF	Dr. B	Thoracotomy	Gen.	TF	Dr. T	AV fistula	local
Rm03				**Rm10**			
7:00	Dr. A	Cystoscopy	MAC	7:00	Dr. K	Fem-pop	Gen.
TF	Dr. A	Cystoplasty	Gen.	TF	Dr. K	Choledocholithotripsy	MAC
12:30	Dr. F	Pyleogram	MAC	TF	Dr. K	Hepatic resection	Gen.
3:00	Dr. F	Cystocele repair	Gen.				
Rm04				**Rm11**			
7:00	Dr. Y	Carotid Endarterectomy	MAC	7:00	Dr. L	Colposcope	Gen.
TF	Dr. Y	AAA	Gen.	12:00	Dr. L	Mastectomy	Gen.
Rm05				**Rm12**			
7:00	Dr. G	Trans-sphenoidal Adenectomy	Gen.	7:00	Dr. W	Trans-metatarsal amputation	Gen.
TF	Dr. G	Trans-urethral resection of the prostate	Gen	TF	Dr. W	Osteotomy	Gen.
TF	Dr. G	Bletharoplasty	Gen.	TF	Dr. W	Arthrocentesis	Gen.
Rm06				**Rm13**			
7:00	Dr. R	Lumbar Laminectomy	Gen.	7:00	Dr. O	Hysterectomy	Gen.

The following questions should be answered using the surgery schedule above

1. During the carotid endarterectomy, the surgeon wants to use a shunt. Which instrument should the Surgical Technologist have ready for the surgeon?

   A. Javid
   B. Greenfield
   C. Potts –smith scissors
   D. Angled DeBakey

2. Which instrument should the Surgical Technologist have ready to hand the surgeon to clamp the aorta during the AAA in Room 4?

   A. Statinsky
   B. Herrick
   C. Angled DeBakey
   D. Bulldog

3. During the femoro-popliteal graft in Room 10, the Surgical Technologist can expect the bypass to be composed of

   A. The in-situ popliteal vein
   B. The in-situ femoral vein
   C. The in-situ cephalic vein
   D. The in-situ Saphenous vein

4. Once the in-situ vein in Room 10 has been decided upon, what should the Surgical Technologist expect next?

   A. The surgeon to request a valvatome to strip valves
   B. The surgeon will reverse the vein
   C. The surgeon will place a Gore-Tex graft around the vein to reinforce it
   D. The surgeon will request the Surgical Technologist to prepare Protamine sulfate for injection in the vein

5. Dr. M has scheduled a patient for a CABG at 7:00. The patient will be placed on bypass for this procedure. What does the Surgical Technologist have to ensure when Cannulas are placed?

   A. That no air is allowed into the vascular system
   B. That the perfusionist is scrubbed in and sterile for the procedure
   C. The tubing leading to the heart has been securely clamped
   D. The pressure between the heart and the tubing is equalized

6. Room 9 has two AV fistulas scheduled. Dr. T wants to use the patient's saphenous vein in the first procedure. What should the Surgical Technologist be prepared for?

   A. A separate prep and drape on the lower calf from ankle to knee
   B. A separate prep and drape on the arm from wrist to axilla
   C. A separate prep and drape on the upper thigh to groin
   D. A separate prep and drape on the outer leg from groin to lower leg

7. A chest drain will be necessary for the Lobectomy in Room 1. Where should the Surgical Technologist or circulator place the drainage system after the tubes have been connected?

   A. Above the patients head, on the affected side
   B. Bed level
   C. Below the chest level
   D. On the patient's chest

8. The surgeon needs to grasp lung tissue during the pneumonectomy in Room 1. What instrument should the Surgical Technologist hand to the surgeon?

   A. DeBakey forceps
   B. Duvall forceps
   C. Crawford clamp
   D. Sarot clamp

9. The surgeon in Room 2 needs a self-retaining retractor to see into the cavity.
   What should the Surgical Technologist hand the surgeon?

   A. Finochetto
   B. Lebsche
   C. Richardson
   D. Volkman

10. The surgeon in Room 2 needs to check for air leaks after the Thoracotomy.
    What should the Surgical Technologist have on hand?

    A. Cold saline
    B. Talc powder
    C. Warm saline
    D. Water-seal unit

Answers & Rationales

1. **A.** **Rationale:** A Javid carotid artery clamp secures the shunt, allowing blood to be diverted during the procedure. This allows more time to perform the procedure without compromising blood circulation to the brain. A Greenfield is a filter, and potts-smiths are scissors.

2. **A.** **Rationale:** Generally, the surgeon will place a large vascular clamp, like a Statinsky, above the aneurysm while using angled clamps on the iliac vessels.

3. **D.** **Rationale:** The in-situ vein most commonly used during a femoral-popliteal bypass is the Saphenous vein. In situ means in the original position or place. As the surgery is being done on the femoral and popliteal arteries, the veins are major structures that should be left in place if possible. The cephalic vein could not be used in situ. The Saphenous vein is a superficial vein in the leg, and is the most common vein used for both grafting and in-situ bypasses.

4. **A.** **Rationale:** Veins have valves to prevent the backflow of blood. These veins must be stripped for the vessel to be used as an arterial bypass. Generally, the surgeon will request a valvatome to strip the valves.

5. **A.** **Rationale:** Air must not be allowed to be present in the cannulas that are placed into the heart. The surgeon may aspirate air with a 19 G hypodermic and a 10-cc syringe.

6. **D.** **Rationale:** The greater Saphenous vein is a long vein that is located superficially on the outer leg. The prep for harvesting this vein will generally incorporate the leg from groin to below the knee, ensuring that a large portion of the vein is exposed. The vein will be isolated with tapes, irrigated with a heparin saline irrigation and ligated.

7. **C.** **Rationale:** Once the chest tubes have been connected to the drain, the drain should be kept below the patient's chest level. The Surgical Technologist may connect the drain and pass it to the circulator to place below the chest level.

8. **B.** **Rationale:** The Duvall is a specialty instrument designed to grasp delicate lung tissue. The Sarot is used to grasp and clamp broncus, and the DeBakey and Crawford are vascular clamps.

9. **A.** **Rationale:** The Finochetto is a commonly used self-retaining retractor used in cardio-thoracic procedures. The Richardson and Volkmann are not self-retaining retractors, and the Lebsche is a sternal knife.

10. **C.** **Rationale:** The surgeon will check for air leaks following thoracic lung cases by filling the cavity with irrigation fluid. This fluid must be warm to prevent a fall in the core body temperature of the patient.

Use this address to access the interactive Companion Website created for this book. Simply select "Surgical Technology" from the choice of disciplines. Find this book and click to enter.

chapter 21

Practice Test

The following practice test will allow you to understand which areas you need to concentrate on when studying to take the certification exam. The questions are in multiple-choice format with one best answer. Read each question fully and carefully before deciding on the best possible answer for the question. Although these are not actual questions from the certification exam, they will cover the areas that you may encounter on the test. The answers following the exam do not give rationales. The questions are not separated into topics; but if you struggle with questions regarding a specific topic, you may want to review that information.

1. Nissen fundoplication is performed to treat
   A. Malignancy
   B. Congenital anomaly of the stomach
   C. Gastroesophageal reflux
   D. Lesions in the pylorus

2. A lumbar puncture removes cerebral spinal fluid from
   A. The subarachnoid space
   B. The epidural space
   C. The lateral ventricle of the brain
   D. The space between C-1 and C-2

3. Cold, clammy skin may be a symptom of
   A. Hypothermia
   B. Hyperthermia
   C. Hypertension
   D. Shock

4. Which of the following is an atraumatic clamp?
   A. Kocher
   B. Allis
   C. Heaney
   D. Babcock

5. The ophthalmic medication which causes pupils to constrict is
   A. Mydriatic
   B. Miotic
   C. Cycloplegic
   D. Corticosteroid

6. A fracture of the frontal process of the maxilla. Nasal bones and orbital floor would be classified as a(n)
   A. LeFort I
   B. LeFort II
   C. LeFort III
   D. Malar Fracture

7. Crushing urinary stones is commonly referred to as
   A. Lithotripsy
   B. Nephrolithotomy
   C. KUB
   D. TURL

8. A procedure performed to correct urinary incontinence is
   A. Wertheim
   B. Cerclage

C. Marshall-Marchetti

D. D&E

9. The CBD joins the duodenum at this juncture

A. Ampulla of Vater

B. Sphincter of Oddi

C. Duct of Wirsung

D. Biliary duct

10. The active electrode in a Monopolar unit is located

A. At the dispersal pad

B. At the tip of the bovie pencil

C. In the generator

D. In the insulated wire

11. The stapling unit that produces a double staggered row of staples and cuts through tissue is a(n)

A. TA

B. EEA

C. GIA

D. Ligating clip

12. The type of suture that loses tensile strength in 5 to 10 days is

A. Vicryl

B. Surgical gut

C. Chromic gut

D. Surgical silk

13. The position with the patient supine and the head tilted down is

A. Trendelenburg

B. Reverse trendelenburg

C. Modified fowlers

D. Kraske

14. For a cesarean section, the patient is positioned

A. Supine, with the feet elevated

B. Lithotomy

C. Supine with the right side slightly elevated

D. Supine with the left side slightly elevated

15. An example of res ipsa loquitor would be

A. Unsigned consent

B. Patient record given to an unauthorized person

C. Leaving the patient alone in a hallway

D. Leaving a raytec in the patient

16. The pathway around the nucleus that electrons follow is called the

A. Valence shell

B. Conduit

C. Atomic current

D. Frequency cycle

17. An expression of the relationship that one property has to another is

A. Proportion

B. Ratio

C. Percentage

D. Fraction

18. During a sentinel node biopsy, the surgeon will inject

A. Hypaque

B. Methylene Blue

C. Lymphazurin

D. Isovue

19. Which structure(s) are removed during a tonsillectomy?

A. Palatine tonsils

B. Adenoid tonsils

C. Pharyngeal tonsils

D. Laryngeal and pharyngeal tonsils

20. A burn that involves epidermis and part of the dermis is classified as

A. First degree

B. Second degree

C. Third degree

D. Fourth degree

21. The proximal and distal ends of a long bone are

A. Diaphysis

B. Metaphysic

C. Epiphysis

D. Condyle

22. The type of saw used for limb amputation is a(n)

A. Oscillating saw

B. Reciprocating saw

C. Skeeter saw

D. Dubousset saw

23. A Keller procedure is used to correct

A. Hammer toe

B. Hallux Valgus

C. Bakers cyst

D. Colles fracture

24. Nearsightedness is

A. Hyperopia

B. Astigmatism

C. Myopia

D. Microtia

25. When preparing ratcheted instruments for sterilization, what should the Surgical Technologist do

A. Close ratchets

B. Soak instrument in normal saline for 10 minutes prior to assembling

C. Place grossly contaminated instruments into the ultrasonic cleaner

D. Leave ratchets open

26. Which connective tissue connects bone to bone?

A. Tendon

B. Ligament

C. Fascia

D. Cartilage

27. Volvulus is a condition describing
    A. Prolapsed of the uterus
    B. Telescoping of the intestine
    C. Twisting of the bowel
    D. Herniation of the bowel

28. An agent used to identified diseased tissue in the cervix is
    A. Lugols solution
    B. Methylene blue
    C. Tannic acid
    D. Conization

29. The surgical removal of a fluid filled sac in the tunica vaginalis is
    A. Bartholin's cyst excision
    B. Hydrocelectomy
    C. Varicocelectomy
    D. Hydrocystectomy

30. A patient suffering from prognathism has a(n)
    A. Receding chin
    B. Imbalance between the sides of the face
    C. Projecting jaw
    D. Open bite

31. Microtia can be corrected with which surgical procedure
    A. Mentoplasty
    B. Palatoplasty
    C. Cheiloplasty
    D. Otoplasty

32. The spleen is located in the
    A. Right hypochondriac region
    B. Right epigastric region
    C. Left hypochondriac region
    D. Left epigastric region

33. The medical term denoting rupture is
    A. –rrhexis
    B. –pexy
    C. –rrhagia
    D. –rrhaphy

34. The gland that is both endocrine and exocrine is the
    A. Spleen
    B. Liver
    C. Pituitary
    D. Pancreas

35. The medication used to treat malignant hyperthermia is
    A. Diprovan
    B. Protamine sulfate
    C. Dantrolene
    D. Lidocaine

36. The second phase of wound healing is
    A. Lag phase
    B. Maturation
    C. Proliferation
    D. Granulation

37. Polygalactin 910 is
    A. Monocryl
    B. Vicryl
    C. Maxon
    D. PDS II

38. The instrument that uses ultrasonic energy to cut and coagulate simultaneously is the
    A. CUSA
    B. LASER
    C. Harmonic Scalpel
    D. Cryotherapy Unit

39. A Billroth II is a(n)
    A. Gastrojejunostomy
    B. Gastroduodenostomy
    C. Total Gastrectomy
    D. Biliopancreatic diversion

40. Endoscopic visualization of the peritoneal cavity is a(n)
    A. colonoscopy
    B. laparoscopy
    C. Arthroscopy
    D. Cystoscopy

41. A rotator cuff tear occurs in the
    A. Knee
    B. Elbow
    C. Shoulder
    D. Ankle

42. Bacteria that lives and grows best in decreased oxygen is classified as
    A. Aerobic
    B. Anaerobic
    C. Bacilli
    D. Clostridium

43. Putti-Platt is a procedure to correct
    A. Rotator cuff tear
    B. AC joint separation
    C. Humeral fracture
    D. Recurrent anterior shoulder dislocation

44. The Galea is located in the
    A. Abdomen
    B. Scalp
    C. Upper leg
    D. Back

45. The eighth Cranial Nerve is the
    A. Vagus
    B. Vestibulocochlear

C. Trigeminal

D. Abducens

46. Continuous suture is also referred to as a(n)

A. Running stitch

B. Purse string

C. Retention suture

D. Buried suture

47. A mayo needle

A. Is swaged

B. Is less traumatic than an eyeless suture

C. Is closed eyed

D. Is a control release

48. During an inguinal hernia repair, the vas deferens is retracted with a(n)

A. Army- Navy

B. Red Robinson Catheter

C. Silastic tubing

D. Penrose drain

49. The most common site for hernia formation is at this anatomical site

A. Hesselbach's triangle

B. Umbilicus

C. Poupart's ligament

D. Diaphragm

50. Pneumoperitoneum is created with this gas

A. Carbon monoxide

B. Nitrous

C. Carbon dioxide

D. Oxygen

51. A simple Mastectomy involves

A. Removal of the entire breast and associated lymph nodes

B. Removal of the breast without lymph node dissection

C. Removal of breast and axillary contents

D. Removal of only affected breast tissue with preservation of the remaining tissue

52. The position for a patient undergoing excision of Zenker's diverticulum will be

A. Spine

B. Prone

C. Lateral

D. Semi-fowlers

53. The hormone that is present in as few as 10 days after conception is

A. Human Chorionic Gonadotropin

B. Luteinizing Hormone

C. Progesterone

D. Prolactin

54. Protamine Sulfate reverses the effects of

A. Epinephrine

B. Narcotics

C. Metabolic acidosis

D. Heparin

55. A Jackson Pratt is a(n)

A. Sump Drain

B. Closed vacuum drain

C. Gravity drain

D. Cigarette drain

56. What is the most likely LASER to be used in conjunction with a Cystoscope?

A. Holmium:YAG

B. Xenon

C. Krypton

D. YAG

57. Atelectasis is

A. Inflammation of mucous membranes

B. Stasis of peristalsis post operatively

C. Collapsed lung

D. Dehiscence of a wound

58. A common post operative complaint after laparoscopic procedures is

A. Size of incision

B. Chest pain

C. Back pain

D. Shoulder pain

59. The patient position for a perineal prostatectomy is

A. Supine

B. Lithotomy

C. Exaggerated lithotomy

D. Kraske

60. The creation of a nasoantral window in the maxillary bone to remove diseased tissue an drain sinuses is a(n)

A. Caldwell Luc

B. Submucosa Resection

C. FESS

D. UPPP

61. An example of a nonadherent dressing is

A. Adaptic

B. Cloth tape

C. Tegaderm

D. Steri-strips

62. Club foot is a condition known as

A. Coxa vera

B. Talipes equinovarus

C. Exostosis

D. Dupuytrens Contracture

63. A hip cast from waist to toes on the affected side and from the waist to knee on the unaffected side is a(n)

A. Cylinder cast

B. Long limb cast

C. Body cast

D. Spica

64. A double bowl shaped glass evacuator used in bladder surgery is a(n)

A. Toomey

B. Ellik

C. Closed vacuum drain

D. Iglesias

65. Hair-like extensions responsible for movement of fluid around cells are

A. Flagella

B. Pili

C. Cilia

D. Pseudopods

66. The only bone in the body that does not articulate with another bone is the

A. Patella

B. Mandible

C. Incus

D. Hyoid

67. The valve separating the right atrium and the right ventricle is the

A. Tricuspid

B. Mitral

C. Pulmonary

D. Semi-lunar

68. The first phase of general anesthesia is

A. Recovery

B. Maintenance

C. Induction

D. Emergence

69. All of the following are factors influencing chemical disinfection EXCEPT

A. Exposure time

B. Pounds of steam pressure (psi)

C. Amount of Bioburden present

D. pH

70. A positioning device for modified prone position is a(n)

A. Wilson frame

B. Bean bags

C. Adhesive tape

D. Kidney rest

71. Which of the following is a non-absorbable synthetic monofilament suture?

A. Polygalactin 910

B. Monocryl

C. Prolene

D. PDS

72. The instrument not commonly found on a D&C set is

A. Randall stone forceps

B. Dilators

C. Sound

D. Weitlaner

73. The congenital defect where the vertebrae do not close leaving the spinal cord unprotected is

A. Myleomengocele

B. Spina Bifida

C. Arteriovenous malformation

D. Meniere's Disease

74. Which instrument is a urethral sound?

A. Hegar

B. Sims

C. Van Buren

D. Mason Judd

75. Whipple procedure is done to treat

A. Pancreatic cancer

B. Obesity

C. Stomach cancer

D. Enlarged spleen

76. Which structure is not ligated and divided during a cholecystectomy?

A. Cystic duct

B. Cystic artery

C. Hepatic duct

D. Cystic vein

77. Anectine is a(n)

A. Non-depolarizing muscle relaxant

B. Depolarizing muscle relaxant

C. Neuroleptanalgesic

D. Sedative

78. Bakers cysts are found

A. In the stomach

B. Behind the patella

C. In the elbow

D. In the popliteal fossa

79. The most common incision for cesarean section is

A. Pfannenstiel

B. Transverse

C. Midline

D. McBurneys

80. A component of effective communication is

A. Speaking for others

B. Defending a stance

C. Using open ended sentences

D. Working independently

81. The common approach for a simple mastoidectomy is

A. Transnasal

B. Anterior neck

C. Postaural

D. Transmaxillae

82. The sequence for screw placement is

A. Drill, tap, measure, insert screw

B. Measure, drill, tap insert screw

C. Drill, insert screw
D. Drill, measure, tap, insert screw

83. Cadaver bone is considered
A. Autograft
B. Homograft
C. Allograft
D. Heterograft

84. PDS is a(n)
A. Absorbable, synthetic monofilament suture
B. Nonabsorbable, synthetic monofilament suture
C. Absorbable, synthetic multifilament suture
D. Nonabsorbable, synthetic multifilament suture

85. Cheyne-stokes respiration is
A. Wheezing sounds due to obstruction
B. Deep, gasping respiration indicative of diabetic coma
C. Irregular breathing due to apnea or hyperpena
D. Rattling or bubbling sounds while breathing

86. Which surgical procedure would be performed with the patient in the lateral position?
A. Pilonidal cystectomy
B. Lumbar laminectomy
C. Hiatal hernia repair
D. Total hip Arthroplasty

87. A contaminated case with an infection rate of 15% to 20% would be classified as
A. Class I
B. Class II
C. Class III
D. Class IV

88. Which side of a sterile wrapper is opened first?
A. The far side
B. The left side
C. The right side
D. The near side

89. The instrument that measures intraocular pressure is a(n)
A. Wicker caliper
B. Schiotz tonometer
C. Taylor sphygmomanometer
D. Wescott keratometer

90. The condition where there is a separation of the retina from the choroid is
A. Retinopathy
B. Retinal detachment
C. Retinol deficiency
D. Retinal layer idiopathic syndrome

91. The innermost layer of the uterus is the
A. Myometrium
B. Perimetrium
C. Endometrium
D. Mucous membrane

92. An example of a hinge joint is the
A. Elbow
B. Hip
C. Wrist
D. Thumb

93. The body's first line of defense against microbial infection is
A. White Blood Cells
B. Lymph
C. Antigen/Antibody reaction
D. Unbroken Skin

94. To reduce the risk of fire when using LASERs, what precaution should be used?
A. Use an alcohol prep that dries quickly
B. Use an open oxygen system
C. Moisten sponges around target tissue
D. Have a class A extinguisher available

95. A solid state has
A. A fixed volume
B. Will expand to fit space
C. Has a solvent
D. Has no fixed shape

96. A single robotic arm is used to
A. Translate surgeons hand movements
B. Perform remote surgery
C. Manipulate endoscopic telescopes
D. Control room functions

97. How are permanent specimens sent to pathology?
A. Dry
B. In 10% formalin
C. Without solution
D. On a sponge

98. The thoracic lymphatic duct drains into
A. The right jugular vein
B. The left jugular vein
C. The right subclavian vein
D. The left subclavian vein

99. An agent given to combat metabolic acidosis is
A. Sodium bicarbonate
B. Magnesium sulfate
C. Potassium Chloride
D. Albumin

100. A patient in the prone position without proper padding is at risk for
A. Lower leg emboli
B. Hyperextension of the head
C. Pressure on the vena cava and abdominal aorta
D. Compartment syndrome

101. Steam sterilizers are tested with the spore forming bacteria called

    A. Bacillus subtilis
    B. Bacillus stearothermophilus
    C. Bacillus palladium
    D. Bacillus shingellosis

102. Which of the following is true about prepping?

    A. Prep "dirty" areas first
    B. Prep "clean" areas first
    C. Use one prep kit for two clean areas
    D. Do not use prep solutions on the face

103. In Robotics, Roll refers to

    A. Movement to the right
    B. Movement to the left
    C. Rotation
    D. Movement upward

104. Which statement is true about microinstrumentation?

    A. They have a dull finish
    B. They are straight
    C. They cannot be flashed
    D. They cannot be placed in the ultrasonic cleaner

105. Hepatitis B is a

    A. Staphylococcal bacterium
    B. Streptococcal bacterium
    C. Vibrios
    D. Virus

106. The masseter muscle is used when

    A. Flexing the head
    B. Abducting the arm
    C. Chewing
    D. Closing the eyes

107. Which of the following is a thoracic retractor?

    A. Davidson
    B. Greenburg
    C. Sauerbruch
    D. Sarot

108. The medication administered after eye surgery to rapidly constrict the pupil is

    A. Miostat
    B. Miochol
    C. Mydriacyl
    D. Diamox

109. The Leyla-yasergil retractor is used in which specialty surgery

    A. Orthopedics
    B. Ophthalmic
    C. Pediatrics
    D. Neurosurgery

110. Which of the following is a bone holding forcep?

    A. Chandler
    B. Lowman
    C. Murphy
    D. Hibbs

111. A possible complication of radical prostatectomy is

    A. Impotence
    B. Testicular torsion
    C. Uremia
    D. Kidney stones

112. Wilms' tumors occur in the

    A. Abdomen
    B. Popliteal fossa
    C. Kidneys
    D. Testes

113. Intussusceptions may require

    A. Gastrectomy
    B. Hemicolectomy
    C. Small bowel resection
    D. Pyloroplasty

114. The incision that is made between two rectus abdominis muscles, continues down the linea alba and curves around the umbilicus is a

    A. Transverse
    B. Midline
    C. Paramedian
    D. Kocher

115. Wertheim procedure with abdominoperineal resection is called

    A. Anterior exenteration
    B. Radical hysterectomy
    C. Posterior exenteration
    D. Vesicourethral exenteration

116. According to Erickson's developmental stages, trust versus mistrust occurs at

    A. 0-1 yrs
    B. 12-18 yrs
    C. 18-30 yrs
    D. 2-5 yrs

117. An institutional accreditation for allied health programs is

    A. JCAHO
    B. AMA
    C. ANSI
    D. CAAHEP

118. The causative agent of thrush is

    A. Mold
    B. Yeast
    C. Bacteria
    D. Parasites

119. Injury sustained by the patient due to activity of health care providers is called

    A. Iatrogenic injury
    B. Assault

   C. Negligence
   D. Contributory injury

120. Surgical patients recover in

   A. The ICU
   B. Pre-op holding areas
   C. PACU
   D. Critical care unit

121. Surgical Stainless Steel would most likely be used for

   A. Abdominal closures
   B. Cardiovascular procedures
   C. General closures
   D. Sternal closures

122. The most likely needle for use in the liver would be

   A. Cutting
   B. Blunt
   C. Taper
   D. Reverse cutting

123. Water for plaster cast application should be

   A. Warm
   B. Cool
   C. Room temperature
   D. Hot

124. The suture line used to close the appendix stump is

   A. Purse string
   B. Continuous
   C. Interrupted
   D. Mattress

125. A FESS is

   A. Abdominal surgery
   B. Orthopedic surgery
   C. Sinus surgery
   D. Oral surgery

126. Rhotons are used in

   A. Vascular surgery
   B. Neurosurgery
   C. Ophthalmic surgery
   D. Plastic surgery

127. The middle layer of the meninges is

   A. Pia
   B. Dura
   C. Neurilemma
   D. Arachnoid

128. –malacia is the medical tern for

   A. Softening
   B. Condition
   C. Enlargement
   D. Break down, dissolve

129. Removal of the parathyroid glands may cause

   A. Muscle weakness
   B. Tetany

   C. Graves disease
   D. Hyperthyroidism

130. The gland that helps develop the immune system is the

   A. Pituitary
   B. Thyroid
   C. Pineal
   D. Thymus

131. Colles fractures occur

   A. In the femur
   B. In the ankle
   C. In the wrist
   D. In the ankle

132. Which in-situ vein is used for femoral popliteal bypass?

   A. Radial
   B. Femoral vein
   C. Popliteal vein
   D. Saphenous vein

133. Arteriotomies are extended with

   A. 11 blade
   B. Potts smith scissors
   C. Metzenbaum scissors
   D. Stevens tenotomy scissors

134. A common site for cerebral aneurysms is

   A. Circle of wills
   B. Temporal lobe
   C. Frontal lobe
   D. Occipital lobe

135. An osteosarcoma is a(n)

   A. Begnin bone tumor
   B. Malignant tumor of cartilage
   C. Malignant tumor of periosteum
   D. Malignant bone tumor

136. Z-plasty may be performed to correct

   A. Dupuytren's contracture
   B. Syndactyly
   C. Rhytidectomy
   D. Cheiloplasty

137. A verruca is a(n)

   A. Mole
   B. Boil
   C. Wart
   D. Skin Ulcer

138. Which anesthetic agent may be used in ENT surgeries?

   A. Levophed
   B. Dantrium
   C. Fentanyl
   D. Cocaine

139. Scar tissue caused by fibrous collagen is
   A. Cicatrix
   B. Granulation
   C. Keloid
   D. Granuloma

140. Sterilization by ethylene oxide takes
   A. 2-3 hours
   B. 24 hours
   C. 30 minutes
   D. 4 minutes

141. A metal or plastic device that holds a carpule of medication is a(n)
   A. Toomey
   B. Tubex
   C. Leur loc
   D. Ampoule

142. Para- is the root word for
   A. Behind
   B. Through
   C. Beside
   D. Beneath

143. A gunshot wound to the bowel would be closed with
   A. First intention wound healing
   B. Granulation
   C. Second intention wound healing
   D. Third intention wound healing

144. Bowel technique involves
   A. Two set ups
   B. Isolation of contaminated instruments
   C. Passing contaminated instruments off the field
   D. Creating a "safe zone" for contaminated instruments

145. A patient undergoing a AAA would be placed in
   A. Supine position
   B. Lateral position
   C. Modified beachchair
   D. Lithotomy position

146. Arterial embolectomy will be cleared with a(n)
   A. Syringe
   B. Foley
   C. T-tube
   D. Fogarty

147. A Javid shunt may be used when performing
   A. CABG
   B. Carotid ensrterectomy
   C. AV shunt
   D. Peritoneojugular shunt

148. There are ___ pair of extrinsic eye muscles
   A. 4
   B. 5
   C. 6
   D. 7

149. The temperature of a prevacuum sterilizer should be
   A. 250 degrees
   B. 270 degrees
   C. 200 degrees
   D. 280 degrees

150. Reglan is a(n)
   A. Histamine blocker
   B. Anesthetic
   C. Antiemetic
   D. Anticholinergic

151. The series of fluid filled canals located in the temporal bone is the
   A. Vestibule
   B. Cochlea
   C. Osseous labyrinth
   D. Semicircular canals

152. Elevated white blood cell count is referred to as
   A. Leukocytosis
   B. Leukopenia
   C. Leukoragia
   D. Leukemia

153. An example of a narcotic antagonist agent is
   A. Lidocaine
   B. Dantrolene
   C. Narcan
   D. Anectine

154. The loss of heat due to collisions of molecules at different temperatures is called
   A. Conduction
   B. Convection
   C. Radiation
   D. Gas diffusion

155. A footboard may be required of patients placed in the _____ position
   A. Lithotomy
   B. Trendelenburg
   C. Kraske
   D. Reverse trendelenburg

156. The purpose of an indwelling urethral catheter for surgical procedures includes all of the following EXCEPT
   A. Monitoring urine production
   B. Keep bladder irrigated
   C. Collect sterile specimens
   D. Keep bladder deflated

157. Abnormal fibrous tissues that bind organs together are
   A. Cohesions
   B. Epithelial granulation

C. Adhesions

D. Keloids

158. Suture gauge refers to

A. Diameter of suture strand

B. Needle size

C. Multifilament suture

D. Tensile strength

159. X-ray visualization of the bladder using contrast media is a(n)

A. Cystoscopy

B. Cystogram

C. Cystometrogram

D. KUB

160. Which of the following is an orthopedic instrument?

A. Fogarty clamp

B. Serrefines

C. Bennett

D. McPherson tying forcep

161. Bleeding between the dura mater and the arachnoid is

A. Epidural hematoma

B. Subdural hematoma

C. Sub arachnoid hematoma

D. Intracerebral hematoma

162. The association that develops medical device standards is

A. AMA

B. ASPAN

C. NIOSH

D. AAMI

163. The term that is used when an infant's head is too large to pass through the pelvis of the mother is

A. Cephalopelvic disproportion

B. Cephalodystocia

C. Cephalophalic disproportion

D. Hyperemisis gravidarum

164. Bougies and balloon dilators may be used to treat

A. Hypospadia

B. Urethral stenosis

C. Vesicourethral reflux

D. Phimosis

165. The highest level of Maslow's Hierarchy is

A. Self-esteem

B. Love and belonging

C. Self-actualization

D. Social affiliations

166. The instrument used to grasp the cervix during a D&C is

A. Sims uterine sound

B. Tenaculum

C. Auvard

D. Bozeman

167. A FESS is

A. A sinus procedure

B. An ear procedure

C. Prostate procedure

D. A procedure to remove a condyloma

168. A three lumen tube is for

A. Irrigation, aspiration and urine

B. Aspiration, escape of air and suction

C. Aspiration, irrigation and escape of air

D. Irrigation, urine and escape of air

169. The second stage loop colostomy is performed how long after the first stage

A. 24 hours

B. 48 hours

C. 72 hours

D. 1 week

170. What should be done before patient catheterization?

A. Test balloon

B. Surgical prep

C. Secure catheter to patient with tape

D. Place patient in lithotomy position

171. Which statement is true regarding lateral positioning?

A. Patient is placed on operative side

B. Lower leg is flexed

C. Arms are tucked

D. A minimum of 3 people must be present

172. Aeger Primo means

A. First, do no harm

B. Negligence

C. The thing speaks for itself

D. Patient first

173. The reason a specific drug should not be used is a(n)

A. Side effect

B. Indication

C. Contraindication

D. Adverse effect

174. The flow of electrons back and forth along a single pathway due to changes in polarity is

A. AC current

B. DC current

C. Voltage

D. Conductivity

175. A common complication of Diabetes Mellitus is

A. Obesity

B. Infection

C. Malnourishment

D. Decreased blood clotting time

176. The psi for gravity air displacement sterilization is

A. Between 20 and 25

B. 27

C. Between 12 and 15
D. Between 15 and 17

177. The biologic test for EO sterilization involves

A. Bacillus stearothermophilus
B. Bacillus tetani
C. Bacillus subtilis
D. Clostridium difficile

178. Distention during hysteroscope is commonly attained by

A. Dextran
B. Sterile water
C. Saline
D. Albumin

179. The series of canals found in compact bone that allows blood vessels and nerves to enter is called the

A. Bursa system
B. Sharpeys fibers
C. Haversian system
D. Elysian system

180. Gtt is the abbreviation for

A. Epiglottis
B. Grain
C. Drop
D. Tongue

181. The stapler which places a double row of staggered staples and has a cutting blade is a(n)

A. Skin stapler
B. TA
C. GIA
D. ILS

182. The common bile duct joins the pancreatic duct at this anatomical structure

A. Sphincter of Oddi
B. Duct of Wirsung
C. Ampulla of Vader
D. Pancreatic fundus

183. Which of the following instruments would be used for a kidney removal?

A. Bailey
B. Kerrison
C. Woodson
D. Davidson

184. Bletharochalasis is defined as

A. Loss of elasticity of the skin of the eyelids
B. Lazy eye
C. Cross eyes
D. Peri-orbital fracture

185. Intracranial aneurysms may be approached in all of the following ways EXCEPT

A. Frontal
B. Bifrontal

C. Frontotemporal
D. Trans sphenoidal

186. When performing a lumpectomy, what should be removed?

A. The entire mass
B. The mass and the lymph nodes
C. The mass and non-affected tissue margins
D. A small amount of tissue for pathology

187. Temporalis fascia taken for tympanic membrane graft should

A. Be placed on a drying block
B. Remain moist
C. Be cut by the ST to the surgeons specifications
D. Taken 24 hours prior to the surgery

188. A self-retaining intracranial retractor is a(n)

A. Beckman
B. Leyla
C. Israel
D. Omni

189. A case where there is a major break in aseptic technique has the designation of

A. Class I
B. Class II
C. Class III
D. Class IV

190. A flat latex drain used to retract the spermatic cord during inguinal repair is

A. Sump drain
B. Penrose drain
C. Red Robinson
D. Tenkhof drain

191. The normal heat rate for infants is

A. 70 beats per minute
B. 100 beats per minute
C. 120 beats per minute
D. 130 beats per minute

192. Movement in and around the sterile field should be

A. Out of normal traffic flows
B. Kept to a minimum
C. Done freely
D. Constricted to the anesthesia personnel

193. During a laparoscopic procedure, who manipulates the tower settings

A. The surgeon
B. The anesthesiologist
C. The circulator under direction from the surgeon
D. The scrub under direction of the surgeon

194. Helminths are

A. Fungal infections
B. Rickettsial agents

C. Protozoan parasites

D. Parasitic worms

195. Muscle irritability may be caused by a buildup of

A. Lactic acid

B. Carbon dioxide

C. Calcium ions

D. Acetylcholine

196. How many carpals are in each wrist?

A. 5

B. 8

C. 10

D. 16

197. Which of the following is a blood thinner?

A. Thrombin

B. Ephedrine

C. Aspirin

D. Purodigin

198. Which of the following is true about surgical masks?

A. They should be worn either on or off, not around the neck

B. Two masks should be worn in active TB cases

C. Masks should be worn in semi-restricted areas

D. Masks should be put on before the bouffant

199. Which tendon will be used as graft when repairing the flexor tendon

A. Achilles

B. Palmaris longus

C. Extensor pollicis

D. Extensor carpi

200. KTP LASERS are produced when Nd:YAG light is passed through a(n)

A. Ruby particulate plasma filter

B. Garnet crystal

C. Argon particle filter

D. Potassium titanium phosphate crystal

201. Which of the following is not true about materials for gowns and drapes?

A. Material should provide microbial barrier

B. Material should be resistant to tears

C. Non-woven material should be laundered and sterilized after each procedure

D. Woven material should be repaired with heat sealed patches

202. The device that is used to measure blood pressure or pulse using ultrasonic high-frequency sound waves is a(n)

A. Doppler

B. Spirometer

C. Insufflators

D. ECHO

203. Glutaraldehyde requires an exposure time of _____ to achieve sterilization.

A. 20 minutes

B. 10 hours

C. 10 minutes

D. 5 hours

204. The suture most likely to be used on slow healing wounds where there is a need for wound support is

A. Polygalactin 910

B. Chromic Gut

C. Polypropylene

D. Polydioxanone

205. A total Abdominal Hysterectomy would remove which anatomical structure(s)

A. Uterus, fallopian tubes and ovaries

B. Uterus and ovaries

C. Uterus

D. Uterus, fallopian tubes, ovaries and upper third of the vaginal vault

206. If a surgical blade is broken during a procedure, how should the Surgical Technologist handle the count?

A. The ST should discard the sharp in the sharps container

B. The count should reflect all parts of the broken blade

C. The count should remain the same, with the pieces counted as one

D. The circulating nurse will remove the blade from the room

207. Which of the following instruments would likely be found in a general set?

A. Gerald forceps

B. Bethune

C. Duvall

D. Curved Kocher

208. A portocaval shunt creates an anastomosis between the inferior vena cava and this structure

A. Portal vein

B. Splenic vein

C. Superior mesenteric vein

D. Renal vein

209. Which of the following procedures is likely to require a drain post operatively?

A. Hysterectomy

B. Marsupialization of Bartholin's cyst

C. D&C

D. Inguinal hernia repair

210. The valve that separates the small intestine from the large intestine is the

A. Pyloric valve

B. Ileocecal valve

C. Cardiac valve

D. Ampulla of Vater

211. A common site of cerebral aneurysms is

A. Circle of Wills

B. External carotid

C. Vertebral artery

D. Basilar artery

212. Cowpers Glands are associated with which anatomical structure

A. Kidneys

B. Uterus

C. Bladder

D. Prostate

213. Gore-tex grafts are made of

A. Knitted polyester

B. Knitted velour

C. Polytetrafluoroethylene

D. Knitted polyester

214. Packages of surgical instruments should not weigh more than

A. 15 lb

B. 16 lb

C. 18 lb

D. 20 lb

215. An example of a surgically clean, but not sterile, endoscopic procedure is

A. Laparoscopic cholecystectomy

B. Thoracoscopy

C. Cystoscopy

D. Mediasinoscopy

216. A liver biopsy would most likely be done with a

A. Toomey syringe

B. Jamshidi needle

C. Silverman

D. Tubex syringe

217. Premature closure of cranial sutures is a condition called

A. AV malformation

B. Hydrocephalus

C. Spina bifida

D. Craniosynostosis

218. When anastomosing the renal vein during living donor procedures, which suture would most likely be used?

A. 5-0 double armed vascular suture

B. 7-0 double armed vicryl

C. 3-0 chromic

D. 6-0 single armed nylon

219. In the event of an incorrect count, which action should be taken immediately?

A. X-rays should be taken to located the item

B. Anesthesia should be informed as the procedure will be delayed

C. Documentation must be completed

D. Inform the surgeon

220. The generic form of Marcaine is

A. Xylocaine

B. Bupivicaine

C. Mepivicaine

D. Tetracaine

221. The toxins that are produced by bacteria and are released upon destruction of the cell are considered

A. Exotoxins

B. Myotoxins

C. Endotoxins

D. Fibrinolysins

222. The fold of peritoneum that hangs like an apron over the abdominal organs is called

A. Mesentery

B. Omentum

C. Visceral peritoneal folds

D. Parietal peritoneal folds

223. Which statement is true of patient positioning for cesarean section?

A. The right side should be elevated

B. The left side should be elevated

C. The patient will be placed in lithotomy

D. Padding will be placed in the lower back

224. A begnin cyst of the ovary containing contents from old blood is called a(n)

A. Carcinoma in situ

B. Dermoid cyst

C. Cystocele

D. Chocolate cyst

225. An example of a motor driven dermatome is a(n)

A. Padgett

B. Hudson brace

C. Reese

D. Padgett-hood

226. Burns are classified as electrical, thermal, chemical, and

A. Dermal

B. Mechanical

C. Solid

D. Accelerant

227. When transporting a patient on a stretcher, you should

A. Push from the feet

B. Push from the sides

C. Push from the head

D. Pull from the head

228. Which of the following is a cephalosporin?

A. Garamycin

B. doxycycline

C. Omnipen

D. Ancef

229. Which of the following is not true about activated glutaraldehyde?

A. Items must be damp when placed in solution
B. It must be monitored for concentration
C. It must be stored in a closed container
D. Gloves and goggles must be worn when working with Glutaraldehyde

230. A non-invasive method to measure anesthesia levels is

A. Urinary output
B. Blood pressure
C. Bispectral index
D. Pulmonary artery pressure

231. A seamless tubular cotton dressing/drape is a(n)

A. Tubex
B. Ace
C. Coban
D. Stockinette

232. The three parts of a needle are point, body, and

A. Diameter
B. Eye
C. Size
D. Code

233. A common intestinal suture is

A. 3-0 silk
B. 4-0 vicryl
C. 6-0 double armed prolene
D. 2 PDS II

234. During a Nissen Fundoplication, the fundus of the stomach is anchored against which anatomical structure?

A. 8th rib
B. Xyphoid process
C. Diaphragm
D. Esophagus

235. A contraindication for hysteroscopy is

A. Lost IUD
B. Pregnancy
C. Infertility
D. Abnormal uterine bleeding

236. Which surgical procedure may be done while sitting?

A. Carpal tunnel release
B. Craniotomy
C. SMR
D. Excision of pressure sores

237. The daily test used to check the veracity of Pre-vacuum sterilizers is

A. Spore strip
B. Chemical indicator
C. Bowie dick
D. Schillers test

238. A common suture used for subcuticular closure is

A. Monocryl
B. Nylon
C. Mersilene
D. Polydek

239. Factors that determine whether an individual will contract a disease post-exposure include all of the following EXCEPT

A. Virulence
B. Duration of exposure
C. Resistance of host
D. Weight of host

240. The space between the cochlea and the semicircular canals of the inner ear is the

A. Labyrinth
B. Anterior cavity
C. Vestibule
D. Auricle

241. A pressure point for someone placed in the prone position is the

A. Sacrum
B. Lesser trochanter
C. Scapula
D. Lateral knee

242. The curette commonly used for endocervical scrapping is a(n)

A. Kevorkian
B. Thomas
C. Bozeman
D. Loop

243. The stage of osteogenisis that creates a fibrous tissue and cartilage mesh is the

A. Remodeling stage
B. Osteoid stage
C. Hematoma formation
D. Callus stage

244. Demerol is an example of a(n)

A. Inhalation anesthetic
B. Narcotic sedative
C. Antianxiety medication
D. Neuromuscular blocker

245. Failure of an organ to develop properly is called

A. Atresia
B. Hypoplasia
C. Aplasia
D. Anaplasia

246. The chemical produced by a cell infected with viral particles that protects other cells is

A. Interferon
B. Interlukin
C. Antitoxin
D. Antiserum

247. Relative humidity in the OR should be maintained at
    A. 55% to 60%
    B. 50% to 55%
    C. 60% to 65%
    D. 45% to 50%

248. The suture line for inner layers of bowel mucosa is
    A. Pursestring
    B. Limbert
    C. Halstead
    D. Connel

249. The gas used to inflate the peritoneum during laparoscopic procedures is
    A. Carbon dioxide
    B. Oxygen
    C. Carbon monoxide
    D. Nitrous oxide

250. A common drain used for cholecystostomy is
    A. Fogarty
    B. Pezzar
    C. Foley
    D. Penrose

Answers

1. C	28. A	55. B	82. D
2. A	29. B	56. A	83. B
3. D	30. C	57. C	84. A
4. D	31. D	58. D	85. C
5. B	32. C	59. C	86. D
6. B	33. A	60. A	87. C
7. A	34. D	61. A	88. A
8. C	35. C	62. B	89. B
9. A	36. C	63. D	90. B
10. B	37. B	64. B	91. C
11. C	38. C	65. C	92. A
12. B	39. A	66. D	93. D
13. A	40. B	67. A	94. C
14. C	41. C	68. C	95. A
15. D	42. B	69. B	96. C
16. A	43. D	70. A	97. B
17. B	44. B	71. C	98. D
18. C	45. B	72. D	99. A
19. A	46. A	73. B	100. C
20. B	47. C	74. C	101. B
21. C	48. D	75. A	102. B
22. A	49. A	76. C	103. C
23. B	50. C	77. B	104. A
24. C	51. B	78. D	105. D
25. D	52. D	79. A	106. C
26. B	53. A	80. C	107. A
27. C	54. D	81. C	108. B

109. D	145. A	181. C	217. D
110. B	146. D	182. B	218. A
111. A	147. B	183. A	219. D
112. C	148. C	184. A	220. B
113. C	149. B	185. D	221. C
114. B	150. C	186. C	222. B
115. C	151. C	187. A	223. A
116. A	152. A	188. B	224. D
117. D	153. C	189. C	225. A
118. B	154. A	190. B	226. B
119. A	155. D	191. D	227. C
120. C	156. B	192. B	228. D
121. D	157. C	193. C	229. A
122. B	158. A	194. D	230. C
123. C	159. B	195. A	231. D
124. A	160. C	196. B	232. B
125. C	161. B	197. C	233. A
126. B	162. D	198. A	234. C
127. D	163. A	199. B	235. B
128. A	164. B	200. D	236. A
129. B	165. C	201. C	237. C
130. D	166. B	202. A	238. A
131. C	167. A	203. B	239. D
132. D	168. C	204. D	240. C
133. B	169. B	205. C	241. D
134. A	170. A	206. B	242. A
135. D	171. B	207. D	243. D
136. A	172. D	208. A	244. B
137. C	173. C	209. B	245. C
138. D	174. A	210. B	246. A
139. B	175. B	211. A	247. B
140. A	176. D	212. D	248. D
141. B	177. C	213. C	249. A
142. C	178. A	214. B	250. B
143. D	179. C	215. C	
144. B	180. C	216. C	

PEARSON
myhealthprofessionskit™

Use this address to access the interactive Companion Website created for this book. Simply select "Surgical Technology" from the choice of disciplines. Find this book and click to enter.

Index